Encyclopedia of Exercise Medicine in Health and Disease

Frank C. Mooren (Ed.)

Encyclopedia of Exercise Medicine in Health and Disease

Volume 1

A–H

With 254 Figures and 92 Tables

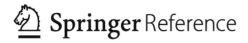
Springer Reference

Editor
Frank C. Mooren
Department of Sports Medicine
Institute of Sports Sciences
Justus-Liebig-University
Am Kugelberg 62
35393 Giessen
Germany

ISBN 978-3-540-36065-0   e-ISBN 978-3-540-29807-6
DOI 10.1007/978-3-540-29807-6
ISBN Bundle 978-3-540-36066-7
Springer Heidelberg Dordrecht London New York

Library of Congress Control Number: 2011944334

Printed on acid-free paper

Springer is part of Springer Science+Business Media (www.springer.com)

Preface

Life expectancy and disease prevalence vary considerably in the different countries and places around the world. They show a strong relationship to the countries' socio-economic status and the cultural development of their societies. Only about one century ago, life expectancy in western Europe was about 46 and 52 years for men and women, respectively. Most common causes of death were infectious diseases, especially of the lungs, such as tuberculosis. Likewise, in 1900 tuberculosis was the most frequent cause of death even in the United States. But nowadays life expectancy and disease prevalence in western countries has changed dramatically. In Germany, life expectancy of new-born children has been calculated at about 82 and 88 years for men and women, respectively. Moreover, a significant shift of disease pattern has occured. Today the most important diseases include cardiovascular diseases such as ischemic heart disease and hypertension, metabolic diseases such as diabetes mellitus type II and hypercholesterinemia, pulmonal diseases such as chronic obstructive pulmonary disease, and malignant diseases. In contrast, infectious diseases are now responsible for less than 1% of all deaths.

These shifts of life expectancy and disease prevalence have several reasons. One important reason is the improvement of the health care systems, including the establishment of better hygienic standards and the development and availability of novel pharmaceutical tools such as mcrobicidal drugs. The next important reason concerns nutritional aspects. In western countries, malnutrition is rare, as food is available at any time in high amounts and quality. Instead, many people ingest more food than necessary for their energy balance leading to overweight and obesity. And finally, developed countries are characterized by a modern infrastructure showing high standards of spatial mobility and communicative devices. This leads, however, to a progressive reduction in people's individual mobility, also called a sedentary lifestyle. Consequently, sedentary lifestyle has been recognized as an independent risk factor for many wealth-related diseases, such as coronary heart disease, hypertension, diabetes etc.

Sedentary lifestyle is an uncommon condition for the human body, a condition which it isn't used to. On the contrary, the human body is designed for movement and activity. Genomic analyses proved that the genome of modern man is nearly identical to that of our prehistoric ancestors, the hunter-gatherer. His survival depended on both – his speed and his endurance. Fast movements during fight-and-flight responses ensured survival against enemies. Long endurance runs were important for his success as a hunter. Therefore, exercise was a question of survival for our ancestors. Today there are ample studies demonstrating the manifold benefits of regular exercise, ranging from physical and psychological well-being, prevention and therapy of cardiovascular, metabolic, proliferative, and neurodegenerative diseases, to a decrease of overall mortality.

The aim of the *Encyclopedia of Exercise Medicine in Health and Disease* is therefore to address these different issues in a comprehensive reference book for both basic and clinical scientists as well as students and lecturers in sport and life sciences. First, it should demonstrate the various and fascinating adaptational responses of the human body towards exercise. These responses are not limited to certain tissues or organs such as muscles or heart. Instead, it has been shown that the exercise stimulus is able to address nearly every cell type, thereby inducing a harmonized systemic adaptational response. Based on tissue plasticity, the adaptation may allow the development of enormous capabilities and capacities, as regularly demonstrated by the records and excellent performances of elite athletes. But these adaptational responses are equally important for both prevention as well as therapy of many diseases. Interestingly, there are manifold relationships between high-performance sports and sports therapy. Several recent developments of training regimes in rehabilitation sports initially originated from protocols of elite sports. And this is the second aim of the Encyclopedia, to highlight the evidence-based effects of an active lifestyle and regular exercise on numerous wealth-related diseases. Exercise is an important therapeutic tool which in many cases shows effects in the same order of magnitude as medicamentous approaches. Consequently, Exercise is Medicine™ as an initiative managed by the American College of Sports Medicine was founded some years ago to inform health care professionals and patients about the potentials of exercise in disease prevention and therapy and to support the inclusion of exercise into therapeutic regimes.

Next, increased life expectancy and longevity doesn't necessarily mean a life without limitations. Often aging is associated with frailty, loss of autonomy, and obstacles. Therefore the encyclopedia also addresses the role of exercise in delaying and hindering the concomitant loss of functional capacities during aging.

And finally, several essays address the molecular mechanisms underlying the beneficial exercise effects. Using various techniques from molecular biology and cellular physiology, scientists were more and more successful in elucidating how different exercise stimuli, e.g. duration, intensity, frequency etc., are sensed and transduced into a cellular response. This molecular dimension opens new horizons and gives us an in-depth understanding of the underlying working mechanisms of the exercise stimulus. And by elucidating the molecular components, new targets for future drug development may be identified.

Together, the *Encyclopedia of Exercise Medicine in Health and Disease* aims to integrate these various aspects of exercise and tries to build bridges – from high-performance sports to leisure-time physical activity, from prevention to sports therapy as well as from system physiology to molecular physiology. In order to meet these challenges, more than 200 authors have contributed their expertise by preparing in-depth essays and keyword definitions. All of them are renowned specialists in their fields and reputable members of the international scientific community. It has been a marvellous experience for me to work with them and I wish to thank every single author for the excellent and constructive collaboration. Furthermore, I would like to thank Ilke Krumholz for her excellent and competent secretarial assistance and my colleagues Karsten Krüger and Christian Pilat for fruitful and interesting discussions. It was a great pleasure to work with the Springer crew. In particular I wish to thank Andrew Spencer who patiently and untiringly managed the multiple aspects associated with manuscript handling and processing.

Finally, I would like to ask the reader for indulgence in case of any lack of clarity or even incorrectness of any contribution. Substantial efforts have been made to avoid these deficits, however, they can never be excluded entirely. All authors look forward to receiving the reader's suggestions and/or possible corrections which should help to improve the scientific standard of this reference work continuously. The parallel publication of the *Encyclopedia of Exercise Medicine in Health and Disease* in an online version allows permanent updating and adaptation to relevant novel scientific findings if necessary.

Giessen, March 2012   Frank C. Mooren

List of Contributors

MATTHEW R. ALLEN
Department of Anatomy & Cell Biology
Indiana University School of Medicine
Indianapolis, IN
USA

STANLEY ANDRISSE
Department of Biology
Saint Louis University
St. Louis, MO
USA

STAVROS APOSTOLAKIS
Haemostasis Thrombosis and Vascular Biology Unit
University of Birmingham Centre for Cardiovascular
Sciences
City Hospital
Birmingham
UK
and
Department of Cardiology
Democritus University of Thrace
Alexandroupolis
Greece

ADAMANTIOS ARAMPATZIS
Department of Training and Movement Sciences
Humboldt-University Berlin
Berlin
Germany

DUARTE ARAÚJO
Technical University of Lisbon
Cruz Quebrada
Portugal

LAWRENCE E. ARMSTRONG
Human Performance Laboratory
University of Connecticut
Storrs, CT
USA

NEIL ARMSTRONG
Children's Health and Exercise Research Centre
Sport and Health Sciences
College of Life and Environmental Sciences
University of Exeter
Exeter
UK

DIDIER ATTAIX
Institut National de la Recherche Agronomique
UMR 1019
Unité de Nutrition Humaine
CRNH Auvergne, Clermont Université
Université d'Auvergne
Clermont-Ferrand
France

MICHEL AUDRAN
Biophysics & Bio-Analysis Laboratory
Montpellier
France

JOSÉ A. AZNAR
Haemostasis and Thrombosis Unit
University Hospital La FE
Valencia
Spain

MARLEEN A. VAN BAAK
NUTRIM School for Nutrition, Toxicology and
Metabolism
Department of Human Biology
Maastricht University Medical Center+
Maastricht
The Netherlands

KEITH BAAR
Department of Neurobiology
Physiology and Behavior
University of California
Davis, CA
USA

Damian M. Bailey
Neurovascular Research Laboratory
University of Glamorgan
Pontypridd, Wales
UK

Julien S. Baker
Health & Exercise Science
School of Science
University of the West of Scotland
Hamilton, Scotland
UK

R. Bals
Dept. Pulmonology
University Giessen and Marburg
Marburg
Germany

Ruben Barakat
Universidad Politécnica de Madrid
Madrid
Spain

Tom Baranowski
Children's Nutrition Research Center
Department of Pediatrics
Baylor College of Medicine
Houston, TX
USA

Tiago M. Barbosa
Department of Sport Sciences
Polytechnic Institute of Bragança
Bragança
Portugal

Alan R. Barker
Children's Health and Exercise Research Centre
Sport and Health Sciences
College of Life and Environmental Sciences
University of Exeter
Exeter
UK

Lukas Beis
College of Medicine
Veterinary and Life Sciences
Institute of Cardiovascular and medical Sciences
University of Glasgow
Glasgow, Scotland
UK

M. G. Bemben
Department of Health and Exercise Science
University of Oklahoma
Norman, OK
USA

Ralph Beneke
Bereich Medizin
Training und Gesundheit
Institut für Sportwissenschaft und Motologie
Philipps Universität Marburg
Marburg
Germany

Istvan Berczi
Department of Immunology
The University of Manitoba
Winnipeg, MB
Canada

Aloys Berg
Medizinische Universitätsklinik
Abt. Rehabilitative und Präventive Sportmedizin
Freiburg
Germany

Elliot M. Berry
Dept of Human Nutrition & Metabolism
The Braun School of Public Health and
Community Medicine
Hebrew University – Hadassah Medical Center
Jerusalem
Israel

Yagesh Bhambhani
University of Alberta
Edmonton, AB
Canada

FIN BIERING-SØRENSEN
Clinic for Spinal Cord Injuries
The NeuroScience Centre Rigshospitalet
Copenhagen
Denmark

GEORGE E. BILLMAN
Department of Physiology and Cell Biology
The Ohio State University
Columbus, OH
USA

DAVID J. BISHOP
School of Sport and Exercise Science
Institute of Sport, Exercise and Active Living (ISEAL)
Victoria University
Melbourne, VIC
Australia

NICOLETTE C. BISHOP
School of Sport Exercise and Health Sciences
Loughborough University
Loughborough
UK

ALESSANDRO BLANDINO
Cardiology Division
Department of Internal Medicine
San Giovanni Battista Hospital
University of Turin
Turin
Italy

WILHELM BLOCH
Department of Molecular and Cellular Sport Medicine
German Sport University Cologne
Institute of Cardiovascular Research and Sport Medicine
Cologne
Germany

DIETER BÖNING
Sports Medicine
Charité – Universitätsmedizin Berlin
Berlin
Germany

JULIUS BOGOMOLOVAS
Klinikum Mannheim GmbH Universitätsklinikum
Universitätsmedizin Mannheim
University of Heidelberg
Mannheim
Germany

MARTIN D. BOOTMAN
Laboratory of Signalling and Cell Fate
Babraham Institute
Cambridge
UK

A. N. BOSCH
Human Biology
University of Cape Town MRC Research Unit for Exercise
Science and Sports Medicine
Sports Science Institute of South Africa
Newlands
South Africa

LAURENT BOSQUET
Faculté des sciences du sport
Université de Poitiers
Poitiers
France

FABIO BREIL
Department of Anatomy
University of Bern
Bern
Switzerland

KLARA BRIXIUS
Department of Molecular and Cellular Sport Medicine
German Sport University Cologne
Institute of Cardiovascular Research and Sport Medicine
Cologne
Germany

ULF G. BRONAS
University of Minnesota
School of Nursing
Minneapolis, MN
USA

PETER H. BRUBAKER
Department of Health and Exercise Science
Wake Forest University
Winston-Salem, NC
USA

ROSA MARIA BRUNO
Department of Internal Medicine
University of Pisa
Pisa
Italy

THIERRY BUSSO
Université de Lyon, Laboratoire de Physiologie
de l'Exercice
Saint-Etienne
France

CHRIS BUTTON
School of Physical Education
University of Otago
Dunedin
New Zealand

WIM A. BUURMAN
Department of General Surgery
Maastricht University Medical Center
Maastricht
The Netherlands

W. TODD CADE
Program in Physical Therapy and Department of
Medicine
Washington University School of Medicine
Saint Louis, MO
USA

MARISSA K. CALDOW
Molecular Nutrition Unit, School of Exercise
and Nutrition Sciences
Deakin University
Burwood, VIC
Australia

DAVID CAMERON-SMITH
University of Auckland
Auckland
New Zealand

C. CAPELLI
Department of Neurological, Neuropsychological,
Morphological and Movement Sciences
School of Exercise and Sport Sciences
University of Verona
Verona
Italy

KAI-HÅKON CARLSEN
Oslo University Hospital, Rikshospitalet
Deptartment of Paediatrics
University of Oslo, Norwegian School of Sport Sciences
Oslo
Norway

C. CASTAGNA
Football Training and Biomechanics Laboratory
Technical Department Italian Football Federation (FIGC)
Coverciano (Florence)
Italy

L. M. CASTELL
University of Oxford
Green Templeton College
Oxford
UK

YOUNG-HUI CHANG
Comparative Neuromechanics Laboratory
School of Applied Physiology
Georgia Institute of Technology
Atlanta, GA
USA

BÉNÉDICTE CHAZAUD
Institut COCHIN INSERM U1016 CNRS UMR8104
Paris
France

YAJUN CHEN
Faculty of Public Health
Sun Yat-sen University
Guangzhou
China

MARTIN K. CHILDERS
Department of Neurology and Institute for
Regenerative Medicine
Wake Forest University
Winston-Salem, NC
USA

PHIL CHILIBECK
College of Kinesiology
University of Saskatchewan
Saskatoon, SK
Canada

LI-SHAN CHOU
Department of Human Physiology
University of Oregon
Eugene, OR
USA

NIELS JUEL CHRISTENSEN
Endocrine Research Laboratory
Department of Medicine
Herlev Hospital
University of Copenhagen
Herlev
Denmark

ANDREW L. CLARK
Hull York Medical School
Hull
UK

TORBEN CLAUSEN
Institute of Physiology and Biophysics
Aarhus University
Universitetsparken, Århus
Denmark

PHILIPPE CONNES
Laboratoire ACTES (EA 3596)
Département de Physiologie
Université des Antilles et de la Guyane
Pointe-à-Pitre, Guadeloupe
French West Indies

STEVEN W. COPP
Departments of Kinesiology
Anatomy and Physiology
Kansas State University
Manhattan, KS
USA

KEITH DAVIDS
School of Human Movement Studies
Queensland University of Technology
Queensland
Australia

STEPHEN H. DAY
MMU Cheshire Sports Genetics Laboratory
Institute for Performance Research
Manchester Metropolitan University
Crewe
UK

MARY JANE DE SOUZA
Women's Health and Exercise Laboratory
Noll Laboratory
Department of Kinesiology
Penn State University
University Park, PA
USA

CATHERINE F. DECKER
Division of Infectious Diseases
National Naval Medical Center
Uniformed Services University of the Health Sciences
Bethesda, MD
USA

LOUISE DELDICQUE
Department of Biomedical Kinesiology
Research Centre for Exercise and Health
K.U.Leuven
Leuven
Belgium

LUÍS DELGADO
Department of Immunology, and Immuno-allergology
division
Faculty of Medicine
Hospital São João, E.P.E.
University of Porto
Porto
Portugal

VINCENZO DENARO
Department of Orthopaedic and Trauma Surgery
Campus Biomedico University
Rome
Italy

JARED M. DICKINSON
Department of Nutrition & Metabolism
Division of Rehabilitation Sciences
University of Texas Medical Branch
Galveston, TX
USA

AMIE J. DIRKS-NAYLOR
School of Pharmacy
Wingate University
Wingate, NC
USA

JAMES R. DOCHERTY
Department of Physiology
Royal College of Surgeons in Ireland
Dublin
Ireland

PAUL VAN DONKELAAR
School of Health and Exercise Science
University of British Columbia – Okanagan Campus
Kelowna, BC
Canada

GAL DUBNOV-RAZ
Exercise, Nutrition and Lifestyle Clinic
The Edmond and Lily Safra Children's Hospital
Sheba Medical Center
Tel Hashomer
Israel

DAVID J. DYCK
Department of Human Health and Nutritional Sciences
University of Guelph
Guelph, ON
Canada

KLAUS EDER
Justus-Liebig-University Giessen Interdisciplinary
Research Center (IFZ)
Institute of Animal Nutrition and Nutrition Physiology
Giessen
Germany

ØYVIND ELLINGSEN
Department of Circulation and Medical Imaging
Norwegian University of Science and Technology
Trondheim
Norway

ROGER M. ENOKA
Department of Integrative Physiology
University of Colorado
Boulder, CO
USA

KIRK I. ERICKSON
Department of Psychology
University of Pittsburgh
Pittsburgh, PA
USA

JOANNA ERION
Physiology Department
Georgia Health Sciences University
Augusta, GA
USA

ANDREA ERMOLAO
Department of Medical and Surgical Sciences
University of Padova
Padova
Italy

KATRIN ESEFELD
Department of Prevention
Rehabilitation and Sports Medicine
Zentrum für Prävention und Sportmedizin im
Olympiapark, Klinikum rechts der Isar
Technische Universität München
Munich
Germany

GERTJAN ETTEMA
Department of Human Movement Science
Faculty of Social Sciences and Technology Management
Norwegian University of Science and Technology
Trondheim
Norway

R. H. FAGARD
Hypertension and Cardiovascular Rehabilitation Unit
Hypertension Unit
University of Leuven K.U. Leuven
U.Z. Gasthuisberg
Leuven
Belgium

AVERY FAIGENBAUM
Department of Health and Exercise Science
The College of New Jersey
Ewing, NJ
USA

FRANCESCO FALLO
Department of Medical and Surgical Sciences
University of Padova
Padova
Italy

RICHARD N. FEDORAK
Division of Gastroenterology
University of Alberta
1–10 Zeidler Ledcor Centre
Edmonton, AB
Canada

JONATHAN S. FISHER
Department of Biology
Saint Louis University
St. Louis, MO
USA

AGNES FLÖEL
Department of Neurology
Charité Universitätsmedizin Berlin
Berlin
Germany

MARC FRANCAUX
Research group in muscle and exercise physiology
Institute of Neuroscience
Université catholique de Louvain
Louvain-la-Neuve
Belgium

CHRISTINE M. FRIEDENREICH
Department of Population Health Research
Alberta Health Services – Cancer Care
Calgary, AB
Canada

TIM J. GABBETT
The University of Queensland
School of Human Movement Studies
Brisbane
Australia

FIORENZO GAITA
Cardiology Division
Department of Internal Medicine
San Giovanni Battista Hospital
University of Turin
Turin
Italy

ANDREW W. GARDNER
CMRI Hobbs-Recknagel Professor
General Clinical Research Center
University of Oklahoma Health Sciences Center
Oklahoma City, OK
USA

MAX GASSMANN
Zurich Center for Integrative Human Physiology (ZIHP)
Institute of Veterinary Physiology
University of Zürich
Zürich
Switzerland
and
Universidad Peruana Cayetano Heredia
Lima
Peru

BERNARD GENY
Département de Physiologie
EA 3072, Hôpitaux Universitaires de Strasbourg
Strasbourg
France

GEORGE GIANNAKOULAS
Cardiology Department
AHEPA University Hospital
Thessaloniki
Greece

MARTIN J. GIBALA
Department of Kinesiology
McMaster University
Hamilton, ON
Canada

L. BRUCE GLADDEN
Department of Kinesiology
Auburn University
Auburn, AL
USA

MICHAEL GLEESON
School of Sport Exercise and Health Sciences
Loughborough University
Loughborough
UK

SONIA GOMEZ-MARTINEZ
Department of Metabolism and Nutrition,
Immunonutrition Research Group
Institute of Food Science and Technology and
Nutrition (ICTAN)
Spanish National Research Council (CSIC)
Madrid
Spain

JOSÉ GONZÁLEZ-ALONSO
Centre for Sports Medicine and Human Performance
Brunel University
Uxbridge
UK

FERGAL GRACE
Health & Exercise Science
School of Science
University of the West of Scotland
Hamilton, Scotland
UK

ROBERT W. GRANGE
Department of Human Nutrition
Foods and Exercise
Virginia Polytechnic Institute and State University
Blacksburg, VA
USA

HENK GRANZIER
Department of Physiology and the Sarver Molecular
Cardiovascular Research Program
University of Arizona
Tucson, AZ
USA

BRUNO GRASSI
Dipartimento di Scienze Mediche e Biologiche
Università degli Studi di Udine
Udine
Italy

STÉPHANE GRÉCIANO
Service de cardiologie
Hôpitaux Civils de Colmar
Colmar, Cedex
France

TRACY L. GREER
Department of Psychiatry
University of Texas Southwestern Medical Center
at Dallas
Dallas, TX
USA

TIMOTHY M. GRIFFIN
Free Radical Biology and Aging Research Program
Department of Biochemistry and Molecular Biology
Department of Geriatric Medicine
Oklahoma Medical Research Foundation
University of Oklahoma Health Sciences Center
Reynolds Oklahoma Center on Aging
Oklahoma City, OK
USA

CHANDAN GUHA
Department of Radiation Oncology
Albert Einstein College of Medicine
Bronx, NY
USA

THOMAS GUSTAFSSON
Department of Laboratory medicine
Karolinska Institutet
Stockholm
Sweden

BERNARD GUTIN
Department of Nutrition
School of Public Health
University of North Carolina
Chapel Hill, NC
USA

RAMIRO L. GUTIÉRREZ
Division of Infectious Diseases
National Naval Medical Center
Uniformed Services University of the Health Sciences
Bethesda, MD
USA

ANTHONY C. HACKNEY
Endocrine Section – Applied Physiology Laboratory
Department of Exercise & Sports Science
University of North Carolina
Chapel Hill, NC
USA

HIDDE J. HAISMA
Pharmaceutical Gene Modulation
Groningen Research Institute of Pharmacy
Groningen University
Groningen
The Netherlands

MARTIN HALLE
Department of Prevention
Rehabilitation and Sports Medicine
Zentrum für Prävention und Sportmedizin im
Olympiapark, Klinikum rechts der Isar
Technische Universität München
Munich
Germany

GREGORY A. HAND
Arnold School of Public Health
Department of Exercise Science
University of South Carolina
Columbia, SC
USA

B. HANDS
Institute for Health and Rehabilitation Research
University of Notre Dame
Fremantle
Australia

HEINZ W. HARBACH
Department of Anaesthesiology
Intensive Care Medicine
Pain Therapy
University Hospital Giessen & Marburg
Campus Giessen
Giessen
Germany

MARK HARGREAVES
Department of Physiology
The University of Melbourne
Melbourne
Australia

DAVID G. HARRISON
Cardiology Division
Department of Medicine and Biomechanical
Engineering
Emory University School of Medicine
Atlanta Veterans Administration Hospital
Atlanta, GA
USA

FRED HARTGENS
Departments of Epidemiology and Surgery
Maastricht University Medical Centre
Research school CAPHRI
Sports Medicine Centre Maastricht
Maastricht
The Netherlands

PETER HASSMÉN
Department of Psychology
Umeå University
Umeå
Sweden

HANS CHRISTIAN HAVERKAMP
Department of Environmental and Health Sciences
JSC Hodgepodge
Johnson State College
Johnson, VT
USA

THOMAS J. HAWKE
Department of Pathology and Molecular Medicine
McMaster University
Hamilton, ON
Canada

JOHN A. HAWLEY
Exercise Metabolism Group, School of Medical Sciences
Health Innovations Research Institute
RMIT University
Bundoora, VIC
Australia

HERMANN HECK
Lehrstuhl für Sportmedizin
University of Bochum
Institute of Sportmedicine and Nutrition
Bochum
Germany

HEIN HEIDBÜCHEL
Cardiology – Electrophysiology
University Hospital Gasthuisberg
University of Leuven
Leuven
Belgium

JAN HELGERUD
Department of Circulation and Medical imaging
Norwegian University of Science and Technology
Trondheim
Norway
and
Department of Sports and Outdoor Life Studies
Bø Telemark University College
Bø
Norway
and
Hokksund Medical Rehabilitation Centre
Hokksund
Norway

MATTHIJS HESSELINK
Department of Human Biology
Maastricht University Medical Center
Maastricht
The Netherlands

TAMARA HEW-BUTLER
Exercise Science School of Health Science
Oakland University
Rochester, MI
USA

KEITH HILL
Musculoskeletal Research Centre
La Trobe University and Northern Health
Bundoora, VIC
Australia

MARNI HILLINGER
Department of Rehabilitation Medicine
Columbia University College of Physicians and Surgeons
New York, NY
USA

CHARLES H. HILLMAN
Department of Kinesiology and Community Health
University of Illinois
Urbana, IL
USA

DANIEL M. HIRAI
Departments of Kinesiology
Anatomy and Physiology
Kansas State University
Manhattan, KS
USA

ANGELA HO
Texas Obesity Research Center
Health & Human Performance
University of Houston
Houston, TX
USA

JORIS HOEKS
Department of Human Biology
Maastricht University Medical Center
Maastricht
The Netherlands

JAN HOFF
Department of Circulation and Medical imaging
Norwegian University of Science and Technology
Trondheim
Norway
and
Department of Physical Medicine
St Olav's University Hospital
Trondheim
Norway

DAVID A. HOOD
Muscle Health Research Centre
School of Kinesiology & Health Science
York University
Toronto, ON
Canada

HANS HOPPELER
Department of Anatomy
University of Bern
Bern
Switzerland

JEFFREY F. HOROWITZ
School of Kinesiology
The University of Michigan
Ann Arbor, MI
USA

GANG HU
Chronic Disease Epidemiology Laboratory
Population Science
Pennington Biomedical Research Center
Baton Rouge, LA
USA

MONICA J. HUBAL
Research Center for Genetic Medicine
Children's National Medical Center
Washington, DC
USA

PETER A. HUIJING
Research Institute Move
Faculteit Bewegingswetenschappen
Vrije Universiteit
Amsterdam
The Netherlands

REED HUMPHREY
School of Physical Therapy & Rehabilitation Science
College of Health Professions & Biomedical Sciences
The University of Montana
Missoula, MT
USA

FERDINANDO IELLAMO
Internal Medicine
University Tor Vergata
Rome
Italy

OMRI INBAR
Department of Life Sciences
Zinman College Wingate Institute
Netania
Israel

OLLIE JAY
Thermal Ergonomics Laboratory
School of Human Kinetics
University of Ottawa
Ottawa, ON
Canada

WOLFGANG JELKMANN
Institute of Physiology
University of Luebeck
Luebeck
Germany

ASKER JEUKENDRUP
School of Sport and Exercise Sciences
The University of Birmingham
Edgbaston, Birmingham
UK

LI LI JI
Department of Kinesiology
Interdepartmental Program of Nutritional Sciences
Institute on Aging
University of Wisconsin-Madison
Madison, WI
USA

HANJOONG JO
Cardiology Division
Department of Medicine and Biomechanical Engineering
Emory University School of Medicine
Atlanta Veterans Administration Hospital
Atlanta, GA
USA

D. A. JONES
Institute for Biomedical Research into Human Movement and Health
Manchester Metropolitan University
Manchester
UK

LEE W. JONES
Department of Surgery
Duke University Medical Center
Duke Cancer Institute
Durham, NC
USA

CARSTEN JUEL
Department of Biology
Copenhagen Muscle Research Centre
University of Copenhagen
Copenhagen
Denmark

Y. PETER JUNG
Exercise & Sport Nutrition Lab
Department of Health and Kinesiology
Texas A & M University
College Station, TX
USA

JAYNE M. KALMAR
Wilfrid Laurier University
Waterloo, ON
Canada

KAMELJIT KALSI
Centre for Sports Medicine and Human Performance
Brunel University
Uxbridge
UK

JIE KANG
Human Performance Laboratory
Department of Health and Exercise Science
The College of New Jersey
Ewing, NJ
USA

HARALAMBOS KARVOUNIS
Cardiology Department
AHEPA University Hospital
Thessaloniki
Greece

ANDREAS N. KAVAZIS
Department of Kinesiology
Mississippi State University
Mississippi State, MS
USA

KEVIN G. KEENAN
Neuromechanics Lab
Department of Human Movement Sciences
College of Health Sciences University of
Wisconsin-Milwaukee
Milwaukee, WI
USA

OLE JOHAN KEMI
Institute of Cardiovascular and Medical Sciences
University of Glasgow
Glasgow, Scotland
UK

MAXIMILIAN KEMPER
Department of Prevention
Rehabilitation and Sports Medicine
Zentrum für Prävention und Sportmedizin im
Olympiapark
Klinikum rechts der Isar
Technische Universität München
Munich
Germany

K. KENN
Klinikum Berchtesgadener Land
GmbH & Co. KG
Prien am Chiemsee
Germany

LON KILGORE
Health & Exercise Science
School of Science
University of the West of Scotland
Hamilton, Scotland
UK

WILFRIED KINDERMANN
Institute of Sports and Preventive Medicine
University of Saarland
Saarbrücken
Germany

RALF KINSCHERF
Head of the Department of Anatomy and Cell Biology
Philipps-University of Marburg
Marburg
Germany

MICHAEL KJÆR
Institute of Sports Medicine and Centre for Healthy
Ageing
Bispebjerg Hospital
University of Copenhagen
Copenhagen
Denmark

CHRISTOPHER E. KLINE
Department of Psychiatry
University of Pittsburgh School of Medicine
Pittsburgh, PA
USA

BEAT KNECHTLE
Institute of General Practice and for Health Services
Research
University of Zurich
Zurich
Switzerland

A. R. KOCZULLA
Dept. Pulmonology
University Giessen and Marburg
Marburg
Germany

PETER KOKKINOS
Cardiology Department
Veterans Affairs Medical Center
Washington, DC
USA
and
George Washington University School of Medicine and
Health Sciences
Washington, DC
USA

PAAVO V. KOMI
Neuromuscular Research Center
University of Jyväskylä
Jyväskylä
Finland

DANIEL KÖNIG
Medizinische Universitätsklinik
Abt. Rehabilitative und Präventive Sportmedizin
Freiburg
Germany

WILLIAM J. KRAEMER
Department of Kinesiology
University of Connecticut Human
Performance Laboratory
Storrs, CT
USA

MATTHEW P. KRAUSE
Department of Pathology and Molecular Medicine
McMaster University
Hamilton, ON
Canada

KIM A. KRAWCZEWSKI CARHUATANTA
Metabolic Disease Institute
University of Cincinnati
Cincinnati, OH
USA

RICHARD B. KREIDER
Exercise & Sport Nutrition Lab
Department of Health and Kinesiology
Texas A & M University
College Station, TX
USA

KARSTEN KRÜGER
Department of Sports Medicine
University of Giessen
Giessen
Germany

SIEGFRIED LABEIT
Klinikum Mannheim GmbH Universitätsklinikum
Universitätsmedizin Mannheim
University of Heidelberg
Mannheim
Germany

TIMO A. LAKKA
Department of Physiology
Institute of Biomedicine
University of Eastern Finland
Kuopio
Finland
and
Kuopio Research Institute of Exercise Medicine
Kuopio
Finland

G. PATRICK LAMBERT
Department of Exercise Science
Creighton University
Omaha, NE
USA

MIKE I. LAMBERT
MRC/UCT Research Unit for Exercise Science and Sports
Medicine, Department of Human Biology
University of Cape Town
Newlands, Cape Town
South Africa

REBECCA E. LEE
Texas Obesity Research Center
Health & Human Performance
University of Houston
Houston, TX
USA

STIG LEIRDAL
Department of Human Movement Science
Faculty of Social Sciences and Technology Management
Norwegian University of Science and Technology
Trondheim
Norway

RENATE M. LEITHÄUSER
Biomedical Science
Department of Biological Sciences
University of Essex
UK

ARTHUR S. LEON
Laboratory of Physiological Hygiene and
Exercise Science
School of Kinesiology
Minneapolis, MN
USA

DANIEL J. LEONG
Department of Orthopaedic Surgery and Radiation
Oncology
Albert Einstein College of Medicine and Montefiore
Medical Center
Bronx, NY
USA

RICHARD LEPPERT
Department of Neurology
Charité Universitätsmedizin Berlin
Berlin
Germany

MICHAEL I. LINDINGER
Department of Human Health and Nutritional Sciences
University of Guelph
Guelph, ON
Canada

DAVID M. LINDSAY
University of Calgary
Calgary, AB
Canada

GREGORY Y. H. LIP
Haemostasis Thrombosis and Vascular Biology Unit
University of Birmingham Centre for Cardiovascular
Sciences
City Hospital
Birmingham
UK

HERBERT LÖLLGEN
Sana-Klinikum Remscheid
Johannes-Gutenberg-University, Mainz
Remscheid
Germany

RUTH LÖLLGEN
Soins intensifs pédiatriques
Département médico-chirurgical de pédiatrie- DMCP
Bâtiment hospitalier
Lausanne
Switzerland

UMILE GIUSEPPE LONGO
Department of Orthopaedic and Trauma Surgery
Campus Biomedico University
Rome
Italy

STEPHEN R. LORD
Falls and Balance Research Group
Neuroscience Research Australia
University of New South Wales
Sydney, NSW
Australia

BRITTA LOREY
Institute for Sport Science
Justus Liebig University
Giessen
Germany

ANNE B. LOUCKS
Department of Biological Sciences
Ohio University
Athens, OH
USA

G. WILLIAM LYERLY
Arnold School of Public Health
Department of Exercise Science
University of South Carolina
Columbia, SC
USA

BRIGID M. LYNCH
Department of Population Health Research
Alberta Health Services – Cancer Care
Calgary, AB
Canada

GORDON S. LYNCH
Basic and Clinical Myology Laboratory
Department of Physiology
The University of Melbourne
Melbourne, VIC
Australia

SCOTT K. LYNN
Department of Kinesiology
California State University
Fullerton, CA
USA

BRIAN R. MACINTOSH
University of Calgary
Calgary, AL
Canada

LIDA MADEMLI
Department of Sports Science
Serres
Aristotle University of Thessaloniki
Thessaloniki
Greece

NICOLA MAFFULLI
Centre for Sports and Exercise Medicine
Barts and The London School of Medicine and Dentistry
Mile End Hospital
Queen Mary University of London
London
UK

FAIDON MAGKOS
Department of Nutrition and Dietetics
Harokopio University
Athens
Greece
and
Center for Human Nutrition
Washington University School of Medicine
St. Louis, MO
USA

ROBERT J. MAJESKA
Department of Biomedical Engineering
The City College of New York
New York, NY
USA

ROBERT M. MALINA
Department of Kinesiology and Health Education
University of Texas at Austin
Stephenville, TX
USA
and
Department of Kinesiology
Tarleton State University
Stephenville, TX
USA

FABIO MANFREDINI
Department of Biochemistry and Molecular Biology
Section of Biochemistry of Physical Exercise Center
Biomedical Studies Applied to Sport
Vascular Diseases Center
University of Ferrara
Ferrara
Italy

ROBERTO MANFREDINI
Department of Biochemistry and Molecular Biology
Section of Biochemistry of Physical Exercise Center
Biomedical Studies Applied to Sport
Vascular Diseases Center
University of Ferrara
Ferrara
Italy

MELINDA M. MANORE
Department of Nutrition and Exercise Sciences
Oregon State University College of Health and Human
Sciences
Corvallis, OR
USA

ASCENSION MARCOS
Department of Metabolism and Nutrition
Immunonutrition Research Group
Institute of Food Science and Technology and Nutrition
(ICTAN)
Spanish National Research Council (CSIC)
Madrid
Spain

CHAD D. MARKERT
Wake Forest Institute of Regenerative Medicine
Wake Forest University
Winston-Salem, NC
USA

GORAN MARKOVIC
School of Kinesiology
University of Zagreb
Zagreb
Croatia

DAVID MARTINEZ-GOMEZ
Department of Metabolism and Nutrition
Immunonutrition Research Group
Institute of Food Science and Technology and
Nutrition (ICTAN)
Spanish National Research Council (CSIC)
Madrid
Spain

ANTONIOS MATSAKAS
Institute of Molecular Medicine
The University of Texas Health Science Center
Houston, TX
USA

MARK P. MATTSON
Laboratory of Neurosciences
National Institute on Aging Intramural Research
Program
Biomedical Research Center Room 05C214
Baltimore, MD
USA

R. J. MAUGHAN
School of Sport, Exercise and Health Sciences
Loughborough University
Loughborough
UK

ROBERT S. MAZZEO
Department of Integrative Physiology
University of Colorado
Boulder, CO
USA

JAMES R. MCDONALD
Department of Kinesiology
Auburn University
Auburn, AL
USA

GEMMA A. MCLEOD
School of Physical Education and Department of
Human Nutrition
University of Otago
Dunedin
New Zealand

ROMAIN MEEUSEN
Department of Human Physiology and Sports Medicine
Faculty of Physical Education and Physical Therapy
Lotto Sports Science Chair
Vrije Universiteit Brussel
Brussels
Belgium

BERTRAND METTAUER
Service de cardiologie
Hôpitaux Civils de Colmar
Colmar, Cedex
France
and
Département de Physiologie
EA 3072, Hôpitaux Universitaires de Strasbourg
Strasbourg
France

MARIE-LAURE MILLE
Université du Sud
Toulon–Var
La Garde
France
and

Institut des Sciences du Mouvement
Aix–Marseille University & CNRS
UMR 6233
Marseille cedex 9
France

BENJAMIN F. MILLER
Department of Health and Exercise Science
Colorado State University
Fort Collins, CO
USA

LINDSEY E. MILLER
Cardioprotection Laboratory
Department of Kinesiology
Auburn University
Auburn, AL
USA

KEVIN MILNE
Department of Kinesiology
The University of Windsor
Windsor, ON
Canada

TOBY MÜNDEL
School of Sport and Exercise
Massey University
Palmerston North
New Zealand

FRANK C. MOOREN
Department of Sports Medicine
Justus-Liebig-University
Giessen
Germany

ANDRÉ MOREIRA
Department of Immunology, and Immuno-allergology
division
Faculty of Medicine
Hospital São João, E.P.E.
University of Porto
Porto
Portugal

DAVID L. MORGAN
Department of Physiology
Electrical & Computer Systems Engineering
Monash University
Clayton, VIC
Australia

SOPHIA-ANASTASIA MOURATOGLOU
Cardiology Department
AHEPA University Hospital
Thessaloniki
Greece

TIMOTHY I. MUSCH
Departments of Kinesiology
Anatomy and Physiology
Kansas State University
Manhattan, KS
USA

KATHRYN H. MYBURGH
Department Physiological Sciences
Fellow of the American College of Sports Medicine
Stellenbosch University
Stellenbosch
South Africa

JONATHAN N. MYERS
VA Palo Alto Health Care System
Stanford University
Palo Alto, CA
USA

GUSTAVO A. NADER
Department of Medicine
Center for Molecular Medicine L8:04
Karolinska Institute
Stockholm
Sweden

NEERAJ NARULA
Department of Medicine (Division of Gastroenterology)
and, Farncombe Family Digestive Health Research
Institute
McMaster University
Hamilton, ON
Canada

CHRISTOPHER L. NEWMAN
Department of Anatomy & Cell Biology
Indiana University School of Medicine
Indianapolis, IN
USA

P. NEWSHOLME
School of Biomolecular and Biomedical Science
Conway Institute and Health Sciences Complex
University College Dublin
Dublin
Ireland

CAROLINE NICOL
Aix-Marseille University
UMR 6233
Marseilles
France

JOSEF NIEBAUER
University Institute of Sports Medicine, Prevention and
Rehabilitation
Institute of Sports Medicine of the State of Salzburg
Sports Medicine of the Olympic Center Salzburg-Rif
Paracelsus Medical University
Salzburg
Austria

DAVID C. NIEMAN
Department of Health, Leisure and Exercise Science
Appalachian State University Fischer Hamilton/Nycom
Biochemistry Laboratory
Boone, NC
USA

EARL G. NOBLE
Department of Kinesiology
The University of Western Ontario
London, ON
Canada

GUILLERMO J. NOFFAL
Department of Kinesiology
California State University
Fullerton, CA
USA

FRANS NOLLET
Department of Rehabilitation
Academic Medical Centre
University of Amsterdam
Amsterdam, AZ
The Netherlands

STEPHEN R. NORRIS
Canadian Sport Centre - Calgary
University of Calgary and Mount Royal University
Calgary, AB
Canada

BLAKESLEE E. NOYES
School of Medicine
St. Louis University at SSM Cardinal Glennon Children's
Medical Center
St. Louis, MO
USA

LOUISE ØSTERGAARD
Zurich Center for Integrative Human Physiology (ZIHP)
Institute of Veterinary Physiology
University of Zürich
Zürich
Switzerland

LOUIS R. OSTERNIG
Department of Human Physiology
University of Oregon
Eugene, OR
USA

KETAN PATEL
School of Biological Sciences
University of Reading
Whiteknights, Reading
UK

KEVIN DE PAUW
Department of Human Physiology and Sports Medicine
Faculty of Physical Education and Physical Therapy
Lotto Sports Science Chair
Vrije Universiteit Brussel
Brussels
Belgium

SOFIA PÉREZ-ALENDA
Department of Physiotherapy
University of Valencia
Spain
and
Haemostasis and Thrombosis Unit
University Hospital La FE
Valencia
Spain

LINDA S. PESCATELLO
Department of Kinesiology U-1110
Human Performance Laboratory
Neag School of Education
University of Connecticut
Storrs, CT
USA

DIRK PETTE
Department of Biology
University of Konstanz
Konstanz
Germany

ANDREW PHILP
Department of Neurobiology, Physiology and Behavior
University of California
Davis, CA
USA

YANNIS PITSILADIS
College of Medicine, Veterinary and Life Sciences
Institute of Cardiovascular and Medical Sciences
University of Glasgow
Glasgow, Scotland
UK

GUY PLASQUI
Department of Human Biology
NUTRIM School for Nutrition, Toxicology & Metabolism
Maastricht University Medical Centre +
Maastricht
The Netherlands

DAVID C. POOLE
Departments of Kinesiology, Anatomy and Physiology
Kansas State University
Manhattan, KS
USA

NICOLE PROMMER
Department of Sports Medicine
University of Bayreuth
Bayreuth
Germany

UWE PROSKE
Department of Physiology
Electrical & Computer Systems Engineering
Monash University
Clayton, VIC
Australia

FELIPE QUEROL
Department of Physiotherapy
University of Valencia
Spain
and
Haemostasis and Thrombosis Unit
University Hospital La FE
Valencia
Spain

JOHN C. QUINDRY
Cardioprotection Laboratory
Department of Kinesiology
Auburn University
Auburn, AL
USA

BLAKE B. RASMUSSEN
Department of Nutrition & Metabolism
Division of Rehabilitation Sciences
University of Texas Medical Branch
Galveston, TX
USA

NICHOLAS A. RATAMESS
Department of Health and Exercise Science
The College of New Jersey
Ewing, NJ
USA

NANCY J. REHRER
School of Physical Education and Department of
Human Nutrition
University of Otago
Dunedin
New Zealand

THOMAS REILLY
Research Institute for Sport and Exercise Sciences
Liverpool John Moores University Henry Cotton
Campus
Liverpool
UK

CHAD D. RETHORST
Department of Psychiatry
University of Texas Southwestern Medical Center at
Dallas
Dallas, TX
USA

JEAN-PAUL RICHALET
EA2363 "Réponses cellulaires et fonctionnelles
à l'hypoxie"
UFR SMBH
Université Paris 13
Bobigny Cedex
France

M. C. RIDDELL
School of Kinesiology and Health Science
Physical Activity and Chronic Disease Unit
Faculty of Health
Muscle Health Research Centre
York University
York
Canada

ROBERT RINGSEIS
Justus-Liebig-University Giessen Interdisciplinary
Research Center (IFZ)
Institute of Animal Nutrition and Nutrition Physiology
Giessen
Germany

HANNU RINTAMÄKI
Finnish Institute of Occupational Health
Oulu
Finland
and
Department of Physiology
Institute of Biomedicine
University of Oulu
Oulu
Finland

LINDSAY E. ROBINSON
Department of Human Health and Nutritional Sciences
University of Guelph
Guelph, ON
Canada

MATTHEW M. ROBINSON
Endocrine Research Unit
Mayo Clinic
Rochester, MN
USA

H. LLEWELYN RODERICK
Laboratory of Signalling and Cell Fate
Babraham Institute
Cambridge
UK
and
Department of Pharmacology
University of Cambridge
Cambridge
UK

MARK W. ROGERS
University of Maryland Claude D. Pepper Older
American Independence Center
University of Maryland School of Medicine
Baltimore, MD
USA

ØIVIND ROGNMO
K.G. Jebsen Center of Exercise in Medicine
Department of Circulation and Medical Imaging
Norwegian University of Science and Technology
Trondheim
Norway

JAVIER ROMEO
Department of Metabolism and Nutrition,
Immunonutrition Research Group
Institute of Food Science and Technology and
Nutrition (ICTAN)
Spanish National Research Council (CSIC)
Madrid
Spain

ERIC RULLMAN
Department of Laboratory medicine
Karolinska Institutet
Stockholm
Sweden

ROBERT L. SAINBURG
Departments of Kinesiology and Neurology
The Pennsylvania State University
Pennsylvania, PA
USA

MICHELE SAMAJA
University of Milan – San Paolo
Milan
Italy

THOMAS G. SANDERCOCK
Department of Physiology M211
Ward 5–295
Feinberg School of Medicine
Northwestern University
Chicago, IL
USA

WILHELM SCHÄNZER
German Sport University Cologne
Institute of Biochemistry – Center for Preventive Doping
Research
Cologne
Germany

ZACHARY J. SCHLADER
School of Sport and Exercise
Massey University
Palmerston North
New Zealand

WALTER SCHMIDT
Department of Sports Medicine
University of Bayreuth
Bayreuth
Germany

PATRICK SCHRAUWEN
Department of Human Biology
Maastricht University Medical Center
Maastricht
The Netherlands

CHRISTOPHER B. SCOTT
Department of Exercise, Health and Sport Sciences
University of Southern Maine
Gorham, ME
USA

DAVID L. SCOTT
Department of Rheumatology
King's College Hospital
Kings College London School of Medicine Weston
Education Centre
London
UK

CHARLES SEARLES
Cardiology Division
Department of Medicine and Biomechanical
Engineering
Emory University School of Medicine
Atlanta Veterans Administration Hospital
Atlanta, GA
USA

MICHAEL SEIMETZ
Excellence Cluster Cardio-Pulmonary System (ECCPS)
University of Giessen Lung Center (UGLC)
Medizinische Klinik II
Giessen
Germany

KAREN SØGAARD
Institute of Sports Science and Clinical Biomechanics
University of Southern Denmark
Odense M
Denmark

ROY J. SHEPHARD
University of Toronto
Toronto, ON
Canada
and
University of Toronto
Brackendale, BC
Canada

JEREMY M. SHEPPARD
Department of Biomedical, Health, and Exercise
Sciences
Edith Cowan University
Joondalup
Australia

CATHERINE SHERRINGTON
Musculoskeletal Division
The George Institute for Global Health, University of
Sydney
Sydney, NSW
Australia

S. M. SHIRREFFS
School of Sport, Exercise and Health Sciences
Loughborough University
Loughborough
UK

MARLENE N. SILVA
Department of Sports and Health
Faculty of Human Kinetics
Technical University of Lisbon
Lisbon
Portugal

RICHARD J. SIMPSON
Laboratory of Integrated Physiology
Department of Health and Human Performance
University of Houston
Houston, TX
USA

KAUSTABH SINGH
Muscle Health Research Centre
School of Kinesiology & Health Science
York University
Toronto, ON
Canada

SEBASTIAN SIXT
Herz-Zentrum Bad Krozingen
Deparment of Angiology
Bad Krozingen
Germany

GISELA SJØGAARD
Institute of Sports Science and Clinical Biomechanics
University of Southern Denmark
Odense M
Denmark

DAVID J. SMITH
Human Performance Laboratory
University of Calgary
Calgary, AB
Canada

ASHLEY J. SMUDER
Department of Applied Physiology and Kinesiology
University of Florida
Gainesville, FL
USA

IOANNIS SMYRNIAS
Department of Cardiology
The James Black Centre
King's College London
London
UK

DANIEL SOFFER
University of Pennsylvania
Philadelphia, PA
USA

ESPEN E. SPANGENBURG
Department of Kinesiology
School of Public Health
University of Maryland
College Park, MD
USA

FILIPPO SPIEZIA
Department of Orthopaedic and Trauma Surgery
Campus Biomedico University
Rome
Italy

NINA S. STACHENFELD
The John B. Pierce Laboratory
New Haven, CT
USA
and
Department of Obstetrics, Gynecology and
Reproductive Sciences
Yale University School of Medicine
New Haven, CT
USA
and
Yale School of Public Health
Yale University School of Medicine
New Haven, CT
USA

ROBERT S. STARON
Department of Biomedical Sciences
College of Osteopathic Medicine
Ohio University
Athens, OH
USA

JOEL STEIN
Department of Rehabilitation Medicine
Columbia University College of Physicians and Surgeons
New York, NY
USA

C. E. STEWART
Institute for Biomedical Research into Human
Movement and Health
Manchester Metropolitan University
Manchester
UK

ALEXIS M. STRANAHAN
Physiology Department
Georgia Health Sciences University
Augusta, GA
USA

ANNA STRÖMBERG
Department of Laboratory medicine
Karolinska Institutet
Stockholm
Sweden

DAINA L. STURNIEKS
Falls and Balance Research Group
Neuroscience Research Australia
University of New South Wales
Sydney, NSW
Australia

HUI B. SUN
Department of Orthopaedic Surgery and Radiation
Oncology
Albert Einstein College of Medicine and Montefiore
Medical Center
Bronx, NY
USA

KATSUHIKO SUZUKI
Waseda University
Tokorozawa, Saitama
Japan

STEFANO TADDEI
Department of Internal Medicine
University of Pisa
Pisa
Italy

HIROFUMI TANAKA
Department of Kinesiology and Health Education
Cardiovascular Aging Research Laboratory
University of Texas at Austin
Austin, TX
USA

PEDRO TAULER RIERA
Departament de Biologia Fonamental i Ciències de la
Salut
Universitat de les Illes Balears
Palma de Mallorca
Spain

HENRY L. TAYLOR
Laboratory of Physiological Hygiene and Exercise
Science
School of Kinesiology
Minneapolis, MN
USA

PEDRO J. TEIXEIRA
Department of Sports and Health
Faculty of Human Kinetics
Technical University of Lisbon
Lisbon
Portugal

MARIO THEVIS
German Sport University Cologne
Institute of Biochemistry – Center for Preventive Doping
Research
Cologne
Germany

ANNE TIEDEMANN
Musculoskeletal Division
The George Institute for Global Health
University of Sydney
Sydney, NSW
Australia

REBECCA J. TOOMBS
Women's Health and Exercise Laboratory
Noll Laboratory
Department of Kinesiology
Penn State University
University Park, PA
USA

ELISABETTA TOSO
Cardiology Division
Department of Internal Medicine
San Giovanni Battista Hospital
University of Turin
Turin
Italy

KARIN E. TRAJCEVSKI
Department of Pathology and Molecular Medicine
McMaster University
Hamilton, ON
Canada

JOSÉ LUIS TREJO
Department of Molecular, Cellular and Developmental
Neurobiology
Cajal Institute
CSIC Consejo Superior de Investigaciones Cientificas
Madrid
Spain

MADHUKAR H. TRIVEDI
Department of Psychiatry
University of Texas Southwestern Medical Center at
Dallas
Dallas, TX
USA

JAAKKO TUOMILEHTO
South Ostrobothnia Central Hospital
Seinäjoki
Finland
and
Red RECAVA Grupo RD06/0014/0015
Hospital Universitario La Paz
Madrid
Spain
and
Centre for Vascular Prevention
Danube-University Krems
Krems
Austria

AXEL URHAUSEN
Centre de l'Appareil locomoteur
de Médecine du Sport et de Prévention
Laboratoire de Recherche en Médecine du Sport
Centre Hospitalier de Luxembourg
CRP-santé
Luxembourg
Luxembourg

ANTHONY A. VANDERVOORT
School of Physical Therapy
University of Western Ontario
Ontario
Canada

LUIGI VARESIO
Laboratory of Molecular Biology
Giannina Gaslini Institute
Genova
Italy

RENÉE VENTURA-CLAPIER
Faculté de Pharmacie
U-769 Inserm
Université Paris-Sud
Châtenay-Malabry
France

C. FRANZ VOGELMEIER
Dept. Pulmonology
University Giessen and Marburg
Marburg
Germany

MICHAEL VOGT
Department of Anatomy
University of Bern
Bern
Switzerland

STELLA LUCIA VOLPE
Department of Nutrition Sciences
Drexel University
Philadelphia, PA
USA

MAURIZIO VOLTERRANI
UO di Riabilitazione Cardiologica
IRCCS San Raffaele Pisana
Rome
Italy

JÜRGEN VORMANN
Institute for Prevention and Nutrition
Ismaning
Germany

PETER WAGNER
Department of Medicine
University of California
San Diego, CA
USA

CLAUDIA WALTHER
Department of Cardiology
Kerckhoff Clinic
Bad Nauheim
Germany

KARLMAN WASSERMAN
Respiratory and Critical Care Physiology and Medicine
David Geffen School of Medicine
University of California at Los Angeles
Los Angeles Biomedical Research Institute
Harbor-UCLA Medical Center
Torrance, CA
USA

CORA WEIGERT
Division of Endocrinology, Diabetology, Angiology,
Nephrology, Pathobiochemistry and Clinical Chemistry
Department of Internal Medicine
University of Tuebingen
Tuebingen
Germany
and
Paul Langerhans Institute Tuebingen
Tuebingen
Germany

MEGAN M. WENNER
The John B. Pierce Laboratory
New Haven, CT
USA
and
Department of Obstetrics, Gynecology and
Reproductive Sciences
Yale University School of Medicine
New Haven, CT
USA

KLAAS R. WESTERTERP
Department of Human Biology
NUTRIM School for Nutrition, Toxicology & Metabolism
Maastricht University Medical Centre +
Maastricht
The Netherlands

KIM VAN WIJCK
Department of General Surgery
Maastricht University Medical Center
Maastricht
The Netherlands

ALUN G. WILLIAMS
MMU Cheshire Sports Genetics Laboratory
Institute for Performance Research, Manchester
Metropolitan University
Crewe
UK

NANCY I. WILLIAMS
Department of Kinesiology
Penn State University 108 Noll Laboratory
University Park, PA
USA

ULRIK WISLØFF
K.G. Jebsen Center of Exercise in Medicine
Department of Circulation and Medical Imaging
Norwegian University of Science and Technology
Trondheim
Norway

STEPHEN C. WOODS
Internal Medicine and Psychiatry
University of Cincinnati
Cincinnati, OH
USA

DAVID C. WRIGHT
Department of Human Health and Nutritional Sciences
University of Guelph
Guelph, ON
Canada

JULIA WÄRNBERG
Department of Metabolism and Nutrition
Immunonutrition Research Group
Institute of Food Science and Technology and Nutrition
(ICTAN)

Spanish National Research Council (CSIC)
Madrid
Spain
and
Department of Preventive Medicine and Public Health
School of Medicine
University of Navarra
Pamplona
Spain

KEVIN E. YARASHESKI
Program in Physical Therapy and Department of
Medicine
Washington University School of Medicine
Saint Louis, MO
USA

JASPER T. YEN
Comparative Neuromechanics Laboratory
School of Applied Physiology
Georgia Institute of Technology
Atlanta, GA
USA

P. ZAMPARO
Department of Neurological, Neuropsychological
Morphological and Movement Sciences
School of Exercise and Sport Sciences
University of Verona
Verona
Italy

JERZY A. ZOLADZ
Department of Physiology and Biochemistry
Faculty of Rehabilitation
University School of Physical Education
AWF-Kraków
Kraków
Poland

A

αB crystalline

Ubiquitously expressed molecular chaperone from the small heat shock protein family. Mutations in this protein are associated with the familial cardiomyopathies.

Abnormal Cardiac Electrical Activity

▶ Cardiac Arrhythmias

Absorption

Movement of a substance into the internal environment of the body by transport through an epithelial membrane.

Acceleration

Acceleration should not be confused with speed. Acceleration is the rate of change of velocity that allows an athlete to reach maximum speed in the minimum amount of time.

Accelerometers

Accelerometers are electronic motion sensors that consist of piezoresistive or piezoelectric sensors. Motion sensors are probably the oldest tools available to measure body movement or physical activity. They have evolved from mechanical pedometers to electronic uniaxial and triaxial accelerometers.

Accessory Pathway

Accessory pathways (AP) are extra nodal pathways that connect the atrial myocardium to the ventricle across the AV groove. Typical APs usually exhibit rapid, non decremental, anterograde and retrograde conduction, demonstrating delta wave on a standard surface ECG. WPW is defined as PR interval <0.12 s, delta wave and supraventricular tachycardia. Among patients with WPW syndrome, atrioventricular reciprocating tachycardia is the most common arrhythmia, followed by atrial fibrillation.

Acclimation

Phenotypic adaptive physiological or behavioral changes occurring within an organism, which reduces the strain or enhances endurance of strain caused by experimentally induced stressful changes in particular climatic factors such as ambient temperature in a controlled environment.

Cross-References

▶ Cold

Acclimatization

Physiological (or behavioral) changes that occur within an individual's lifetime that reduce the physiological strain associated with a particular naturally occurring stressful climatic environment. A phenotypic adaption.

Cross-References

▶ Cold

Frank C. Mooren (ed.), *Encyclopedia of Exercise Medicine in Health and Disease*, DOI 10.1007/978-3-540-29807-6,
© Springer-Verlag Berlin Heidelberg 2012

Acid–Base Buffering Systems

DIETER BÖNING

Sports Medicine, Charité – Universitätsmedizin Berlin, Berlin, Germany

Synonyms

Stabilization of hydrogen ion activity or concentration

Definition

pH is the negative decadic logarithm of hydrogen ion (H^+) activity in a solution. Water dissociates into equal amounts of H^+ and OH^-, the reaction is neutral (10^{-7} mol H^+ per kg water, pH 7.0 at 25°C, 6.8 at 37°C). Acids (Ac) dissociate to H^+ and the negatively charged rest of the acid (Ac^-) or conjugate base, bases to OH^- and the positively charged base rest or conjugate acid. Strong acids or bases dissociate nearly completely. The tendency to dissociate is smaller in weak acids and bases because of the molecular structure and distribution of charges; it is described by the dissociation constant $K = ([H^+] \times [Ac^-])/[Ac]$, pK being the negative logarithm. If pH = pK, the acid is half-dissociated. This can be artificially obtained by mixing one part of a weak acid (e.g., CH_3COOH, acetic acid) with one part of its salt with a strong base (e.g., $Na^+\ CH_3COO^-$, sodium acetate), since salts are fully dissociated in water. For another set point of pH, the proportion of acid and salt may be changed. When mixing a strong acid with such a solution, part of the added H^+ is bound to the conjugate base of the weak acid, thus the increase in $[H^+]$ is attenuated, "buffered". Equal effects, but into the opposite direction, occur when adding a strong base.

Buffer capacity β is defined according to Van Slyke (1922) as

$$\beta = \Delta[\text{base}] \times \Delta pH^{-1} = -\Delta[\text{acid}] \times \Delta pH^{-1}$$

The usual unit in biology (often denominated as Slyke) is mmol l^{-1}, because pH is a dimensionless logarithm.

β can be measured by titration with strong acids or bases; the slope of the curve is largest at the pK value (maximal value 0.576 mol mol^{-1}) with an effective range at pH = pK ± 1 (Fig. 1). Under in vivo conditions (pH values between 6.2 and 7.6 at 30–41°C in various tissues), buffers with pK around 7 are most effective. Actual β depends additionally on the concentration of the buffer. Measurements of buffer capacities in an organism can be either performed in vitro in samples (e.g., blood, tissue samples, cell cultures) or in vivo using implanted electrodes

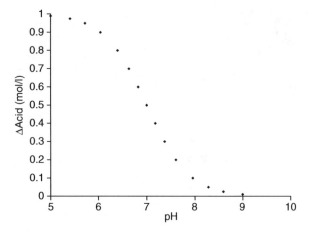

Acid–Base Buffering Systems. Fig. 1 Change of pH in a solution of weak acid (1 mol l^{-1}) with a pK value of 7.0 by addition of strong acid. The dissociation of the pure weak acid is about 1% (pH = 9). Against convention, the y-axis is used for the independent quantity ΔAcid to demonstrate buffer capacity as slope of the curve (multiplied by −1)

or indirect methods like nuclear magnetic resonance. The total amount of bound H^+ is calculable as $\beta \times \Delta pH$.

In biology, the meaning of buffering has to be extended: besides physicochemical buffering (described above) respiration (excretion of the volatile acid H_2CO_3), metabolic effects (consumption or production of nonvolatile acids) and transmembrane fluxes of H^+ or corresponding molecules like HCO_3^- play an important role for pH stability and are considered as special forms of buffering. When evaluating titrations, the different components cannot always be discerned. On a long term also excretion of acid or base by kidney, gut, and sweat glands plays a role.

Since hydrogen ions produced in large amounts by metabolism (especially as carbonic and lactic acid) take part in many chemical reactions and influence the charges and thus the conformation of proteins, stabilization of their concentration by the above-mentioned mechanisms is essential for the organism.

Basic Mechanisms

Physicochemical Buffering

In the body, two general types of physicochemical buffers exist: non-bicarbonate (nb) and bicarbonate (b) buffers.

Non-bicarbonate Buffers

The second dissociation constant of inorganic phosphoric acid ($H_3PO_4 <-> H_2PO_4^- + H^+ <-> HPO_4^{2-} + 2H^+ <-> PO_4^{3-} + 3H^+$) fits to the physiological pH range

$(pK_2 = 6.84$ at $37°C)$, the concentration varying between 1 (extracellular fluid) and 13 (muscle cell water) mmol l^{-1} at rest. The amount of organic phosphates (creatine phosphate, glucose phosphates, adenosine phosphates, nucleic acids, phospholipids, etc.) is larger especially within cells, but because of the repelling forces among neighboring charges, often dissociation is complete at physiological pH. ATP looses its buffering power by complexing with Mg^{++} and proteins. This group of buffers may therefore change their buffer effect markedly and rapidly, if phosphate groups are transposed or liberated.

Most carboxyl and NH_3^+ groups in proteinic amino acids possess pK values outside of the pH range in the body or disappear by peptide formation. Only histidine (imidazole group) and to a lower extent cystein (SH group) are effective buffers (pK approximately 6 and 8, respectively, in the free amino acids). Their dissociation varies if neighboring charged groups move as a result of allosteric effects. Best known is the increase of pK values in hemoglobin with deoxygenation. In muscle, histidine is found mainly in proteins (between 15 and 37 mmol l^{-1}) and the dipeptide carnosine (pK = 6.83, 2.5–3.5 mmol l^{-1}), with highest levels in sprinters [4].

Bicarbonate Buffers
The pair H_2CO_3/HCO_3^- possesses a pK value of approximately 4, far outside the biological pH range. Because of its instability, however, most H_2CO_3 decays to CO_2 and H_2O within minutes in absence and within milliseconds in presence of carboanhydrase, reducing the acidifying effect; traditionally the sum of H_2CO_3 and CO_2 is considered as acid with a pK_1 of 6.1 at $37°C$. But even this pK is slightly outside the physiological pH range. The bicarbonate buffer works, however, very effectively in an open system, that is, with contact to a gas phase where the liberated CO_2 can escape; this may be exaggerated by hyperventilation. At a constant CO_2 pressure (PCO_2), the buffer capacity of bicarbonate is very high at pH 7.4 (2.3 mol mol^{-1}) but decreases with acidification because of a flattening of the titration curve; an average value for physiological pH changes during exercise in plasma and interstitial fluid is about 2 mol mol^{-1} [1]. In a closed system without excretion of CO_2 (apnea or static contraction with stopped blood flow), this buffer has little importance. It is important to state that a buffer salt cannot buffer against its own acid, that is, bicarbonate cannot buffer against CO_2. However, the given changes of PCO_2 (e.g., $\Delta = 20$ mmHg) are relatively larger at low values of this quantity (e.g., 30 mmHg) than at high ones (e.g., 60 mmHg) and cause, therefore, larger pH changes in the former case.

Metabolic Effects
Splitting of creatine phosphate (CrP) for production of ATP finally yields inorganic phosphate, thus increasing the amount of nb buffers. Consumption of lactic acid by aerobic metabolism, for example, in the heart or slow-twitch skeletal muscle fibers or by resynthesis of glucose in the liver is an effective means to reduce the acid load.

Transmembrane Fluxes of H^+ or Corresponding Molecules
There are a lot of transporters allowing excretion from cells to the extracellular space or into the opposite direction. Excretion by kidney or sweat glands reduces the acid load of the body; in the case of substances like lactic acid this means a loss of energy and seems not to play a significant role. Movement between body compartments is only helpful, if a more sensitive tissue (e.g., the brain) has to be protected by shifting H^+ into cells with high physicochemical buffer capacity as observed during severe respiratory acidosis (cf. from [4]).

Exercise Intervention

Acute Effects

General
Changes markedly influencing acid–base equilibrium during exercise are production of CO_2 and increase of lactic acid concentration (other acids like pyruvic acid and fatty acids are negligible); the former occurs always, the latter only if in some tissues aerobic and anaerobic-alactic synthesis of ATP is not sufficient and if the production of lactic acid is larger than its consumption in the rest of the body. Oxygen delivery to the muscle is retarded at the beginning of work because of delay in cardio-pulmonary activation; anaerobic-alactic generation of ATP occurs initially by splitting of CrP with liberation of secondary phosphate, which binds H^+. Thus, alkalinization within the fiber happens always during the first seconds. With intense exercise, lactic acid concentration in muscle fibers rapidly begins to increase up to maximal values of approximately 30 mmol l^{-1}; large amounts of lactic acid leave the cells, but the extracellular concentration maximum is always lower because of distribution to the rest of the body and consumption in other tissues. PCO_2 rises proportionally to intensity in muscle and venous blood while remaining approximately constant in arterial blood during moderate exercise. If, however, acidification by lactic acid becomes remarkable, the rise is attenuated by hyperventilation; in arterial blood, the values are even lowered. After exercise, the return of high lactic acid levels to control values lasts

about 1 h with continuing hyperventilation. Little investigated is the effect of the rising temperature in the body, which in general intensifies the dissociation of acids.

Buffering in Muscle Fibers

Phosphates. The pK of CrP (4.5) is much lower than cell pH, therefore it does not buffer. The production of ATP by the reaction between CrP and ADP consumes one H^+, which is again liberated during the splitting of ATP:

$$CrP^{2-} + ADP^{3-} + H^+ \rightarrow Cr + ATP^{4-}$$

$$ATP^{4-} + H_2O \rightarrow ADP^{3-} + HPO_4^{2-} + H^+$$

But now, the buffer HPO_4^{2-} (pK = 6.84) binds H^+. Consequently, pH rises; there is no contribution to exercise acidosis.

During exhausting exercise with 30 mmol l^{-1} cell water of lactic acid pH decreases from 7.0 to 6.4 (−0.6 units) exploiting 60% of the nb buffer capacity related to 1 pH unit according to Sahlin [5]. He calculates binding of 15 mmol H^+ per liter by liberation of inorganic phosphates from CrP (β = 26 mmol l^{-1}). Already present inorganic phosphate (β = 7 mmol l^{-1}) binds the additional 4 mmol H^+. Changes in other phosphates (binding of H^+ by ATP and ADP, ATP degraded to AMP and lost after deamination to the extracellular fluid, formation of glucose 6-P and α-glycerol-P) in total, decrease H^+-binding by only 1 mmol. Immediately after stopping exercise, CrP is resynthesized, consequently cellular pH drops temporarily before recovery.

Proteins and related substances. According to Sahlin, histidine in proteins (β = 15 mmol l^{-1}) and carnosine (β = 2 mmol l^{-1}) bind 11 mmol H^+ in his experiments. Together with the preexisting inorganic phosphates, the total amount of non-bicarbonate buffers at rest is 25 mmol l^{-1}, being lower than the range of β_{nb} in mammalian muscle tissue (between 40 and 100 mmol l^{-1} cell water supplied by histidine-related compounds and inorganic phosphates, with the higher values in fast fibers [4]). The difference can be explained by splitting of CrP during processing of the samples.

Bicarbonate buffers. Sahlin [5] calculates a buffer capacity of 12 mmol l^{-1} for $[HCO_3^-]$ during exhaustive bicycle exercise (decrease from 10 to 3 mmol l^{-1}), since CO_2 may leave the cells. In any case, the importance of the bicarbonate buffers is reduced compared to the extracellular space because of the low concentration.

Total buffers. Summarizing all exploited buffers (15 + 4 − 1 +11 + 7) yields 36 mmol l^{-1}, which is reasonable because the rise in PCO_2 and minor amounts of organic acids add H^+ to the 30 mmol of lactic acid.

Buffering in Interstitial Fluid and Blood

The interstitial fluid without appreciable protein and phosphate content can only buffer against fixed acids using the CO_2–HCO_3^- system. Its capacity amounts to approximately 55 mmol l^{-1} before exercise (24 mmol l^{-1} $HCO_3^- \times 2.3$), but decreases with consumption of bicarbonate when approaching exhaustion. Thus, the average value for physiological pH changes in plasma and interstitial fluid during hard dynamic exercise is about 47 mmol l^{-1} [1]. However, capillary wall and erythrocyte membrane are permeable for CO_2, HCO_3^-, Cl^-, La^-, and H^+ (both latter ions enter the red cells somewhat retarded); therefore blood nb buffers (approximately 30 mmol l^{-1}) are available also for the interstitial fluid. The average β_{nb} for the combined volumes of interstitial fluid and blood amounts to ca. 10–15 mmol l^{-1} at rest. During exercise, it rises temporarily up to approximately 30 mmol l^{-1} in untrained subjects. This is mainly caused by increasing extracellular buffer concentrations, because of a water shift to the interior of muscle fibers resulting from osmotic effects of metabolites [1].

Training Effects

The total amount of buffers in the body is larger in athletes than in nonathletes because of more muscle mass (especially after resistance training) or a higher blood volume (endurance training). There are some indications that also nb buffer concentration rises in muscle fibers after training (more after high intensity than endurance training). Some increase of carnosine and CrP contents seems to play a role. Finally, upregulation of La^- and H^+ transporters might accelerate the defense against acidosis.

Paradoxically, extracellular β_{nb} is attenuated in endurance-trained subjects, the cause being the dilution of Hb in a larger plasma and interstitial volume. Clear differences in bicarbonate concentrations between untrained and trained subjects have never been detected.

Altitude

Reduction of bicarbonate concentration by renal regulation (nonrespiratory compensation of respiratory alkalosis) and also of muscle mass at extreme altitude decreases the amount of buffers in the whole body. Transport mechanisms for relevant ions (Na^+, H^+, HCO_3^-, La^-, Cl^-), however, are improved in muscle and red cell membranes. In contrast to the traditional view, extracellular β is not reduced in altitude dwellers because Hb mass is increased and the extracellular volume is decreased [3]. After training related to moderate hypoxia (living high – training low model as well as classical altitude training) β_{nb} of muscle slightly increases.

References

1. Böning D, Klarholz C, Himmelsbach B, Hütler M, Maassen N (2007) Extracellular bicarbonate and non-bicarbonate buffering against lactic acid during and after exercise. Eur J Appl Physiol 100:457–467
2. Böning D, Maassen N (2008) Point: counterpoint "Lactic acid is/is not the only physicochemical contributor to the acidosis of exercise". J Appl Physiol 105:358–359
3. Böning D, Rojas J, Serrato M, Reyes O, Coy L, Mora M (2008) Extracellular pH defense against lactic acid in untrained and trained altitude residents. Eur J Appl Physiol 103:127–137
4. Parkhouse WS, McKenzie DC (1984) Possible contributions of skeletal muscle buffers to enhanced anaerobic performance: a brief review. Med Sci Sports Exer 16:328–338
5. Sahlin K (1978) Intracellular pH and energy metabolism in skeletal muscle of man. With special reference to exercise. Acta Physiol Scand Suppl 445:1–56

Acidosis

MICHAEL I. LINDINGER
Department of Human Health and Nutritional Sciences, University of Guelph, Guelph, ON, Canada

Synonyms

Exercise acidosis; Lactacidosis; Lactic acidosis

Definition

Acidosis specifically refers to an increase in the hydrogen ion concentration ($[H^+]$; decrease in pH) of the systemic circulation. There are two main types of acidosis that are associated with exercise and recovery from exercise, and these typically occur together with the contributions of each dependent on where the acidosis is assessed, e.g., contracting skeletal muscle, venous blood draining contracting muscle, and arterial blood [4]. A respiratory acidosis is defined as in increase in $[H^+]$ caused by or associated with an increase in the partial pressure of carbon dioxide (▶ PCO_2).With a respiratory acidosis there typically occurs an increase in the bicarbonate concentration ($[HCO_3^-]$) as described by the Henderson–Hasselbalch equation:

$$K_c \cdot PCO_2 = [H^+] \cdot [HCO_3^-]$$

A metabolic acidosis is defined as an increase in $[H^+]$ caused by or associated with an increase in acid anions, whether they be strong (>90% dissociated in body fluids, e.g., lactate$^-$) or weak (e.g., albumin and phosphate). A metabolic acidosis is typically associated with a decrease in $[HCO_3^-]$ because the increase in $[H^+]$, in the absence of increase in PCO_2, shifts the equilibrium of the CO_2 system as follows:

$$H^+ + HCO_3^- \leftrightarrow CO_2 + H_2O$$

Increases in acid anion concentrations and PCO_2 produce an acidosis because, physically, they cause an increased dissociation of H^+ from water ($H^+ - {}^-OH$) [1].

Basic Mechanisms

With moderate to high intensity exercise, the systemic (within blood) acidosis of exercise results from three nearly simultaneously occurring events occurring within contracting skeletal muscle. These are: (a) the increased production, accumulation, and release of lactate$^-$; (b) the influx of fluid from the blood, thus raising plasma [protein]; and (c) the increased production and release of CO_2 (Fig. 1). The lactate$^-$ and CO_2 produced in muscle rapidly enters venous blood draining muscle, and together with the increase in plasma [protein], results in a marked increase in venous plasma $[H^+]$.

The ▶ physicochemical approach is the most useful method for assessing acid–base state and for determining the origins of acid–base disturbances [2, 4, 5]. This approach recognizes three independent variables that determine the concentrations of the dependent variables $[H^+]$ and $[HCO_3^-]$. These are the strong ion difference (▶ [SID]), the total concentration of ▶ weak acid anions (▶ [Atot]), and the PCO_2. Decreases in [SID], increases in [Atot], and increases in PCO_2 independently contribute to the acidosis (increased $[H^+]$). Lactate$^-$ is a ▶ strong acid anion because it is nearly fully dissociated in solution due to its strong acid pK_A of 3.86.

With moderate to high intensity exercise, the acidosis within contracting muscle arises from a pronounced decrease in intracellular [SID] that is due to: (1) a decrease in intracellular [SID] and (2) an increase in the PCO_2 (2). The decrease in intracellular [SID] is nearly equally due to the increase in [lactate$^-$] and the loss of intracellular $[K^+]$ (due to repolarization of action potentials). The increase in PCO_2 occurs as a result of increased mitochondrial CO_2 production (aerobic metabolism) and from the titration of CO_2 stored within the cells.

Within venous blood draining contracting skeletal muscle, the plasma acidosis is due to a decrease in [SID], an increase in PCO_2, and an increase in [Atot] (Fig. 1). We will use a literature study of four repeated, 30-s bouts of very high intensity leg bicycling exercise to exemplify the contributions of these variables to the acidosis in both femoral venous plasma and in arterial plasma [3]. Femoral venous plasma [lactate$^-$] peaked at 21 ▶ mEq/L and contributed to the 18 mEq/L decrease in [SID]. Plasma PCO_2 increased by 50 mmHg to peak at 97 mmHg and [Atot]

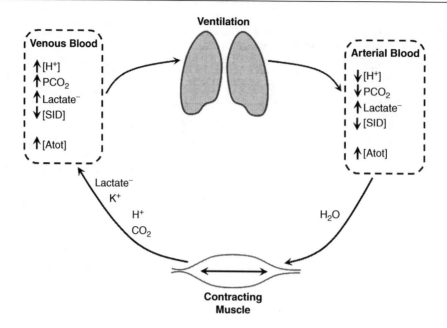

Acidosis. Fig. 1 Representation of the major acid–base events occurring within the body during exercise that contribute to the acidosis within venous blood draining contracting muscle and in arterial blood

increased by 4 mEq/L to 20.4 mEq/L. The increase in [Atot] is due to the next osmotic flux of fluid into contracting muscle cells. Using the physicochemical approach, it was determined that this decrease in [SID] contributed only ~15% to the 54 nEq/L increase in [H^+]. In comparison, the increase in PCO_2 contributed ~75% to the increase in [H^+], while the balance was due to the increase in [Atot].

Within arterial plasma, the picture of acid–base status is very different from that in muscle and in femoral venous plasma. As venous blood perfuses the lungs, and in association with the hyperventilation of exercise, the CO_2 is eliminated. In this study, this resulted in a marked lowering of plasma PCO_2 to 29 mmHg (from as high as 97 mmHg in femoral venous plasma) and in [H^+] to 70 nEq/L (compared to [H^+] of 100 nEq/L in femoral venous plasma). The elimination of all of the "excess" CO_2 at the lungs, and the reduction of PCO_2 to below pre-exercise values, helped to restore [H^+]. This leaves primarily decreased [SID] and secondarily increased [Atot] contributing to the arterial acidosis. With cessation of exercise, the plasma acidosis gradually resolves due mainly to the restoration of fluid balance, which restores [Atot], and metabolism of lactate⁻, which restores [SID]. Within skeletal muscle, restoration of [SID] also involves the re-accumulation of K^+ by the action of the sodium-potassium pump.

Exercise Intervention

Exercise intensity. In the example provided above, the intensity of exercise was very high, with power outputs 3.5–5 times greater than achieved at VO_2 max. This type of exercise produces a very large acidosis that, with repeated exercise bouts, can persist for 90 min of post-exercise recovery. When exercise is performed at an intensity below the lactate⁻ threshold, then there may be no acidosis associated with exercise. As exercise intensity increases above the lactate⁻ threshold, and continues to the point of voluntary exhaustion, there is a proportional increase in the magnitude and duration of the acidosis.

Exercise duration. At submaximal exercise intensities above the lactate⁻ threshold, the magnitude of the acidosis is primarily dependent on the intensity. With increasing duration, a new steady state will often be achieved, which can result in a decreasing acidosis as exercise continues, with proportionate decreases in the contributions from PCO_2 and lactate⁻.

Passive versus active recovery. Recovery of the acidosis of exercise can often be enhanced maintaining low levels of activity, compared to inactivity. Maintaining a low level of activity of the exercised muscle groups during the recovery periods helps to maintain a higher rate of muscle blood flow, cardiac output, and ventilation. Together, these serve to reduce the time needed to achieve a new, post-exercise steady state facilitating transmembrane ion, water, and gas movements between muscle, blood, and other tissues.

References

1. Edsall JT, Wyman J (1958) Biophysical chemistry. Academic, New York, p 669
2. Lindinger MI, Heigenhauser GJ (1991) The roles of ion fluxes in skeletal muscle fatigue. Can J Physiol Pharmacol 69:246–253
3. Lindinger MI, Heigenhauser GJF, McKelvie RS, Jones NL (1992) Blood ion regulation during repeated maximal exercise and recovery in humans. Am J Physiol Regul Integr Comp Physiol 262: R126–R136
4. Lindinger MI, Kowalchuk JM, Heigenhauser GJF (2005) Applying physicochemical principles to skeletal muscle acid-base status. Am J Physiol Regul Integr Comp Physiol 289:R891–R894, author reply R904
5. Lindinger M, Waller A (2008) Muscle and blood acid–base physiology during exercise and in response to training. In: Hinchcliff K, Kaneps AJ, Geor RJ (eds) Equine exercise physiology. Saunders Elsevier, Toronto, pp 350–381

Acquired Immune Deficiency Syndrome (AIDS)

▶ HIV

Actigraphy

A method of estimating sleep/wake patterns, accomplished by wearing a monitor that continuously records movements, with each epoch of data classified as sleep or wake based upon algorithms that incorporate movement counts for the epoch in question and the epochs immediately surrounding; for sleep/wake assessment, most commonly worn on the wrist; algorithms used by actigraphy to establish sleep/wake status are typically validated against polysomnography.

Actin

Actin is a protein that is a major component of the thin filaments. It is a part of the contractile apparatus in muscle cells. Muscles contract by sliding the thin (actin) and thick (myosin) filaments along each other. Actin has the binding sites for the myosin crossbridges.

Action Potentials

Action potentials are transient depolarizations of the membrane potential of excitable cells, including neurons and muscle fibers. They play a key role in communication between cells.

Action Simulation

Action simulation defines cognitive motor states like action observation, motor imagery and action verbalization. These states are not observable, covert stages of action that contain a representation of the action goal, the means to reach the action goal, as well as the consequences of the respective action.

Cross-References
▶ Mental Training

Activation Induced Cell Death (AICD)

AICD occurs in T lymphocytes through previous activation and Fas induced apoptosis. AICD can occur in a cell-autonomous manner and is influenced by the nature of the initial T-cell activation events. It plays essential roles in both central and peripheral lymphocyte deletion events involved in tolerance and homeostasis, although it is likely that different forms of AICD proceed via different mechanisms.

Active Heating

Forced hyperthermia induced by elevating heat production beyond the capacity for heat loss. Achieved via the production of external work, such as during exercise.

Activity Dependent Potentiation

Activity dependent potentiation is the generic term that has been used to describe all forms of enhanced contractile response that can be attributed to prior activation: staircase, posttetanic potentiation and postactivation potentiation (PAP). The cellular mechanism that allows more force for a given activation is thought to be phosphorylation of the regulatory light chains of myosin. Phosphorylation of the light chains increases calcium sensitivity, which means there can be more force for a given level of submaximal calcium concentration. Maximal force is not enhanced, but the peak rate of force development is increased. Posttetanic potentiation, the electrical analogue of PAP, is an enhanced contractile response following an electrically induced tetanic contraction. Staircase is an enhanced contractile response during identical sequential submaximal activations, usually with single pulses of stimulation. However, staircase is also evident during sequential brief incompletely fused tetanic contractions. It is important to realize that in most experimental work on PAP, electrical stimulation has been used to evaluate the enhanced contractile response with a given stimulation; otherwise, it would be difficult to know if the enhanced response was due to extra activations, or a true enhancement of force for a given stimulation. The term complex training has also been used to refer to a high intensity effort, leading in the short-term (minutes) to a subsequent better performance. It is believed that the mechanism contributing to this improvement is the same as the mechanism for PAP, but this has not been confirmed.

▶ Postactivation Potentiation

Acute Febrile Illness

▶ Acute Phase Reaction

Acute Mountain Sickness

DAMIAN M. BAILEY
Neurovascular Research Laboratory, University of Glamorgan, Pontypridd, Wales, UK

Synonyms

Altitude illness; Altitude sickness; Hypobaropathy

Definition

Acute mountain sickness (AMS) describes a collection of nonspecific vegetative symptoms that include headache, anorexia, nausea, vomiting, fatigue, dizziness, and insomnia experienced by non-acclimatized mountaineers within 6–12 h of arrival to altitudes above 2,500 m. It is considered a primary disorder of the central nervous system since headache, indistinguishable from that encountered during migraine without aura, is the most common feature. AMS is generally benign though may progress to high-altitude cerebral edema (HACE) in more severe cases or during continued ascent when symptoms of AMS are present. HACE typically occurs above 4,000 m and leads, if left untreated, to death due to brain herniation [1, 2].

Complicated by differences in the clinical definition of AMS, individual susceptibility, rate of ascent and prior exposure have been identified as the major independent risk factors that determine prevalence. In susceptible individuals exposed to 4,559 m, the prevalence of AMS was 7% assuming prior exposure and slow ascent, 29% with prior exposure only, 33% with slow ascent only, and 58% following rapid ascent and no prior exposure. In non-susceptible individuals, the corresponding prevalence was estimated at 4%, 11%, 16%, and 31%, respectively. The overall odds-risk-ratio for developing AMS in susceptible versus non-susceptible individuals was estimated to be 2.9 [2].

Pathophysiological Mechanisms

While it is well established that patients with HACE exhibit extracellular (vasogenic) edema subsequent to disruption of the blood–brain barrier (BBB) [1, 2], the situation with AMS is more complex, due in large part to the difficulties associated with clinical diagnosis. Traditionally, AMS has been considered a mild form of HACE and that both syndromes share a common pathophysiology linked by vasogenic edematous brain swelling and intracranial hypertension at opposing ends of a clinical continuum. However, recent studies employing diffusion-weighted (DW)-magnetic resonance imaging (MRI) have questioned this paradigm and since provided insight into alternative mechanisms [1]. The subsequent discussion will critically appraise each of the traditional and newly emerging components currently implicated in the pathophysiology of AMS. These are summarized schematically in Fig. 1 and will take the form of Phases I–III.

Phase I: The Stimulus

Hypoxia: Although ▶ hypoxia is not the immediate cause of AMS since symptoms typically take 6 h to evolve, it is the primary stimulus since symptoms typically become worse with increasing altitude and relieved by normalizing the inspiratory PO_2. Furthermore, it has been suggested that AMS-susceptible subjects are systemically more

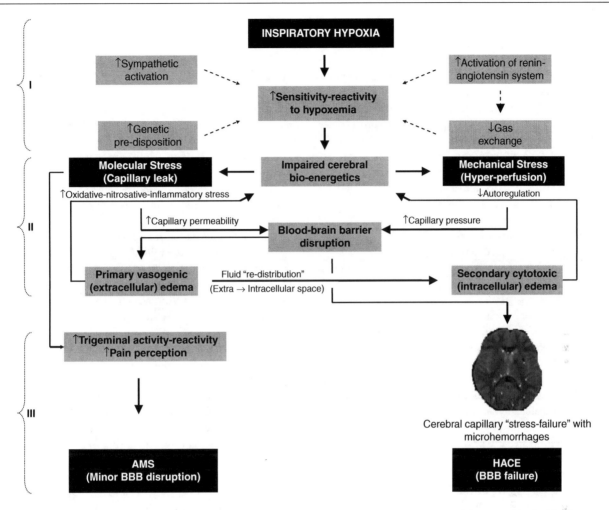

Acute Mountain Sickness. Fig. 1 Schematic of the major pathways involved in acute mountain sickness and high-altitude cerebral edema

hypoxemic or equally, more reactive to hypoxemia for any given inspirate during wakefulness and sleep compared to their healthier counterparts. Tentative evidence suggests that a blunted hypoxic ventilatory response and sympathetic activation leading to activation of the renin-angiotensin system, fluid retention, and subclinical interstitial pulmonary edema may prove additional risk factors that further compound hypoxia subsequent to impaired gas exchange and thus account for the increased sensitivity-reactivity. However, evidence of interstitial pulmonary edema in AMS is at best indirect and inconsistent, while fluid retention might prove the consequence rather than the direct cause of AMS [2].

Since a previous history has been identified as one of the most reliable predictors of illness during subsequent ascent, there may be some innate predisposition to AMS. Subsequent investigations have focused on candidate gene polymorphisms in an attempt to identify potential genetic variants underlying susceptibility. Recent interest has focused on the angiotensin-converting enzyme (ACE) gene since the insertion (I) allele has previously been associated with elite mountaineering status and successful ascent to 8,000 m peaks. However, studies have failed to support any association between ACE genotype and susceptibility to AMS.

While the current evidence has failed to identify a genetic contribution to AMS, it is important to emphasize that the sample sizes of all the aforementioned studies are too small for genetic association studies. Furthermore, "genetophysiology" is very much in its infancy with only 20 out of ≈25,000 genes in the human genome and only 50 out of ≈millions of polymorphisms currently assessed for roles in hypoxic (mal)-adaptation and altitude illness.

Phase II: The Response

Impaired cerebral bioenergetics: While existing measurement techniques have failed to identify any evidence for a "global" cerebral O_2 deficit in the severely hypoxic-hypocapnic human [3], positron-emission tomography studies have revealed striking spatiotemporal differences in the brain's "regional" energy consumption. Furthermore, neurotransmitters, the ubiquitous regulators of neuronal activity, are particularly vulnerable to hypoxia in light of their correspondingly high Michaelis constant for O_2. Thus, it is conceivable that even mild arterial hypoxemia could result in focal cerebral deoxygenation and impaired bioenergetic/neuronal communication with further decrements expected due to the "additional" deoxygenation associated with AMS.

Molecular-mechanical stress: Focal impairments in cerebral oxygenation have the potential to promote capillary leakage (molecular stress) and hyper-perfusion (hemodynamic stress), established risk factors that conspire to disrupt the BBB. Much interest has focused on the hemodynamic pathway since increased cerebral blood flow (CBF) occurs in response to hypoxia and impaired autoregulation has recently been documented in AMS [4]. These findings suggest that the AMS-brain is less capable of "buffering" rapid surges in arterial pressure and thus potentially more vulnerable to hyper-perfusion. A pressure-passive rise in regional CBF could translate into increased capillary hydrostatic pressure, though this is yet to be confirmed in humans. Elevated intravascular pressure could cause vasogenic edema subsequent to hydrostatic disruption of the BBB.

Oxidative-nitrosative-inflammatory stress constitutes an alternative, albeit complementary, pathway that can further compound barrier disruption through its (molecular) impact on capillary permeability. A recent study provided direct electron paramagnetic resonance (EPR) spectroscopic evidence for an increased release of lipid-derived alkoxyl-alkyl ($LO^\bullet$-$LC^\bullet$) radicals and associated reactive oxygen-nitrogen species (ROS-RNS) across the hypoxic human brain in direct proportion to AMS symptom scores [3]. Furthermore, dietary antioxidant vitamin supplementation provided some, albeit mild, prophylactic benefit, though further research employing larger sample sizes with improved methods of delivering novel antioxidant vehicles across the BBB to the brain parenchyma is warranted [1].

These findings indicate that the AMS-brain is especially vulnerable to molecular attack by free radicals which is not surprising given its modest antioxidant defenses, abundance of transition metals, auto-oxidizable neurotransmitters, and neuronal membrane lipids rich in polyunsaturated fatty acid side-chains exposed to a disproportionately high O_2 flux [1]. The $LO^\bullet$-$LC^\bullet$ species detected in hypoxia are associated with the impaired autoregulation observed in AMS [4], and they are thermodynamically capable of causing direct structural damage to the BBB microvascular endothelium, neurons, and glia and promoting cell swelling through down-regulation of Na^+/K^+-ATPase, Ca_2^+-ATPase, calmodulin-associated Ca_2^+-ATPase, and Na^+–Ca_2^+ exchanger activities [1].

Since free radicals are so reactive with lifetimes ($t_{1/2}$) in the order of $\approx 10^{-3}$–10^{-9} s, they may prove the "upstream" initiators of comparatively longer-lived inflammatory biomolecules. Indeed, current evidence suggests that hypoxia is associated with mild inflammation as indicated by a systemic increase in Pro-inflammatory cytokines. Inflammatory "priming" prior to exposure to hypoxia with exercise, heat, and intravenous endotoxin infusion has been shown to increase susceptibility to AMS (Bailey et al., unpublished findings). These observations may also help explain the link between obesity and AMS since the former is characterized by chronic vascular oxidation-inflammation.

Animal models have demonstrated that hypoxia stimulates vascular endothelial growth factor (VEGF) resulting in vascular leakage and cerebral edema tempting speculation that it's expression may predispose to high-altitude illness. Human studies have since failed to demonstrate any relationship between blood and/or cerebrospinal fluid concentrations of "total" VEGF and AMS [5]. However, this may be due to the fact that differences in the "free" concentration of VEGF mediated largely by its soluble receptor (sFlt-1) which serves to bind VEGF thus reducing vascular leak and angiogenesis were not evaluated. Hence, a recent study demonstrated a greater increase in "free" VEGF and "blunted" rise in sFlt-1 at high altitude in subjects with AMS compared to controls suggesting that it may well prove a molecular risk factor.

BBB integrity and vasogenic edema: Figure 1 describes how this combination of molecular-mechanical stress "arrives" at the brain, ultimately compromising barrier integrity and encouraging the formation of extracellular (vasogenic) edema. This was recently confirmed by DW-MRI which established the "signature" rise in brain volume, T_2-relaxation time, and apparent diffusion coefficient during hypoxia characteristic of mild vasogenic edematous brain swelling [6]. These changes were particularly pronounced in the splenium and genu of the corpus callosum, the same predilection site to that observed in HACE, likely the result of its unique vascular anatomy; densely packed horizontal fibers characterized by short arterioles that lack adrenergic tone may render it more susceptible to hyper-perfusion edema in the setting of hypoxic cerebral vasodilatation.

In contrast, previous studies have failed to detect any changes in the cerebrospinal fluid (CSF)-blood protein concentration quotients [5] and trans-cerebral release of the astrocytic protein S100β, a surrogate biomarker of BBB integrity [3]. In combination, these studies imply that the extent of barrier disruption in hypoxia is so subtle that it is beyond standard biomolecular detection limits. Follow-up studies employing gadolinium-enhanced MRI will provide a more accurate assessment of the extent of barrier disruption in hypoxia.

Traditional opinion suggests that AMS is the direct consequence of elevated intracranial pressure (ICP) caused by more pronounced vasogenic edematous brain swelling in hypoxia [7]. Intracranial hypertension has been implicated as the primary stimulus responsible for cephalalgia through mechanical activation of the trigeminovascular system (TVS). However, DW-MRI has consistently failed to support this concept with no relationships observed between the hypoxia-induced increases in brain volume or T_2rt and cerebral AMS scores. Mild vasogenic edematous brain swelling therefore appears to be an incidental finding that occurs in all brains exposed to the hypoxia of high-altitude [5, 6].

Furthermore, the observation that intracranial volume (ICV) is not increased to any greater extent in the AMS-brain argues against intracranial hypertension as a significant event. The recent increases observed in optical disc swelling and optical nerve sheet density as measured by ultrasound were often minor and not consistently related to AMS scores. Thus, there is no convincing human evidence to date to suggest that ICP is raised in AMS [1, 2].

Intracranial-intraspinal buffering capacity: Borne out of an original hypothesis developed over 20 years ago, the lack of correlation between brain swelling and AMS symptoms has since been ascribed to anatomical differences that determine how effectively the human skull can accommodate swelling through displacement of cranial CSF to extracranial compartments [7]. Thus, individuals characterized by a smaller ratio of cranial CSF to brain volume (popularized as the "tight-fit" brain) would be expected to be more prone to intracranial hypertension and thus by consequence AMS, since they are less capable of "buffering" the volume increase through changes in CSF dynamics due to an inadequate cranio-spinal axis CSF reserve.

To date, only one human study has provided indirect evidence to support the "tight-fit" hypothesis with AMS-susceptible subjects identified as having comparatively larger brain to intracranial volume ratios that was apparent even at sea level [6]. However, we are not entirely convinced that this has any bearing on the pathophysiology of AMS. It would seem highly unlikely that the minor volumetric changes of 0.6–0.8% of total brain volume would translate into any physiologically meaningful changes in the mechanical displacement of pain-sensitive structures capable of activating the trigeminovascular system (TVS) [1]. The small increases in ICV documented in the literature likely occupy the flat part of the ICP-volume curve and eminently well buffered by semielastic membranes and changes in CSF dynamics.

Cytotoxic edema: To date, the "only" defining morphological feature that distinguishes the AMS-prone from the healthy brain as revealed by DW-MRI is a selective decrease in apparent diffusion coefficient (ADC) scores [6] taken to reflect (secondary) intracellular (cytotoxic) edema "superimposed" upon preexisting (primary) extracellular vasogenic edema. Since both studies failed to provide any evidence for additional edema or swelling, the attenuation of the ADC likely reflects "fluid redistribution" from within the extracellular space (ECS) as intracellular (astrocytic) swelling proceeds without any additional increment in brain volume, edema, or ICP [1]. The cause of this is unknown, but may reflect "pump failure" subsequent to a down-regulation of Na^+/K^+-ATPase activity triggered by the prevailing oxidative-nitrosative-inflammatory milieu [1].

However, the critical question is whether the symptoms of AMS are caused by such a "minor" translocation of water from the ECS into the cells of the corpus callosum that entered as a result of mild vasogenic edema in hypoxia. This is highly unlikely since edema of the corpus callosum would typically give rise to a disconnection syndrome (e.g., associative agnosia). Headache, its leading symptom, is more likely associated with functional alterations in alternative structures, notably the brainstem.

Phase III: The Phenotype

Thus, the current findings suggest that AMS and HACE share similar features in that there is an underlying vasogenic component ranging from mild to severe. However, Phase III of Fig. 1 represents the point of "departure" from traditional theory since the edema cannot be held responsible for the symptoms of AMS. Furthermore, the clinical observation that HACE can develop rapidly in the "absence" of preceding AMS, and that in a large cohort of 66 cases with HACE, 33% had no headache, further questions the concept that the AMS-to-HACE symptom complex can be explained by this continuum of mild to severe cerebral edema [2].

Pain and the trigeminovascular system (*TVS*): Preliminary evidence suggests that AMS may be the result of altered pain perception and trigeminovascular nociceptive input from the meningeal vessels during hypoxia. Direct inhibition of TVS activity with oral sumatriptan, a selective 5-hydroxytryptamine (HT)$_1$ receptor subtype agonist, was shown to reduce the relative risk of AMS by as much as 50% in the largest randomized trial to date. In addition to its ability to attenuate cell excitability in trigeminal nuclei via stimulation of 5-HT$_{1B/1D}$ receptors within the brainstem and vasoconstriction of meningeal, dural, cerebral, or pial vessels, sumatriptan can also scavenge nitric oxide, superoxide, and hydroxyl radicals. Thus, direct activation of the TVS through oxidative-nitrosative-inflammatory stress may prove the final common pathway since, consistent with the current evidence, it does not rely on any volumetric changes to the brain.

The recent observation that AMS did not influence the (steady-state) cerebral metabolism of the "migraine-molecule" calcitonin gene related peptide (CGRP) [8] argues against "sustained activation" of the TVS as an important event. However, this finding does not exclude acute release from trigeminal perivascular nerve fibers, the site of nociception during the early phase of hypoxia and the lack of major breach in the BBB may have also prevented intrathecally formed CGRP from entering the extracranial circulation in sufficient amounts to permit molecular detection. This finding also argues a need to focus on the cerebral metabolism of alternative redox-reactive biomarkers that are equally capable of activating the TVS in the acute term [3].

The link to HACE: While HACE has traditionally been ascribed to vasogenic edema [7], it is reasonable to assume that a cytotoxic component may also be present since hypoxemia is likely more severe compared to AMS. Therefore, cell swelling should be even more pronounced in HACE. However, ADC mapping has not been performed immediately following evacuation from altitude in patients with HACE.

A recent study combined conventional T$_2$* with a novel, highly sensitive susceptibility-weighted MRI technique to reveal multiple "microbleeds" detected as hemosiderin deposits confined to the genu and splenium of the corpus callosum of patients with a history of HACE that had occurred up to 3 years ago [1]. Erythrocyte extravasation was taken to reflect cerebral capillary "stress failure" subsequent to cerebral hyper-perfusion and severe BBB disruption. The failure to detect any hemosiderin deposits in subjects diagnosed with severe AMS reinforces the fundamental concept that vasogenic edema is minor in AMS and is unlikely to account for symptoms and points

to a novel diagnostic feature that further discriminates AMS from HACE.

Diagnostics/Treatment

Headache is the cardinal symptom of AMS and is associated with, if not the primary trigger for, anorexia, nausea, vomiting, fatigue, dizziness, and insomnia. There are no diagnostic physical findings in benign AMS, although the onset of ataxia and altered consciousness signal clinical progression to HACE. The Lake Louise (LL) and Environmental Symptoms Questionnaire Cerebral (ESQ-C) scoring systems are the subjective tools most commonly employed to rate AMS. A LL score of ≥ 5 points and ESQ-C score of ≥ 0.7 points in the presence of headache and following a recent gain in altitude signals the presence of clinically significant (i.e., moderate-to-severe) AMS [2].

AMS can be prevented by gradual ascent thus ensuring adequate time for acclimatization. Analgesics for the symptomatic relief of headache and day of rest are recommended for mild to moderate AMS. If no improvement is observed, the individual should descend. Severe AMS can be managed through immediate descent or the administration of low-flow oxygen (1–2 L/min). If descent and oxygen are unavailable, dexamethasone (4 mg every 6 h) is advised. Acetazolamide (250 mg twice daily) might be considered for mild to moderate AMS in a setting where further ascents must be made as a mixed therapeutic and prophylactic intervention. Prophylaxis is recommended in individuals with a history of AMS when slow ascent is not possible or for those with unknown susceptibility who plan to ascend above 3,000–4,000 m (sleeping altitude) within 1–2 days [2].

References

1. Bailey DM, Bartsch P, Knauth M, Baumgartner RW (2009) Emerging concepts in acute mountain sickness and high-altitude cerebral edema: from the molecular to the morphological. Cell Mol Life Sci 66(22):3583–3594
2. Bartsch P, Bailey DM, Berger MM, Knauth M, Baumgartner RW (2004) Acute mountain sickness: controversies, advances and future directions. High Alt Med Biol 5:110–124
3. Bailey DM, Taudorf S, Berg RMG, Lundby C, McEneny J, Young IS, Evans KA, James PE, Shore A, Hullin DA, McCord JM, Pedersen BK, Moller K (2009) Increased cerebral output of free radicals during hypoxia: implications for acute mountain sickness? Am J Physiol Regul Integr Comp Physiol 297(5):R1283–R1292
4. Bailey DM, Evans KA, James PE, McEneny J, Young IS, Fall L, Gutowski M, Kewley E, McCord JM, Moller K, Ainslie PN (2009) Altered free radical metabolism in acute mountain sickness: implications for dynamic cerebral autoregulation and blood-brain barrier function. J Physiol 587(1):73–85
5. Bailey DM, Roukens R, Knauth M, Kallenberg K, Christ S, Mohr A, Genius J, Storch-Hagenlocher B, Meisel F, McEneny J, Young IS, Steiner T, Hess K, Bartsch P (2006) Free radical-mediated damage

to barrier function is not associated with altered brain morphology in high-altitude headache. J Cereb Blood Flow Metab 26(1):99–111

6. Kallenberg K, Bailey DM, Christ S, Mohr A, Roukens R, Menold E, Steiner T, Bartsch P, Knauth M (2007) Magnetic resonance imaging evidence of cytotoxic cerebral edema in acute mountain sickness. J Cereb Blood Flow Metab 27(5):1064–1071
7. Hackett PH, Roach RC (2001) High-altitude illness. N Engl J Med 345:107–114
8. Bailey DM, Taudorf S, Berg RMG, Jensen LT, Lundby C, Evans KA, James PE, Pedersen BK, Moller K (2009) Transcerebral exchange kinetics of nitrite and calcitonin gene-related peptide in acute mountain sickness: evidence against trigeminovascular activation? Stroke 40(6):2205–2208

Acute Phase Proteins (APPs)

During the acute phase reaction, the liver expresses rapidly new proteins named APPs. APPs recognize infectious agents, tissue breakdown products, and numerous other homotopes. Some APPs activate innate immune cells, mediate neutralization, and cytotoxicity; others are enzyme inhibitors or anti-inflammatory agents. Thus, the liver is a key organ in acute illness by providing APPs on a very short notice.

Acute Phase Reaction

ISTVAN BERCZI
Department of Immunology, The University of Manitoba, Winnipeg, MB, Canada

Synonyms

Acute febrile illness; Acute phase response; General adaptation syndrome

Definition

Acute phase reaction (APR) is a systemic host defense response against infectious agents, and to a great variety of noxious insults that are harmful to the host. During APR innate immune mechanisms are activated, which induce APR, a highly coordinated and very effective defense reaction against the initiating insults. Neuroendocrine and metabolic changes, catabolism, and fever are the hallmarks of APR. APR may be regarded as a host defense response whereby the adaptive immune system (ADIM) failed to control a problem (e.g., infection) so it became necessary for the innate immune system (INIM) to mount an emergency host defense response, which is APR [1,2].

Characteristics

Hans Selye discovered that rats develop a specific syndrome when exposed to various "nocuous" agents: The adrenal glands were enlarged, the thymus and other lymphoid tissues developed atrophy, and there were bleedings in the gastrointestinal tract [2]. Selye called the noxious agents stressors, which elicited the stress response. Later Selye realized that stressed animals can resist damaging agents with elevated resistance. He argued that this resistance was a defense reaction and named it the general adaptation syndrome [3]. Selye also defined the stress reaction, which is the first and a fairly accurate description of the acute phase reaction as we know it today [2].

Historically fever has been regarded as a healing reaction. So Boivin purified bacterial LPS for the purposes of fever therapy. LPS is a very effective pyrogen. Today we know that detoxified LPS is in fact a very effective stimulant of the innate immune system and indeed, it is capable of increasing host immunity in animals and in man in critical illness [2].

The Immune System

We distinguish specific or adaptive immunity and innate or natural immunity [4].

Adaptive Immunity

The adaptive immune system is also known as thymus dependent, or T lymphocyte dependent immunity. T lymphocytes mature in the thymus gland. We distinguish helper (Th1, Th2) killer or cytotoxic (Tk, CTL) and suppressor/regulatory (Tsr Treg) lymphocytes [4].

Helper T lymphocytes (Th1) generate CTL and delayed type hypersensitivity reactions, which are classified as cell-mediated immunity. Th2 helper cells stimulate bone marrow–derived (B) lymphocytes to secrete antibodies, which mediate humoral immunity. Suppressor regulatory cells are a heterogeneous group of cells, which include several types of Tsr, suppressor monocyte/macrophages. Suppressor antibodies and cytokines, such as interleukin (IL)-10, and transforming growth factor-beta [(TGF)-beta] also regulate immune function.

T and B lymphocytes develop antigen-specific surface receptors, which undergo somatic mutation and clonal selection after stimulation by the specific antigenic determinant (epitope). The B and T cells bearing such receptors show exquisite specificity to the epitope that stimulated their maturation. The T cells develop into mature effector cells (e.g., helper, killer, regulatory), whereas B lymphocytes secrete antigen-specific antibodies [4].

Specific immune responses are initiated by antigen presenting cells (APCs), which could be a macrophage or dendritic cells (DCs), which are "professional" APCs. APCs are phagocytic cells, they ingest the antigen and digest (process) it and peptides of the antigen (epitopes) are expressed in the grooves of the surface MHC-I (MHC-I-Ag) molecules of APC, which are recognized by Th1 cells. B lymphocytes also present antigen to helper Th2, via MHC II-Ag on their surface. Helper T lymphocytes then stimulate the proliferation and maturation of immature T and B cells into mature effector cells that mediate cell-mediated and humoral immunity. Such T cells recognize the MHC-Ag complexes and secrete interleukins (e.g., IL2, -4, -6, etc.), which are growth and differentiation signals for the immature lymphoid cells [4].

Adaptive immune reactions may be induced by injection of the antigen by various routes to animals and humans. Immunity will develop within a week or more because cell proliferation is necessary for clonal expansion, which takes time, and then the cells must differentiate into mature effector cells that mediate the specific immune responses [4].

Innate or Natural Immunity

Traditionally it was held that INIM was initiated by monocytes and macrophages that recognize foreign material in general and induced nonspecific immunity, or natural immunity via stimulating leukocytes to eliminate the invader organism or insult. This latter term indicates that this immunity could not be induced but was always there naturally. Indeed, we are born with this form of immunity; it is always with us until our last moment of life, protecting us for a lifetime. INIM has the capacity to protect us instantaneously, no immunization is necessary [3].

LPS turned out to be an excellent stimulator of natural antibodies, which could not be stimulated by traditional immunization. LPS was also a potential stimulant of host resistance in general. When natural antibodies were examined, it was clear that they recognize highly cross-reactive antigens specifically. LPS is also present in all gram-negative bacterium species, regardless of pathogenicity. We proposed that evolutionarily highly conserved cross-reactive (homologous) epitopes (homotopes) are recognized by INIM. LPS is one such homotope. Others emphasized the pattern nature of recognition. Natural killer cells recognize "missing self" and kill cells without surface MHC proteins. So the term "nonspecific immunity" had to be replaced with poly-specific immunity. Toll-like receptors and a number of other cell surface molecules function as INIM receptors (INIRs) for antigen [3].

Recently it has been discovered that toll-like receptors, which are the best studied INIR, are expressed by neurons, glia cells, in all leukocytes, in the pituitary gland, in the adrenal gland, in the liver, in mucosal epithelial cells, in endothelial cells, in vascular smooth muscle, and also in the cornea. These facts suggest that the entire body, including the CNS, endocrine organs, the liver, epithelium, and endothelium, and possibly even more, participate in innate immune host defense. The CNS is capable of directly sensing infectious agents through TLR, and react instantaneously by causing inflammation, the final effector response of all immune compartments. Similarly the pituitary produces proopiomelanocortin (POMC) in response to LPS (TLR4 is involved), mucosal epithelial TLR participates in inflammation and responds to pathogens, corneal TLR was found to fight infection, and endothelial TLR was observed to play important roles in homeostasis of the heart. Therefore, in addition to participating in NATIM, TLR fulfills important physiological functions [5]. Cytokines show similar poly-specific action, especially IL-1, -6 and tumor necrosis factor (TNF)-alpha, which have a prominent role in the induction of APR [2].

Neuroendocrinology of APR

The Central Nervous System (CNS)

The CNS is able to sense directly infectious and noxious agents via innate immune receptors, such as TLR. Nerves have also such receptors as well as receptors for cytokines, so sensory nerves will carry the signals of infection/insult to the paraventricular nucleus in the hypothalamus. Moreover, the cytokines that induce APR (IL-1, -6; TNF-alpha) are able to signal the brain directly. Several mechanisms have been proposed for this direct signaling pathway. The hypothalamic centers regulating the HPA axis, and the sympathetic nervous system are activated. Fever develops [2].

The Hypothalamus-Pituitary-Adrenal (HPA) Axis

Corticotrophin-releasing hormone (CRH) and vasopressin (VP) are the hypothalamic regulators of adrenocorticotropic hormone (ACTH), which is secreted by the pituitary gland and it stimulates glucocorticoid (GC) production in the adrenal cortex. This axis is activated invariably during APR. GC catecholamine (CAT) productions are increased (sympathetic outflow) during APR. The HPA axis has an immunoregulatory and anti-inflammatory role during APR. GC and CAT amplify INIM mechanisms, and stimulate Tsr cells, which in turn suppress ADIM. ADIM reactions need a long time to develop, so this system is not capable of instantaneous host defense. ADIM is suppressed in a reversible fashion. The INIM system takes over host defense entirely during APR [1].

Growth hormone and prolactin (GLH) rise quickly for a few hours during APR, which temporarily amplify ADIM mechanisms. If this does not resolve the problem, GLH become suppressed, and the HPA axis will coordinate the next phase of host defense.

Insulin, glucagon, and leptin are elevated during APR. There is insulin resistance.
Epinephrine, norepinephrine, and aldosterone are also elevated.
Thyroid and sex steroid hormones are suppressed [2].

Immune Activation in APR

The bone marrow is activated and produces elevated amounts of monocytes and granulocytes. B cells producing natural antibodies are also activated.

The thymus is involuted [2].

Monocyte/macrophages are the key cells that recognize the infection/insult by their INIR and secrete the cytokines IL-1, IL-6, and TNF-alpha which act on the CNS, activate leukocytes, stimulate bone marrow function, induce acute phase production in the liver, increase complement and the coagulation system [2].

Pathophysiology of APR

Cytokines

In addition to the cytokines that initiate APR, leukemia inhibitory factor (LIF), IL-8, -10, interferon (IFN)-gamma, TNF synthesis inhibitor, interleukin receptor antagonist, platelet activating factor, colony stimulating factors, prostaglandins, and thromboxanes were shown to play a role in APR [2].

Natural Antibodies

A special subset of B lymphocytes (CD5+) belong to INIM. They respond directly to infection and insults by natural antibody production. Such antibodies typically recognize highly cross-reactive homotopes on microbes and provide protection in a poly-specific manner [3].

Acute Phase Proteins

Liver proteins change significantly during APR. Very rapidly under the influence of IL-6 and glucocorticoids, the liver will synthesize the so-called acute phase proteins (APPs). APPs consist of molecules serving host defense, such as C-reactive protein, endotoxin binding protein,

and mannose binding lectin. Enzymes and enzyme inhibitors, antioxidants, anti-apoptotic and anti-inflammatory proteins, and other bioactive molecules, such as complement components, coagulation factors, fibrinogen, etc. During APR, C-reactive protein and serum amyloid A may increase over 1,000-fold in the serum within 24 h [2].

Systemic Inflammatory Response

APR may be regarded as a systemic inflammatory response. Bone marrow–derived white blood cells are the effectors, equipped with natural antibodies, supported by the complement system and by a myriad of cytokines. Phagocytosis and cytotoxicity are the main mechanisms of clearance of noxious agents. Blood coagulation also plays a role, perhaps to localize pathogens. During APR, the CNS, the bone marrow, WBC, and the liver are activated. The other tissues undergo catabolism, which is essential for fueling the immune system. Treatment with anabolic hormones, such as growth hormone, interferes with the catabolic process, and consequently with host defense [2].

Healing, Recovery

The hypothalamic regulators of APR are CRH and VP. However when APR is subsiding CRH becomes inactive and VP will regulate healing and recovery. VP regulates the HPA axis, and also PRL, it is capable to create the homeostatic conditions, which lead to recovery and restoration of normal immune function [1].

Clinical Relevance

Clinically APR is characterized by fever, inactivity, somnolence, loss of appetite, and weight loss. If there is no recovery, multiple organ failure and death will follow. However most individuals encounter febrile illness on numerous occasions during their lifetime and survive. This experience makes it very clear that APR is very efficient in protecting the host.

Much information is available about the biology and medical significance of CRP.

Serum levels of CRP are used clinically for diagnosing inflammatory disease. In Crohn's disease (CD) serum levels of CRP correlate well with disease activity and with other markers of inflammation. CRP is a valuable marker for predicting the outcome of certain diseases as coronary heart disease and hematological malignancies. An increased CRP (>45 mg/L) in patients with inflammatory bowel disease predicts with a high certainty the need for colectomy, and this by reflecting severe ongoing and uncontrollable inflammation in the gut. CRP is also a diagnostic marker in systemic lupus erythematosus [2].

Strenuous exercise increased plasma levels of TNF-alpha, IL-1, IL-6, IL-1 receptor antagonist, TNF receptors, IL-10, IL-8, and macrophage inflammatory protein-1. IL-6 increased up to hundredfold after a marathon race and the increase was tightly related to the duration and intensity of the exercise. IL-6 is produced in the skeletal muscle in response to exercise. Exercise induces immune changes and also alters neuroendocrinological factors including catecholamines, growth hormone, cortisol, beta-endorphin, and sex steroids. Exercise-associated muscle damage initiates the inflammatory cytokine cascade. LPS enters the circulation in athletes after ultra-endurance exercise and may, together with muscle damage, be responsible for the increased cytokine response and hence GI complaints [2].

Cachexia is the clinical consequence of a chronic, systemic inflammatory response. There is redistribution of the body's protein content, with preferential depletion of skeletal muscle and an increase in the synthesis of APP involved in APR [2].

The anorexia of infection is part of the host's APR and is beneficial in the beginning, but deleterious, if long lasting. Bacterial cell wall compounds (e.g., LPS, peptidoglycans), microbial nucleic acids and viral glycoproteins trigger the APR and anorexia by stimulating the production of proinflammatory cytokines (e.g., interleukins, TNF, interferons), which serve as endogenous mediators. The central mediators of the anorexia during infection appear to be neurochemicals involved in the normal control of feeding, such as serotonin, dopamine, histamine, CRF, neuropeptide Y, and MSH. Reciprocal, synergistic, and antagonistic interactions between various pleiotropic cytokines, and between cytokines and neurochemicals, form a complex network that mediates the anorexia during infection [2].

Aging is associated with increased inflammatory activity, increased circulating levels of TNF, IL-6, cytokine antagonists, and acute phase proteins. Chronic low-grade inflammation in aging promotes an atherogenic profile and is related to age-associated disorders (e.g., Alzheimer's disease, atherosclerosis, type 2 diabetes, etc.) and enhanced mortality risk. A dysregulated production of inflammatory cytokines, delayed termination of inflammatory activity, and a prolonged fever response suggest that the acute phase response is altered in aging [2].

The metabolic syndrome is characterized by cardiovascular and diabetes risk factors generally linked to insulin resistance, and obesity. Cross-sectional analysis demonstrated that markers of inflammation and endothelial dysfunction predict the development of diabetes mellitus and weight gain in adults. There is biological evidence to suggest that chronic activation of the innate immune system may underlie the metabolic syndrome [2].

In allergic patients, increased IL-6 levels correlated with greater erythema extent, lower mean arterial blood pressure, and a longer duration of symptoms. There was an inverse relationship between CRP and histamine levels [2].

In patients with rheumatoid arthritis (RA), IL-6 correlated closely with CRP and with erythrocyte sedimentation rate (ESR). These three parameters correlated well with serum cortisol, which is increased in active RA [2].

CRP and C3a levels were significantly higher in patients with IgA nephropathy as compared with healthy controls and with patients with hypertension or nonimmune renal diseases. Mean CRP but not C3a levels were significantly higher in IgA nephropathy patients with disease progression than in those with stable renal function [2].

References

1. Berczi I, Quintanar-Stephano A, Kovacs K (2009) Neuroimmune regulation in immunocompetence, acute illness, and healing. Ann N Y Acad Sci 1153:220–239
2. Berczi I, Szentivanyi A (2003) The acute phase response. In: Berczi I, Szentivanyi A (eds) Neuroimmune biology, vol 3, The immune-neuroendocrine circuitry. History and progress. Elsevier, Amsterdam, pp 463–494
3. Bertok L, Chow DA (2005) Natural immunity. In: Berczi I. Szentivanyi A, Series (eds) Neuroimmune biology, vol 5. Elsevier, Amsterdam
4. Janeway CA, Travers P, Walport M, Schlomchik MJ (2005) Immunobiology. Galand science. Taylor and Francis Group, New York/London
5. Berczi I (2010) Antigenic recognition by the brain. The brain as an immunological organ. In: Berczi I (ed) New insights to neuroimmune biology. Elsevier, Amsterdam, pp 145–154 Elsevier Insights, www.amazon.com

Acute Phase Response

▶ Acute Phase Reaction

Acute Polio

Infection of the Central Nervous system by the polio virus, leading to acute flaccid paralysis of muscles by destruction of the motor neurons in the spinal cord.

Acute Program Variables

The features of a resistance training protocol that impact its physiological stimuli to the body, i.e., choice of exercises, order of exercises, amount of rest between sets and exercises, number of sets, and the intensity of the resistance used.

Adaptability

▶ Neural Plasticity

Adaptation

Refers to any beneficial, or presumably beneficial, change to the structure or function of an organ or the whole body in response to chronic exercise training.

Cross-References
▶ Cold
▶ Training, Adaptations

Adaptive Immune Cells

▶ Lymphocytes

Adaptive Immune System (ADIM)

The adaptive immune system is also known as thymus dependent, or T lymphocyte dependent immunity. T lymphocytes mature in the thymus gland. We distinguish helper (Th1, Th2) killer or cytotoxic (Tk, CTL) and suppressor/regulatory (Tsr, Treg) lymphocytes. T cells mediate antigen-specific cellular immunity and regulate immune function. Bone marrow–derived (B) lymphocytes produce antigen-specific antibodies.

Cross-References
▶ Lymphocytes

Adaptive Movement Variability

Also known as functional or compensatory variability, this type of neurobiological system variability emerges in coordination of a performer during attempts to satisfy changing task constraints during sport performance. The traditional idea of variability representing "noise" in a neurobiological system is eschewed in ecological dynamics in favor of a more functional role for movement pattern variability in adapting to changes in the performance environment, due to factors like changes in ambient temperature, performance conditions, and fatigue. Whilst this idea is understandable in coordination of multi-articular actions in dynamic environments such as team games, adaptive movement variability have also been observed to play a functional role in helping athletes adjust coordination patterns in more stable task environments such as pistol shooting, archery, and diving.

Adaptive Physical Activity (APA)

Physical activity for fitness and aerobic conditioning that has been modified to meet the needs of individuals with physical limitations.

Adenine Nucleotides

The adenine nucleotides are forms of adenosine that are phosphorylated, or contain one or more phosphate groups. The adenine nucleotides include adenosine $5'$-triphosphate (ATP), adenosine $5'$-diphosphate (ADP), and adenosine $5'$-monophosphate (AMP).

Cross-References
▶ Adenosine Triphosphate

Adenosine

Adenosine is an endogenous purine nucleoside comprised of adenine and a ribose sugar that modulates many physiological processes via G protein coupled adenosine receptors. It contributes to energy exchange as a component of adenosine triphosphate (ATP), adenosine diphosphate (ADP), and adenosine monophosphate (AMP). It also plays a role in cellular signaling as a component of cyclic adenosine monophosphate (cAMP). Adenosine is a vasodilator and a central nervous system inhibitor. Pharmacologically, it is also used as a cardiac antiarryhythmic.

Adenosine 5′-Monophosphate-Activated Protein Kinase

▶ AMP-Activated Protein Kinase

Adenosine Triphosphate

Kameljit Kalsi, José González-Alonso
Centre for Sports Medicine and Human Performance, Brunel University, Uxbridge, UK

Synonyms

Adenosine triphosphoric acid; Nucleotide

Definition

▶ ATP is an adenosine-derived nucleotide, $C_{10}H_{16}N_5O_{13}P_3$, that has a dual role as an ▶ energy source and a ▶ signaling molecule recognized by ▶ purinergic receptors. It contains high energy phosphate bonds and is used to transfer energy to cells for biochemical processes, including muscle contraction and enzymatic metabolism, through its hydrolysis to its diphosphate, ADP. ATP is hydrolyzed to its monophosphate, AMP, when it is incorporated into DNA or RNA.

Basic Mechanisms

The role of ATP as a direct energy source for biological systems was first proposed by Lipmann and Kalckar in 1941. Earlier experiments had shown that there was a decline in phosphocreatine (▶ PCr) levels with muscle contraction. It was therefore believed that PCr played this role. It was not until the 1960s when it was discovered that the high energy phosphate bond of PCr is first transferred into ATP before it could be utilized in biochemical reactions requiring energy. ATP is first generated by the glycolytic pathway in the cytoplasm outside the mitochondria where glucose is converted to pyruvate by the process of anaerobic metabolism. The majority of ATP is formed within the mitochondria by the second pathway known as the citric acid cycle or Kreb's cycle by the oxidation of pyruvic acid to carbon dioxide. Coupled to this is the third method of generating ATP from the electron transport chain found on the inner mitochondrial membrane, where the efflux of protons from the mitochondrial matrix creates an electrochemical gradient (proton gradient). This gradient is used by the F_OF_1 ATP synthase complex to make ATP via oxidative phosphorylation [1].

During exercise, the mechanism of muscle contraction involves the contractile proteins actin which combines with myosin and ATP to produce force, ADP, and inorganic phosphate (Pi), a phenomenon known as the "Cross Bridge Cycle." Evidence provided from protein crystallography and electron microscopy proposes a model whereby ATP causes a conformational change in the actin-binding site for myosin resulting in movement of the muscle fibers. A constant source of ATP relies on the availability of substrates for oxidation mainly in the form of muscle glycogen, blood glucose, and free fatty acids. The use of these various substrates depends on the intensity and duration of the exercise but would also be influenced by the training and nutritional status before and during exercise. Inadequate ATP production in patients with mitochondrial myopathy predisposes the individual to increased incidence of myalgia, fatigue, dyspnea, and muscular cramping during exercise [2].

ATP can also be synthesized by precursors within the body by the de novo and salvage pathways. The major site for purine synthesis is in the liver; however, these pathways are energy consuming. In contrast, the exercising muscle triggers the purine nucleotide cycle which synthesizes AMP from inosine monophosphate (IMP), a by-product of this cycle is the generation of fumarate an essential substrate for the Kreb's cycle and hence the regeneration of more ATPs.

ATP also has important roles outside of the cell acting as an extracellular signaling molecule by activating specific ATP receptors on cells lining the arteries, nerve endings, and various organs. As a result, extracellular ATP regulates many physiological responses including vascular, heart, and skeletal muscle functions. In the vasculature it has been proposed that the erythrocyte releases ATP out the cell as a response to stimuli such as low oxygen, mechanical deformation, changes in pH [3], and more recently demonstrated by increasing physiological temperatures. The mechanism by which ATP leaves the ▶ erythrocytes remains contentious, but inhibitor studies have described a regulatory role for the membrane bound ion transporter cystic fibrosis transmembrane regulator (▶ CFTR), a member of the ATP-binding cassette proteins (ABC-proteins).

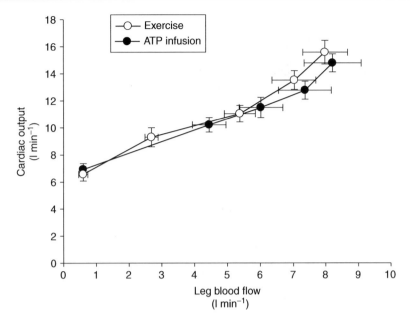

Adenosine Triphosphate. Fig. 1 Cardiac output and leg blood flow changes with incremental exercise and graded intrafemoral artery ATP infusion (Adapted from González-Alonso (2008))

ATP is a potent ▶ vasodilator when infused in intact humans or when infused locally in vessel preparations. To demonstrate the influence of ATP on the regulation of ▶ blood flow in humans, intra-luminal infusion of ATP produces an increase in flow similar to levels found with exercise hyperemia (7–8 L min^{-1} from resting values of $\sim$0.5 L min^{-1}) (Fig. 1) [4]. This is due to the interaction of ATP with the endothelium P_{2y} receptors triggering the release of nitric oxide (NO), endothelium-derived hyperpolarization factor (EDHF), and prostaglandins mostly prostacyclin (PGI_2) as well as non-NO, non-prostacyclin induced vasodilation [5] (Fig. 2).

Yet again, ATP is also known to act as a sympathetic neurotransmitter where it activates P_{2x} receptors on the vascular smooth muscle causing vasoconstriction. Thus, circulatory and interstitial ATP is essential in regulating and controlling blood flow in exercising and non-exercising limbs.

Exercise Intervention

To improve exercise performance, the key requirements are the exercise regimen and proper nutrition. Access to a continuous supply of ATP for energy is of continual interest in the sporting world. However, most legal sports supplements do not improve exercise performance except for three legal supplements creatine, carnitine, and sodium bicarbonate. Increasing the intake of creatine enhances the levels of creatine and PCr in the muscle and provides a good reserve of high energy phosphates for ATP regeneration. Carnitine supplementation should in principle augment the oxidation of fats by the mitochondria; however, the benefits have been inconclusive. Lastly, sodium bicarbonate reduces the acidosis associated with exercise, but again the results have been varied and some negative effects have been described. Another key regulator at the center of muscle bioenergetics is the enzyme AMPK (AMP-kinase) which is activated when ATP is used for energy and the by-product AMP is formed. Activation of AMPK by AMP generates more ATP, but is also involved in lowering blood sugar, sensitizing cells to insulin, and suppressing inflammation. All of these benefits are stimulated with exercise itself and research into drugs that simulate this response is emerging. A drug that mimics AMP, AICAR (aminoimidazole carboxamide ribonucleotide) combined with a gene activating drug GW1516 is currently been tested with promising results such that they have been included on the prohibited list by the World Anti-Doping Agency.

The best method of stimulating ATP synthesis in skeletal muscle is by increasing the frequency and intensity of exercise. This is proven by studies using ^{31}P magnetic resonance spectroscopy where they demonstrate an increase in ATP synthase flux and an increase in the rate

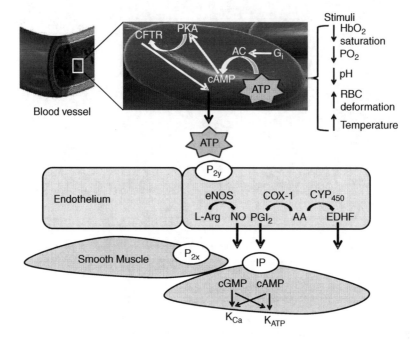

Adenosine Triphosphate. Fig. 2 Mechanism of ATP release from erythrocytes and ATP-mediated vasodilatation. ATP is released from erythrocytes which interact with the endothelium by releasing vasoactive mediators which stimulate vasodilation of the smooth muscle lining the vessel walls. List of abbreviations: Gi, heterotrimeric G protein; AC, adenylyl cyclase; cAMP, 3'5'-adenosine monophosphate; PKA, protein kinase A; CFTR, cystic fibrosis transmembrane conductance regulator; P_{2y} and P_{2x}, purinergic receptor subtypes; NO, nitric oxide; eNOS, endothelial NO synthase; COX-1, cyclooxygenase-1; CYP_{450}, cytochrome P_{450}; L-Arg, L-arginine; PGI_2, prostacyclin; AA, arachidonic acid; EDHF, endothelium-derived hyperpolarizing factor; IP, prostacyclin receptor; K_{Ca}, calcium sensitive K^+ channel; K_{ATP}, ATP-sensitive K^+ channel.

of PCr recovery. Endurance training is accompanied by a number of physiological adaptations that include improvements in oxidative metabolism, increased capillary density and glycogen storage, and enhanced insulin sensitivity. But the most apparent change is the increased number of mitochondria within the muscle. This ensures that there is an adequate production of ATP for muscle contraction during exercise and reduction in the incidence of early fatigue.

Since ATP can regulate blood flow, enhancing ATP release from erythrocytes may aid patients with vascular disease, heart failure, COPD, or spinal cord injury that are unable to participate in physical activity to a level that would improve circulation to the peripheral limbs. In this way, increasing blood flow could deliver more oxygen and nutrients to the muscle. Currently, there does not seem to be a good pharmacological alternative for improving circulation in these patients. Promoting the release of ATP from red blood cells, that is, with heat, could elicit blood flow changes that would be beneficial to patient populations is an attractive non-pharmacological remedy [6].

References

1. Baker JS, McCormick MC, Robergs RA (2010) Interaction among skeletal muscle metabolic energy systems during intense exercise. J Nutr Metab 2010:905612
2. Testa M, Navazio FM, Neugebauer J (2005) Recognition, diagnosis, and treatment of mitochondrial myopathies in endurance athletes. Curr Sports Med Rep 4(5):282–287
3. Ellsworth ML et al (2009) Erythrocytes: oxygen sensors and modulators of vascular tone. Physiology (Bethesda) 24:107–116
4. González-Alonso J et al (2008) Haemodynamic responses to exercise, ATP infusion and thigh compression in humans: insight into the role of muscle mechanisms on cardiovascular function. J Physiol 586(9):2405–2417
5. Mortensen SP et al (2009) ATP-induced vasodilation and purinergic receptors in the human leg: roles of nitric oxide, prostaglandins, and adenosine. Am J Physiol Regul Integr Comp Physiol 296(4): R1140–R1148
6. Kalsi KK, González-Alonso J (2010) Temperature-dependent release of ATP from human erythrocytes: mechanism for the control of local tissue perfusion. Circ 122:A13005

Adenosine Triphosphate–Binding Cassette A1 (ABCA1)

Is the membrane-bound enzyme responsible for transfer of cholesterol from peripheral cells to apoA1/immature HDL in the first step of reverse cholesterol transport. This enzyme and others are upregulated by exercise.

Adenosine Triphosphoric Acid

▶ Adenosine Triphosphate

Adherence (Regimen Adherence)

The change in behavior in comparison to the prescribed regimen, sometimes suggesting making the changes due to an internal desire to change.

Cross-References
▶ Behavioral Changes

Adhesion Molecules

They are proteins located on the cell surface involved with the binding with other cells or with the extracellular matrix (ECM) in the process called cell adhesion. The increase of these molecules is used as a signal of cardiovascular disease risk.

Adipocytokines

▶ Adipose-Tissue-Derived Hormones
▶ Adipokines

Adipogenesis

Is the process of cell differentiation by which preadipocytes become adipocytes.

Adipokines

Adipokines (also called adipocytolines) are polypeptides that are secreted from and/or produced by the adipocytes. They include leptin, adiponectin, resistin, and many cytokines of the immune system, such as tumor necrosis factor-alpha (TNF-α), interleukin-6 (IL-6), and complement factor D (also known as adipsin). They have potent autocrine, paracrine, and endocrine functions.

Cross-References
▶ Adipose-Tissue-Derived Hormones

Adiponectin

Adiponectin is produced largely by the adipocyte, and like leptin, has effects on numerous metabolic parameters including glucose and lipid metabolism. However, the effects of adiponectin on appetite/food intake are not nearly as pronounced as that of leptin. In contrast to leptin, circulating adiponectin concentrations generally decrease in obesity. Resistance of tissues such as liver and muscle to adiponectin also seems to occur in obesity.

Adipose Tissue

Adipose tissue includes adipocytes, along with other associated tissues such as connective tissue, vascular supply, as well as other infiltrating cells such as macrophages. Adipose tissue has classically been considered as a storage depot, but is now well recognized as having an important endocrine role.

Adipose-Tissue-Derived Hormones

David J. Dyck, Lindsay E. Robinson, David C. Wright
Department of Human Health and Nutritional Sciences, University of Guelph, Guelph, ON, Canada

Synonyms
Adipocytokines; Adipokines; Cytokines

Definition

Cytokines are defined as cell-to-cell signaling proteins (or peptides) that confer an immunomodulatory effect. Adipocytokines (usually abbreviated as adipokines) were first defined as cytokines specifically produced and secreted by adipocytes. However, this definition of adipokines is generally considered to be insufficient as many proteins that were originally defined as such, e.g., leptin and adiponectin, are now known to be produced by adipocytes as well as other cells within adipose tissue. Other so-called adipokines such as resistin may in fact not be secreted by adipocytes at all (at least in humans), but rather by macrophages that have infiltrated adipose tissue. In this regard, adipokines might better be defined as proteins that are secreted by adipose *tissue*, which would include adipocytes along with the associated connective tissue, vasculature, and immune cells such as macrophages. Even so, numerous proteins currently defined as adipokines, such as leptin, adiponectin, and chemerin, are also produced within unrelated tissues such as skeletal muscle, placenta, bone, etc., further complicating the definition of adipokines. Furthermore, many proteins originally classified as adipokines (leptin, adiponectin, resistin) were not known to have an immunomodulatory role, although in some cases this has been later identified. Nonetheless, despite the imprecision with its definition, the term "adipokines" generally refers to the collection of well over 100 identified proteins and hormones produced and secreted by adipose tissue.

Basic Mechanisms

Adipose tissue, an endocrine organ, produces a myriad of adipokines that contribute to various metabolic abnormalities, such as insulin resistance, a hallmark feature of obesity. Adipokines can act locally within adipose tissue itself and/or systemically, interacting with numerous peripheral tissues, including skeletal muscle, heart, liver, endothelial cells of blood vessels, other adipocytes, etc., to affect many metabolic and inflammatory processes [1]. Of the more than 100 identified adipokines, several are notably related to insulin responsiveness in skeletal muscle, including leptin, adiponectin, tumor necrosis factor-alpha (TNFα), interleukin-6 (IL-6), and apelin. Skeletal muscle is the largest sink for insulin-stimulated glucose uptake in the body and is therefore an important contributor to glucose homeostasis. Thus, the communication or "cross talk" between adipose tissue and muscle, and the role that adipokines might serve in this cross talk has been a point of considerable interest in recent years (Fig. 1). Specifically, leptin and adiponectin improve insulin response, an effect that is generally ascribed to their ability to increase fatty acid oxidation and reduce intramuscular lipid content. TNFα is a pro-inflammatory cytokine secreted from numerous cells including macrophages, adipocytes, and skeletal muscle, and has been implicated as a critical mediator of insulin resistance, particularly in relation to obesity. Perhaps, most controversial of the major adipokines associated with insulin response is IL-6. IL-6 is produced by adipocytes, immune cells, and contracting muscle and was the first identified myokine. There is evidence to implicate IL-6 both as a mediator of impaired insulin action in obesity, and also as a facilitator of increased fuel metabolism during exercise.

Leptin and Adiponectin

Leptin and adiponectin are generally considered to be important adipokines for the maintenance of insulin responsiveness. Certainly, their near absence in conditions such as lipoatrophy is accompanied by severe insulin resistance, as well as massive accumulations of lipid in numerous peripheral tissues (liver, muscle, etc.). Since lipid accumulation is strongly associated with insulin resistance, it is believed that leptin and adiponectin are important in the prevention of lipotoxicity and the subsequent impairment of insulin response. It is widely accepted that the ability of leptin and adiponectin to prevent or minimize lipid accumulation in tissues is achieved by their ability to stimulate AMP-activated protein kinase (AMPK) and fatty acid oxidation. However, other mechanisms including lipolysis, fatty acid uptake and trafficking are also involved, some of which do not involve AMPK. The obese condition is typically characterized by increased fatty acid uptake and accumulation, and a decline in the responsiveness to insulin in peripheral tissues such as muscle. This may in part be due to the onset of leptin and adiponectin resistance, leading to reduced protection against lipid accumulation [2]. Leptin and adiponectin resistance are evident in muscle from both rodents and humans, and have been shown to be inducible by the consumption of high-saturated fat diets in rodents. The mechanisms underlying this resistance have not been elucidated, but may in part involve an increase in suppressor of cytokine signaling (SOCS3). Feeding a diet high in polyunsaturated fatty acids delays the onset of leptin and adiponectin resistance; furthermore, including fish-oil-derived long-chain omega-3 fatty acids in a high-fat diet prevents/delays the development of leptin and adiponectin resistance. The exact mechanisms underlying these fatty acid effects are unknown but might involve modulation of toll-like receptor-4 (TLR4) content and downstream inflammatory signals. However, the role of

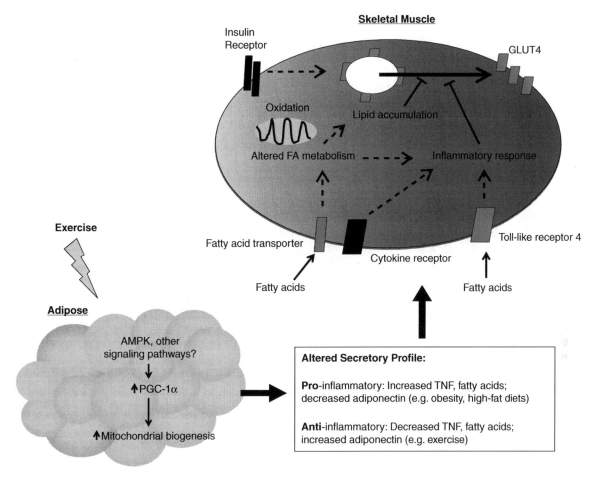

Adipose-Tissue-Derived Hormones. Fig. 1 Fatty acids, particularly saturated species, and pro-inflammatory adipokines are generally believed to induce lipid accretion, as well as an inflammatory response ultimately leading to the impairment of insulin-stimulated translocation of GLUT4 (glucose transporter 4). Anti-inflammatory and insulin-sensitizing adipokines are thought to reduce lipid accumulation and protect against inflammation

inflammation as a cause of leptin and adiponectin resistance has not yet been established.

TNFα and IL-6

Tumor necrosis factor-α is an inflammatory cytokine that is produced by numerous tissues that include skeletal muscle and adipose tissue. However, its chief source is immune cells, such as monocytes and macrophages. TNFα concentrations in plasma, muscle, and adipose tissue are often increased in cases of insulin resistance and type 2 diabetes, although this is not always the case. Its receptors, TNFR1 and 2, are located in most tissue and are also typically elevated in obesity. The deletion of TNFα receptors in mice conveys protection against the diet-induced induction of insulin resistance. TNFα may impair insulin response through several mechanisms, including (1) the stimulation of p38 mitogen-activated protein kinase (MAPK) and c-Jun-terminal kinase (JNK) leading to Ser307/312 phosphorylation and inhibition of the insulin receptor substrate-1 (IRS-1), and (2) increased formation of diacylglycerol and ceramides which are believed to impair insulin signaling through the inhibition of IRS-1 (via activation of novel PKC isoforms) and Akt. Interleukin-6 (IL-6) is produced by numerous tissues in the body, including various immune cells, fibroblasts, and adipose tissue. It was also the first identified myokine and is produced by contracting muscle. There has been considerable controversy regarding the role of IL-6 as it has been shown to be proinflammatory and impair glucose tolerance (when secreted by macrophages, for example), but also promotes glucose utilization during exercise.

Apelin

Apelin is a recently identified adipokine that has been reported to have a host of salutary effects on skeletal muscle and systemic carbohydrate and lipid metabolism [3]. Glucose tolerance and insulin sensitivity are reduced in apelin-deficient mice whereas increasing circulating apelin levels in severely insulin-resistant mice through the use of mini-osmotic pumps partially restores systemic insulin action. From a cellular perspective this effect is likely mediated through the activation of 5′AMP activated protein kinase (AMPK), an energy-sensing enzyme and master regulator of cellular metabolism that stimulates insulin-independent skeletal muscle glucose disposal, enhances insulin sensitivity, and increases fatty acid oxidation. Apelin would also appear to regulate the oxidative capacity of skeletal muscle. For example, repeated daily injections of apelin for several weeks increase mitochondrial enzyme content and activity in rat skeletal muscle. Similarly, apelin-over-expressing mice have increased skeletal muscle mitochondrial content when fed a high-fat diet relative to control animals. It is interesting to note that the effects of apelin are strikingly similar to that of exercise and would perhaps imply a role for apelin in mediating the effects of exercise on skeletal muscle metabolism.

Exercise Intervention

The effects of chronic exercise training as a means to improve glucose tolerance and insulin responsiveness are well characterized. While there are potentially several mechanisms that may underlie this effect, an increase in mitochondrial content leading to greater rates of fatty acid oxidation is often cited as an important contributor. However, it is also noteworthy that a single bout of exercise can improve insulin response for 12–24 h prior to any increases in mitochondrial content or capacity to oxidize fat. Although there are numerous speculations as to the possibility that exercise might confer some of its benefits on insulin response by altering the secretion of adipokines, or by changing the sensitivity of their target tissues, this has generally been poorly documented.

Leptin and Adiponectin

Both the acute and chronic effects of exercise on plasma leptin and adiponectin concentrations have been examined, with inconsistent findings. In general, acute exercise can decrease circulating levels of leptin if the intensity and duration are sufficiently intense, i.e., significant energy deficit. However, the provision of sufficient calories to meet the energy needs of the exercise can prevent the decrease in leptin. Chronic exercise training has been shown to lower leptin and increase adiponectin. In the case of leptin, this seems to be largely dependent on reductions in body fat. In the absence of changes in body mass/fat, changes in leptin are generally not evident. There is recent evidence that adiponectin concentrations can be increased by intense exercise independent of changes in body fat [4]. There is also evidence based on rodent models that intense treadmill exercise can protect skeletal muscle from becoming both leptin- and adiponectin-resistant during the administration of a high-fat diet.

TNFα

There is evidence that chronic exercise, in combination with dietary restriction, can reduce circulating TNFα concentrations. However, dietary restriction alone also reduces TNFα and other markers of inflammation, suggesting that it is the reduction in body fat that is the important factor, rather than the exercise per se. Moreover, the effect of exercise on TNFα production has largely focused on circulating immune cells. Thus, the degree to which adipose-tissue-derived TNFα is reduced is less well characterized, as is the responsiveness of peripheral tissues to TNFα following chronic exercise.

Apelin

Apelin, similar to adiponectin, has been shown to increase with exercise. Exercise, possibly working via catecholamines, activates AMPK in adipose tissue. In cell culture models, the pharmacological activation of AMPK with a compound called AICAR leads to increases in the expression of PPARγ coactivator 1 alpha (PGC-1α), a transcriptional coactivator that controls the expression of apelin. PGC-1α also increases adipose tissue mitochondrial content, an event that is required in adiponectin synthesis and secretion. In this regard, a catecholamine-AMPK-PGC-1α axis may be critical in the exercise-mediated regulation of adipose tissue metabolism and adipokine profile.

References

1. Schaffler A, Scholmerich J (2010) Innate immunity and adipose tissue biology. Trends Immunol 31:228–235
2. Mullen KL, Pritchard J, Ritchie I, Snook LA, Chabowski A, Bonen A, Wright D, Dyck DJ (2009) Adiponectin resistance precedes the accumulation of skeletal muscle lipids and insulin resistance in high-fat-fed rats. Am J Physiol Regul Integr Comp Physiol 296: R243–251
3. Xu S, Tsao PS, Yue P (2011) Apelin and insulin resistance: another arrow for the quiver? J Diabetes 3:225–231
4. Garekani ET, Mohebbi H, Kraemer RR, Fathi R (2011) Exercise training intensity/volume affects plasma and tissue adiponectin concentrations in the male rat. Peptides 32:1008–1012

Adiposity

The accumulation of adipose (fat) tissue; the state of being overweight.

Cross-References
▶ Obesity

Adiposity Signal

Hormone that circulates in the blood in proportion to the amount of fat stored in the body and which provides a signal to other organs such as the brain. A decrease in adiposity signals may elicit hyperphagia (increased energy intake) and decreases in energy expenditure, while an increase results in decreased energy intake and increased energy expenditure. Insulin and leptin are adiposity signals that are secreted primarily from the pancreas and adipose tissue, respectively.

ADMA

Asymmetric dimethylarginine (ADMA) is an endogenous inhibitor of NO-synthase. It is generated during proteolysis of methylated proteins. ADMA is removed either by renal excretion or metabolic degradation by the enzyme dimethylarginine dimethylaminohydrolase. ADMA can be produced and degraded by several cell types including human endothelial and tubular cells. Elevated ADMA concentrations in the blood are found in a number of chronic diseases associated with endothelial dysfunction such as hypercholesterolemia, hypertension, arteriosclerosis, chronic renal failure, and chronic heart failure.

Adolescence

A transitional stage of human development occurring between puberty and adulthood. The term adolescence includes girls aged 12–18 years and boys aged 14–18 years.

Adrenergic Receptors

James R. Docherty
Department of Physiology, Royal College of Surgeons in Ireland, Dublin, Ireland

Synonyms
Adrenoceptors; Sympathetic response mediators

Definition
▶ Adrenergic receptors are cell membrane receptors belonging to the seven transmembrane spanning G-protein-linked superfamily of receptors [1]. They respond to the sympathetic neurotransmitter noradrenaline and to the hormone adrenaline (and to various exogenous agonists) by producing a response within the cell, involving a second messenger, or ion channel. Adrenergic receptors can be divided into three major types, each with three subtypes [2, 3] (see Table 1). ▶ Alpha1-adrenergic receptors are linked to the enzyme phospholipase C (PLC), ▶ alpha2-adrenergic receptors are linked to inhibition of the enzyme adenylate cyclase (AC) and to opening of potassium (K^+) channels, and ▶ beta-adrenergic receptors are linked to stimulation of AC (see Table 1).

Basic Mechanisms
Adrenergic receptors are classically the receptors involved in the "fight or flight" reaction, the mobilization of resources caused by activation of the sympathetic nervous system that prepares the body for bouts of severe activity. This involves the release of the hormone adrenaline from the adrenal medulla into the bloodstream and an increase in sympathetic nerve activity mediated by the neurotransmitter noradrenaline. Adrenaline and the sympathetic nerves act to cause cardiac stimulation, increasing both heart rate and force of ventricular contraction to increase cardiac output and get more blood to exercising muscle. Adrenaline acts on vascular beta2-adrenergic receptors to dilate particularly muscle arterioles to deliver more of this increased cardiac output to skeletal muscle. Adrenaline mobilizes glucose and free fatty acids as energy sources. Sympathetic activation will also cause vasoconstriction in less vital vascular beds, particularly splanchnic and skin (although the skin vasculature may dilate later to dissipate heat), to divert blood to skeletal muscle. Sympathetic activation also mobilizes blood from the reservoir in the large veins (the capacitance vessels) by veniconstriction. Adrenaline also causes bronchodilatation to aid in getting

Adrenergic Receptors. Table 1 Subtypes of the adrenergic receptor family, important G protein and second messenger linkages (enzyme or ion channel), and major actions

Subtype	G protein	Linkage	Major actions
Alpha1A	Gq/11	PLC	sm contraction
Alpha1B	Gq/11	PLC	sm contraction
Alpha1D	Gq/11	PLC	sm contraction
Alpha2A	Gi/o	ACI/K$^+$	Nerve inhibition/sm contraction
Alpha2B	Gi/o	ACI/K$^+$	Nerve inhibition/sm contraction
Alpha2C	Gi/o	ACI/K$^+$	Nerve inhibition/sm contraction
Beta1	Gs	ACS	Cardiac stimulation/lipolysis
Beta2	Gs	ACS	sm dilatation/metabolic
Beta3	Gs	ACS	sm dilatation/metabolic/cardiac inhibition

ACI inhibition of enzyme adenylate cyclase, *ACS* stimulation of enzyme adenylate cyclase, *K$^+$* opening of potassium (K$^+$) channels, *PLC* stimulation of enzyme phospholipase C, *sm* smooth muscle (e.g., vascular, bronchial)

oxygen into the blood. Ocular effects involve alpha1-adrenergic receptor mediated dilatation of the pupil, and beta-adrenergic receptor mediated paralysis of accomodation, increasing the amount of light reaching the retina and setting the lens for wider vision. Sweating is also an adrenergic response, but the neurotransmitter is acetylcholine and beyond the scope of this article.

Genito-urinary actions of the adrenergic system are also important, and alpha- receptors are involved in contraction the smooth muscle of the vas deferens, in contracting the neck of the bladder and involved in prostate function. Adrenergic receptors are also present in the spinal cord and brain mediating diverse functions from control of blood pressure to mediating analgesia.

We can now consider the subtypes of adrenergic receptor that mediate these many physiological actions.

Alpha1-Adrenergic Receptors

Alpha1-adrenergic receptors are the classical adrenergic receptors mediating smooth muscle contraction, but we do not know the exact physiological role of each of the three subtypes. Alpha1A-receptors are widespread in many smooth muscles and are activated by administered agonists, but alpha1D or alpha1B may be more important physiologically for neurotransmission.

Alpha1-adrenergic receptors in the vascular system have a major role in the control of blood pressure and the response to falls in blood pressure. A fall in blood pressure due to causes such as hemorrhage will activate the baroreceptor reflex and cause sympathetic activation to vasoconstrict less vital vascular beds, especially splanchnic and skin. However, profound falls in blood pressure resulting in a decreased blood flow to the brain activates

a stronger reflex due to brain ischemia. This is the CNS Ischemic Reflex which is a last-ditch reflex to maintain brain blood flow at the expense of all other vascular beds by causing widespread vasoconstriction involving alpha1-adrenergic receptor activation.

Another important role of vascular alpha1-adrenergic receptors is temperature control. as vasoconstriction of superficial blood vessels is an important mechanism to conserve heat. Alpha1-adrenergic receptors are also involved in the hyperthermia to amphetamine derivatives such as ▶ methylenedioxymethamphetamine (MDMA), which produces a dangerous hyperthermia in hot conditions, such as found at a "Rave."

In nonvascular smooth muscle, alpha1-adrenergic receptors mediate inhibition of micturition, but the density of alpha1-adrenergic receptors in the neck of the bladder is greater in males, suggesting a sexual function to prevent retrograde ejaculation into the bladder. Alpha1-adrenergic receptors mediate contraction of the vas deferens and seminal vesicles and have an important role in ejaculation.

Alpha1-adrenergic receptor agonist mediated vasoconstriction can be used to treat hypotension, and can be used in nasal decongestion. Alpha1-adrenergic receptor agonists also act on the eye to dilate the pupil by contracting the dilator pupillae muscle, and also have actions to reduce intraocular pressure, presumably by restricting blood flow. Alpha1-adrenergic receptor antagonists lower blood pressure in hypertension and are used in the treatment of Benign prostatic hypertrophy.

Alpha2-Adrenergic Receptors

Like alpha1-adrenergic receptors, alpha2-adrenergic receptors are involved in vasoconstriction, but their exact role, and the role of each of the subtypes, in the control of blood pressure has not been fully established. They are not as widespread in the vascular system as alpha1-adrenoceptors, but they may have a role particularly on veins (possibly alpha2C-receptors) to cause veniconstriction. In addition, alpha2A-receptors on endothelial cells mediate relaxation of vascular smooth muscle.

Alpha2A-adrenergic receptors are involved in the central control of blood pressure, mediating a profound fall in blood pressure, and this explains the antihypertensive actions of alpha2-receptor agonists such as clonidine. Alpha2-adrenergic receptors also mediate analgesia centrally.

Alpha2-adrenergic receptors, particulary alpha2A and to a lesser extent alpha2C, are also present on the prejunctional nerve terminal of adrenergic and other nerves, where they mediate inhibition of neurotransmitter release. In adrenergic nerves, this is a negative feedback to modulate release. Although the exact importance of these receptors is unclear, there is evidence that absence of the prejunctional alpha2-adrenergic receptor in animal models increases susceptibility to heart failure, presumably by allowing excess release of noradrenaline neurotransmitter. Alpha2-adrenergic receptors on non-adrenergic nerves act to inhibit function in those nerves. Sympathetic activation inhibits the cholinergic and other nerves involved in digestion and so causes inhibition of gastrointestinal function.

Beta1-Adrenergic Receptors

Beta1-adrenergic receptors are the major receptors involved in cardiac stimulation. Like all beta-receptors, the main signaling pathway is by activation of the enzyme adenylate cyclase, resulting in increased levels of the second messenger cAMP (Table 1). Beta1-receptor activation depolarizes the unstable pacemaker cells of the ▶ Sinoatrial (SA) node so that the threshold for generation of action potentials is reached faster, resulting in a faster heart rate. At the ▶ atrioventricular (AV) node, beta-receptor mediated depolarization allows faster conduction of the impulse from the atria to ventricles, allowing a fast atrial rate to pass from atria to ventricles. In the atrial and ventricular muscle fibers, beta1-receptor stimulation increases calcium entry during depolarization, increasing the force of contraction, thus increasing stroke volume.

Cardiac output (CO) is defined as the volume of blood pumped per minute, and depends both on heart rate (HR) (per minute) and stroke volume (SV) (volume pumped per beat), by the equation: $CO = HR \times SV$. Resting cardiac output is around 5 L/min. In exercise, we can increase cardiac output by increasing either HR or SV, or both. In light exercise, HR tends to increase markedly, with a smaller effect on SV, but in severe exercise there are also larger increases in SV. HR may reach 200 beats/min in severe exercise in a young healthy adult, from a resting of around 70 beats/min, and stroke volume may increase from 70 to 125 ml, giving a change in CO from 5 to 25 l. Trained athletes, who may have an enlarged ventricle, will increase their CO further by increasing SV further. Cardiac transplant patients who have a functional denervation of the heart, can increase their CO by the intrinsic properties of the heart and by the actions of the hormone adrenaline.

Beta1-adrenergic agonists are employed as cardiac stimulants. ▶ Beta-blockers, or beta1-adrenergic receptor antagonists, are used for a wide variety of cardiovascular indications including hypertension, angina, and even heart failure. A number of beta-adrenergic receptor antagonists exhibit partial agonism, that is, they produced some beta-adrenergic stimulation while acting mainly as antagonists. The mode of action may involve actions at two forms of the beta1-adrenergic receptor: antagonist at beta1 high affinity receptors and agonist in higher concentrations at beta1 low affinity receptors.

Beta2-Adrenergic Receptors

Beta2-adrenergic receptors mediate relaxation of vascular smooth muscle and the smooth muscle of the bronchus, gut, bladder, urethra, uterus, etc. Beta-2 adrenergic receptors are generally thought to be non-innervated receptors, far from nerve endings, acting as targets for circulating adrenaline since noradrenaline is a poor agonist at these receptors. In the vascular system, beta2-adrenergic receptors are the main mediators of adrenergic relaxation, acting to stimulate the enzyme adenylate cyclase and increase cAMP production, although all beta-receptor subtypes mediate relaxation. Interestingly, in the coronary artery, relaxation is mediated by the beta1-receptor, perhaps allowing nerve-released noradrenaline to dilate these crucial arteries. Beta-adrenergic receptor mediated relaxation of the vascular system can be direct by actions on the smooth muscle or indirect by causing release of nitric oxide from the endothelium. Another important site of beta2-adrenoceptor relaxation is bronchial smooth muscle and beta2-adrenergic agonists are widely used in asthma as bronchodilators.

Beta3-Adrenergic Receptors

The Beta3 is a controversial beta-adrenergic receptor, with difficulties in positive identification due to lack of truly selective antagonist drugs. Beta3-adrenergic receptors, like beta2- and even beta1-, are involved in metabolic effects, particularly lipolysis in adipose tissue. Beta3-adrenergic receptors also mediate smooth muscle relaxation of vascular and nonvascular smooth muscle, and may be particularly important in the bladder. The most surprising effect mediated by beta3-adrenergic receptors is an action to decrease myocardial contractility by stimulation of nitric oxide synthase in cardiac muscle cells to produce nitric oxide, and this may be a protective mechanism to prevent overstimulation of the heart by the adrenergic system as these receptors would be activated by high concentrations of noradrenaline and adrenaline to partly counteract their beta1-mediated stimulant actions.

Exercise Intervention

Adrenergic Drugs and Sport

The beta2-adrenergic receptor is the main beta-adrenergic receptor targeted in sport since beta2-adrenergic receptor activation has bronchodilator and anabolic actions [4]. A large number of athletes are classed as asthmatic, perhaps caused by continual exposure to allergens and to cold air in winter. Inhaled beta2-adrenergic receptor agonists have been reported to be effective against exercise-induced bronchospasm. Beta2-adrenergic receptor agonists also have growth promoting (anabolic) actions to improve muscle regeneration and function after injury.

A second class of adrenergic agents relevant in sport belong to the class of stimulants. Stimulants are banned only in competition, as any advantage would be transient, and a total ban would be difficult since many over the counter medicines contain stimulants [5]. For example, nasal decongestants are alpha1-adrenergic receptor agonists which produce vasoconstriction of the nasal mucosa, reducing mucosal swelling, and mucosal mass to reduce congestion [5]. Stimulants that have actions centrally in the brain would be likely to increase alertness or increase motivation, and those with beta1-adrenoceptor actions would produce cardiac stimulant effects. For these reasons, most stimulants are banned in competition.

Training and Adrenergic Responses

Training may increase an athlete's ability to release ▶ catecholamines from the adrenal medulla during bouts of exercise [6]. Although increased release of catecholamines in exercise might be predicted to cause downregulation of adrenergic receptors and so largely counteract the effects of increased release, there is evidence that training may also result in increased metabolism of catecholamines [7]. Hence, a greater release coupled with a more rapid metabolism of catecholamines would allow increased acute response to catecholamines (for instance, cardiac

stimulation) but less chronic desensitization of adrenergic receptors, as the exposure time to elevated catecholamines is reduced, resulting in a training related increase in adrenergic responsiveness.

References

1. Alexander SP, Mathie A, Peters JA (2008) Guide to receptors and channels (GRAC). Br J Pharmacol 153(Suppl 2):S1–S209 3rd edition
2. Docherty JR (1998) Subtypes of functional alpha1- and alpha2-adrenoceptors. Eur J Pharmacol 361(1):1–15
3. Guimarães S, Moura D (2001) Vascular adrenoceptors: an update. Pharmacol Rev 53(2):319–356
4. Davis E, Loiacono R, Summers RJ (2008) The rush to adrenaline: drugs in sport acting on the beta-adrenergic system. Br J Pharmacol 154(3):584–597
5. Docherty JR (2008) Pharmacology of stimulants prohibited by the World Anti-Doping Agency (WADA). Br J Pharmacol 154(3):606–622
6. Zouhal H, Jacob C, Delamarche P, Gratas-Delamarche A (2008) Catecholamines and the effects of exercise, training and gender. Sports Med 38(5):401–423
7. Bracken RM, Brooks S (2010) Plasma catecholamine and nephrine responses following 7 weeks of sprint cycle training. Amino Acids 38(5):1351–1359

Adrenoceptors

▶ Adrenergic Receptors

Adult Hippocampal Neurogenesis

It consists of the generation of new neurons in the adult brain, specifically, the neurons born during adult life in the subgranular zone of the hippocampal dentate gyrus (generating granule neurons that populate the granule cell layer). These neurons differentiate into mature neurons becoming integrated in adult networks. They may play roles both during differentiation and after maturation.

Aerobic Activity

Aerobic activity is any form of rhythmic muscular activity where the cardio-respiratory system is able to supply sufficient oxygen to meet metabolic demand without the accumulation of significant quantities of lactate. If the intent is to use such aerobic activity to maintain cardiovascular health, sufficient of the large body muscles must be activated to use 50–70% of the individual's maximal oxygen consumption (for example, by jogging, treadmill running or exercising on a cycle ergometer).

Aerobic Capacity ($\dot{V}O_{2\,max}$)

The maximal amount of oxygen that can be consumed and utilized per time unit.

Cross-References

▶ Maximal Oxygen Update ($\dot{V}O_{2\,max}$)

Aerobic Endurance

Aerobic endurance represents the capacity to sustain a high fraction of maximal oxygen consumption through the entire effort duration. It is mainly determined by oxidative enzymes activity and muscle fiber composition.

Aerobic Energy System

▶ Aerobic Metabolism

Aerobic Exercise Energy Expenditure

Exercise energy demands that are met by aerobic metabolism and measured as the amount or rate of O_2 consumed.

Aerobic Fitness

The ability to deliver oxygen to the exercising muscles and to utilize it to generate energy during exercise.

Cross-References

▶ Aerobic Power, Tests of

Aerobic Glycolysis

The catabolism of glucose or glycogen to CO_2 and H_2O.

Aerobic Metabolism

Antonios Matsakas[1], Ketan Patel[2]
[1]Institute of Molecular Medicine, The University of Texas Health Science Center, Houston, TX, USA
[2]School of Biological Sciences, University of Reading, Whiteknights, Reading, UK

Synonyms

Aerobic energy system; Aerobic respiration; Cellular oxidation; Oxidative metabolism; Oxygen system

Definition

Metabolism is defined as the sum of chemical reactions taking place in a live organism to maintain life. Aerobic means *oxygen dependent* and aerobic metabolism refers to an energy-generating system under the presence of oxygen as opposed to anaerobic, i.e., oxygen independent metabolism. Aerobic metabolism uses oxygen as the final electron acceptor in the electron transport chain and combines with hydrogen to form water [1]. In essence, the vast majority of adenosine triphosphate (ATP) synthesis takes place via aerobic breakdown of energy substrates through the coupling of respiratory chain and oxidative phosphorylation. Aerobic metabolism includes in terms of energy sources carbohydrates and lipids and to a less extent proteins. In exercise, aerobic metabolism predominates supplying a large amount of energy at low power during exercise exceeding 1 min in duration regardless of intensity (e.g., the 800 m run and upward, the 200 m swim and upward; [2]). In terms of enzymes, aerobic metabolism includes pyruvate dehydrogenase, the enzymes of lipolysis, fatty acid degradation, the citric acid cycle, and the electron transport chain and the ATP synthase.

Characteristics

Dietary macronutrients containing carbohydrates, fats, and proteins are biochemically processed to give rise to cellular energy substrates such as glucose, fatty acids and glycerol, as well as amino acids. The different metabolic pathways of glucose, fatty acid, and protein catabolism are integrated in the form of acetyl coenzyme A (coA) in the mitochondria. Glucose is broken down to pyruvate through the anaerobic process of glycolysis and enters the mitochondria where it is converted to acetyl coA and cellular energy is generated in the citric acid cycle, electron transport chain, and oxidative phosphorylation via the removal and transfer to oxygen of energy-rich electrons (Fig. 1).

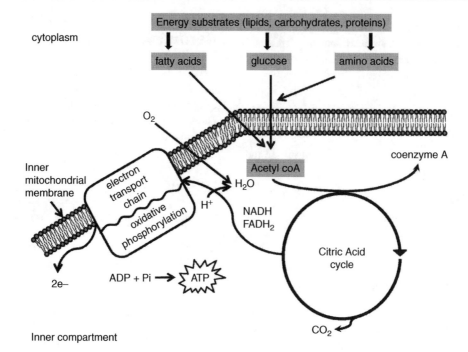

Aerobic Metabolism. Fig. 1 Schematic overview of aerobic metabolism. Acetyl coenzyme A, the activated carrier that transfers the acetyl group into the citric acid cycle, interconnects the metabolic pathways of lipid, carbohydrate, and protein catabolism. A significant amount of energy can be generated during aerobic metabolism by means of citric acid cycle, electron transport chain, and oxidative phosphorylation during light to moderate endurance exercise

There are two major electron carriers in the oxidation of substrates that provide energy-rich molecules by carrying electrons with a high energy-transfer potential: the nicotinamide adenine dinucleotide (NAD^+) and flavin adenine dinucleotide (FAD). NAD is derived from niacin and FAD is derived from riboflavin, both are members of the vitamin B family. In the substrate oxidation two protons (H^+) and electrons are removed. NAD^+ receives the two electrons and one H^+ (the other H^+ is carried in the cell fluid), while FAD accepts both the H^+ and electrons are reduced to NADH and H^+ ($NADH.H^+$) and $FADH_2$, respectively. Acetyl coenzyme A, the common intermediate compound in carbohydrate, lipid and protein breakdown releases carbon dioxide and for one CO_2 removed one NAD^+ is reduced. The gaining of electrons known as the process of reduction aims at capturing most of the substrate energy, which can be further transferred to oxygen and thus release energy that can be used to phosphorylate ADP and give rise to ATP. Oxidation of one glucose in muscle yields six CO_2, four ATP, eight NADH, and four $FADH_2$. NADH and $FADH_2$ are oxidized in electron transport chain by oxygen providing the energy for ATP synthesis in oxidative phosphorylation. Thus the net energy

Aerobic Metabolism. Table 1 Energy amount in aerobic metabolism

Net energy (ATP) yield from glucose oxidation	
	Blood glucose
Glycolysis	2
Citric acid cycle	2
Electron transport chain	26
Total	30[a]

[a]Assumption: Based on more recent calculations the oxidation of 1 mol of $NADH.H^+$ or $FADH_2$ produces 2.5 or 1.5 ATP, respectively (although in older textbooks the energetic yields for $NADH.H^+$ and $FADH_2$ are traditionally reported as 3 and 2 ATP, respectively)

yield in ATP from glucose oxidation through pyruvate oxidation, the citric acid cycle, the electron transport chain, and oxidative phosphorylation is 30 ATP (Table 1). In addition, fatty acids represent a significant source of energy in light and moderate-intensity exercise stimuli. However, since the rate of ATP resynthesis through the oxidation of fatty acids derived from either the myocellular triacylglycerol depots or the adipose tissue is relatively low (0.2–0.3 mmol/kg/s), they cannot support hard exercise. Exercise is known to accelerate the glycolysis (the breakdown of glucose to pyruvate), pyruvate oxidation, lipolysis (the breakdown of triacylglycerols), fatty acid oxidation, citric acid cycle, and the oxidative phosphorylation in skeletal muscle [2].

Measurements/Diagnostics

A product of anaerobic metabolism, the lactate, can be useful in estimating aerobic endurance and indirectly aerobic metabolism, since there is a strong relationship between performance in endurance events and the moderate exercise intensity corresponding to a given blood lactate concentration. Thus, the higher endurance performance, the lower the blood lactate concentration. Higher endurance performance indicative of higher aerobic metabolism capacity can be developed through exercise. A plot of blood lactate concentration versus exercise intensity for an untrained individual shifts to the right as a consequence of training adaptation. Therefore an untrained individual will produce more lactate for a given intensity of exercise compared to a trained individual (Fig 2a). Exercise intensities that maintain blood lactate levels below 4 mmol/L are considered the most effective for improvements in aerobic metabolism, cardiovascular system, and lipidemic profile. At the histological level, succinate dehydrogenase activity (SDH) is another useful indicator of mitochondrial oxidative potential reflecting the metabolic properties of the cell. Slow- and fast-twitch muscle fibers have high and low SDH activity, respectively, and can be identified on a muscle section (Fig. 2b). Skeletal muscle fiber SDH activity can be modulated by regular endurance exercise [3].

Regular endurance exercise promotes aerobic metabolism and has been considered to be beneficial in both health and disease triggering the transition of skeletal muscle toward an oxidative phenotype by regulating slow-twitch contractile machinery, mitochondrial biogenesis, and fatty acid oxidation. Such remodeling of the skeletal muscle is brought about by a wide signaling network of transcriptional regulators that boost aerobic metabolism. An overview of power metabolic regulators and their downstream targets are summarized in Table 2. In brief, peroxisome-proliferator-activated receptor δ (PPARδ) is a member of the nuclear receptor super-family of transcriptional regulators that has been shown to regulate oxidative metabolism and slow-twitch fiber phenotype. AMP-activated protein kinase (AMPK) is a cellular energy sensor that is activated robustly in skeletal muscle by both acute and chronic exercise boosting muscle transcriptional activity and inducing aerobic metabolism. Sirtuins are known to regulate cell differentiation, metabolism and inflammation. Silent information regulator two protein 1 (SIRT1) is the most extensively studied sirtuin and is expressed predominantly in oxidative slow-twitch muscle. SIRT1 induces oxidative genes and mitochondrial biogenesis in skeletal muscle, leading to an increase in oxygen consumption, running endurance, and protection against metabolic diseases. Peroxisome-proliferator-activated receptor γ coactivator-1 alpha (PGC-1α) is a well-characterized transcriptional coactivator that regulates a fast-to-slow muscle fiber shift leading to an improved aerobic metabolism. Recent interest has emerged for pharmacological targeting of such key molecules that stimulate aerobic metabolism mimicking exercise-mediated changes and exhibiting potential therapeutic effects against metabolic disorders [4].

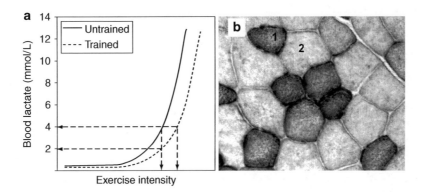

Aerobic Metabolism. Fig. 2 Examples of measurements for aerobic metabolism. (**a**) Estimation of aerobic capacity by using the lactate-intensity plot, (**b**) SDH activity of skeletal muscle; 1 and 2: muscle fibers with high and low SDH activity, respectively

Aerobic Metabolism. Table 2 Powerful metabolic regulators of aerobic metabolism and their gene targets in skeletal muscle (Due to space limitations references have been omitted)

PPARδ	PGC-1α	AMPK	SIRT1
Fatty acid oxidation: *HFBP, FAT/CD36, m-CPT1, PDK4, HMGCS2, thiolase, LCAD*	Fatty acid oxidation: *m-CPT1*	Fatty acid oxidation: *PPARδ, PDK4, SCD1*	Fatty acid oxidation: *MCAD, PDK4, FAT/CD36*
Oxidative metabolism: *Succinate dehydrogenase, citrate synthase*	Oxidative metabolism: *Nrf1, ERRγ*	Oxidative metabolism: *PPARδ, FASN, SCD1*	Oxidative metabolism: *NDUFB8, CoxVa*
Mitochondrial respiration and thermogenesis: *Cytochrome C, cytochrome oxidase II/IV, UCP-2/3, PGC-1α*	Mitochondrial respiration and thermogenesis: *Cytochrome C, cytochrome oxidase II and IV, UCP-2/3, Nrf1*	Mitochondrial respiration and thermogenesis: *PPARδ, PGC-1α*	Mitochondrial biogenesis: *PPARs(α/γ/δ/PGC-1α), ERRα, Nrip1, Tfam, Nrf1, UCP3*
Fiber type shift: Myoglobin, troponin I slow	Slow-twitch fiber program: *Myoglobin, troponin I slow, Mef2*	Fiber type shift: *PPARδ*	Fiber type shift: *PGC-1α, Myoglobin, troponins*
		Energy expenditure: *NAD⁺, SIRT1*	Energy metabolism: *PGC-1α/β, FOXO 1/3, ERRα, Nrip1 ATP5G3*

AMPK AMP-activated protein kinase; *ATP5G3* ATP synthase, H + transporting, mitochondrial F0 complex, subunit C3; *CoxVa* cytochrome c oxidase subunit V; *ERRα/γ* estrogen related receptor α/γ; *FASN* fatty acid synthase; *FAT/CD36* fatty acid translocase protein/(CD36); *FOXO* Forkhead box class O; *H-FABP* Heart fatty acid-binding protein; *HFBP* high-affinity folate-binding protein; *HMGCS2* 3-hydroxy-3-methylglutaryl coenzyme A synthase; *LCAD* long-chain acyl-coenzyme A dehydrogenase; *MCAD* Medium-chain acyl-coenzyme A dehydrogenase; *m-CPT1* muscle carnitine palmitoyl-transferase 1; *Mef2* myocyte enhancer factor-2; *NAD⁺* Nicotinamide Adenine Dinucleotide; *NDUFB8* NADH dehydrogenase (ubiquinone) 1 beta subcomplex, 8; *Nrf1* Nuclear respiratory factor 1; *Nrip 1* Nuclear receptor interacting protein 1; *PDK4* pyruvate dehydrogenase kinase 4; *PGC-1α* peroxisome-proliferator-activated receptor γ coactivator 1α; *PPARδ* peroxisome-proliferator-activated receptor δ; *SCD1* stearoyl-CoA desaturase 1; *SIRT1* Silent information regulator two protein 1; *Tfam* transcription factor A, mitochondrial; *UCP-2/3* uncoupling protein-2/3

References

1. McArdle WD, Katch FI, Katch VL (2007) Exercise physiology: energy, nutrition and human performance. Lippincott Williams and Wilkins, Baltimore
2. Mougios V (2006) Exercise biochemistry. Human Kinetics, Champaign
3. Matsakas A, Mouisel E, Amthor H, Patel K (2010) Myostatin knock-out mice increase oxidative muscle phenotype as an adaptive response to exercise. J Muscle Res Cell Motil 31:111–1125
4. Matsakas A, Narkar V (2010) Endurance exercise mimetics in skeletal muscle. Curr Sports Med Rep 9:227–232

Aerobic Power, Tests of

ALAN R. BARKER, NEIL ARMSTRONG
Children's Health and Exercise Research Centre, Sport and Health Sciences, College of Life and Environmental Sciences, University of Exeter, Exeter, UK

Synonyms

Aerobic fitness; Cardiorespiratory fitness; Maximal aerobic power; Maximal O₂ uptake; Peak O₂ uptake

Definition

Aerobic power, otherwise known as maximal O_2 consumption ($\dot{V}O_{2\ max}$), can be defined as the maximal rate at which O_2 can be consumed during whole body exercise at sea level. According to the Fick equation, $\dot{V}O_{2\ max}$ is the product of ▶ cardiac output ($\dot{Q}$) and the arteriovenous O_2 content difference ($C_aO_2 - C_vO_2$):

$$\dot{V}O_2 = \dot{Q} \cdot (C_aO_2 - C_vO_2)$$

where $\dot{Q}$ is the product of heart rate and ▶ stroke volume.

As the direct determination of $\dot{V}O_{2\ max}$ using cardiac catheterization combined with serial arterial and venous blood samples is highly invasive, its use in humans is limited for specific research purposes only. Consequently, whole body $\dot{V}O_{2\ max}$ is routinely measured using indirect calorimetry based on respiratory measurements of the volume of expired air and its fractional O_2 content. This is performed using either the classical Douglas bag technique providing a $\dot{V}O_2$ sample every 30–60 s, or on a breath-by-breath basis using an automated gas analysis system. However, due to the presence of large inter-breath fluctuations in $\dot{V}O_2$ during exercise in humans, the breath-by-breath response is typically averaged over 10–30 s to establish $\dot{V}O_{2\,max}$.

Based on the physiological determinants of the Fick equation, $\dot{V}O_{2\,max}$ can be viewed as the functional upper limit for the cardiovascular, pulmonary, and muscular systems to transport and utilize O_2 during exercise. Since its original description in 1923 by the Nobel Laureate A.V. Hill and colleagues, $\dot{V}O_{2\,max}$ has become one of the most measured variables in exercise physiology and is widely considered as the best single measure of cardiorespiratory fitness. For example, a high $\dot{V}O_{2\,max}$ is known to reduce the risk of all-cause mortality and cardiovascular disease in adults and is considered a prerequisite for successful endurance performance in elite athletes.

Description

The traditional paradigm for $\dot{V}O_{2\,max}$ requires that during progressive exercise to exhaustion, $\dot{V}O_2$ will no longer increase linearly with increasing exercise intensity, but display a plateau (Fig. 1). Therefore, if $\dot{V}O_2$ fails to increase by a predetermined amount despite an increase in exercise intensity, a valid $\dot{V}O_2$ max is achieved. In practice, however, only 20–50% of adults and children performing exhaustive exercise display a $\dot{V}O_2$ plateau

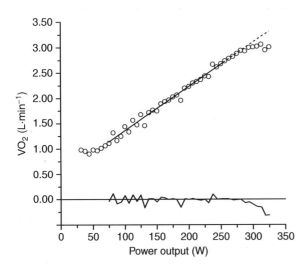

Aerobic Power, Tests of. Fig. 1 The $\dot{V}O_2$ response during incremental cycling exercise using a ramp rate of 25 W min^{-1} in a healthy adult female. The *solid line* represents a simple linear regression that was plotted between 75 and 250 W and extrapolated to end exercise (denoted by the *dotted line*). The departure ($\sim$250 mL min^{-1}) in $\dot{V}O_2$ from that expected based on the submaximal $\dot{V}O_2$-power output relationship indicates a clear $\dot{V}O_2$ plateau in this participant

[3, 4]. The term peak $\dot{V}O_2$ ($\dot{V}O_{2\,peak}$) is more appropriate here, reflecting the highest $\dot{V}O_2$ obtained during an exercise test to exhaustion in the absence of a plateau.

Due to the failure to consistently observe a $\dot{V}O_2$ plateau during exhaustive exercise, secondary criteria are often used to verify a $\dot{V}O_{2\,max}$. These include the measurement of heart rate and ▶ respiratory exchange ratio at exhaustion, and the assessment of post-exercise blood lactate accumulation. While there is no universal agreement for which set of criteria (or single criterion) and the specific cutoff values that should be used, they remain commonplace when measuring $\dot{V}O_{2\,max}$ [4]. However, recent research has shown that secondary criteria produce a significantly lower $\dot{V}O_{2\,max}$ by up to 30% in some cases, or falsely reject a "true" $\dot{V}O_{2\,max}$ during cycling exercise [3]. The authors cautioned against using secondary criteria and championed the use of a supramaximal exercise bout to exhaustion following the initial incremental test to confirm the measurement of a "true" $\dot{V}O_{2\,max}$ (Fig. 2). By plotting the composite $\dot{V}O_2$ profile from both tests (incremental and supramaximal), the $\dot{V}O_2$ plateau criterion can be obtained within a single testing session despite the absence of a plateau during the initial incremental test in the majority of cases. If the highest $\dot{V}O_2$ during the supramaximal exercise bout is greater than a predetermined amount (usually the within-participant reproducibility for $\dot{V}O_{2\,max}$), say 5%, then the supramaximal bout will need to be repeated at a higher exercise intensity following a short rest. This will be repeated until the increase in $\dot{V}O_2$ is less than 5%. The highest $\dot{V}O_2$ across the incremental and supramaximal tests is then taken as the participant's $\dot{V}O_{2\,max}$.

Clinical Use/Application

Maximal Exercise Testing

The most widely used protocol to measure $\dot{V}O_{2\,max}$ is the progressive incremental test to exhaustion, otherwise known as the graded exercise test. Such tests are extremely powerful in profiling an individual's ▶ aerobic fitness, as in addition to determining $\dot{V}O_{2\,max}$, "submaximal" parameters of aerobic function (e.g., O_2 cost of exercise, ▶ blood lactate threshold) can be obtained (see [5] for further discussion). Such tests are routinely performed on a cycle ergometer or motorized treadmill. Although $\dot{V}O_{2\,max}$ is typically $\sim$5–10% higher during treadmill running and treadmill exercise allows for a more common form of physiological stress (e.g., walking, jogging), it does not permit accurate quantification of power output, unlike cycling. When testing athletes or sport performers,

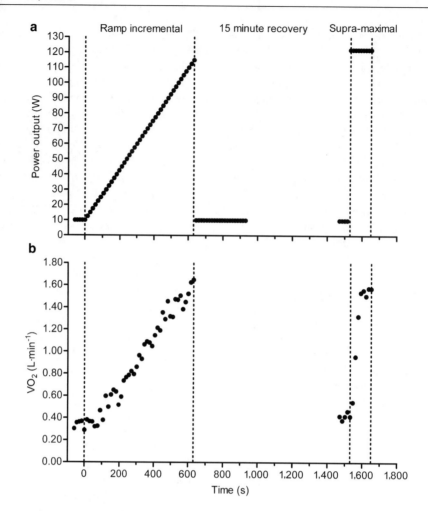

Aerobic Power, Tests of. Fig. 2 A combined ramp incremental and supramaximal cycle test to establish $\dot{V}O_{2\,max}$ in a 9-year-old boy. The protocol is shown in A where a 10 W min^{-1} increment was used for the ramp test, and following a 15 min of recovery, a supramaximal bout to exhaustion at 105% of the ramp test peak power was used. The resultant $\dot{V}O_2$ response is shown in B. The highest $\dot{V}O_2$ from the ramp test was 1.65 L min^{-1}. Despite the increase in power output during the supramaximal bout, the highest $\dot{V}O_2$ recorded was 1.57 L min^{-1}, indicating the achievement of a $\dot{V}O_2$ plateau. The child's $\dot{V}O_{2\,max}$ was taken to be 1.65 L min^{-1}. The *vertical dotted lines* represent the start and end of the incremental and supramaximal bouts

however, it is important to establish $\dot{V}O_{2\,max}$ on a sport-specific ergometer to monitor their modality-specific training adaptations and maximize training prescription.

The choice of testing protocols to establish $\dot{V}O_{2\,max}$ are numerous and vary on whether the increments in exercise intensity (e.g., power output, running speed, and/or gradient) are made continuously or discontinuously (each stage is separated with a 1–10 min rest), or in a ramp or stepwise function (Fig. 3). Studies have shown no differences in $\dot{V}O_{2\,max}$ between continuous and discontinuous protocols, or protocols employing either a ramp function or 1–3 min step increments. However, due to the shorter

test duration and the avoidance of large increments in exercise intensity, which may result in premature fatigue especially in participants with low fitness and physical activity levels, there is increasing popularity toward using continuous incremental protocols employing either a ramp or 1 min step increments in exercise intensity [1, 5]. If steady-state conditions are required to quantify physiological variables in relation to exercise intensity though (e.g., O_2 cost of exercise), longer stage durations of ~3 min may be required.

For cycle ergometry the protocol usually begins with a brief period of unloaded or very light pedaling

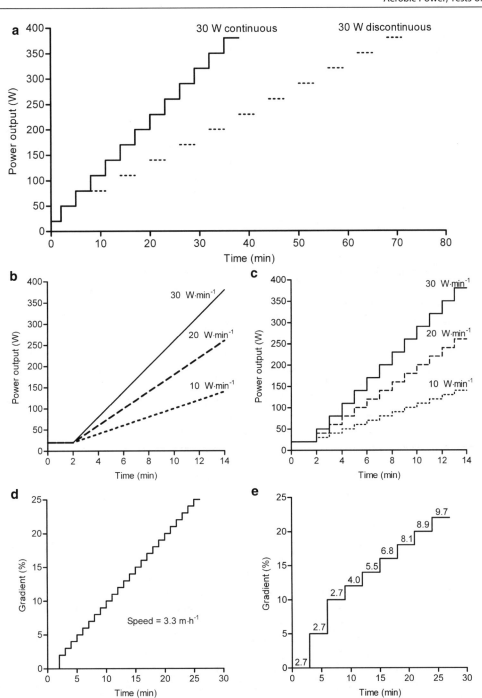

Aerobic Power, Tests of. Fig. 3 Example incremental protocols for cycle ergometry (**a–c**) and treadmill running (**d–e**). In (**a**) power output is increased by 30 W every 3 min using either a continuous or discontinuous protocol (note the markedly increased test duration for the discontinuous protocol). In **b** and **c** power output is increased using three different increments (10, 20, or 30 W min^{-1}) in a ramp (**b**) or stepwise (**c**) fashion. In **d** the treadmill protocol has a fixed belt speed at 5.3 km h^{-1} but the gradient increases 1% every minute until exhaustion (Balke protocol). In contrast, in **e** both the belt speed (2.7–9.7 km h^{-1}) and gradient (0–22%) are increased in a stepwise fashion until exhaustion (Bruce protocol)

(e.g., 10–20 W) followed by an individualized (see below) or predetermined power output increment until exhaustion. This is typically defined as a fall in pedal cadence of ~10 rev min^{-1} below that prescribed (usually between 60 and 80 rev min^{-1}). Alternatively, treadmill protocols typically start at a fixed speed and the exercise intensity is increased by altering the gradient until exhaustion (e.g., Harbor protocol), or until a given gradient is reached and the exercise intensity is further enhanced by increases in treadmill belt speed (e.g., Balke test), or a combination of both (e.g., Bruce protocol). Such tests are more routinely used in the clinical environment or in the general population (see [1, 5] for an overview). For athletic or highly active participants, such tests may end at a very high gradient (>20%) caused by lower limb fatigue and/or discomfort, rather than a cardiorespiratory limitation. Therefore, a protocol that increases in treadmill belt speed initially until the achievement of ~80% their heart rate predicted maximum (220 − age), after which the gradient can be increased 1–2% each stage until exhaustion, may be more appropriate.

It has been suggested that providing the incremental exercise test is between ~8 and 12 min in duration, a valid $\dot{V}O_{2\,max}$ can be obtained [5]. To achieve this test duration, the rate at which the exercise intensity is increased can be tailored to each participant based on their predicted $\dot{V}O_{2\,max}$ and $\dot{V}O_2$ during unloaded cycling [5]:

$$\text{Predicted } \dot{V}O_2 \text{ during unloaded cycling} = 510 + (6 \times \text{weight [kg]})$$

$$\text{Predicted } \dot{V}O_{2\,max} \text{ for males} = (\text{height[cm]} - \text{age [y]}) \times 20$$

$$\text{Predicted } \dot{V}O_{2\,max} \text{ for females} = (\text{height [cm]} - \text{age [y]}) \times 14$$

For example, a 30-year-old male (weight = 75 kg, height = 178 cm) has a predicted $\dot{V}O_2$ during unloaded cycling of 600 mL min^{-1} and a predicted $\dot{V}O_{2\,max}$ of 2,960 mL min^{-1}. Assuming an O_2 cost of cycling of 10 mL min^{-1} W^{-1} and a target test duration of 10 min, a ramp rate of a 23.6 W min^{-1} is recommended ((2,960 − 600)/100 = 23.6 W). In reality however, a ramp rate of 25 W min^{-1} would be used resulting in a test duration <10 min. It should be noted that these calculations are "broad brush" estimates and that the experience of the investigator combined with knowledge of the participant's medical history and physical activity status is likely to result in modifications to the power output increment. The advantage of this cycling protocol, however, is that only the power output increment needs to be manipulated and typically ranges from 10 W min^{-1} for patients with cardiopulmonary disease and young children, up to 50 W min^{-1} for elite athletes.

Submaximal Exercise Testing

Although direct determination of $\dot{V}O_{2\,max}$ or a symptom-limited $\dot{V}O_{2\,peak}$ using an incremental exercise test to exhaustion is considered the "gold standard" approach, such tests are not always feasible due to the requirement for specialized equipment and trained personnel. Therefore, there has been a great interest in developing submaximal protocols, largely based on heart rate responses obtained under steady-state conditions, to estimate $\dot{V}O_{2\,max}$. While submaximal protocols offer a less strenuous and technically simplified protocol to estimate $\dot{V}O_{2\,max}$, care must be taken when interpreting the outcome in the context of the error that is associated with the prediction. The reasons for this error are likely to be related to the assumed linearity between heart rate, $\dot{V}O_2$ and power output during incremental exercise, the error in predicting an age adjusted maximal heart rate (up to ±15 beats min^{-1}), the assumption that mechanical efficiency during cycling is relatively fixed across all participants, and the method used to quantify heart rate (e.g., palpation vs. short-range telemetry) [2]. In addition, environmental (e.g., ambient temperature), dietary (e.g., caffeine), and behavioral (e.g., anxiety) factors can all influence the heart rate response to exercise and should be adequately controlled for [1]. Finally, prediction equations should only be used with participants that reflect closely the specific characteristics (e.g., age, sex, and physical activity status) of the original sample. Failure to do so will introduce further error in the predicted $\dot{V}O_{2\,max}$.

Perhaps the most popular submaximal prediction of $\dot{V}O_{2\,max}$ is the Åstrand-Rhyming nomogram which is recommended by the American College of Sports Medicine (ACSM) [1]. The test is relatively straightforward as it requires a steady-state heart rate between 125 and 170 beats min^{-1} to be obtained during 6 min of cycling at 50 rev min^{-1} at a single power output. The heart rate at a given power output is then used to estimate the participant's $\dot{V}O_{2\,max}$ using a nomogram following correction for the age-related decline in maximal heart rate [2]. Alternatively, multiple submaximal power outputs, such as the YMCA cycle test, also recommended by the ACSM, may be used to predict $\dot{V}O_{2\,max}$ [1]. Using 3 min stages, between two and four submaximal heart rates are recorded within the range of 110 beats min^{-1} and 85% age-predicted maximum and plotted against power output. A linear regression is then used to extrapolate to the power output that corresponds to their age-predicted maximum heart rate. By entering the participant's predicted maximal power output and body mass into standard formulae, $\dot{V}O_{2\,max}$ can be estimated [1]:

$\dot{V}O_{2\,max}\ (mL \cdot min^{-1})$
$= (1.8 \times$ power output $[kg \cdot m \cdot min^{-1}])/$body mass $[kg]$

Note: to convert W to kg·m·min^{-1} use the conversion factor 6.12.

While not as popular as submaximal cycling tests, treadmill and stepping protocols are available for estimating $\dot{V}O_{2\,max}$ [1]. Likewise, indirect predictions of $\dot{V}O_{2\,max}$ can be obtained using field-based tests, including the 20 m shuttle running test, or time (e.g., 1 mile test) and distance (e.g., 6 min test)-based tests [1]. While requiring a maximal effort, such tests are useful for estimating the aerobic power of large groups of healthy participants in a time-efficient manner.

References
1. ACSM (2010) ACSM's guidelines for exercise testing and prescription. Lippincott Williams and Wilkins, Baltimore
2. Astrand P-O, Rodahl K, Dahl HA, Stromme SB (2003) Textbook of work physiology: physiological bases of exercise. Human Kinetics, Champaign
3. Barker AR, Williams CA, Jones AM, Armstrong N (2011) Establishing maximal oxygen uptake in young people during a ramp cycle test to exhaustion. Br J Sports Med 45:498–503
4. Howley ET, Bassett DR Jr, Welch HG (1995) Criteria for maximal oxygen uptake: review and commentary. Med Sci Sports Exerc 27:1292–1301
5. Wasserman K, Hansen J, Sue D, Stringer W, Whipp B (2005) Principles of exercise testing and interpretation: including pathophysiology and clinical application. Lippincott Williams & Wilkins, Philadelphia

Aerobic Respiration
▶ Aerobic Metabolism

Aerobic Training
▶ Endurance Training

Aerobic Work Capacity
▶ Maximal Oxygen Uptake ($\dot{V}O_{2\,max}$)

Aerobic–Anaerobic Threshold (AAT)

Is defined as a transition zone in which the metabolism of a working muscle shifts from purely aerobic to partially anaerobic lactacid in a given exercise situation.

Cross-References
▶ Anaerobic Threshold
▶ Lactate Threshold

Age
Usually measured in humans by number of years.

Aged Athlete
▶ Aging Athlete

Agility

Jeremy M. Sheppard[1], Tim J. Gabbett[2]
[1]Department of Biomedical, Health, and Exercise Sciences, Edith Cowan University, Joondalup, Australia
[2]The University of Queensland, School of Human Movement Studies, Brisbane, Australia

Synonyms
Change of direction speed

Definition
Classically, agility has been defined as the ability to change direction rapidly and accurately. However, this definition and similar definitions fail to recognize that cognitive skills such as anticipation and decision making are generally involved in most movements in the sport setting. The difficulty in finding an accepted definition of agility may be due to the multiple factors from the various sport science disciplines that influence agility performance. Bloomfield et al. [1] suggested that the difficulty in defining agility stems from the multiple individual skills involved in performing a task that is seen as an agile

movement. A comprehensive definition of agility would recognize the technical skills, cognitive processes, and physical demands involved in agility performance.

An agility task may be best described as a rapid, whole-body change of direction or speed in response to a stimulus [5]. As noted by Young et al. [7], agility can be separated into subcomponents that are comprised of both physical qualities as well as cognitive abilities (Fig. 1). These more exclusive descriptions and definitions differ from previous uses of the term agility that have generally been described as solely dependent on physical components such as "rapid change of direction." In other words, agility is an open skill that requires physical action (change of direction or speed) in response to a domain-specific stimulus.

Characteristics

In many sports, athletes perform sprints, as well as sprints with rapid deceleration and changes of direction. As such, speed and speed in changing direction is a clear determinant of performance in many sports and therefore should be an emphasis in the preparation of these athletes. However, speed qualities such as acceleration and acceleration with changes of direction are somewhat distinct from each other, and likely require individual attention to maximize performance application to the sporting context [8]. Furthermore, the speed and change of direction qualities of an athlete are underpinned by a multifactorial model of strength qualities, techniques, and other related variables that also need to be addressed [5, 7]. Preplanned changes in direction often occur in the sport setting. However, speed and directional changes in the sporting context are also often performed in response to a stimulus, such as an opposing player's movements or the movement of a ball (e.g., from an opponent's racquet). As such, cognitive skills are highly important to agility performance.

Perceptual qualities (e.g., reduced decision-making time) have been shown to discriminate between higher and lesser-skilled performers despite similarities in physical abilities (e.g., speed and change of direction speed) [4, 6]. It therefore can be asserted that "agile" athletes require well-developed physical qualities to move and execute skills within the field of play, as well as highly trained domain-specific cognitive abilities to attend to appropriate cues and execute rapid and accurate decisions [2, 4, 6].

Considering the multifactorial nature of agility and its sub-qualities (Fig. 1), it is important for the practitioner to attend to the qualities most relevant to the sport in question, and also to the individual athlete. It has been well established that speed and its specific subqualities (e.g., acceleration, change of direction speed) are highly trainable [8]. Generally, this has been observed by employing a low-volume, that is, training regimen (<500 m, 2–3 sessions/week) of sprint and change of direction speed activities.

However, not to be overlooked is the profound impact of speed's underpinning qualities on overall performance in speed and agility tasks. For example, if an athlete is limited in their strength, and they improve this quality, they will most certainly improve their acceleration and likely their performance in change of direction tasks [7]. Using the model illustrated in Fig. 1, this could in theory lead to improvements in agility by broadly improving the physical components of the athlete.

Perceptual (e.g., anticipation) and decision-making skills appear to be trainable through integrating cognitive and physical components into the training regimen. In other words, by incorporating sport-relevant open skill tasks, agility performance can be improved. This is generally accomplished through combined "speed-agility" training sessions where athletes perform not only closed skill

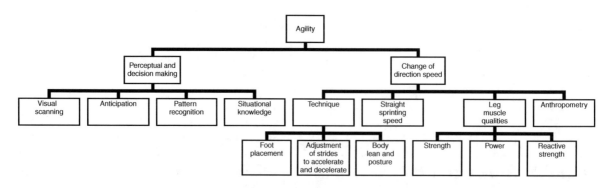

Agility. Fig. 1 Theoretical model of agility components [7]

speed and change of direction speed training, but also open skill reactive tasks of a general but sport-relevant nature (e.g., 1 on 1 tagging games) and also of a highly specific nature (e.g., 1 on 1, 2 on 2 offensive–defensive drills).

In addition, domain-specific perceptual and decision-making skills can be enhanced through video-based occlusion techniques [3]. Video-based occlusion techniques generally involve a sport-relevant sequence on display to the athlete, with this video sequence occluded prior to the execution of the task of interest. For example, a tennis serve might be displayed until 50 ms prior to ball contact, and the athlete is required to either physically respond to the "serve" or describe the serve (i.e., direction and type). After this occurs, the complete and un-occluded sequence can be played in its entirety to reinforce correct perception or incorrect responses. Using a variety of clips, the practitioner can increase the temporal stress of the training over time by occluding the skill earlier in the execution of the task (e.g., 50, 75, 100 ms prior to contact in the serve). This and other implicit learning methods have been successful in several sports. Importantly, the skills developed in this manner appear to offer a robust learning stimulus, with some studies reporting a direct transfer of the competitive environment, and the retention of anticipatory skill even when the training stimulus is removed for a period [3].

Measurements

While the majority of agility testing has been devoted to preplanned change of direction speed tests, researchers have recently begun to investigate the perceptual components of agility, with particular focus on the ability of team sport athletes to "read and react" to a game-specific stimulus in the testing protocol [2, 4, 6]. Sheppard et al. [6] demonstrated that a test of agility, called the Reactive Agility Test, that included the measurement of an athlete's movement speed in changing direction in response to the change of direction of an "opponent," was reliable and able to discriminate higher and lesser skilled Australian football players [6], with similar findings observed in rugby league [4], netball [2], and softball [3]. These findings may reflect the fact that effective agility performance is limited by both physical (e.g., linear speed, strength, change of direction speed) and perceptual/decision-making (visual scanning, anticipation, pattern recognition, and situational knowledge) factors. It is suggested that agility be developed and assessed with training and testing that involves both movement speed and decision-making speed and accuracy [4, 5]. The results of these assessments would allow the practitioners to profile and create an individual-needs analysis of their athletes, as suggested by Gabbett et al. [4], and outlined in Table 1.

Agility. Table 1 Interpretation and training prescription for four players with different results on the reactive agility test. Gabbett, Kelly, and Sheppard (2008)

Player	Decision time (ms)	Movement time (s)	Interpretation	Prescription
Fast mover–fast thinker	58.75	2.31	Speed and fast decision time contribute to above-average anticipation skills.	Continue to develop change of direction speed and decision-making skills.
Fast mover–slow thinker	148.75	2.33	Has speed but slow decision time contributes to below-average anticipation skills.	Needs more decision-making training on (e.g., reactive agility training) and off (e.g., video-based perceptual training) the field.
Slow mover–fast thinker	28.75	2.85	Perceptually skilled, but lacks change of direction speed.	Needs more speed/change of direction speed training to improve physical attributes.
Slow mover–slow thinker	112.50	2.86	Poor speed and slow decision time contributes to below average anticipation skills.	Needs more decision-making and speed/change of direction speed training to improve physical attributes and perceptual skill.

Fast movers/fast thinkers = good change of direction speed and good perceptual skill
Fast movers/slow thinkers = good change of direction speed and below average perceptual skill
Slow movers/fast thinkers = below average change of direction speed and good perceptual skill
Slow movers/slow thinkers = below average change of direction speed and below average perceptual skill

Using the results of the speed and decision-making times in the examples in Table 1, the practitioner can allocate athletes into groups according to their differing training requirements. For example, the "slow mover–fast thinker" would devote a larger percentage of training time to physical components of agility performance, while the "fast mover–slow thinker" would devote a larger percentage of training time to perceptual training and/or training that was "open skill" (i.e., including a high perceptual demand) in nature. For the "fast mover–slow thinker," a combination of open skill agility tasks and small-sided games could be performed in conjunction with implicit video-based perceptual training and other domain-specific anticipation and decision-making tasks. Finally, for the "slow mover–slow thinker," training would include an emphasis on sprint-running, change of direction speed, and its underpinning qualities such as technique coaching, strength development, etc., as well as game-specific perceptual (decision-making) training.

References

1. Bloomfield J, Ackland TR, Elliot BC (1994) Applied anatomy and biomechanics in sport. Melbourne, Blackwell Scientific, p 374
2. Farrow D, Young W, Bruce L (2005) The development of a test of reactive agility for netball: a new methodology. J Sci Med Sport 8:52–60
3. Gabbett T, Rubinoff M, Thorburn L, Farrow D (2007) Testing and training anticipation skills in softball fielders. Int J Sport Sci Coach 2:15–24
4. Gabbett TJ, Kelly JN, Sheppard JM (2008) Speed, change of direction speed, and reactive agility of rugby league players. J Strength Cond Res 22:174–181
5. Sheppard JM, Young W (2006) Agility Literature Review: classifications, training and testing. J Sport Sci 24:919–932
6. Sheppard JM, Young WB, Doyle TLA, Sheppard TA, Newton RU (2006) An evaluation of a new test of reactive agility and its relationship to sprint speed and change of direction speed. J Sci Med Sport 9:342–349
7. Young WB, James R, Montgomery I (2002) Is muscle power related to running speed with changes of direction? J Sports Med Phys Fit 43:282–288
8. Young WB, McDowell MH, Scarlett BJ (2001) Specificity of sprint and agility training methods. J Strength Cond Res 15:315–319

Aging

The process of growing old associated with deteriorative changes with time that renders organisms vulnerable to challenge and a decreased ability to survive. It covers natural changes in function that occur across the lifespan, which are not caused by disease. Aging can result from a failure of body cells to function normally or to produce sufficient new cells to replace those that have died or malfunctioned. With respect to deteriorative changes, "senescence" is a synonym and describes the state or process of aging.

Aging Athlete

HIROFUMI TANAKA
Department of Kinesiology and Health Education, Cardiovascular Aging Research Laboratory, University of Texas at Austin, Austin, TX, USA

Synonyms

Aged athlete; Master's athletes; Old competitor; Senior athlete; Veteran athlete

Definition

There is no general agreement on the age at which an athlete becomes a masters or aging athlete. This is similar to a lack of definition for an older or elderly person. Although most organizations and agencies have accepted the chronological age of 65 years as a definition of elderly, chronological ages of 50, 55, and 60 years have also been used. In the masters sports, because of a lack of an accepted definition, the age at which an athlete became eligible for the senior or veteran competitions has become the default definition. However, the starting age varies widely among different athletic events; 25 years in masters swimming, 30 years in track and field, 35 years in weightlifting, 40 years in long distance running, and 50 years in senior games. In this entry, the masters athletes are defined as exercise-trained individuals who compete in athletic events at a high level well beyond a typical athletic retirement age.

Characteristics

It is apparent that the demographics of age in most industrialized countries, including the United States, is changing dramatically. The percentage of older adults will continue to rise for the foreseeable future. This would create potentially unmanageable situations from both economical and societal standpoints since older adults demonstrate the highest rates of morbidity, functional disability, loss of independence, and mortality. A unique group of older adults that are situated at the completely opposite end of the functional capacity spectrum is masters athletes (Fig. 1). In contrast to the high prevalence of

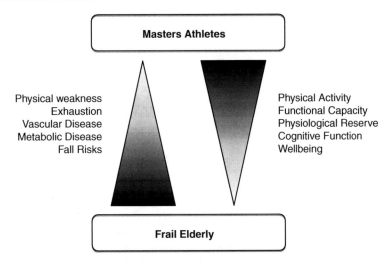

Aging Athlete. Fig. 1 Contrasting positions of masters athletes and frail elderly in the functional and disease spectrum

sedentary lifestyle and frailty in the overall aging population, the masters athletes comprise an extremely small portions of older adults. These groups of athletes are challenging the prevalent notion that aging is an inevitable process of deterioration that not much can be done to retard or minimize it.

Observing young elite runners finishing marathon races in little over 2 h is certainly amazing. But a 73-year-old masters athlete who breaks 3-h mark in marathon is equally marvelous. It is simply amazing or even amusing to observe a 95-year-old sprinter exerting maximal effort to sprint 100 m. This tiny Japanese runner who stood 146 cm and weighed 38 kg (Kozo Haraguchi) ran 22.04 s. Two months later, he broke the record again by running 21.69 s. These exceptional individual athletic achievements are fascinating not only to the aging individuals but also to those of us who study the effects of aging [2]. Aging athletes continue to improve and shutter age-group records in most athletic events ranging from sprint to endurance events. Indeed, yearly improvements in athletic records are substantially greater in older age groups, rapidly closing the gap between younger and older athletes. In these days, masters athlete over the age of 60 can run faster in 100 m sprint than the gold medal winner in the first Olympic games in Athens [1]. In marathon, the time achieved by 75-year-old man is faster than the time of the gold medalist in the first Olympics [1]. In conjunction with the remarkable improvements in athletic performance in older senior athletes, increasing number of elite athletes are remaining in the athletic events way past the typical athletic retirement age and are experiencing success against much younger counterparts. In some cases,

they compete against the opponents half of their age. Some particularly noteworthy examples of such success are listed below.

- Dara Torres, Olympic swimming silver medalist at age 41
- Hilde Pedersen, Olympic cross-country skiing silver medalist at age 41
- Carlos Lopez, Olympic marathon gold medalist at age 42
- Randy Couture, UFC mixed martial arts champion at age 44
- Nolan Ryan, baseball pitcher throwing no hitter at age 44
- George Foreman, Boxing heavy weight champion at age 45
- Jack Nicklaus, Masters golf tournament winner at age 46
- Martina Navratilova, US Open tennis champion at age 49
- Gordie Howe, all-star NHL ice hockey player at age 52
- Albert Beckles, body building Mr. Olympia title at age 52
- Willie Shoemaker, the Kentucky Derby winner at age 54

These exceptional performances may be considered unreachable for most individuals. But it sets the upper limit or a barometer of what is possible for aging adults in general and aging athletes in particular. Masters athletes continue to raise the ceilings of what aging humans can accomplish and break the barriers of physical limitations of older adults.

Training/Exercise Response

Peak athletic performance decreases with advancing age in a curvilinear fashion [2]. In general, peak athletic performance is maintained until a given age (~35 years in endurance events) followed by modest decreases with progressively steeper reductions thereafter. A recently published longitudinal study indicates that maximal aerobic capacity may also decline curvilinearly with advancing age. There is no question that declines in the exercise training "stimuli" with advancing age play an important role in reductions in athletic performance and functional capacity [1]. In a study that evaluated 24 senior track athletes between the ages of 50 and 82 years, about half of them quit competing and reduced training and the other half remained very competitive. The senior athletes who remained competitive and continued to train hard maintained their maximal aerobic capacity over a 10-year period whereas those athletes who became noncompetitive demonstrated a large decline in maximal aerobic capacity [3]. Although exercise training volume and intensity can be maintained up to 10 years, there is no evidence that exercise training volume and intensity can be maintained for longer periods, especially in older adults (e.g., 20 years) [3]. Jobs, family responsibilities, injuries, and reduced motivation all appear to contribute to the reductions in training stimuli in older athletes. When the aforementioned senior track athletes were followed up another 10 years later (over a 20-year period), all the runners reduced their training intensity and volume and experienced substantial declines in maximal aerobic capacity [3].

Improvements in training and conditioning techniques, and cares provided by athletic training and sports medicine, appear to have contributed to better preservation of athletic ability and athletic records with advancing age. Indeed, many aging athletes can surround them with an army of athletic trainer, physiologist, nutritionist, biomechanist, and massage therapist. Could masters athletes maintain exercise training and athletic performance in these surroundings? Certainly, this "racing car" approach is becoming a common practice among elite aging athletes. However, exact role and contribution of these supporting staff have not been evaluated, especially in the context of masters athletes.

In marked contrast to the prevalent presumptions that masters athletes are life-long trained athletes and that their high athletic performance was acquired from years of accumulated exercise training since they were youth, most of the currently successful masters athletes inherited the exercise training habit and emerged in the competition very late in life. In the case of the aforementioned Japanese sprinter Kozo Haraguchi, he started jogging at 65 years of age for health reasons after the retirement from his job and turned to 100 m sprint when he was 75 years of age. It is of great interest if current world-class athletes were to continue to train and compete as hard, as frequent, and as long as when they were young, what athletic records can be achieved at older age. Recently, Joan Benoit, who won the gold medal at the 1984 Olympic games in Los Angeles, recorded the fastest ever performance by a woman over 52 years of age at the Chicago marathon.

Clinical Relevance

Human aging is associated with arterial dysfunction and an increased risk of clinical cardiovascular disease. Advancing age is now a major risk factor for cardiovascular disease. In general, a physically active lifestyle is associated with more favorable risk factors and reduced incidence of cardiovascular disease. There is accumulating evidence indicating that masters athletes demonstrate more favorable levels of risk factors for cardiovascular disease than their sedentary counterparts [4]. In many cases, age-related deteriorations of vascular function as well as elevations in vascular risk factors that typically observed in sedentary adults are substantially attenuated or even absent in masters athletes. For example, progressive increases in arterial stiffening with age observed in sedentary adults are markedly attenuated in endurance-trained masters athletes. Additionally, the elevations in systolic blood pressure and pulse pressure seen with age in sedentary adults are absent in those who participate in high-level athletic competition [4]. Furthermore, compared with that observed in sedentary adults, the age-related increases in body weight and in body fatness are smaller or even absent in masters athletes, due in part to the elevated levels of basal metabolic rate.

In addition to much lower prevalence of cardiovascular disease, the masters athletes possess greater levels of functional capacity than sedentary adults (Fig. 1). They are also capable of performing physical tasks with much more reserve and much less exertion than their sedentary peers. The "masters athlete model" will continue to be a rich source of insight into our strategy to maintain physiological function and minimize disease risks with advancing age. Achieving and maintaining physical activity levels are one of the most difficult elements of exercise prescription as ~50% of adults who initiate exercise programs quit within 6 months. For one, we can attempt to reveal the secret of masters athletes as to how they are motivated to continue exercising vigorously into older ages. These exceptional aging athletes will also be an inspiration for ever growing elderly population who often suffer from chronic degenerative diseases and functional disability.

▶ He's soft and he's fat and he's wearing my clothes and he's getting too old and he was born on my birthday and I'm afraid if I stop running, he'll catch up with me. (The Nike poster depicting an aging athlete)

References

1. Tanaka H, Seals DR (2008) Endurance exercise performance in masters athletes: age-associated changes and underlying physiological mechanisms. J Physiol 586(Pt 1):55–63
2. Tanaka H, Seals DR (2003) Dynamic exercise performance in masters athletes: insight into the effects of primary human aging on physiological functional capacity. J Appl Physiol 95(5):2152–2162
3. Pollock ML, Mengelkoch LJ, Graves JE et al (1997) Twenty-year follow-up of aerobic power and body composition of older track athletes. J Appl Physiol 82(5):1508–1516
4. Seals DR, Desouza CA, Donato AJ, Tanaka H (2008) Habitual exercise and arterial aging. J Appl Physiol 105(4):1323–1332

Aging, Adaptations to Training

M. G. Bemben
Department of Health and Exercise Science, University of Oklahoma, Norman, OK, USA

Definition

Aging defies an easy definition, at least in biological terms, since not all organ systems age in the same way or at the same rate or extent in any individual in a given species. However, a few things are certain; aging is developmental or progressive, and aging is a gift of twentieth century technology and scientific advancements. Historically, old age was based on government determined social policies that created social security to begin at 65 years of age; however, it is not uncommon for individuals to reach into their 90s or even 100s since the fastest growing population in the United States are those 85 years and older. Based on these facts, aging can be described as a decreased ability to respond to a changing environment [1].

Adaptation to training implies a semi permanent improvement to a physiological system as the result of attending successive bouts of structured exercise sessions that have been developed based on sound training guidelines that incorporate the following principles: Specificity; Overload, Adaptation, Progression, Retrogression, Maintenance, Individualization; and Warm-up and Cool-down.

Mechanisms

The most obvious result that occurs from resistance training is an increase in strength. Increases in muscular strength have been differentiated into different phases of development. Early phase adaptations occurring during the first 2 weeks of training are usually attributed to a learning phase. This phase is often characterized by improved motor skill coordination and an improvement in motivational levels of the participants. The next phase of development that occurs over the next couple of weeks of training usually results in strength increases without a concomitant increase in muscle size and therefore has been attributed to neural adaptations. These neural adaptations can include increased activation of muscle from an increased number of ▶ motor units being activated, an increased firing rate for the motor units, or an improved synchronization of the motor units contracting together. Other factors can also include a better coordination of synergistic and antagonistic muscles, increased neural drive from the central nervous system, decreased electromyographic activity (EMG) in the antagonistic muscles, increased M-wave potentials which might reflect an increase in muscle membrane excitability, selective increases in Type II muscle fiber areas, alterations in muscle architecture, and increases in tendon stiffness. The final phase associated with strength increases following at least 6 week of training are due to muscle hypertrophy [2].

Increases in muscle size or hypertrophy occur as the result of increased rates of protein synthesis. The improved rates of protein synthesis for the elderly following resistance training are similar to that rates exhibited by young people; and have been documented in as short as 2 weeks following the beginning of a resistance training program. This suggests that muscle proteins retain the ability to respond to an overload stimulus and are not limited by advanced age. In addition to the increased rates of protein synthesis, resistance training might also reduce the gene expression and protein levels of Tumor Necrosis Factor alpha (TNFα), a marker of chronic inflammation and an initiator of cell death [3]. In order for hypertrophied muscle to maintain an appropriate ratio between nuclear control and increased mass, it appears that satellite cells are activated during the regenerative phase of skeletal muscle growth [4]. Other factors that have been implicated in satellite cell proliferation and increased muscle cell size are a number of ▶ myogenic regulatory factors that include MyoD, myf-5, myf-6, and myogenin [4].

Ultrasound methodologies have found that increases in strength attributable to muscle hypertrophy can also be explained by an increased length of the muscle fascicles and an increased pennation angle, both of which may indicate an increased number of sarcomeres that occur in series to the myofibril, and in parallel to the myofibrils [5]. In other words, there can be an increase in the number of myofibrils within a single muscle fiber, but there are no increases in the number of muscle fibers (hyperplasia) resulting from resistance training adaptations.

Increases in muscle power, or the ability to exert force quickly, following training are also reported. Improved muscular power is due to increases in the cross-sectional area of Type II muscle fibers and the increased shortening velocity of these muscle fibers. The increase in power can also be attributable to an earlier activation of motor units and an enhanced motor unit firing rate [2].

Improved muscle endurance can also be the result of muscular adaptation to training. Improved muscle endurance is often evidenced by a decrease in the number of motor units that need to be activated in order to complete a submaximal task, a decreased coactivation of antagonist muscles, increased substrate availability, like adenosine triphosphate (ATP) and phosphocreatine (PC), and increases in mitochondrial density and improved oxidative capacity [6].

Adaptations also occur in the tendons that connect muscle to bone. There is an increase in tensile stiffness due to changes in the material properties of the tendons which might be due to changes in the fibrous structure or the extracellular matrix. This can often cause an increase in the rate of force transmission and a decreased chance of tension injury during exercise. The increase in tendon stiffness may also be associated with the improved development of torque about an axis of rotation which might benefit an older person's ability to respond to a loss of balance [7].

Exercise Response/Consequences

Muscular strength in older adults can significantly increase from 25% to over 100% following properly designed resistance training programs, but increases are often dependent on several complex factors that can include the gender of the subjects training, the duration of the training intervention, the muscle groups being trained, initial fitness levels of those participating in the training program, health status of those training, and the nutritional status of those training.

The increase in muscle strength and power following training are often times greater than would be expected if only based on muscle mass changes and are probably indicative of changes in ▶ muscle quality. These strength and power improvements are often associated with a decreased risk of falling, lower risks of hip fractures, and a lower risk for developing osteoporosis in the elderly.

The improvements in muscular endurance that can arise as a training adaptation allow older individuals to maintain muscular forces and power over extended periods of time. These adaptations can then improve the ability to carry out normal activities of daily living with less fatigue and help maintain a sufficient energy reserve that might allow an individual to increase their physical activity by engaging in a structured exercise program or to pursue a new recreational activity.

Improvements in muscular endurance are facilitated by a number of changes in the vascular network that supplies nutrients and oxygen to the exercising muscle. Adaptations to the cardiovascular system often include improved muscle capillarity as demonstrated by significant increases in the number of capillary contacts per fiber and the capillary to muscle fiber ratio [8].

Diagnostics

Assessing Muscle Quantity

Estimating Regional Changes to Muscle Mass

Anthropometric measures such as limb circumferences corrected for subcutaneous adipose tissue have been used to estimate muscle plus bone cross-sectional areas, although there is substantial error associated with this technique. Muscle plus bone cross-sectional area can be estimated from the following equation: $A = (C - \pi s)^2/4\pi$; where A is the estimated muscle plus bone cross-sectional area corrected for subcutaneous adipose tissue, C is the limb circumference, and s is the subcutaneous adipose tissue calculated as the average of half of the skinfold thickness at two opposite locations from the respective limb (anterior and posterior or dorsal and ventral) [9].

Muscle Metabolites

Creatinine: Creatinine is formed when creatine is broken down. Creatine is found primarily in skeletal muscle (about 98%) in the form of creatine phosphate. Urinary creatinine excretion is related to the fat-free body mass and skeletal muscle mass, since 1 g of creatinine excreted in a 24 h period is equivalent to about 18–20 kg of muscle tissue, although dependent on factors that include age, gender, and training status and reflects whole body measures of muscle [9].

3-Methylhistidine: 3-Methylhistidine is an amino acid that is located mostly in skeletal muscle, and the urinary excretion of 3-methylhistidine has been used to estimate whole body muscle mass. Problems with this assessment arise because of different protein consumptions of individuals and the fact that it can also reflect nonskeletal muscle protein turnover (i.e., smooth muscle and connective tissue) [3, 9].

Ultrasound
Muscle thickness can be assessed by B-mode ultrasound with an electronic linear array probe (usually 5.0 MHz wave frequency). The frequencies used in diagnostic ultrasound usually range between 2 and 18 MHz. The choice of frequency results in a compromise between spatial resolution of the image and the imaging depth, with lower frequencies producing less resolution but an increased ability to image deeper into the tissues [7].

Radiographic Methods
Computed Tomography (*CT*): Computed tomography is based on the attenuation of x-ray intensities relative to water and is dependent on tissue density. Problems with this technique are a lack of accessibility to very expensive equipment, unnecessary exposure to fairly high doses of ionizing radiation due to the high energy photons associated with x-rays, the high cost of the analyses, and the large variation in the attenuation of different muscle groups [7, 10].

Nuclear Magnetic Resonance (*NMR*): Nuclear magnetic resonance can provide images of tissue known as MRI (Magnetic Resonance Imaging) or information about the chemical composition of the tissue (NMR Spectroscopy). This technique is based on the concept that the nuclei of atoms act like magnets and when an external magnetic field is applied to the tissue, it absorbs the energy and then emits a radio signal that can be used to develop an image of the chemical composition of the tissues. It can detect the abundance of ^{31}P containing components like ATP, inorganic phosphate, and PC. Many of the problems with this technique are similar to the CT scanning – a lack of accessibility to very expensive equipment, cost of the analyses, etc. [9, 10].

Dual Energy X-Ray Absorptiometry (*DXA*): Dual energy X-ray absorptiometry is also based on the attenuation of two different energy sources of X-rays which can be used to assess fat and bone-free lean tissue (lean tissue mass). This equipment is also very expensive, but much less than CT and MRI equipment; there is greater accessibility to this type of equipment, and it is much safer than CT scans since it has lower doses of radiation exposure [9].

Peripheral Quantitative Computed Tomography (*pQCT*): pQCT is restricted to peripheral measurements of the arms and legs but uses very low radiation doses compared to whole body CT scanning. pQCT was originally designed to evaluate both trabecular and cortical

bone mineral densities as a volumetric density (gm/cm^3) but has also been used to estimate muscle volumes or muscle cross-sectional areas. Different scan analyses are used to estimate muscle cross-sectional area and involve different thresholds and modes (i.e., contour detection mode or peel mode). Generally, coefficients of variation for muscle cross-sectional areas with this technique are about 1.5%.

Muscle Biopsy
There are basically two types of muscle biopsies needle biopsies and open biopsies. A needle biopsy involves inserting a needle into the muscle with no previous incision being made. When the needle is removed, a small piece of tissue remains in the needle. An open biopsy involves making a small cut in the skin and into the muscle. The muscle tissue is then removed with a Bergström needle facilitated with suction. Samples are then usually frozen in isopentane, cooled to $-160°C$ before being sectioned and analyzed.

Fractional Protein Synthesis Rates of Skeletal Muscle
The fractional protein synthesis rates of skeletal muscle can be determined by the incorporation of an intravenously administered stable isotope-labeled amino acid (^{13}C-leucine) into skeletal muscle protein. Gas chromatography-mass spectroscopy then measures muscle cytosolic ^{13}C-leucine, plasma ^{13}C-leucine, and plasma $\alpha^{13}C$- ketoisoceproil acid enrichment, and gas chromatography-combustion-isotope ratio mass spectroscopy is then used to measure ^{13}C-leucine enrichment in mixed, MCH, and actin proteins [3].

Assessing Muscle Quality

Muscle Strength
Muscular strength, or the maximal voluntary force generating capabilities of a muscle or muscle group, can be assessed by three different modalities: isometrically, dynamically, and isokinetically.

Isometric Strength: Maximal voluntary isometric strength is usually assessed with load cells or force transducers that allow a muscle or muscle group to exert force while no external movement of the limb or limb joint takes place. Typically, values for maximal forces from this technique are greater than those obtained with dynamic assessments or isokinetic assessments since the nature of the tension development during an isometric contraction maximizes the ability for greater motor unit synchronization to take place since no limb movement is occurring.

Dynamic Strength: Dynamic strength is the maximal load that can be lifted or moved. This type of assessment usually involves free weights or plate loaded machines, and the standard terminology for this assessment is referred to as 1-RM, or one-repetition maximum. The term 1-RM implies the greatest amount of weight that can be lifted successfully with proper form.

Isokinetic Strength: Isokinetic strength or maximal torque is the maximal force about an axis of rotation that can be exerted against a pre-set rate-limiting device. This type of assessment requires specially designed equipment that can control the velocity of the contraction while maximal effort is being generated into a force dynamometer. In other words, no matter how much effort is exerted, the movement takes place at a pre-set constant speed that can range from 0°/s (isometric) to 450°/s. This type of assessment is often used to test and improve muscular strength during rehabilitation from an injury.

Muscle Power

The term power implies the application of a force as quickly as possible. It can be calculated as force multiplied by the velocity of the movement or the force applied over a given distance divided by time taken to complete the task. Some laboratory methods used to assess muscular power include the vertical jump (Lewis Power Jump) or a timed stair run (Margaria-Kalamean Power Stair Run) and is expressed as $kg \cdot m \cdot s^{-1}$, $kg \cdot m \cdot min^{-1}$, or watts.

Muscle Endurance

Muscle endurance is often described as the ability of a muscle or muscle group to maintain a force or to do repeated submaximal contractions over a given period of time. Muscular endurance can be thought of as the opposite of muscular fatigue, in other words, the greater the endurance capacity of muscle the less fatigue that is exhibited in terms of a declining force output. Most activities of daily living require good muscle endurance and seldom require maximal effort or maximal strength. These types of activities can include shopping, carry groceries, and gardening, for example. Muscular endurance can be assessed by evaluating the number of submaximal repetitions that can be completed before total or partial fatigue occurs.

References

1. Smith EL (1981) Age: the interaction of nature and nurture. In: Smith EL, Serfass RC (eds) Exercise and aging: the scientific basis. Enslow Publishers, New Jersey, pp 11–17
2. Macaluso A, De Vito G (2004) Muscle strength, power, and adaptations to resistance training in older people. Eur J Appl Physiol 91:450–472
3. Yarasheski KE (2003) Exercise, aging and muscle protein metabolism. J Gerontol A Biol Sci Med Sci 58A:918–922
4. Hunter GR, McCarthy JP, Bamman MM (2004) Effects of resistance training on older adults. Sports Med 34:329–348
5. Folland JP, Williams AG (2007) The adaptations to strength training. Morphological and neurological contributions to increased strength. Sports Med 37:145–168
6. Chodzko-Zajko WJ et al (2009) Exercise and physical activity for older adults. Position stand for the American College of Sports Medicine. Med Sci Sports Exerc 41(7):1510–1530
7. Narici MV, Maganaris CN, Reeves ND (2005) Myotendinous alterations and effects of resistance loading in old age. Scand J Med Sci Sports 15:392–401
8. Harris BA (2005) The influence of endurance and resistance exercise on muscle capillarization in the elderly: a review. Acta Physiol Scand 185:89–97
9. Lukaski HC (1996) Estimation of muscle mass. In: Roche AF, Heymsfield SB, Lohman TG (eds) Human body composition. Human Kinetics, Champaign, IL, pp 109–128
10. Lang T, Streeper T, Cawthon P, Baldwin K, Taaffe DR, Harris TB (2010) Sarcopenia: etiology, clinical consequences, intervention. Osteoporos Int 21:543–559

Aging, Motor Performance

Scott K. Lynn[1], Guillermo J. Noffal[1], David M. Lindsay[2], Anthony A. Vandervoort[3]
[1]Department of Kinesiology, California State University, Fullerton, CA, USA
[2]University of Calgary, Calgary, AB, Canada
[3]School of Physical Therapy, University of Western Ontario, Ontario, Canada

Synonyms

Gerontology; Master's athletes; Movement control in older people; Neuromuscular aging

Definition

It is well known from the results of masters competitions throughout the world that motor performance of the athletes declines with ▶ age. Furthermore this gerontological effect can also be observed longitudinally by following the changes in scores, speed or distance achieved of elite sportspersons who continue their participation over several decades, sometimes into very old age [1]. Thus to ensure a fair competition, events are organized into various age groupings across the adult ▶ lifespan, and these categories depend upon each sport's requirements. Most tissues and systems of the body experience an age-related loss of physiological capacity to some degree, although it can be debated whether such effects are maladaptive under all circumstances. For example, there is conclusive evidence that the typical mixture of fast and slow myosin fibers that comprises human muscles shifts in favor of the latter type in old age, which reduces speed of response but enhances aerobic metabolism. In this entry, we will first discuss the general mechanisms of ▶ aging within the motor performance system, and then utilize the sport of golf to illustrate how such age-related changes affect the exercise response.

Mechanisms

Functions of the neuromuscular, sensory, skeletal, and cardiorespiratory systems are each integral to performance of physical activity, and all affected significantly by the aging process [2–4]. The age-related trends for nerve, muscle, and bone tissues that directly affect motor performance are summarized for the reader in the Table.

Muscle strength is one of the more obvious examples of how physical parameters are influenced by age. Absolute strength increases through the growth years of childhood and adolescence up to one's early 20s, has a general plateau phase until the fifth decade, and then decreases by about 10% per decade thereafter [4, 5]. The decline in strength is primarily the result of decreased muscle mass (age-related ▶ sarcopenia), due to the loss of functioning ▶ motor units consisting of motor neurons and the family of fibers they innervate. Total muscle cross sectional area declines by 10% between the ages 24 and 50, then drops another 30% between ages 50 and 80 years and beyond. Equal amounts of both type 1 (slow twitch) and type 2 (fast twitch) muscle fibers are lost with old age. However, in addition to overall fiber loss, type 2 fibers also undergo a much greater decrease in size compared to their type 1 counterparts, and thus the older athlete has an even further reduced capacity for generating muscle power.

The resultant pattern of the sarcopenic strength loss is such that a middle-aged golfer would not be expected to have any significant decrease in maximum isometric or concentric strength compared to a young player, but an 80-year-old would have only about half the overall strength level of the young adult. It is quite interesting to note that golf performance tends to follow the same pattern, as evidenced by comparisons of average ▶ golf "handicaps" versus age – handicap being a sport-specific, standardized way of monitoring a golfer's scores, and hence ability. Recreational golfers tend to reach their prime in the third decade and then begin to experience some loss of performance after their forties. However, they can still continue to play well and even compete with other age groups via the handicap system for the rest of their lives. For example, adolescents who are learning the game are expected to have higher scores than young adults at the peak of their performance years, but then players in older age groups would also have more of a benefit on average from the handicap index factor. Thus the older golfer's "net" score can be adjusted statistically to compare expected performance on a more equal basis.

Exercise Response

It is important to note that the aging muscular system remains quite adaptable to exercise programming [2, 3, 5] and so there are definite benefits for senior golfers who decide to take up a ▶ resistance training program that trains the appropriate patterns of movement that can help to optimize the ability to generate effective muscle forces for the golf swing. These types of programs can also be valuable for the prevention of musculoskeletal injuries and degenerative joint changes. Furthermore, our recent research has shown that older individuals can take advantage of the muscle strengthening benefits of eccentric overload resistance training principles, and that this mode of exercise also causes less cardiovascular stress compared to concentric exercises [4]. Finally, it is useful to take advantage of any motor learning associated with the training exercises, especially those involving coordinated ballistic movements among several muscles. Therefore, it would seem logical to design some of the exercises to simulate the golf swing with its various concentric and eccentric activation muscle patterns, thereby stimulating adaptation within the appropriate musculature and neural pathways.

Another common complaint of older golfers is generalized stiffness in several of the key joints involved in the golf swing. From a physiological standpoint, much of this stiffness relates to connective tissue changes within the body, due to the significant water loss with age that contributes to a reduction in this tissue's plasticity. There may also be osteoarthritic changes in the joints that affect the older golfer's ability to assume the desirable athletic posture and movements for a full, powerful swing [6]. Clinically, age-related changes in connective tissue are manifested by losses in flexibility from key joints of the body that generate power for the swing such as the trunk and shoulders.

As an example study, Thompson and Osness [7] examined muscle strength and flexibility in older male recreational golfers (mean age = 65.1 years), and determined that both ▶ resistance training and flexibility exercises emphasizing trunk rotation were related to improvements in clubhead speed and flexibility for golf. Even though this gain in rotational flexibility increases clubhead speed, one must be careful to avoid excessive spinal motion because it can actually be a risk factor for future back troubles. This risk is thought to arise from

---

twisting of the annulus fibrosis, which combined with spinal flexion greatly increases the chances of posterior disk herniation [8].

To summarize, all golfers continually hope to improve their game, however the older golfer is also dealing with age-related changes and may be content with simply not having their performance decline. For example, typical club head speed decreases as the golfer ages but there are encouraging examples from studies of exercise programs after which increases in clubhead speed are likely a result of the cumulative impact of increasing flexibility of key muscles, along with the benefits of increasing overall muscle strength. Even simply following a maintenance program as one ages is a good strategy for some if it

Aging, Motor Performance. Table 1 Effects of training and warm-up on age-related changes in aspects of motor function

System	Changes with aging	Effects of warm-up	Effects of activity
Muscle	– Max strength 25–50 years, then decline of 1.5%/year after 60 – ↓ Number of motor units – ↓ Number of muscle fibers – ↓ The size of Type II fibers – Some lean muscle replaced with fat and connective tissue	– General body warm-up increases blood flow and body temperature, which speeds up muscle contraction – Static and Dynamic stretching alter the biomechanical length-tension relationship of shortened "tight muscles	– Plays a key role in maintenance of muscle mass – Overload training ↑ muscular strength – Changes in cross sectional area ↑ with training – Early strength gains primarily by neurological adaptation then some hypertrophy possible
Nervous system	– Muscle atrophy contributed to by neurological changes – 37% ↓ Number of spinal cord axons – 10% ↓ Nerve conduction velocity in older adults – ↓ Sensory and proprioception function – ↓ Reflex speed when responding to stimuli	– General body warm-up increases blood flow to the brain, which enhances alertness and cognitive function ("getting into the zone") – Dynamic stretching and specific motor rehearsal enhance coordination of muscle activation sequences, plus postural control	– Activity allows rapid response time to remain relatively unchanged in older adults – Balance can be improved with specific strengthening exercises and postural maneuvers
Skeletal	– After third and fourth decade ↓ mineralization of 0.3–0.5%/year – Over lifetime: 35% of cortical and 50% of trabecular bone is lost – Men only lose 2/3 the bone mass which females lose, i.e., notable menopause effect	– General body warm-up, plus and Static and Dynamic Stretching gradually increase range of motion for stiffened joints (e.g., shoulders and wrists) to maximum levels needed for full swing	– Gravitational loading and muscular traction found to affect: bone thickness, strength, calcium concentration – Regular activity found to help counteract demineralization
Connective tissue	– Altered proportions and properties of connective components – ↑ Stability of cross-links in collagen, ↑ strength, become non-adaptive – ↓ Water and ↓ plasticity – Becomes non-pliable, brittle, weak – Predisposition to tendon and ligament injury	– General body warm-up increases blood flow and body temperature, facilitates elongation of connective tissue – Static and dynamic stretching increases flexibility of muscle-tendon units, allowing golfer to obtain desired biomechanical positions for swing	– Physical activity known to increase turnover rate of collagen – ↑ Pliability and ↓ formation nonadaptive connective tissue
Cartilage	– Atrophies with age – Proteoglycan subunits smaller – ↓ Cartilage water content – ↓ Lubrication of joint – Vulnerability to injury	– Weight bearing activity throughout the warm-up facilitates diffusion of lubricating fluid into joint space (but need to avoid excessive stresses)	– Consistent weight bearing activity over time thickens cartilage and facilitates processes for diffusion of fluid into joint space

Note: ↑ increase in variable, ↓ decrease.

Gerontological information in Table is based on research summarized in ACSM et al. [2]; Paterson et al. [3]; Vandervoort [4]; Versteegh et al. [9].

comes from a well-rounded resistance exercise program that trains the appropriate patterns of movement at the correct target level for the individual. Specific focus on certain directions of movement can also be recommended if abnormal patterns of motion are observed.

In terms of age-related changes to cardiovascular performance, cardiac output decreases by about 30% between the ages of 30 and 70 years [2, 3]. In golfers, this decrease in aerobic ▶ endurance may cause premature mental and physical fatigue leading to performance inconsistencies, particularly toward the end of a round. As noted above, there can be a significant demand placed on the cardiorespiratory and metabolic systems by the prolonged duration of a typical round of walking the golf course. The effect of limited cardiovascular capacity on performance may further be compounded by localized muscle ▶ fatigue that can occur during ambulation on uneven terrain. Given that the overall ability of older adults to carry an absolute load over time is reduced compared to younger adults, a common mechanism of many sports injuries – fatigue and associated neuromuscular incoordination – is a likely contributing factor. However, fatigue resistance can be also built up with appropriate exercise strategies.

While golf performance may be compromised by the diminished cardiovascular capacity of senior players, it should also be mentioned that the muscular and cardiovascular requirements of golf can also provide considerable health benefits. These gains can include increased aerobic performance, as well as improved body composition and high-density lipoprotein serum cholesterol levels. Thus, walking the golf course provides a sufficient amount of physical activity that has been shown to aid overall health and well-being, especially for older golfers whose physiological training threshold is lowered by age [9].

Remarkably, the benefits of a ▶ warm-up session before competition for the older athlete can have many of the same effects as training, albeit to a lesser extent [4, 10]. These effects are also summarized in Table 1. For example, the slowed speed of muscle contraction and power generation in older adults can be altered just by increasing body temperature via the initial low-intensity exercise phase of a typical warm-up routine. Then additional benefits can be derived from ensuring that the connective tissue in muscles and tendons is ready to support the required range of motion of full golf swings. Finally, there is the facilitation of motor coordination that results from rehearsal of the specific swings that will soon be used on the course. From the perspective of injury prevention, it is also valuable to practice the desired movements and incorporate any necessary adjustments to accommodate painful or stiff joints [6].

Conclusion

In summary, there are extensive age-related changes in physical functions that affect the motor performance of older athletes. However, there are also worthwhile advantages of a maintained training program and appropriate warm-up routine for this age group as they prepare to engage in skilled movement patterns for their sport. The example of golf was used due to its high popularity and recognized health benefits for seniors from among the physical activity choices that they have. Due to the age-related changes in the motor and skeletal systems that reduce the effectiveness of golf swings with optimal tempo and rhythm, training can be essential for performance. Yet most male and female recreational golfers aged 50 or older fail to stay in good physical condition. Senior athletes should be encouraged to participate in continuing training programs throughout the year that include cardiovascular endurance (i.e., if additional physiological stimulation is necessary beyond the effects of walking the course). Overall reductions in the body's ability to maintain cardiovascular and muscular homeostasis also indicate that older players need to pay close attention to maintaining adequate hydration, nutritional supplementation, and blood electrolytes during their round of golf, particularly in hotter climates.

References

1. Spirduso WW, Francis KL, MacRae PG (2005) Physical dimensions of aging, 2nd edn. Human Kinetics, Champaign, Il
2. ACSM, Chodzko-Zajko WJ, Proctor DN et al (2009) American college of sports medicine position stand. Exercise and physical activity for older adults. Med Sci Sports Exerc 41:1510–1530
3. Paterson DH, Jones GR, Rice CL (2007) Ageing and physical activity: evidence to develop exercise recommendations for older adults. Appl Physiol Nutr Metab 32:S69–S108
4. Vandervoort AA (2009) Potential benefits of warm-up for neuromuscular performance of older athletes. Exerc Sports Sci Rev 37:60–65
5. Aagaard P, Suetta C, Caserotti P, Magnusson SP, Kjaer M (2010) Role of the nervous system in sarcopenia and muscle atrophy with aging: strength training as a countermeasure. Scand J Med Sci Sports 20:49–64
6. Lynn SK, Noffal GJ (2010) Frontal plane knee moments in golf: effect of target side foot position at address. J Sports Sci Med 9:275–281
7. Thompson CJ, Osness WH (2004) Effects of an 8-week multimodal exercise program on strength, flexibility, and golf performance in 55- to 79-year-old men. J Aging Phys Act 12:144–56
8. Marshall LW, McGill SM (2010) The role of axial torque in disc herniation. Clin Biomech 25:6–9
9. Versteegh TH, Vandervoort AA, Lindsay DM, Lynn SK (2008) Fitness, performance and injury prevention strategies for the senior golfer. Ann Rev Golf Coach 2:199–214
10. Fradkin AJ, Sherman CA, Finch CF (2004) Improving golf performance with a warm up conditioning programme. Brit J Sports Med 38:762–765

AI (Adequate Intake)

Term developed by the Food and Nutrition Board (FNB) at the Institute of Medicine of the National Academies (USA). The AI is defined as the average daily recommended intake level based on observed or experimentally determined estimates of nutrient intake that is assumed to be adequate to sustain health. This term is used when an RDA (recommended daily allowance – the average daily nutrient intake level sufficient to meet the nutrient requirements of 97–98% of healthy individuals) cannot be determined from currently available data.

AICAR

5-Aminoimidazole-4-carboxamide-1-β-d-ribofuranoside (AICAR) is an adenosine analog that is taken up by cells and phosphorylated to become 5-Aminoimidazole-4-carboxamide-1-β-d-ribofuranosyl 5′-monophosphate (ZMP), an analog of adenosine 5′-monophosphate (AMP). AICAR is commonly used as a means to activate the AMP-activated protein kinase.

Cross-References

▶ AMP-Activated Protein Kinase

AIDS, Exercise

Gregory A. Hand, G. William Lyerly
Arnold School of Public Health, Department of Exercise Science, University of South Carolina, Columbia, SC, USA

Synonyms

Clinical population; HIV; Infection; Physical activity; Resistance training

Definition

AIDS, acquired immunodeficiency syndrome, is an advanced stage of human immunodeficiency virus (HIV) infection characterized by a CD4 T-cell count below 200 cells/ml of blood and a chronic susceptibility for opportunistic infections. HIV is a retrovirus that targets immune cells that display CD4 surface proteins for infection, then replicates within the cell and kills it. The severe reduction in CD4 lymphocytes, the immune cells most affected by HIV infection, resulting from this infection and replication process is the primary mechanism for HIV-associated immunosuppression [1].

Pathogenetic Mechanisms

Infection by HIV, a retrovirus of the lentivirus group, is mediated by physical binding to the CD4 cell surface protein followed by penetration of the cell. Cells that display CD4 molecules, all of which are targets for HIV infection, include T lymphocytes, macrophages, peripheral blood cells various epithelial cells, peripheral nerve cells, testicular Sertoli cells, and hepatic cells. Immunosuppression, resulting from depletion of CD4 T cells, is the hallmark of HIV infection. T cells play a critical role in regulating the systemic immune response, and loss of this function results in development of opportunistic infections in various organs and tissues.

As highly active antiretroviral therapy (HAART) has increased the life expectancy of individuals infected with HIV, previously unreported conditions have become a critical concern for maintaining functionality in the individual. These newly identified conditions are chronic with accumulating effects, are typically associated with aging in non-infected populations, and include various physiological and psychological diseases including cardiovascular diseases, muscle wasting and deconditioning syndromes, metabolic disorders, and increased levels of depression, anxiety, and stress.

Fatigue, which is a major contributor to physical inactivity, is a commonly reported symptom in those infected with HIV. As a result, HIV-infected individuals usually have lower levels of physical activity, which leads to a reduction in functional capacity and health-related quality of life. This sedentary lifestyle can exacerbate HIV-related symptoms and accelerate the progression of the disease.

Exercise Intervention/Therapeutical Consequences

Emerging evidence demonstrates that health benefits can be obtained in chronically ill populations through implementation of a structured, moderate-intensity exercise regimen. Similar to what has been seen in other clinical populations, the benefits of aerobic and resistance exercise participation are documented in studies of HIV-infected individuals. Exercise is a potential treatment for many of the symptoms associated with the HIV disease and can elicit improvements in body composition, strength, cardiorespiratory fitness, and mood and well-being [2].

Exercise has been shown to be safe in the HIV-infected population with no reports of adverse side effects. Studies involving regimens comprised of low- to moderate-intensity aerobic exercise have shown no increase in prevalence of opportunistic infections, no increase in viral load, and no reduction in CD4+ T-cell count. Some studies have reported enhanced immune function via exercise, especially in asymptomatic individuals. However, these results are controversial. Numerous studies have demonstrated an immunosuppressive effect of large doses of high-intensity exercise training in healthy individuals. Therefore, overtraining should be avoided when prescribing exercise regimens to HIV-infected individuals who are at risk for opportunistic infections.

The majority of studies investigating the effects of exercise in the HIV-infected population have focused on aerobic training. The interventions used in these studies have differed greatly in dosage (intensity × time). Studies have varied in duration from 5 weeks to 6 months and intensity levels from low to high. For this reason, dose response interpretations are controversial. However, the preponderance of evidence indicates that HIV-infected individuals can obtain beneficial results in as little as 6 weeks of aerobic activity of at least 2–3 sessions per week. Important adaptations can be categorized as functional, anthropomorphic, biochemical, and psychological. Numerous studies using various doses of exercise have demonstrated significant gains in functional aerobic capacity (FAC) at both high- and moderate-intensity levels, with greater gains being experienced when working at a higher intensity. Additionally, increases in high density lipoprotein (HDL) cholesterol, as well as significant decreases in total abdominal adipose tissue, total cholesterol, and triglycerides (TG) have been shown. One emerging area of beneficial results includes reductions in anxiety and depression. These psychological gains are particularly important since HIV-infected individuals often suffer from social isolation and depression after learning of their HIV infection. Besides these significant changes with aerobic exercise, some studies have observed beneficial changes in immunological variables, including increases in plasma CD4 T-cell counts. However, numerous studies have failed to replicate these findings. Further, it can be proposed that these changes in blood levels of immune cells are an enhanced mobilization of cells into the blood from lymphoid tissues rather than increased overall quantity of cells.

Only a few studies have examined the effects of resistance training, independent of aerobic exercise, on the health and fitness of HIV-infected individuals. The majority of these investigations has focused primarily on levels of strength and muscle mass rather than overall fitness or immune function. Further, most have incorporated high-intensity programs. Studies of resistance training report beneficial changes in body composition, including

increases in lean tissue mass (LTM) and overall body mass, increases in muscular strength, decreases in TG, and increases in physical functioning. Lean tissue mass increases have been shown to be positively correlated with the slowing of HIV progression and a decrease in HIV-related mortality. Because of these beneficial effects, resistance training has been prescribed to HIV-infected individuals with varying results. Results suggest that high-intensity resistance training may elicit favorable outcomes, while research is needed to elucidate the effects associated with low- to moderate-intensity resistance training.

A growing number of studies are investigating the effects of combined aerobic and resistance exercise training programs that follow the guidelines established by numerous federal agencies and foundations. These combined programs offer several advantages, including enhanced cardiorespiratory function in a population that is typically deconditioned with the additional benefit of strength and muscle mass gains that accompany resistance training. Moderate-intensity combined exercise regimens have been shown to improve total cholesterol, body composition, and psychological well-being as well as increase overall health, and quality of life. Results also demonstrate increases in FAC similar to exercise regimens consisting of only aerobic training, and increases in strength greater than that produced by the aerobic regimens. Thus, combined exercise training likely results in both cardiovascular and musculoskeletal adaptations, making this intervention more appealing than either individual exercise modality. However, the majority of these studies utilized high-intensity resistance training, which often results in poor exercise adherence due to muscle soreness and increased risk of injury in untrained individuals recruited from healthy or clinical populations. As with either mode individually, the optimal dosage of combined training has not been elucidated.

Recent work has begun to address the issue of finding a manageable exercise regimen that will enhance program adherence and optimize health benefits. One study has examined the effects of a 6-week combined program in which the physical activity was performed at a moderate-intensity level [3]. Results showed a significant training effect that included enhanced FAC, decreased heart rate at absolute submaximal workloads (training bradycardia), increases in LTM, and peak strength increases between 14% and 28% on eight resistance exercises. Circulating levels of cytokines and hormones were also investigated, which resulted in increases in growth hormone (GH), interleukin-6 (IL-6), and decreases in cortisol and soluble tumor necrosis factor receptor-2 (sTNFrII). These changes in cytokines and hormones are important as they present potential mechanisms for the increases in LTM resulting from the program. Additionally, HIV-infected individuals adhered well to the low-volume, moderate-intensity training. These findings, as well as those from a number of other studies, indicate that HIV-infected individuals can experience beneficial cardiovascular adaptations from short-duration training combining low-volume aerobic and resistance movements at moderate intensity. Importantly, the results also suggest that the functional limitations common in HIV-infected individuals are due in part to detraining and are reversible through moderate exercise adherence [4].

In summary, the preponderance of data indicate that moderate- and higher-intensity aerobic, resistance, and combined exercise regimens can both be safe and elicit beneficial changes in HIV-infected individuals. Benefits observed in controlled trials include changes in body composition, FAC, muscular strength, total and HDL cholesterol, cognitive function, depression and anxiety, self-reported overall health, and quality of life. Conversely, beneficial effects of exercise training on HIV status, viral load, or immune function are controversial. However, aerobic exercise has been shown to have no negative impact on immunity or disease progression. Further research is required in order to determine the minimal and optimal duration, frequency, and intensity of exercise needed to produce beneficial changes in this population. A confounding factor in the majority of studies has been the lifestyle choices of the participants, which include severe deconditioning that is often confused with HIV-associated wasting or other symptoms evoked by poor diet and exercise participation. Further, most studies have yet to approach the exercise program from the perspective of validating commonly used exercise prescriptions, or from a dose response perspective. Both approaches are critical for a full understanding of the effects of training on the HIV-infected population.

References

1. http://www.cdc.gov/hiv/
2. Dudgeon WD, Phillips KD, Carson JA, Brewer RB, Durstine JL, Hand GA (2006) Counteracting muscle wasting in HIV-infected individuals. HIV Med 7:299–310
3. Hand GA, Phillips KD, Dudgeon WD, Lyerly GW, Durstine JL, Burgess SE (2008) Moderate intensity exercise training reverses functional aerobic impairment in HIV-infected individuals. AIDS Care 20(9):1066–1074
4. Schmitz HR, Layne JE, Humphrey R (2002) Exercise and HIV infection. In: Myers JN, Herbert WG, Humphrey R (eds) ACSM's resources for clinical exercise physiology: musculoskeletal, neuromuscular, neoplastic, immunologic, and hematologic conditions. Lippincott Williams & Wilkins, Philadelphia, pp 206–218

Airway Inflammation

▶ Pulmonary System, Training Adaptation

Algesic Substances

Substances that excite free nerve endings or pain receptors finally eliciting the perception of pain.

Alkaline Earth Metal

▶ Magnesium

Alkaloid

Alkaloids are nitrogenous organic compounds produced by bacteria, fungi, plants, and animals. Many alkaloids are used for therapeutic purposes (e.g., atropine, morphine, caffeine).

Allele

One possible sequence of DNA at a specific location on a specific chromosome. An allele may refer to a single base in the DNA sequence or a sequence of many bases.

Allergy

An altered, hypersensitive reaction to second contact with an antigen that causes an allergic reaction that may be local or systemic. Most allergies are characterized by type 1 hypersensitivity. Initial presentation of the antigen results in the production of large number of IgE secreting plasma cells that release antibodies to mast cells, and these release histamine on subsequent presentation of the antigen, leading to an allergic response.

Allosteric

A molecule allosterically regulates enzyme activity by binding to a non-catalytic site of an enzyme, resulting in either enhancement or inhibition of the catalytic rate.

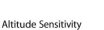

Allosteric Hemoglobin Modifiers

Are substances which increase the deliverance of oxygen by hemoglobin.

All-Out Exercise

Maximal-intensity exercise, longer in duration that a sprint (i.e., >10 s), where there is a considerable decrease in performance.

Alpha1-Adrenergic Receptors

One of the three major subfamilies of adrenergic receptor, divided into alpha1A-, alpha1B-, and alpha1D-adrenoceptors.

Cross-References

▶ Adrenergic Receptors

Alpha2-Adrenergic Receptors

One of the three major subfamilies of adrenergic receptor, divided into alpha2A-, alpha2B-, and alpha2C-adrenoceptors.

Cross-References

▶ Adrenergic Receptors

Alpha-Amylase or Amylase

A digestive enzyme found in saliva that begins the digestion of starches in the mouth (also called ptyalin). It also has an antibacterial action.

ALS

Amyotrophic lateral sclerosis is caused by the degeneration of motor neurons in the spinal cord and brain, resulting in progressive muscle atrophy, paralysis and death.

Alteration in Structure and Function

▶ Training, Adaptations

Altered Modulation of Vasomotor Tone

▶ Endothelial Dysfunction

Alternative Activation

Alternative activation is a macrophage inflammatory state characterized by the secretion of effectors such as TGFbeta and a series of chemokines (CCL13, CCL23...) and growth factors (IGF-1...). They express higher levels of scavenger receptors. Alternative activation can be triggered in vitro by IL-4. Alternatively activated macrophages are associated with chronic inflammation.

Altitude

Refers to the height above sea level and in this setting high altitude is defined as 2,500 m and above.

Altitude Illness

▶ Acute Mountain Sickness

Altitude Sensitivity

Altitude sensitivity is defined as the percent difference of maximal oxygen consumption ($\%\Delta VO_2 max$) when measured at sea level and at a defined altitude. The $\%\Delta VO_2 max$ usually becomes more negative the higher the altitude. $\%\Delta VO_2 max$ is individually different and depends on gender, training state, body fat content, as well as on muscular characteristics.

Altitude Sickness

▶ Acute Mountain Sickness

Altitude Training

Altitude training is a popular training approach among athletes to increase exercise performance at sea level or to acclimatize to competition at altitude. Muscle structural, biochemical, and molecular findings point to a specific role of the altitude-associated hypoxia in combination with training. It has been reasoned that exercising in hypoxia increases the training stimulus. However the effects of training in hypoxia on aerobic and anaerobic performance as well as strength development are controversial. Hypoxia training studies published in the past have varied considerably in altitude (2,200–5,700 m) and training duration (1–8 weeks) as well as in the fitness state of the subjects. Especially frequency and intensity in combination with the level of hypoxia seem to play a major role in the effectiveness of training in hypoxia. Several approaches have evolved during the last few decades, with "live high – train low" and "live low – train high" being the most popular.

Cross-References

▶ Hypoxia, Training
▶ Training, Altitude

Altitude, Physiological Response

Robert S. Mazzeo
Department of Integrative Physiology, University of Colorado, Boulder, CO, USA

Synonyms

High elevation; Hypobaric hypoxia; Low inspired oxygen (O_2) pressure

Definition

The main physiological consequence of exposure to high altitude is hypoxia, which can be defined as a reduction in the partial pressure of oxygen in inspired air (P_IO_2) resulting in hypoxemia (subnormal arterial blood O_2 saturation – S_aO_2). Hypoxia can be induced by decreasing either the ambient barometric pressure (P_B) or the O_2 concentration of the inspired gas. As one ascends to higher altitudes, there is a reduction in P_B known as hypobaria. Accordingly, per Boyle's law (the volume of a gas is inversely proportional to its pressure), as the P_B decreases with increasing elevation, the volume of any given gas will increase. As a result of the expanding volume of ambient air at altitude, the partial pressure of each individual gas declines in proportion to the decline in ambient P_B. Thus, as the elevation increases, the PO_2 (as well as the other gases) decreases resulting in less O_2 per liter of air. Consequently, less O_2 is presented to the lungs, which results in a reduction of O_2 diffusing into the arterial circulation for subsequent utilization by tissues throughout the body.

Obviously, the severity of the hypoxia is dependent upon the eventual altitude elevation achieved. At low altitudes (0–4,900 ft, 760–635 mmHg), resting arterial O_2 saturation (S_aO_2) is generally well maintained imparting only a marginal disruption in homeostasis. As one ascends to more moderate altitudes (4,900–9,800 ft, 635–525 mmHg), a slight but significant decrease in resting S_aO_2 (95–92%) is observed as the inspired P_IO_2 can decrease to 110 mmHg compared to 159 mmHg at sea level. At high altitudes (9,800–16,000 ft, 525–405 mmHg), ambient P_IO_2 will decrease further with resting S_aO_2 approaching 80% and lower. Consequently, the final altitude and degree of hypoxia play a critical role in determining the extent of the physiologic and metabolic responses required to ensure proper tissue oxygenation in response to this environmental disruption to homeostasis.

Mechanisms

Acute Altitude Exposure: The underlying mechanism responsible for the physiological responses observed during acute exposure to high altitude is the direct effect of hypoxia. Adjustments in many physiologic and metabolic systems are necessary to properly respond to the disruption in homeostasis imposed by exposure to high altitude (Fig. 1). These adjustments are regulated, in part, by activation of key components of the neuroendocrine system [4]. Specifically, the autonomic nervous system and the adrenal glands play a major role in both the physiological and metabolic responses. Hypoxia has a direct effect on stimulating epinephrine production and release from the adrenal medulla thereby increasing circulating epinephrine levels. Via β-adrenergic receptors, both heart rate and stroke volume are subsequently increased, both contributing to the increase in cardiac output observed during acute hypoxia. The net result is to increase O_2 delivery to critical tissues when the O_2 content per liter of blood (C_aO_2) is reduced as a result of hypoxia.

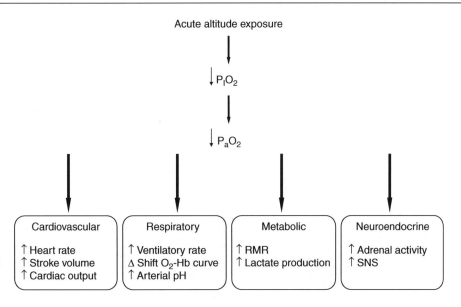

Acute altitude exposure

$\downarrow P_IO_2$

$\downarrow P_aO_2$

Cardiovascular	Respiratory	Metabolic	Neuroendocrine
↑ Heart rate ↑ Stroke volume ↑ Cardiac output	↑ Ventilatory rate Δ Shift O_2-Hb curve ↑ Arterial pH	↑ RMR ↑ Lactate production	↑ Adrenal activity ↑ SNS

Altitude, Physiological Response. Fig. 1 Effect of acute hypoxia (altitude exposure) on arterial oxygen pressure. Adjustments in several key systems are necessary to respond to this disruption in homeostasis to ensure adequate oxygen delivery to tissues

Additionally, epinephrine can contribute to local vasodilation of vascular beds promoting increased blood flow and O_2 delivery to the tissues involved. Further, to improve O_2-carrying capacity, a reduction in plasma volume (by way of increased urination) occurs in an attempt to concentrate existing red blood cells and increase hematocrit.

Activation of both central and peripheral (aortic and carotid bodies) chemoreceptors associated with the respiratory system is the driving force for increases in both ventilatory rate and volume. This response is essential in helping to maintain, as best as possible, O_2 pressure in the lungs, and subsequently, in arterial blood. A side effect of this increase in ventilation is a reduction in the partial pressure of carbon dioxide (PCO_2) as more CO_2 than normal is blown off. This, in turn, results in an increase in arterial pH (alkalosis) initiating a leftward shift in the O_2-hemoglobin (O_2-Hb) dissociation curve facilitating O_2 diffusion and loading from lungs into blood (onto hemoglobin).

Upon ascent to altitude, resting metabolic rate (RMR) is elevated above sea-level values and can persist for an extended period of time while remaining at altitude residence. Consequently, the total energy requirement necessary to maintain a stable body weight increases proportionately. In order to avoid a negative energy balance and remain weight stable, this increase in the energy requirement must be coupled with an equal increase in energy intake. However, cachexia (weight loss) is a commonly reported consequence during the initial weeks of high altitude exposure [1]. The weight loss most likely results from a combination of the increase in total energy requirement at altitude coupled with loss of appetite and lower energy intake. While several mechanisms have been suggested that may contribute, in part or combination, to the suppression of appetite at altitude (e.g., SNS activity, leptin, insulin, IL-6), exact causes for this observation remain to be determined.

Chronic Altitude Exposure: The classic adaptation associated with acclimatization to chronic altitude exposure is the increase in red blood cell (RBC) numbers [3]. This response is a direct result of the hypoxic stimulus and is secondary to the production of erythropoietin (EPO), a hormone produced primarily by the kidneys that promotes the synthesis of new RBCs in the bone marrow. While the time course and magnitude of change in EPO, and eventual RBC numbers, will vary dependent upon altitude elevation (degree of hypoxia) as well as individual differences, initial changes can be seen within the first week of exposure. These changes, in conjunction with the ventilatory adjustments, result in significant improvements in both arterial oxygen saturation (S_aO_2) and content (C_aO_2). Consequently, the physiological stress associated with altitude exposure is partially reduced resulting in a number of physiologic and metabolic adjustments when compared with initial arrival (Fig. 2). Additionally, an increase in RBC 2, 3-diphosphoglycerate (2,3 DPG) coupled with a decrease in bicarbonate (kidney excretion) induce a rightward

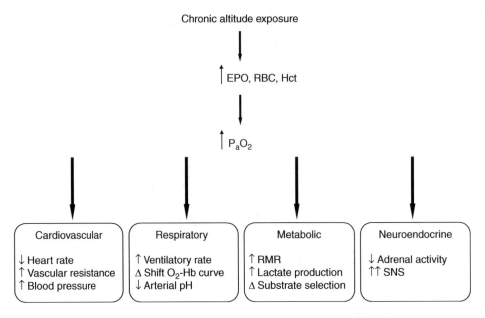

Altitude, Physiological Response. Fig. 2 In response to chronic hypoxia (acclimatization) improvements in oxygen carrying capacity and transport allow for adaptations in various physiologic and metabolic pathways

shift in the O_2-Hb dissociation curve facilitating O_2 unloading from hemoglobin to tissues.

A significant elevation in the sympathetic nervous activity is observed during the first week of chronic altitude exposure. This is thought to be responsible for the increase in systemic vascular resistance (α-adrenergic mechanism) and subsequent elevation in arterial blood pressure. Alterations in the sympathoadrenal pathways also contribute to other adjustments made during the acclimatization process, including changes in substrate selection, continued elevation of RMR, and lactate production (particularly during exercise – see below).

Exercise Response
The physiological responses to exercise at altitude are dependent upon a number of factors. As always, the extent of hypoxia plays a major role in the amount of stress incurred and the extent to which normal homeostasis is disrupted. The addition of the added stress of exercise along with that of hypoxia will have an additive effect that will influence maximal exercise capacity, endurance time until fatigue, and submaximal exercise performance.

It is also important to consider the intensity of the exercise bout while at altitude as the relative intensity of an exercise bout plays a major role in the subsequent physiologic and metabolic adjustments (cardiovascular, respiratory, hormonal, etc.) needed to maintain performance [2]. It is clear that decline $\dot{V}O_{2max}$ progressively declines

with increasing altitude elevation. As a result, a given power output represents a greater relative exercise intensity (i.e., a higher percentage of $\dot{V}O_{2max}$) while at higher elevations. Consequently, a greater adjustment (physiologic, metabolic) to exercise is required when performing similar exercise tasks at an altitude compared to sea level. This is reflected by greater increases in sympathoadrenal responses, heart rate, cardiac output, ventilatory rate, and lactate production for a given power output when compared to sea-level values (Fig. 1).

In individuals that have become acclimatized to altitude, the adaptations made in O_2 carrying capacity, transport, and diffusion (described above) allow for a reduced level of exercise stress when compared to acute altitude exposure. As a result, for a given power output, an acclimatized individual will demonstrate lower sympathoadrenal responses, heart rate, cardiac output, ventilatory rate, and lactate production for a given power output when compared to values during acute exposure.

A number of these adaptations associated with acclimatization to high altitude may be of potential benefit for the endurance athlete in improving performance at sea level. This is the basic premise for the "Live High–Train Low" paradigm that continues to receive considerable attention [5]. Acclimatization to altitude will result in a number of adaptive responses that improve O_2 carrying capacity, transport, and utilization. Specifically, increases in red blood cell volume, total blood volume, and improved oxygen delivery to muscle are well documented. Changes in skeletal muscle capillary density and mitochondrial oxidative capacity with acclimatization, while not as consistent, are possible and could result in improvements in endurance performance. It is important to note that these adaptations occur as a result of simply living at high altitudes independent of a training stimulus. The concept of training "low" relates to the observation that training at lower altitudes allows an individual to exercise at a higher absolute workload and power output than would be possible at higher altitudes. Thus, with live high–train low there are two independent stimuli (hypoxia and training) acting to enhance oxygen delivery and utilization, $\dot{V}O_{2max}$, and endurance performance.

Any performance benefits from altitude adaptations are going to be event specific as participation in events where oxygen delivery and utilization are potentially limiting factors would demonstrate the most benefits to athletes acclimatized to altitude. As there are no changes in key components of anaerobic pathways and an actual reduction in blood bicarbonate levels with altitude acclimatization, very high-intense activities more reliant on non-oxidative fuel sources (power, sprint) would not be expected to show any benefits during return to sea-level performance.

References

1. Butterfield GE, Gates J, Fleming S et al (1992) Increased energy intake minimizes weight loss in men at high altitude. J Appl Physiol 72:1741–1748
2. Mazzeo RS, Reeves JT (2003) Adrenergic contribution during acclimatization to high altitude: perspectives from Pikes peak. Exerc Sport Sci Rev 31:13–18
3. Mazzeo RS, Fulco CS (2006) Physiological systems and their responses to conditions of hypoxia. In: Tipton CM (ed) ACSM's advanced exercise physiology, Ch 7. Lippincott Williams & Wilkins, Baltimore, pp 564–580
4. Mazzeo RS (2008) Physiological responses to exercise at altitude: an update. Sports Med 38:1–8
5. Stray-Gundersen J, Chapman RF, Levine BD (2001) "Living high-training low" altitude training improves sea level performance in male and female elite runners. J Appl Physiol 91:1113–1120

Alzheimer's Disease

A neurodegenerative disorder of aging characterized by progressive memory impairment as the result of the dysfunction and death of nerve cells in the brain, particularly those in the temporal and frontal lobes. The most common form of dementia that results in memory and cognitive impairments during late adulthood. The degenerative disease is currently considered to be progressive and irreversible with behavioral symptoms usually occurring after the age of 65. The causes of the disease are still under debate, but amyloid plaque formation and neurofibrillary tangles in the brain are two putative pathways leading to the disease. Later stages of the disease results in more extensive memory impairments as well as behavioral problems such as agitation, wandering, and irritability.

Cross-References
▶ Neurodegenerative Disease

Amenorrhea
▶ Athletic Amenorrhea

Amide
▶ Glutamine

2-Amino-4-Carbamoylbutanoic Acid
▶ Glutamine

2-Aminoglutaramic Acid
▶ Glutamine

α-amino Carboxylic Acid
▶ Amino Acids

Amino Acid Kinetics
▶ Metabolism, Protein

Amino Acid Oxidation

Amino acid oxidation is the process by which amino acids are used as a fuel source to produce ATP. The amino group is removed to convert the amino acid into an α-keto acid that is incorporated into the tri-carboxylic acid cycle for eventual production of ATP within the mitochondria.

Amino Acids

JARED M. DICKINSON, BLAKE B. RASMUSSEN
Department of Nutrition & Metabolism, Division of Rehabilitation Sciences, University of Texas Medical Branch, Galveston, TX, USA

Synonyms
α-amino carboxylic acid; Protein building blocks

Definition
An amino acid is a molecule in which a central carbon (C) atom is bound by an amino group (NH₂), a carboxyl group (COOH), a hydrogen atom (H), and an organic side chain (R) (Fig. 1). Amino acids are differentiated from one another by the structure of the organic side chain, which is unique to a given amino acid and also defines the specific properties of that amino acid. There are 20 common amino acids that are utilized as the "building blocks" for ▶ protein, such that the linking of amino acids in a precise linear sequence serves as the foundation for the structure and function of a protein. Further, amino acids are categorized as either nonessential or essential. Proper physiological concentrations of nonessential amino acids can be achieved through *de novo* synthesis, whereas physiological concentrations of essential amino acids cannot be maintained through *de novo* synthesis and must be introduced in the diet. Of the 20 common amino acids, 9 are considered essential and 11 nonessential (Table 1). In addition to the 20 common amino acids classified as standard, amino acids can undergo post-translational modifications prior to the formation of a protein. These amino acids are referred to as nonstandard amino acids.

Mechanism of Action
Amino acids most notably serve as the building blocks for protein. Specifically, amino acids are joined together via peptide bonds in a precise linear sequence to form a single polypeptide chain. Through ensuing processes, one or

$$H_2N - \overset{\overset{\displaystyle R}{|}}{\underset{\underset{\displaystyle H}{|}}{C}} - COOH$$

Amino Acids. Fig. 1 Schematic of the general structure of an amino acid

Amino Acids. Table 1 List of essential and nonessential amino acids

Essential	Nonessential
Histidine[a]	Alanine
Isoleucine	Arginine
Leucine	Asparagine
Lysine	Aspartic acid
Methionine	Cysteine
Phenylalanine	Glutamic acid
Threonine	Glutamine
Tryptophan	Glycine
Valine	Proline
	Serine
	Tyrosine

[a]Essential to infants

more of these polypeptide chains can be utilized to construct a protein, and the specific amino acid sequence of each polypeptide chain provides the foundation of the protein's structure and function. In fact, removing or replacing a single amino acid in the precise sequence can substantially interfere with the proper functioning of the protein or even render the protein completely inactive. The sequence of amino acids in a given polypeptide is ultimately determined by the base sequence of specific regions of DNA, referred to as ▶ genes. This genetic information is communicated within the cell through the processes of ▶ transcription and ▶ translation, and the production of a single polypeptide/protein requires collaboration between numerous molecules, including DNA, messenger RNA (mRNA), transfer RNA (tRNA), ▶ ribosomes, and several enzymes.

Not only do amino acids serve as the foundation for protein structure, but changes in amino acid availability have a potent effect on protein turnover, which is the concurrent processes of protein synthesis and breakdown. Specifically, an increase in amino acids availability, such as that experienced during a meal, rapidly and transiently stimulates an increase in the rate of protein synthesis, whereas protein breakdown appears to decrease slightly

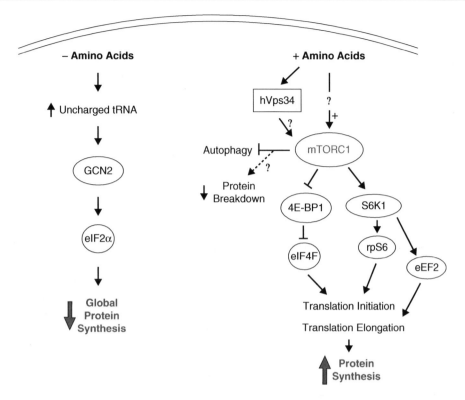

Amino Acids. Fig. 2 Simplified schematic of the effect of amino acid availability on protein metabolism. Low levels of amino acids (*left*) decrease global rates of protein synthesis through increased activity of general control nonrepressed 2 (GCN2). High levels of amino acids (*right*) increase protein synthesis rate by stimulating the activity of mammalian target of rapamycin complex 1 (mTORC1). In addition, stimulation of mTORC1 by high levels of amino acids appears to decrease autophagy, which contributes to a reduction in protein breakdown: tRNA, transfer RNA; eIF2α, eukaryotic initiation factor 2 alpha; hVps34, human vacuolar protein sorting-34; 4E-BP1, 4E binding protein 1; S6K1, p70 ribosomal S6 kinase 1; eIF4F, eukaryotic initiation factor 4F; rpS6, ribosomal protein S6; eEF2, eukaryotic elongation factor 2

(Fig. 2). The increased availability of amino acids (primarily essential amino acids) stimulates an increase in mammalian target of rapamycin complex 1 (mTORC1) activity, which is a key nutrient sensor and regulator of protein metabolism [1, 2]. mTORC1 subsequently phosphorylates two important direct downstream targets, ribosomal protein S6 kinase 1 (S6K1) and 4E binding protein 1 (4E-BP1), that facilitates a variety of downstream effects that ultimately enhance translation initiation and elongation. In addition, mTORC1 activation in response to increased amino acid availability also appears to decrease protein breakdown, and thus the liberation of free amino acids, which may in part be due to a decrease in autophagy as a result of human vacuolar protein sorting-34 (hVps34) signaling to mTORC1 (Fig. 2). On the other hand, a decrease in amino acid availability has been shown to slow the rate of protein synthesis. Specifically, deficient levels of amino acids lead to an increase in uncharged tRNA that in turn bind to and

activate general control nonrepressed 2 (GCN2) kinase. Subsequently, GCN2 kinase phosphorylates eukaryotic initiation factor 2α (eIF2α), which slows the rate of global protein synthesis [3] (Fig. 2). As a consequence of their impact on the regulation of protein metabolism, amino acids have a tremendous role in growth and development.

Amino acids also serve in the maintenance of energy stores and energy substrate within the body. For instance, amino acids are necessary for the production of nucleotides, which not only form the structure of RNA and DNA and serve as cellular signaling molecules, but they also act as chemical energy stores in the form of ATP and GTP. Moreover, the importance of amino acids in terms of bioenergetics becomes severely important during stress, malnutrition, and injury conditions. Under such conditions, the carbon skeleton of many amino acids can be utilized to produce acetyl-CoA, which in turn can be oxidized via the Krebs cycle and electron transport chain for the production of ATP. Additionally, during these conditions several amino acids serve as major hepatic gluconeogenic substrates and can be utilized to provide energy substrate to several tissues including the brain and immune cells.

In addition to those addressed above, amino acids and their metabolites are imperative to numerous other medically relevant biological processes. For instance, glutamine serves as a major energy substrate for cells of the immune system and is involved in reducing inflammation. Arginine serves as the precursor for nitric oxide, an important signaling molecule associated with mitochondrial biogenesis, blood flow regulation, and cardiovascular health. In fact, several amino acids are utilized as biosynthetic molecules for a variety of products that serve a multitude of biological functions, including but not limited to: hormones, coenzymes, oxidative stress response, ammonia detoxification, neurotransmitters, porphyrins, immune function, signaling molecules, reproduction, metabolic intermediates, and energy substrates [4].

Clinical Use

Due to the diversity of metabolic pathways that require the use of one or more amino acids, disturbances in the physiological levels of many amino acids can lead to disruptions in several biological processes. For instance, high physiologic levels of amino acids can induce insulin resistance, which chronically can lead to a multitude of debilitating clinical conditions. Similarly, deficiencies in some amino acids can impair growth, compromise proper immune function, and lead to development of cardiovascular complications. Maintenance of appropriate amino acid levels can be achieved either through the diet or through *de novo* synthesis, dependent upon whether the specific amino acid is classified as essential or nonessential. However, under some circumstances *de novo* synthesis of certain amino acids usually classified as nonessential may not provide optimal levels, and thus supplementation is required. For example, arginine concentration is substantially reduced during various clinical conditions, including burn injury, sepsis, and trauma. Under such circumstances, not only is arginine supplementation necessary to restore proper physiological levels of the amino acid, but supplementation of arginine also appears to improve the healing/immune response. In fact, arginine supplementation has also been suggested as a useful supplement in a variety of conditions such as obesity, diabetes, and cardiovascular disease [4].

It is very well established that numerous clinical conditions are associated with muscle wasting. Not only does this loss of muscle mass impair physical function, but because skeletal muscle serves as the largest reservoir of amino acids in the body, muscle atrophy is also detrimental to a multitude of amino acid dependent biological processes that are imperative for healing, immune function, and recovery. Increasing amino acid availability, either through infusion or ingestion, promotes an anabolic environment in skeletal muscle and therefore represents a potential countermeasure to conditions of muscle wasting that can easily be employed in a majority of clinical settings. The ability for amino acids to increase muscle protein synthesis is driven primarily by an increased availability of essential amino acids. Further, both young and older individuals appear to have a similar increase in muscle protein synthesis when a large dose (>15 g) of essential amino acids is ingested. In contrast, older adults are less sensitive to a lower amount of essential amino acids. The discrepancy between younger and older individuals in their muscle protein anabolic response to amino acid availability is likely to be important since aging itself results in reductions in muscle size and function. Future research is clearly warranted to more precisely define proper guidelines for use of amino acid supplementation with various clinical conditions.

The clinical value of increased amino acid availability is also observed when coupled with exercise. Specifically, ingesting essential amino acids shortly following a bout of resistance exercise stimulates muscle protein synthesis to a much greater extent than that elicited independently by each stimulus [2], suggesting that increased amino acid availability following exercise may aide in muscle recovery and growth. Moreover, coupling amino acid ingestion and exercise may also serve an important role in the maintenance of muscle mass with aging, as the blunted anabolic response following resistance exercise in older adults can be restored by providing essential amino acids shortly after exercise.

Diagnostics

Important insight into the in vivo metabolic kinetics of amino acids can be examined with the use of amino acid tracers. Amino acid tracers are amino acids that contain either a radioactive or a stable ▶ isotope (depending on the specific measurement) that differentiates the tracer from the most common form of the amino acid by mass (and the presence of radiation emission for radioactive isotopes), but does not alter the chemical or functional identify of the amino acid. The difference in mass, and/or the emission of radiation, allows investigators and clinicians to follow the fate of the amino acid in a variety of biological processes, which can serve as a unique diagnostic tool for many diseases/conditions. For instance, a variety of radiolabeled amino acids have been utilized to identify cancerous tumors. Specifically, cancer cells display an accelerated rate of protein synthesis and amino acid transport, which leads to accumulation of an infused radiolabeled amino acid within the cell. The release of emissions from the accumulated radiolabeled amino acid is then measured with positron emission tomography to visualize the tumor [5].

Amino acid tracers can also be utilized to examine muscle protein metabolism following various therapeutic interventions. Monitoring muscle protein metabolism provides useful insight into the anabolic response of skeletal muscle to a given intervention (i.e., exercise or nutrition) and thus provides important information as to the usefulness of a given intervention to promote muscle mass gain or attenuate muscle loss. Such insight is clinically significant due to the loss of muscle mass that is associated with a variety clinical conditions and the importance of muscle mass as an amino acid reservoir for numerous medically relevant biological processes.

References

1. Kimball SR (2007) The role of nutrition in stimulating muscle protein accretion at the molecular level. Biochem Soc Trans 35:1298–1301
2. Drummond MJ, Dreyer HC, Fry CS, Glynn EL, Rasmussen BB (2009) Nutritional and contractile regulation of human skeletal muscle protein synthesis and mTORC1 signaling. J Appl Physiol 106:1374–1384
3. Hundal HS, Taylor PM (2009) Amino acid transceptors: gate keepers of nutrient exchange and regulators of nutrient signaling. Am J Physiol Endocrinol Metab 296:E603–E613
4. Wu G (2009) Amino acids: metabolism, functions, and nutrition. Amino Acids 37:1–17
5. Jager PL, Vaalburg W, Pruim J, de Vries EG, Langen KJ, Piers DA (2001) Radiolabeled amino acids: basic aspects and clinical applications in oncology. J Nucl Med 42:432–445

AMP Kinase

▶ AMP-Activated Protein Kinase

AMP-Activated Protein Kinase

STANLEY ANDRISSE, JONATHAN S. FISHER
Department of Biology, Saint Louis University, St. Louis, MO, USA

Synonyms

Adenosine 5′-monophosphate-activated protein kinase; AMP kinase; AMPK

Definition

AMPK, a trimeric serine/threonine ▶ protein kinase, acts as a cellular energy gauge [1]. Association of AMP with the γ ▶ adenine nucleotide binding subunit ▶ allosterically activates AMPK and appears to make the catalytic α subunit less susceptible to ▶ dephosphorylation of its activation site. The β subunit has been suggested to play a role in sensing of glycogen levels by AMPK [1].

Basic Mechanisms

This review focuses on effects of AMPK activation in skeletal muscle. However, AMPK functions in a wide variety of tissues. For example, AMPK suppresses fatty acid synthesis in ▶ lipogenic tissues, stimulates feeding behavior by actions in hypothalamus, and might play a role in oxygen sensing in the carotid body [1].

Activation of AMPK

Muscle contractions activate AMPK in crucial support of exercise performance. For example, mice that express a ▶ dominant negative form of AMPK (DN-AMPK) that prevents AMPK activation have a substantial reduction in exercise capacity [2]. In resting skeletal muscle, ATP levels are about 800 times higher than AMP concentrations. During metabolic stress such as muscle contractions, the reaction catalyzed by adenylate kinase (2 ADP → ATP + AMP) increases AMP concentration by approximately tenfold. In contrast, ATP levels generally do not fall during exercise except under extreme conditions. Thus, in working muscle, a large increase in the AMP-to-ATP ratio promotes binding of AMP to the γ subunit and activation of AMPK. Calcium- and cytokine-dependent pathways that are independent of changes in cellular energy status also activate AMPK.

Glucose Transport

Since the 1990s, muscle biologists have hypothesized that activation of AMPK in contracting skeletal muscle causes the increase in glucose uptake into muscle during exercise [1]. However, we now know that expression of DN-AMPK in mouse skeletal muscle does not prevent stimulation of glucose transport by treadmill running [2], despite previous findings that DN-AMPK blunts glucose transport after electrically stimulated muscle contractions [3]. It appears that a role of AMPK in regulation of glucose transport depends on the duration of the contraction pattern. For example, glucose transport in mouse muscles expressing DN-AMPK does not increase during the first 15 min of electrically stimulated muscle contractions but then reaches the same levels as in wild-type mice after 20 min of contractions [4]. Using different

▶ transgenic models of AMPK deficiency in skeletal muscle, other groups have found no requirement for AMPK in stimulation of glucose transport by contractions. Taken together, these data suggest that AMPK plays a nonessential part in stimulation of glucose transport in skeletal muscle during exercise. Despite the apparently limited role of AMPK in regulation of glucose transport during muscle contractions, activation of AMPK in the absence of muscle contractions appears sufficient to stimulate glucose transport in skeletal muscle. For example, ▶ AICAR, a precursor of an AMP analog, stimulates glucose transport in skeletal muscle. Likewise, expression of a chronically active form of the AMPK catalytic subunit in cultured skeletal muscle cells increases basal glucose transport. On the other hand, mutations of the γ subunit of AMPK that cause chronic activation of AMPK do not enhance basal glucose transport. Therefore, roles of AMPK in stimulation of glucose transport remain to be worked out. Unresolved issues include the subtle differences in transgenic animal models and the timing of AMPK effects during exercise. In addition, whether activation of AMPK is sufficient to stimulate glucose transport in skeletal muscle needs further clarification.

Fatty Acid Uptake and Oxidation in Skeletal Muscle

Over 15 years of studies have shown an association of AMPK activation with the increase in fatty acid oxidation that occurs during muscle contractions [1]. For example, AICAR stimulates fatty acid oxidation in skeletal muscle. On the other hand, muscle-specific deletion of LKB1, which is an activator of AMPK and a dozen other members of the AMPK-related kinase family, prevents activation of AMPK but does not interfere with contraction-stimulated fatty acid oxidation [3]. Further, expression of DN-AMPK in mouse muscle does not affect whole body fatty acid oxidation during exercise. To complicate matters, DN-AMPK expression in skeletal muscle prevents contraction-stimulated fatty acid oxidation in some studies but not others. Thus, while it seems likely that activation of AMPK suffices to stimulate fatty acid oxidation, the conditions under which AMPK plays a role in fatty acid oxidation in skeletal muscle remain to be defined. Likewise, mixed results exist regarding a possible action of AMPK in regulation of fatty acid uptake during muscle contractions. Using the DN-AMPK model, some groups find no requirement for AMPK for an increase in fatty acid uptake during contractions. However, another group has reported that AMPK plays a necessary role in stimulation of fatty acid uptake during extended contraction protocols but not early in a sequence of contractions [4].

Mitochondrial Biogenesis and Glucose Transporter Abundance

AICAR injections in rats or incubation of isolated skeletal muscle with AICAR causes increases in activity or abundance of marker enzymes of mitochondrial biogenesis and also increased levels of GLUT4, the insulin- and contraction-responsive glucose transporter in skeletal muscle. In contrast, AMPK appears nonessential to exercise training-related increases in mitochondrial gene or protein expression or GLUT4, as these adaptations occur in LKB1-deficient or AMPKα2 knockout mice [3].

Protein Synthesis

In rodents and humans, skeletal muscle protein synthesis is reduced during exercise/muscle contraction and by treatment with AICAR. Protein synthesis is regulated by mammalian target of rapamycin complex 1 (mTORC1), a protein kinase that manages mRNA translation initiation via phosphorylation of key mediators of mRNA translation [1]. The increase in muscle cross-sectional area, also known as hypertrophy, associated with resistance exercise is largely due to enhanced protein synthesis via activation of mTORC1 [1]. AMPK's reduction of mTORC1 activity is one of several proposed mechanisms by which exercise lowers protein synthesis [1]. Oddly enough, AMPK appears to display its inhibitory effects on mTORC1/protein synthesis during both endurance and resistance exercise; however, immediately following resistance exercise, AMPK, although still elevated, does not restrain mTORC1 activity. It has been shown that swimming exercise causes an increase in the sensitivity of ▶ System A amino acid transport to insulin-like growth factor 1 in skeletal muscle. However, it remains unknown whether AMPK plays a role in this process and whether the increased amino acid influx would be sufficient to stimulate mTORC1. Interestingly, in animals expressing DN-AMPK in skeletal muscle, protein synthesis remains suppressed during skeletal muscle contraction, suggesting that AMPK is not required for inhibition of protein synthesis during exercise [3].

Lifespan

Caloric restriction increases maximal lifespan in a variety of organisms, including flies, worms, mice, rats, and dogs. Interestingly, several effects of caloric restriction, such as activation of sirtuins, inhibition of mTOR, and mitochondrial biogenesis, are also effects of AMPK activation [1]. Indeed, worms that lack AMPK do not display a caloric restriction effect on maximal lifespan. Interestingly, wheel running exercise, that would activate AMPK in skeletal muscle, increases average but not maximal life span in rats.

This suggests that if AMPK mediates extension of maximal lifespan during caloric restriction, the effect occurs in a tissue other than skeletal muscle.

Exercise Intervention

Exercise and Increased Insulin Action

Changes in lifestyle over the past several decades, such as a decrease in physical activity and increased consumption of calorie-dense foods, have contributed to a dramatic, world-wide rise in the prevalence of non-insulin-dependent diabetes mellitus, or type II diabetes. Subjects with type II diabetes display impaired insulin-stimulated glucose transport into skeletal muscle. Fortunately, exercise increases both insulin-stimulated glucose transport and glycogen storage [3, 5]. For example, after exercise, a physiological level of insulin produces a twofold higher stimulation of glucose uptake compared to glucose transport into non-exercised muscle. In rat skeletal muscle and cultured skeletal muscle cells, activation of AMPK by AICAR mimics the increased insulin action that occurs after exercise. Moreover, AICAR infusion in humans increases insulin-stimulated glucose uptake. Expression of a constitutively active α1 subunit of AMPK also causes increased insulin action in cultured muscle cells. These data and others suggest that activation of AMPK is sufficient to increase insulin sensitivity in skeletal muscle. Intriguingly, several compounds and ▶ adipokines that activate AMPK, including metformin, rosiglitazone, leptin, and adiponectin, have antidiabetic effects. It remains

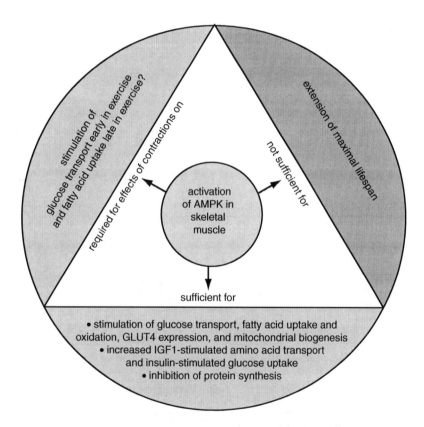

AMP-Activated Protein Kinase. Fig. 1 *AMPK actions in skeletal muscle.* AMPK can be experimentally activated by chemicals such as AICAR or therapeutically activated by drugs such as metformin. AMPK is also activated during muscle contractions by factors including an increase in the AMP:ATP ratio or a rise in cytosolic calcium ion availability. Activation of AMPK in skeletal muscle appears to be sufficient to stimulate glucose transport, fatty acid uptake and oxidation, GLUT4 glucose transporter expression, and mitochondrial biogenesis. Activation of AMPK also is sufficient to increase stimulation of amino acid transport by insulin-like growth factor 1 (IGF1), increase stimulation of glucose uptake by insulin, and inhibit protein synthesis. However, work with transgenic animals lacking AMPK activity in skeletal muscle suggests that AMPK is not required for any of the above actions in response to muscle contractions. Possible exceptions migh-t be time-dependent requirements for AMPK in regulation of glucose transport and fatty acid uptake during exercise

to be determined, however, whether AMPK is required for increased insulin action in skeletal muscle after exercise.

Summary

It seems clear that activation of AMPK can produce healthful effects in skeletal muscle, such as enhanced glucose transport, increased fat oxidation, and mitochondrial biogenesis (see Fig. 1 for summary). However, future study should be done to fully elucidate the sufficiency of and/or requirement for AMPK in the acute and chronic effects of skeletal muscle contraction. It seems that AMPK's role in muscle contractions could be dependent on exercise duration or intensity, but this area needs further examination. While many of the mediators of AMPK's effects in skeletal muscle have been described [1, 3], novel effectors are likely to be discovered. Finally, it needs to be determined which proteins work with – or instead of – AMPK in orchestrating the consequences of skeletal muscle contraction or treatment with AICAR.

Cross-References

▶ Diabetes Mellitus
▶ Diabetes Mellitus, Prevention
▶ Diabetes Mellitus, Sports Therapy
▶ Energy Metabolism
▶ Insulin Resistance
▶ Insulin-like Growth Factor
▶ Metabolism, Carbohydrate
▶ Metabolism, Lipid
▶ Metabolism, Protein
▶ Mitochondrial Biogenesis

References

1. Hardie DG (2011) Energy sensing by the AMP-activated protein kinase and its effects on muscle metabolism. Proc Nutr Soc 70:92–99
2. Maarbjerg SJ, Jorgensen SB, Rose AJ et al (2009) Genetic impairment of AMPKα2 signaling does not reduce muscle glucose uptake during treadmill exercise in mice. Am J Physiol Endocrinol Metab 297: E924–E934
3. Jensen TE, Wojtaszewski JF, Richter EA (2009) AMP-activated protein kinase in contraction regulation of skeletal muscle metabolism: necessary and/or sufficient? Acta Physiol (Oxf) 196:155–174
4. Abbott MJ, Bogachus LD, Turcotte LP (2011) AMPKα2 deficiency uncovers time-dependency in the regulation of contraction-induced palmitate and glucose uptake in mouse muscle. J Appl Physiol 111:125–134
5. Turcotte LP, Fisher JS (2008) Skeletal muscle insulin resistance: roles of fatty acid metabolism and exercise. Phys Ther 88:1–18

AMPK

▶ AMP-Activated Protein Kinase

Amputation

Amputation is a congenital or acquired disability which results in the loss of one or more limbs. Amputations of the upper or lower extremities are performed as a result of trauma, peripheral vascular disease, type II diabetes, tumors, and other medical conditions.

Amyloid

A 40–42 amino acid peptide that aggregates and damages neurons in the brain in Alzheimer's disease.

Amyotrophic Lateral Sclerosis

▶ Neurodegenerative Disease

Anabolic

Metabolic reactions that construct molecules from smaller units and require energy. They tend toward building up organs and tissues by favoring growth and differentiation of cells.

Anabolic Androgens

▶ Anabolic Steroids

Anabolic Hormones

Anabolic hormones are those hormones required to stimulate protein synthesis, either directly or indirectly. This group of hormones includes: testosterone, Growth hormone, insulin and the IGFs. Anabolic processes, triggered by these hormones culminate in the growth and differentiation of tissues, ultimately increasing body size as is the case in skeletal muscle hypertrophy. These hormones may be steroid (testosterone) or peptide (IGF and GH) hormones acting via nuclear or cell surface receptors, respectively. The processes of protein synthesis initiated by anabolic hormones are energy requiring, with the fuel source in the form of adenosine tri-phosphate (ATP). It is not cheap (metabolically) to generate or maintain tissue mass, therefore it is unlikely that an organism will lay down new protein unless it requires that new mass to function. During puberty, males lay down more muscle than females as a consequence of elevated testosterone production. The abuse of anabolic steroids therefore, will culminate in excess hypertrophy of skeletal muscle, beyond what may have occurred naturally.

Anabolic Steroids

FRED HARTGENS

Departments of Epidemiology and Surgery, Maastricht University Medical Centre, Research school CAPHRI, Sports Medicine Centre Maastricht, Maastricht, The Netherlands

Synonyms
Anabolic androgens; Male sex hormones

Definition
Around 1930 androgenic–anabolic steroids (AAS) were developed. AAS are drugs derived from the male sex hormone testosterone. Although many efforts have been undertaken to dissipate the androgenic and anabolic effects, until now this was not successful. Therefore, all AAS still have both androgenic and anabolic effects.

In adults, the androgenic properties stimulate masculinization of the human body including growth of genital size, male body hair distribution, and increase of libido and potency. The anabolic effects refer to building effects on several organ systems, e.g., muscle and bone growth and enlargement of the heart, kidney, and prostate.

Mechanisms of Action
AAS exert their action via several pathways. These substances cross the cell membrane and bind to androgen receptor. The steroid-receptor complex exerts their action in the cell nucleus. Other intracellular routes run via the enzymes 5-α-reductase and aromatase. Under normal circumstances, 5-α-reductase plays an important role in the expression of the sex hormones. The enzyme aromatase converts AAS into female sex hormones and is, therefore, mainly active in the presence of excessive concentrations of AAS (Fig. 1).

Steroids possessing high affinity to these receptors are categorized as (strong) androgens (e.g., metenolone, 19-nortestosterone), whereas others show only low affinity to these receptors (e.g., fluoxymetholone, stanozolol) and therefore are called weak androgens. Moreover, some AAS (e.g., oxymetholone) do not bind to a receptor at all but exert their action via other routes.

Another pathway is mediated by glucocorticoid receptors. AAS may bind to these receptors and exert anti-glucocorticoid actions by counteracting the glucocorticoid-induced breakdown of proteins, resulting in an anti-catabolic effect.

The hematologic system is considered to be influenced by two main pathways: stimulation of erythropoiesis and erythropoietin synthesis in the kidney.

At the muscular level, AAS may induce muscle hypertrophy directly and indirectly via the formation of new muscle fibers. A key role is assigned to satellite cells that are progenitor cells of muscle. AAS increase the number of satellite cells and accelerate the incorporation of these cells in preexisting muscle fibers. The distribution of androgen receptors, that are located predominantly in neck and shoulder girdle muscles resulting in largest muscle growth at these body sites, is also of importance.

The cardiovascular system may be affected by several pathways. Firstly, AAS may enhance the activity of the enzyme hepatic triglyceride lipase. This induces lowering of HDL-cholesterol and elevation of serum LDL-cholesterol serum concentrations, resulting in a decrease of regression of atherogenic plaques in vessel walls. Secondly, AAS affect the haemostatic system unfavorably, especially platelet aggregation, which includes an increased risk for the occurrence of thrombosis. Thirdly, nitric oxide may be of importance. In smooth muscles and arteries, nitric oxide has the property to act as an endothelial-derived relaxing factor. AAS may affect nitric oxide leading to reduced relaxation or induction of vasospasm. Finally, AAS may also directly injure myocardial cells and cause cell death.

Clinical Use

Therapeutic Use of AAS
The main indications for AAS treatment are androgen deficiency states, lichen sclerosis and dystrophy of the vulva, postmenopausal osteoporosis, aplastic anemia and anemia in chronic renal insufficiency. New indications are subject to research yet, and include diseases characterized by catabolic states like COPD, HIV/AIDS, and rheumatic disease conditions.

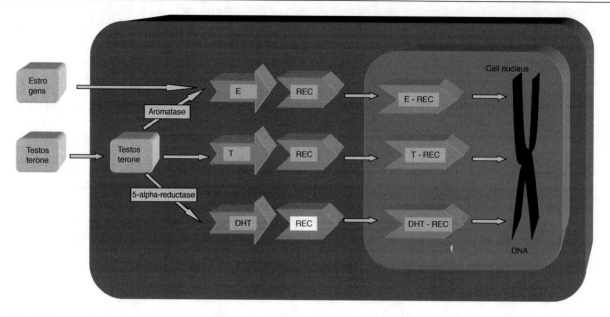

Anabolic Steroids. Fig. 1 Mechanism of action. *T* testosterone, *DHT* dihydrotestosterone, *E* estradiol, *Rec* receptor, *DHT-rec* dihydrotestosterone-receptor complex, *T-rec* testosterone-receptor complex, *E-rec* estradiol-receptor complex

(Mis-)use of AAS in Sport

For many years, the laboratory statistics of the International Olympic Committee (IOC) indicate that AAS are by far the most detected substances at doping analyses. AAS count for over 40% of positive tested urine samples. Moreover, in elite sports not under responsibility of the IOC, many athletes have been found to have used these substances. In some professional sports, especially in strength sports and American football, up to 68% of athletes admitted to have used these drugs during their sports career.

Abuse of AAS by amateur and recreational sportsmen is also widespread. In some sports (especially bodybuilding and power lifting) up to 67% of the athletes used these substances at least once. In addition, in college and high school athletes, misuse of AAS is of great concern, especially in the USA with prevalence rates of 12–15%.

Effects on Body Composition

Body Mass

It is well established that AAS increase body mass. Increments up to 9 kg have been observed after 6 months polydrug AAS abuse in experienced strength athletes. Even in healthy non-training males the administration of testosterone enanthate for 10–20 weeks lead to comparable body mass changes. However, the average mass gain may be considered between 2 and 5 kg, in experienced as well as in novice athletes.

Fat Mass

The fat-reducing properties of AAS are well demonstrated in healthy males. The main sites where fat reduction may be observed are the trunk, limbs, and intermuscular adipose tissue. However, in men under physical training, both novice and experienced, no reduction of fat mass has been observed so far.

Fat-Free Mass

AAS posses strong fat-free mass stimulating properties. For many years, it was assumed that only experienced athletes participating in a strength training program were susceptible. However, recent research revealed that AAS may also stimulate fat-free mass in non-training subjects. Fat-free mass may increase by 2–5 kg, although gains up to 9 kg have been observed. The effects on fat-free mass show a strong dose–response relationship, whereas mode of application and duration of administration seem to be of lesser importance.

Skeletal Muscle

In healthy males, the increase of fat-free mass can be ascribed to stimulation of muscle mass. Examination by ultrasonography and magnetic resonance imaging (MRI) elucidated that muscle mass of selected body parts may increase dramatically under AAS administration. Testosterone enanthate administration (600 mg/week, intramuscularly) for 20 weeks revealed increments up to 15%

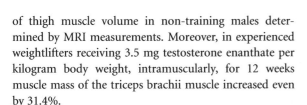
of thigh muscle volume in non-training males determined by MRI measurements. Moreover, in experienced weightlifters receiving 3.5 mg testosterone enanthate per kilogram body weight, intramuscularly, for 12 weeks muscle mass of the triceps brachii muscle increased even by 31.4%.

The muscle mass increments can be attributed to enlargement of muscle fibers, although there are indications that the number of muscle fibers may also increase. The drugs used and methods of administration may influence outcome. In strength athletes participating in their regular strength training program, nandrolone decanoate administered in high therapeutic doses, was not able to affect muscle fiber dimensions. On the other hand, in strength athletes, polydrug administration in supratherapeutic doses lead to the largest alterations of muscle fiber dimensions. Muscle fiber growth after short-term (8–10 weeks) administration was less pronounced compared to long-term administration during 24 weeks, with the longer duration having an advantage of approximately 50%.

In a non-training study in healthy young males, high doses of testosterone enanthate for 20 weeks lead to enlargement of individual muscle fibers in a dose-dependent fashion. Administration of 50 mg/week increased cross-sectional area of slow twitch muscle fibers by 20%, while 600 mg/week counted for an increment of fiber dimension of 50%.

Body Water

Recent investigations showed that the increase of body mass may be attributed to increments of total muscle mass since hydration of fat-free mass was unaffected by AAS. This is in contrast to previous observations indicating that an increase of blood volume and/or water retention was responsible for the body mass increase.

Effects on Performance

Strength

In many sports, muscle strength is an important factor for success. Until recently, it was assumed that AAS might enhance strength only in experienced and well training strength athletes. This was mainly based on the results of two identical studies by the same researchers, in which only the population (experienced strength athletes and non-strength trained students, respectively) under investigation differed. In the last decades, this theory was abandoned when several well-designed studies demonstrated that in novice athletes and even in non-training humans skeletal muscle strength may increase under AAS

treatment. However, in non-training men higher doses of AAS are required to obtain comparable strength improvements than in males receiving AAS and concomitantly participating in a strength training program.

The effects of different drugs on strength may differ, and a dose–response relationship is identified. Duration of drug administration seems of lesser importance.

Endurance

Based on the putative hematological effects it has been proposed that AAS might improve endurance performance. However, all studies in endurance athletes (including runners, cyclists, cross-country skiing) undergoing endurance training were not able to determine any effect of AAS on performance or aerobic capacity. On the contrary, a remarkable observation in two studies was that in strength athletes AAS administration improved aerobic capacity significantly while the subjects did not train their endurance capacity at all. Until now the explanation for this finding remains to be established.

Mixed Strength-Endurance

Only one study investigated the effects of AAS on a combined strength-endurance sports activity, i.e., canoeing, and observed improvements of strength (+6%) and canoeing performance (+9%) after 6 weeks Oral-Turinabol (Dehydrochlormethyltestosterone) usage.

Recovery

Due to the anabolic and anti-catabolic properties of AAS it has been speculated that these substances might enhance recovery in athletes. This effect has been found in animals, but the results in human studies investigating physiological indicators of recovery and performance as well as indirect parameters of recovery (e.g., response of enzymes like creatine phosphokinase and aspartate aminotransferase, heart rate response, steroid hormone responses, lactate response) are inconclusive yet.

Side Effects

AAS have the potential to affect many organs system and therefore may induce untoward effects as well. The most pronounced side effects include the reproductive system, the cardiovascular system, the brain, and liver function.

Reproductive System

AAS exert suppressive effects on the hypothalame-pituitary-gonadal axis. This will lead to lowering of serum levels of testosterone, follicle-stimulating hormone (FSH) and luteinizing hormone (LH). The male athlete may experience alterations of libido and eretile function, testicular athropy, subfertility, gynaecomastia, and prostate dysfunction. Untoward effects in females consist mainly of menstrual irregularities, breast atrophy, clitoris hypertrophy, and masculinization (e.g., hirsutism).

Cardiovascular System
The cardiovascular risk profile may change unfavorably and heart muscle may be affected, partially dependent on the drugs used. AAS suppress serum concentrations of HDL-cholesterol and its subfractions (HDL2- and HDL3-cholesterol), apolipoprotein-B1 levels, and lipoprotein(a), whereas serum levels of LDL-cholesterol and apolipoprotein-A levels increase. AAS do not seem to influence serum triglycerides levels and the effects on serum total cholesterol are inconsistent.

The effects of AAS on blood pressure are inconclusive yet, but indicate that androgenic substances may affect blood pressure more than anabolic agents. Elevation of blood pressure may occur in susceptible persons, but do not exceed medical reference values.

AAS may affect heart function and structure at the cellular level shortly after starting AAS administration as has been well established in animal studies. In male AAS-using athletes, cross-sectional echocardiographic examinations revealed larger left ventricular wall thickness, posterior wall thickness, and interventricular septum thickness compared to non-using counterparts, and additionally, diastolic function may be impaired. However, such alterations could not be observed in short-term prospective studies until now. Therefore, the influence of AAS on heart function remains to be established.

Liver
The hazardous effects of AAS on the hepatic system are well recognized from patient studies. The most pronounced observations include subcelllular changes of hepatocytes, impaired excretion function, cholestasis, peliosis hepatis, hepatocellular hyperplasia, and carcinomata. The most liver toxic substances are the 17-alpha-alkylated steroids, like oxymetholone and methyltestosterone.

On the other hand, in athletic populations such untoward effects on the liver could not be confirmed after short-term (weeks to months) use of AAS. Serum liver function enzyme alterations under AAS seem to be limited. Slight transient elevations of ALAT and ASAT may occur after taking oral AAS, whereas other liver enzymes remain unaffected. Nevertheless, the occurrence of liver disease should be of great concern in athletes abusing AAS, especially in those administering these substances for prolonged periods.

Psyche and Behavior
Psychological state and behavior are affected by AAS use. Most reported are increased irritability, greater drive to train, and several (minor) mood disturbances. Serious psychiatric problems may occur only in a few AAS users and is associated with abuse of higher doses of AAS administration. The most pronounced alterations are increased aggression and hostility, mood disturbances (e.g., mania, psychosis, depression) and criminal behavior, including assault and homicide. Athletes in cosmetic sports are dissatisfied with their body and expose a narcissistic personality that may trigger starting AAS abuse. Moreover, AAS dependence and withdrawal effects are seen in a substantial number of AAS abusers.

Other
In case reports, a large number of side effects have been associated with AAS abuse in athletes, including disturbance of glucose metabolism and thyroid function, occurrence of acne vulgaris and fulminans, sebaceous glands alterations, reduction of immune function, myocardial infarction, suicidal efforts, musculoskeletal injuries, bladder and prostate dysfunction. Furthermore, the formation of tumors (e.g., renal cell carcinoma, Wilm's tumor) has been ascribed to AAS abuse in athletes. However, such reports have to be interpreted with some reservations.

Diagnostics
The use of AAS in sports is prohibited by doping regulations of the national and international sports federations. Since 1976, laboratory techniques to detect AAS are available. For decades, AAS are the most detected substances in doping controls in sports. In athletes, urine samples are obtained for analysis of doping substances, including AAS, by specialized laboratories that are accredited by the International Olympic Committee. Athletes who test positive on AAS will be punished by the sports federations.

References
1. Casavant MJ, Blake K et al (2007) Consequences of use of anabolic androgenic steroids. Pediatr Clin North Am 54(4):677–690, x
2. Friedl K (2000) Effect of anabolic steroid use on body composition and physical performance. In: Yesalis C (ed) Anabolic steroids in sport and exercise, vol 2. Human Kinetics, Champaign, pp 139–174
3. Hall RC, Hall RC (2005) Abuse of supraphysiologic doses of anabolic steroids. South Med J 98(5):550–555
4. Hartgens F, Kuipers H (2004) Effects of androgenic-anabolic steroids in athletes. Sports Med 34(8):513–554
5. Kutscher EC, Lund BC et al (2002) Anabolic steroids: a review for the clinician. Sports Med 32(5):285–296
6. Van Amsterdam J, Opperhuizen A, Hartgens F (2010) Adverse health effects of anabolic androgenic steroids. Reg Pharmacol Toxicol 57:117–123

Anaerobic Activity

Anaerobic activity is a more intense form of muscular activity, where the cardiorespiratory system is unable to supply sufficient oxygen to meet metabolic demand, and there is a significant accumulation of lactate. Anaerobic activity is fuelled only by carbohydrate, and is rapidly fatiguing.

Anaerobic Energy Expenditure

Cellular energy demands that are met by anaerobic metabolism: glycolysis/glycogenolysis and stored ATP/CP.

Anaerobic Glycolysis

The catabolism of glucose or glycogen to lactic acid.

Anaerobic Metabolism

JAMES R. MCDONALD, L. BRUCE GLADDEN
Department of Kinesiology, Auburn University, Auburn, AL, USA

Synonyms
Fermentation; Glycolysis; Phosphagen system

Definition
"▶ Anaerobic metabolism" is the production of adenosine triphosphate (ATP) through energy pathways that do not require oxygen. From early in the twentieth century, anaerobic metabolism implied pathways of energy metabolism that were activated due to a lack of O_2 (dysoxia) [1]. However, it is now clear that the more common condition for faster rates of anaerobic ATP production is simply increased exercise intensity. In other words, neither a complete absence of O_2 (anoxia) nor a relative lack of O_2 (hypoxia) is a prerequisite for the recruitment of anaerobic pathways, and in fact, these pathways are routinely stimulated, both at the onset of exercise in the transition from rest to mild-to-moderate activity and during high-intensity exercise as more Type II muscle fibers are recruited [2].

Basic Mechanisms
What are the anaerobic reactions? The starting point is ATP hydrolysis:

$$ATP + H_2O >>>>>>>>> ADP + Pi + Energy$$

where ADP is adenosine diphosphate and Pi is inorganic phosphate. ATP is of course the universal supplier of energy, the "energy currency" of the cell, i.e., the chemical form that is required for most energy-requiring processes in the body. Foods are ingested and metabolized with a significant portion of the energy release being captured in the form of ATP. In exercise metabolism, the major energy-requiring processes in skeletal muscle are (1) crossbridge cycling to produce force and movement with the catalytic enzyme being myosin ATPase, (2) re-sequestration of Ca^{2+} into the sarcoplasmic reticulum powered by Ca^{2+}-ATPase, and (3) restoration of the membrane potential via the Na^+-K^+-ATPase pump [4].

Although ATP is the required energy form, it is stored only in small quantities within the skeletal muscle [3, 5], only enough for a few seconds (s) of all-out sprinting. Thus, ATP must be replenished rapidly during exercise, or muscle contraction will stop. The pathways to replenish ATP typically keep levels at 70% or more of the resting concentration, and rarely if ever does the ATP concentration decline below 50% of the resting value [2].

Despite these relatively small changes in ATP concentration, cellular stores of ATP are considered part of the "immediate" anaerobic system because they are the first energy source used at the onset of exercise. These stores are replenished by (1) other components of the ▶ immediate energy system, (2) the glycolytic system, and (3) the oxidative system. All of these systems are stimulated at the onset of exercise, but the immediate and glycolytic systems have much, much faster response times. The major reaction of the immediate system involves phosphocreatine (PC):

$$PC + ADP <<<<<>>>>> ATP + C \, (creatine)$$

This reaction is catalyzed by creatine kinase and is so rapid and effective at resupplying ATP that it took nearly 35 years from the identification of ATP and PC until Cain and Davies in 1962 directly demonstrated (by poisoning the creatine kinase reaction) that ATP was the required energy form for muscle contractions [1]. Energy from the ATP and PC stores is delivered, as the name of the system implies, immediately with the start of exercise/muscle contraction. Experimental evidence shows that PC concentration declines by several mM in the first 10 s of heavy exercise with a continued rapid decline to approximately 30 s when PC is below 50% of its resting value, and continues to be depleted by as much as 80% or more as exercise is prolonged. The creatine kinase reaction reverses when there is an abundance of ATP as occurs in recovery [4].

Also part of the immediate energy system and triggered by intense exercise is the reaction catalyzed by adenylate kinase, sometimes referred to as myokinase in skeletal muscle:

$$ADP + ADP <<<<<>>>> ATP + AMP$$

This reaction provides another route for replenishment of ATP, and reduces the concentration of ADP. This is arguably important for maintaining a higher ATP/ADP ratio which helps to maintain a high energy of hydrolysis for ATP breakdown [4]. While the immediate system appears to become fully active within the first 1–2 s after the onset of exercise, ▶ glycolysis, the second anaerobic system, is hypothesized to reach its maximum rate within about 7 s after exercise onset and then become the predominant system for ATP production as all-out exercise continues beyond 10 s [2]. Glycolysis continues to be the major producer of ATP until the aerobic system, ▶ oxidative phosphorylation, takes precedence in activities of longer duration. This has been generally considered to occur at 120 s of exercise but newer evidence has led to a downward revision to approximately 75 s [2].

Glycolysis, the second major anaerobic energy system, begins with glucose or glycogen and then through a series of enzymatic steps, produces two molecules of ATP and two molecules of pyruvate. Pyruvate is rapidly converted to lactate in a reaction catalyzed by lactate dehydrogenase (LDH), the enzyme having the highest activity of any enzyme in the glycolytic pathway. Due to this high activity, the LDH reaction is near-equilibrium, a condition in which the reaction is heavily in the direction of lactate such that lactate concentration is typically 10–200 times greater than pyruvate concentration [2]. Accordingly, lactate can correctly be considered the normal end product of glycolysis, regardless of whether or not lactate is increasing in concentration. At exercise intensities below 100% of maximal O_2 uptake ($\dot{V}O_{2max}$), most of the lactate is reconverted to pyruvate in locations near mitochondria where the pyruvate enters the mitochondrial matrix to be fully oxidized through the pyruvate dehydrogenase reaction and the reactions of the Krebs cycle.

The starting fuels for glycolysis are either glucose or glycogen (via glycogenolysis), but during intense exercise, glycogen becomes the sole fuel source. This is fortuitous given that the net ATP gain from glycogen to lactate is 3 as compared to only 2 ATP when glucose is the fuel.

Figure 1 illustrates the oxygen uptake ($\dot{V}O_2$) response to a submaximal exercise task and clearly shows that all

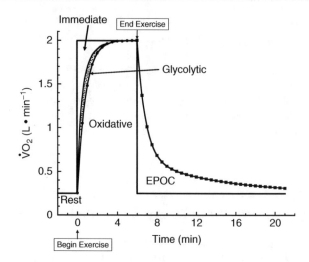

Anaerobic Metabolism. Fig. 1 $\dot{V}O_2$ for 6 min of submaximal exercise followed by 15 min of recovery. Oxidative metabolism is indicated by the area under the $\dot{V}O_2$ on-kinetics curve. Glycolytic metabolism is indicated by the stippled area. The clear area above the glycolytic area, bounded by the steady state VO_2 (min 4–6) at the *top* and the start of exercise on the *left*, is the immediate energy system contribution (primarily PC breakdown). The sum of the glycolytic and immediate areas is the O_2 deficit. In recovery (which begins at min 6), the VO_2 above the pre-exercise resting baseline is the O_2 debt, or EPOC (excess postexercise oxygen consumption). See text for additional discussion

three of the energy systems are activated at exercise onset, but that the oxidative system is slowest to reach its full expression (2–3 min). $\dot{V}O_2$ on-kinetics describe the oxidative response and also reveal that there is an ▶ O_2 deficit in terms of energy equivalents in the early phase of exercise. The oxidative energy equivalents for this deficit are provided by the rapidly activated immediate (primarily PC) and glycolytic energy systems. In recovery, the $\dot{V}O_2$ remains elevated above the pre-exercise level for a considerable period of time, producing what is known as an ▶ O_2 debt or ▶ EPOC (excess postexercise O_2 consumption). There is a general relationship between the EPOC and O_2 deficit mainly because the PC that is broken down at exercise onset is resynthesized early in recovery at an added energy cost above the pre-exercise baseline. However, the contribution of lactate removal to the EPOC is variable, and typically small because most of the lactate accumulated during early exercise is oxidized as a fuel during recovery, a process that does not require extra O_2 consumption [2]. Much of the EPOC (other than that due to PC resynthesis) is caused by elevated cardiovascular and respiratory activity, elevated hormones (particularly epinephrine), elevated body temperature, and fatty acid recycling with an additional small amount for refilling blood and muscle O_2 stores.

Rapid accumulation of lactate in muscle and blood with an accompanying decrease in pH is the hallmark of accelerated glycolysis. At normal body pH values (6.4–7.4) both pyruvic acid and lactic acid are nearly completely dissociated into a proton (H^+) and a pyruvate or lactate anion, respectively. Lactate movement across cell membranes is facilitated by a family of carrier proteins called monocarboxylate transporters (MCTs) of which MCT1, MCT2, and MCT4 appear to be the major isoforms [1, 2]. Currently, there is overwhelming evidence that lactate is not simply a dead-end waste product, but is instead a highly mobile fuel that circulates through the body from lactate-producing tissues to lactate-utilizing tissues [1, 2]. Resting and mild to moderately exercising muscles (particularly oxidative muscle fibers), the heart, and the brain can use lactate as a fuel. The liver and kidney are primary sites for lactate uptake and conversion to glucose (gluconeogenesis). This distribution of lactate and its utilization by most tissues of the body is known as the ► cell-to-cell lactate shuttle, a concept that was formulated by George Brooks at the University of California, Berkeley [2].

Exercise Interventions

The anaerobic systems are involved at the onset of all types of exercise, but are especially prevalent in high-intensity exercise. Therefore, these systems are relevant in short bursts of speed and power that are typically found in sports like football, weightlifting, gymnastics, and basketball, as well as in sprinting, track, swimming, and cycling. Exercises for training the phosphagen and glycolytic systems are generally intense, of short duration, and involve more time in recovery than in the exercise itself [5].

PC concentration in muscles can be elevated by exercise training and creatine supplementation. Exercises to improve this system focus on repeated short sprint activity (e.g., 10 s) with comparatively much longer recovery intervals. "Creatine loading" to elevate resting PC levels elicits improvement in exercise performance in short-duration events and faster gains in muscle mass and strength with resistance training [4]. However, results with highly trained athletes, in particular elite sprint athletes, are sparse and less clear, failing to show clear improvements in performance with creatine loading.

Training the glycolytic system focuses on improving the body's ability to buffer or tolerate high lactate levels and the accompanying acidosis [5]. Events that rely mainly on the glycolytic system and thus create high lactate levels include running and swimming events between 30 s and 2 min. Training usually relies on high-intensity efforts of the same length or slightly longer than the target event with shorter recovery periods. Recovery between intense exercises as in interval training ranges from twice the exercise time, a 1:2 ratio, to half the time it took to complete the exercise, a 1:0.5 ratio.

References

1. Brooks GA, Gladden LB (2003) The metabolic systems: anaerobic metabolism (glycolytic and phosphagen). In: Tipton CM (ed) Exercise physiology: people and ideas. Oxford University Press, New York, pp 322–360
2. Gladden LB (2003) Lactate metabolism during exercise. In: Poortmans JR (ed) Principles of exercise biochemistry, 3rd edn. Karger, Basel, pp 322–360
3. Gollnick PD (1973) Biochemical adaptations to exercise: anaerobic metabolism. Exerc Sport Sci Rev 1:1–44
4. Houston ME (2006) Biochemistry primer for exercise science. Human Kinetics, Champaign
5. Kraemer WJ (1994) General adaptations to resistance and endurance training programs. In: Baechle TR (ed) Essentials of strength training and conditioning. Human Kinetics, Champaign, pp 127–150

Anaerobic Power, Test of

OMRI INBAR
Department of Life Sciences, Zinman College Wingate Institute, Netania, Israel

Synonyms
Short-term power testing

Definition
Anaerobic power testing is the evaluation of the human capacity to perform short-term work at the highest possible rate. Relevant work durations range from a few seconds to about 1 min.

Description

Historical Perspective
Quantification of anaerobic power and fitness did not start taking place until the mid-1960s – nearly a quarter of a century since aerobic power testing began. Despite its role as a major component of physical performance capacity, anaerobic fitness testing is still rarely included in standard fitness evaluations.

Anaerobic Metabolism

Higher organisms use anaerobic metabolism for two primary reasons: (a) to bridge temporary gaps between the slow-responding aerobic metabolism and the immediate energy demands at the onset of physical activity and (b) to supplement aerobic metabolism in attaining short-term power output exceeding that which can be attained by aerobic metabolism alone.

There are two distinct kinds of anaerobic energy sources: (a) *Phospholytic energy,* derived from tapping existing phosphagen (ATP & PCr) stores. While its response to exercise demands and the rate of its release (power) are extremely high, the total energy available from phospholysis is greatly limited by phosphagen stores' size. (b) *Glycolytic energy,* which produces new ATP and replenishes phosphagen stores via glycolysis. The energy available from this source depends on exercise mode and intensity and on hydrogen ion accumulation, but is many times greater than phospholytic energy. Maximal glycolytic power output is intermediate between maximal aerobic power and peak phospholytic power outputs.

Functional Attributes of Anaerobic Power

By its very nature, anaerobic power production is largely independent of circulation and oxygen supply and, therefore, is mostly determined by the metabolic and functional (e.g., neuro-motor control, motor-unit composition) characteristics of the involved muscles. That is, unlike aerobic power, which to a large extent depends on central cardiopulmonary factors, anaerobic power is a local/peripheral phenomenon. This would mean, for example, that training the anaerobic power of a given muscle or muscle group cannot be expected to affect other muscles. While aerobic power is directly related to oxygen consumption, there is no comparable variable by which the anaerobic component of a given exercise can be teased out from the overall power output. Thus, anaerobic power must be evaluated by physical exercise that is sufficiently short so as to limit aerobic contribution and ensure anaerobic dominance of the test.

General Considerations in Anaerobic Testing

General anaerobic fitness. Being muscle-specific, anaerobic performance capacity cannot be whole-body tested. However, in the general untrained or non-specifically trained population, there is a good correlation between the anaerobic fitness of major muscle groups (e.g., legs) and the rest of the body's musculature. General anaerobic fitness, therefore, is typically tested in leg exercise (mainly cycling).

Upper-/lower-body specificity. When lower-body (leg) ergometry is impossible (e.g., in paraplegics, leg amputees), or when specific training is involved (e.g., kayaking vs. cycling, or swimming vs. running), upper-body (arm) ergometry can be performed to best represent the individual's anaerobic fitness.

Specificity of test modality. Anaerobic training effects are specific not only to the involved muscle group but to the specific nature and modality of training. Thus, compared to a runner, a cyclist is expected to have *a priori* advantage in cycle ergometry although nearly identical muscle groups are involved.

Test duration. Determines the proportional contribution of aerobic vs. anaerobic metabolism to the measured work and power output and the relative involvement of anaerobic endurance in the overall performance. Thus, the longer the test, the higher the aerobic contribution and the involvement of anaerobic endurance (enduring increasing acidosis).

Phospholytic power. Can only be estimated by ~5–10-s all-out exertions or from the initial segments of like durations in longer all-out exertions.

Glycolytic power. Fully activated only several seconds into a strenuous exertion, it has a longer effective span than phospholytic power. It is therefore best estimated by maximal exertions of 20–40 s. Shorter durations would be too phospholytic while longer ones too aerobic.

Anaerobic capacity. The kinetics of the phospholytic, glycolytic, and aerobic metabolic pathways do not allow for a single exertion to provide a work- or power-output value representative of the whole-body capacity for anaerobic energy production. This is reflected by the highest attainable lactate concentration, typically following ~2–4 min of maximal whole-body (e.g., rowing, cross-country skiing) or lower-body (e.g., running, cycling) exercise. Lactate, however, is only a rough indicator since lactate is unevenly distributed among the various body compartments and is already actively metabolized during the exertion. The accepted, more valid measure of anaerobic capacity is the maximal oxygen debt (excess post-exercise oxygen consumption) following such an exertion. It should be re-emphasized that in athletes a meaningful test must involve their specific mode of exercise.

Subject population. Anaerobic testing is extremely intense and for reasons of both safety and relevance it should not be administered to the old, the frail, or the cardiovascularly impaired.

Application

Various tests have been used since the mid-1960s for evaluating anaerobic fitness. Some of the most common and significant are described in Table 1.

The nature of anaerobic fitness dictates that no single test can provide the best possible evaluation of all its components.

Anaerobic Power, Test of. Table 1 Comparison of common laboratory tests of anaerobic fitness

Test	Ergometer	Duration	Measures	Reliability	Validity	Comments
Motorized treadmill test (MTT)	Treadmill	80–120 s	Anaerobic capacity	$r = 0.76$–0.84	Low (high aerobic contribution)	
Non-motorized treadmill test (NMT)	Passive, non-motorized treadmill	30 s	GP, PP	$r = 0.82$ – PP, 0.88 – GP	Aerobic contribution not known	Non-standardized computation of power
Isokinetic mono-articular test (IMT)	Isokinetic dynamometer	30 s	GP, PP, FI	No data	$r = 0.94$ for GP. Low r's for PP, FI, and sprinting capacity	Expensive equipment
					Isokinetic contractions are atypical of normal exercise tasks	Difficult to modify for children
Wingate anaerobic test (WAnT)	Cycle-ergometer	30 s	GP, PP, FI	$r = 0.87$–0.98	High with many anaerobic-type performances and physiologic measures	Most validated and researched test
						Simple to perform
						Applicable to both lower and upper extremities
Force-velocity cycling test (FVT)	Cycle-ergometer	4–6 sprints, 5–10 s each	Mainly PP	11.9% test-retest CV for PP 3.5% for adolescents	No data	Time consuming (40–60 min)
						Motivation is likely compromised with duration
Isokinetic cycling test	Cycle-ergometer	6 s	PP only	5.4% test-retest CV for GP	Isokinetic contractions are atypical of normal exercise tasks	Time consuming
						Expensive equipment
Accumulated oxygen deficit test (AOD)	Cycle-ergometer or treadmill	2–4 min	Anaerobic capacity	0.95–0.98 interclass correlations for time to exhaustion	Low correlations with WAnT, but good correspondence with several anaerobic field performances	Time consuming (lengthy pretests to establish VO_2-power relationships)
						Exercise mode specific
						Assumed linearity of VO_2-power relationship below and above AnT

PP phopholytic/peak power, *GP* glycolytic power, *FI* fatigue index (WAnT), *CV* coefficient of variation, *AnT* anaerobic threshold

Particular needs may be met by different tests. Also, anaerobic tests were typically developed on healthy and active young adult populations. Extending the use of such tests to children and other atypical populations may be unwarranted.

Since the mid-1970s, the Wingate Anaerobic Test (WAnT) has been the most researched, validated, reliability-verified, and widely used test on varied populations, and it evaluates three distinct anaerobic fitness components [1, 2]. The WAnT is the universally accepted test of choice and will be described in the following sections.

The WAnT

Ergometers. While electromagnetically braked cycle-ergometers have been a boon to general ergometry, their loading characteristics in WAnT ergometry have not yet been reconciled with those of their mechanically braked counterparts. Only the latter will be referred to here. Upper-body ergometry is facilitated by modified cycle-ergometers or dedicated arm-ergometers with identical test protocols [1].

Setup. Seat height is individually adjusted according to accepted standards, with toe-clips or the equivalent used for securing feet to pedals. A forward leaning posture is attained by proper handlebar adjustments. In arm ergometry the crank axis of rotation should be set at shoulder height. In both leg and arm ergometry, both ergometers and subjects must be secured in a way that prevents undue motion during the test.

Resistance load. Determined according to body mass and composition, age, and fitness level, as recommended in Table 2.

Warm-up. Five to ten minutes of mild to moderate intensity pedalling interspersed in its latter part by three 4- to 7-s all-out sprints against the gradually applied test load; a rest period of 2–3 min follows.

Load application.

(a) Upon the start command, the subject accelerates the unloaded flywheel, *as fast as possible*, against its inertial resistance.
(b) Following ~3 s, as pedal revolution rate starts to plateau the predetermined load is applied.
(c) The actual test begins (monitoring of time and pedal revolutions). The subject continues to pedal, as fast as possible (no pacing), for the entire 30-s duration of the test. Verbal encouragement is continuously given to facilitate maximal effort.

Results. Figure 1 illustrates a typical WAnT output and its three derived variables:

(a) *Mean Power* (MP). Mean power output throughout the test's 30-s duration. It is the WAnT's primary variable (for which the test was optimized) and largely represents glycolytic power. It is calculated as:

$$MP_{(Watt)} = M_{Load} * g * D * n_{30}/30$$

where M_{Load} = resistance (friction) load mass (kg)

Anaerobic Power, Test of. Table 2 Recommended resistance loading

Units: • $J \cdot kg^{-1} BW \cdot rev^{-1}$ [a] • $g \cdot kg^{-1} BW$ (Fleisch) • $g \cdot kg^{-1} BW$ (Monark)		Children		Adolescents and young adults (up to ~30 year)
		Pre-pubescent	Pubescent	
Leg ergometry	♂	3.92	4.41	4.90
		40	45	50
		66.7	75	83.3
	♀	3.92	4.41	4.70
		40	45	48
		66.7	75	80
Arm ergometry	♂	2.65	2.94	3.43
		27	30	35
		45	50	58.3
	♀	2.65	2.65	2.65
		27	27	27
		45	45	45
"Reference" subject		Lean to normal weight, sedentary to mildly active		
Age adjustment		Reduce resistance by ~5% for every 10 years beyond 30		
% Fat adjustment		Reduce resistance by ~10% for every 10% rise in fat percentage above 15%		
Fitness adjustment (anaerobic fitness)		- Reduce resistance by up to 10% for particularly unfit subjects		
		- Raise resistance by ~10% for active, anaerobically fit subjects		
		- Raise resistance by ~20% for elite anaerobically trained subjects		

Electromagnetically braked WAnT ergometers set their own resistance and are not adjustable
[a]Universal loading unit, independent of specific design of the particular mechanically braked ergometer

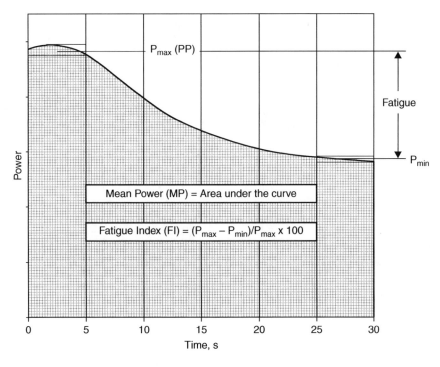

Anaerobic Power, Test of. Fig. 1 WAnT schematics

$g = 9.81$ m/s^2 (gravitational acceleration)

D = flywheel circumference (m) [6 and 10 m for Monark and Fleisch, resp.]

n_{30} = 30-s pedal revolutions count

(b) *Peak Power* (PP). The mean of the highest 5-s power output (typically, the first 5 s). Largely represents pholpholytic power.

$$PP_{(Watt)} = M_{Load} * g * D * n_{max}/5$$

where n_{max} = highest 5-s pedal revolutions count

(c) *Fatigue Index* (FI). The percentage drop in power output from PP to P_{min} (see Fig. 1). FI is typically low in endurance-athletes and high in power-athletes.

Recommended Resistance Loading

Maximal power is the largest attainable product of force (resistance) and velocity ($\propto$ pedal RPM). Since the two components are conversely interrelated, maximal power occurs at the mid-portions of their attainable ranges. Optimal load, therefore, is one that enables maximal power output in most cases of a given subject population. Compared with the normal stature and fitness, subjects of higher relative muscle mass or fitness require higher loads while overweight or under-fit subjects require reduced loads [1, 3].

The WAnT is optimized to maximize MP. Table 2 provides the recommended loads for standard child and adult

populations of both sexes with adjustments for body composition, age, and fitness level.

The use of optimal braking torque based on total body mass assumes that people have a similar relationship between muscle mass and total body mass. While this may be true for the general healthy population, it will be untrue for people with marked obesity, malnourished, muscle atrophy, muscle dystrophy, etc. Further research is required to assess the optimal resistance for such groups.

Limitations/Special Considerations [4]

While the WAnT has been widely used and is the test of choice since the early 1980s, variability in application has affected the universality of results. This must be accounted for in comparing data from different sources or using performance norms (see below). This variability stems from the following:

1. Use of ergometers of different designs, resistance characteristics, and consequent results. Most notable is the use of mechanically braked cycle-ergometers (on which the WAnT was developed and validated) as well as electromagnetically braked ergometers.

2. Use of different application protocols. Most notable are differences in the timing of load application (test onset) and warm-up characteristics.

3. Use of non-optimal loading.

Anaerobic Power, Test of. Table 3 Predictive equations for typical PP/kg and MP/kg during the WAnT

Limb	Gender	Variable		N	R^2
Leg ergometry	♂	MP/kg	$4.378 + 0.263 \times age - 0.005 \times age^2$	180	0.884
		PP/kg	$4.738 + 0.349 \times age - 0.006 \times age^2$		0.846
	♀	MP/kg	$4.476 + 0.099 \times age - 0.002 \times age^2$	45	0.650
		PP/kg	$2.568 + 0.453 \times age - 0.008 \times age^2$		0.972
Arm ergometry	♂	MP/kg	$-1.07 + 0.613 \times age - 0.016 \times age^2$	130	0.994
		PP/kg	$-0.44 + 0.864 \times age - 0.023 \times age^2$		0.997

No sufficient data are available for females' arms and for the fatigue index

4. Use of a single crank length (170 mm) for adults and children of all sizes.
5. Non-standardized saddle height.
6. Use of different algorithms for WAnT data derivation (e.g., Monark and Lode use different algorithms, both deviating from the original).
7. Computerization and high-resolution revolution counting have increased data accuracy and reliability (PP and FI in particular).
8. WAnT's original algorithm did not account for kinetic energy gained in acceleration, prior to load application, resulting in somewhat inflated power values – PP in particular. Some later algorithms (e.g., Monark and Lode) have corrected this.

Norms

Norms are essential for the evaluation and the establishment of performance criteria. The following normative formulae are the result of a judicious compilation of published data from several sources. Based on these results, stepwise regression analysis was performed to create predictive equations and to determine the accuracy with which peak and mean power, for a standard 30-s WAnT, could be predicted (see Table 3). It should be emphasized, however, that the database is limited in size, particularly in some categories (mainly in females). This, in conjunction with the limitations listed above, places the predicted norms in a tentative rather than authoritative category. Also, children's performance data during maturation is best evaluated relative to maturational rather than chronological age. The former, however, is often unavailable and the norms are consequently age based [2, 5].

Nonetheless, the use of such simple predictive equations allow the calculation of normal values for females and males and for arm and leg WAnT performance of a wide range of ages, for comparison of data to published norms.

References

1. Inbar O, Bar-Or O, Skinner JS (1996) The Wingate anaerobic test. Human Kinetics, Champaign
2. Maud PJ, Schultz BB (1989) Norms for the Wingate anaerobic test with comparison to another similar test. Res Q Exerc Sport 60:144–151
3. Dotan R, Bar-Or O (1983) Load optimization for the Wingate anaerobic test. Eur J Appl Physiol 51:409–417
4. Dotan R (2006) The Wingate anaerobic test's past and future and the compatibility of mechanically versus electro-magnetically braked cycle-ergometers. Eur J Appl Physiol 98:113–116
5. Inbar O, Bar-Or O (1986) Anaerobic characteristics in male children and adolescents. Med Sci Sports Exerc 18:264–269

Anaerobic Threshold

KARLMAN WASSERMAN
Respiratory and Critical Care Physiology and Medicine, David Geffen School of Medicine, University of California at Los Angeles, Los Angeles Biomedical Research Institute, Harbor-UCLA Medical Center, Torrance, CA, USA

Synonyms

Individual anaerobic threshold (IAT); Lactate threshold; Lactic acidosis threshold

Definition

The anaerobic threshold (AT) is the exercise O_2 uptake ($\dot{V}o_2$) below which work is sustained totally aerobically, without an increase in arterial blood lactate, and that level of exercise above which ▶ anaerobic glycolysis supplements ▶ aerobic glycolysis, lactate accumulates, lactic acidosis develops, and the lactate/pyruvate ratio increases (the Pasteur effect).

Below the AT, the transport of O_2 to the muscles is sufficient to regenerate the adenosine triphosphate (ATP) to power the muscles, aerobically (mitochondrial respiration). Above the *AT*, the muscle capillary PO_2 falls to a critically low level, so that if exercise level increases, anaerobic glycolysis increases, and lactate accumulates in the systemic circulation (Fig. 1) [1]. The *AT* could be determined by measuring the threshold of arterial lactate increase, bicarbonate decrease, or the onset of increased CO_2 output from HCO_3^- buffering of lactic acid (gas exchange) [2, 3].

Description

The *AT* was developed as a measure of cardiovascular function, i.e., the maximal rate at which the circulation is able to supply O_2 for sustaining a given form of exercise, aerobically. Above the *AT*, anaerobic glycolysis and lactate accumulation are added to the aerobic bioenergetic sources of *ATP* during exercise [4].

Differences Between Aerobic and Anaerobic Glycolysis

Glucose (glycogen) is the primary substrate which undergoes catabolism to regenerate *ATP* for exercise

(Fig. 2) [6]. There is an oxidative step in glycolysis in which coenzyme nicotinamide adenine dinucleotide (NAD^+) accepts two protons, converting it to the reduced form ($NADH + H^+$). To continue the breakdown of glucose to pyruvate, and subsequent decarboxylation to combine with co-enzyme-A for acetate's entry into the mitochondrial tricarboxylic acid cycle and electron transport chain complex, the reduced cytosolic $NADH + H^+$ must be reoxidized back to NAD^+. For this, $NADH + H^+$ must be reoxidized either by the mitochondrial membrane shuttle, aerobically (Fig. 2, pathway A) or, anaerobically by pyruvate (Fig. 2, pathway B). Pathway A consists of dihydroxy acetone phosphate which reoxidizes $NADH + H^+$ back to NAD^+. The resulting saturated molecule is glycerol phosphate, which is apparently readily permeable to the outer mitochondrial membrane. In the mitochondria, glycerol phosphate is reoxidized by flavine adenine dinucleotide (FAD). The reduced $FADH + H^+$ is reoxidized back to FAD by the electron transport chain, with the production of two *ATP* [6]. If the O_2 supply to the mitochondria were insufficient to reoxidize

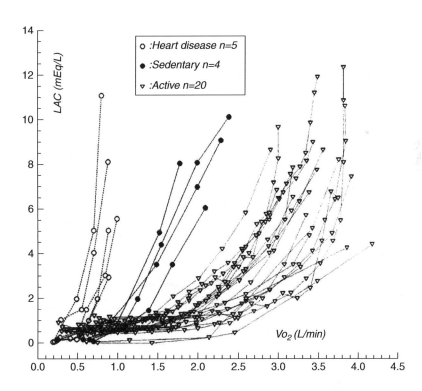

Anaerobic Threshold. Fig. 1 Pattern of increase in arterial lactate in active and sedentary healthy subjects and patients with heart disease as a function of oxygen uptake ($\dot{V}o_2$) during exercise. Arterial lactate (LAC) concentration rises from approximately the same resting value to peak concentration at maximal exercise in each of the three groups. The fitter the subject for aerobic work, the higher the $\dot{V}o_2$ before lactate starts to increase above resting levels. (Modified from [1])

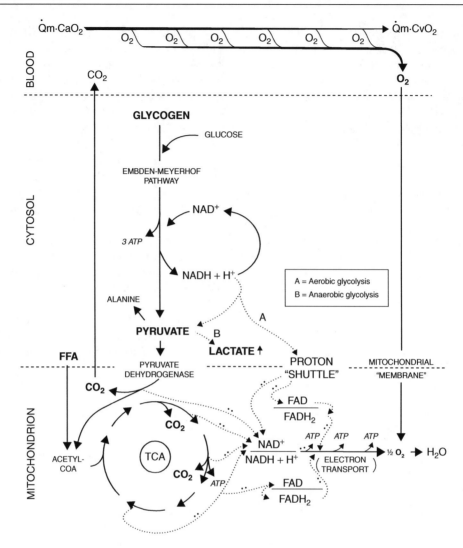

Anaerobic Threshold. Fig. 2 The major biochemical pathways for production of *ATP*. The transfer of H$^+$ and electrons to O$_2$ by the mitochondrial electron transport chain and the "shuttle" of protons from the cytosol to the mitochondrion (*Pathway A*) are the essential components of aerobic glycolysis. This allows the efficient use of carbohydrate substrate in regenerating *ATP* to replace that consumed by muscle contraction. Also illustrated is the important O$_2$ flow from the blood to the mitochondrion, without which the aerobic energy generating mechanisms within the mitochondrion would come to a halt. At the sites of inadequate O$_2$ flow to mitochondria, *Pathway B* serves to reoxidize *NADH + H$^+$* to *NAD$^+$* with a net increase in lactic acid production (lactate accumulation). Lactate will increase relative to pyruvate as *NADH + H$^+$/NAD$^+$* increases in the cytosol [5]

the mitochondrial membrane proton shuttle (glycerol-3 phosphate) back to its unsaturated form (dihydroxy acetone phosphate), pyruvate reoxidizes cytosolic NADH + H$^+$ back to NAD$^+$. By accepting the two protons, pyruvate becomes lactate.

Lactate accumulation is an end reaction of anaerobiosis. It is reversed back to pyruvate when sufficient O$_2$ is available to normalize the cytosolic redox state (NADH + H$^+$/NAD$^+$) [1, 7]. As the cytosolic redox state moves to the reduced state, anaerobic glycolysis accelerates, and the arterial lactate/pyruvate ratio increases (Fig. 3) [7]. The increased lactate/pyruvate ratio reverses at the start of recovery from exercise [7].

Lactate Accumulates During Exercise at a Threshold V̇o$_2$

Careful repeated studies of arterial lactate relative to increasing $\dot{V}o_2$ reveal that lactate concentration increases

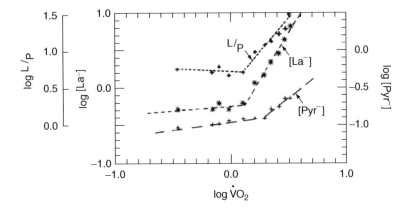

Anaerobic Threshold. Fig. 3 Arterial log lactate [La⁻], log pyruvate [Pyr⁻], and log lactate/pyruvate (L/P) ratio plotted against log $\dot{V}_{O_2}$. The log-log transform of the lactate-$\dot{V}_{O_2}$ and pyruvate-$\dot{V}_{O_2}$ relationships allows easy detection of the lactate and pyruvate inflection points. The pyruvate inflection point is at a higher $\dot{V}_{O_2}$ than the lactate inflection point. Because the pre-threshold pyruvate slope is the same as the lactate slope, the L/P ratio does not increase until after the lactate inflection point [7]

at a threshold $\dot{V}_{O_2}$ [7, 8]. It does not increase as a continuum or exponential function [8], as some authors had speculated. The ▶ lactate threshold increases with fitness and decreases with cardiovascular diseases affecting O_2 transport [1].

Lactate accumulates during exercise as an anion, its negative charge being balanced by H^+. Thus it requires buffering to maintain arterial H^+ homeostasis and avoid physiologically important changes in arterial blood pH. This is done by bicarbonate (HCO_3^-), a ▶ volatile buffer. See equation below:

$$pHa = pK_1 + [Na^+HCO_3^-]/[H_2CO_3]$$
$$= pK_2 + [Na^+Lac^-]/[H^+Lac^-]$$
$$= pK_3 + [Na^+Org^-]/[H^+Org^-]$$

Na^+Org^- represents all salts of weak acids capable of serving as acid buffers and are converted to acids (H^+Org^-) when buffering. These nonvolatile buffers can be activated to buffer H^+ only when the pHa changes, sufficiently. However, pH changes of the aqueous fluids of the body are defended, first and foremost, by the HCO_3^- buffer. Theoretically and experimentally, HCO_3^- is the first buffer used to regulate cell and blood H^+ because the resulting acid, H_2CO_3, dissociates into CO_2 and H_2O. The CO_2 is eliminated by the lungs, while the H_2O is neutral. As long as HCO_3^- buffer is available, nonvolatile buffers could not serve as H^+ buffers because the H^+ concentration increases little. To buffer H^+, the nonvolatile buffer would need to be exposed to a significantly reduced pH and be quantitatively significant relative to HCO_3^-.

Buffering of the Accumulating Lactate

Lactate is the end product of anaerobic glycolysis. Its pK equals 3.8. Therefore, over 99% of the lactate increase during exercise is dissociated, functioning as an anion, its negative charge balanced by H^+ at the pH of blood and cell water. The H_2CO_3 generated during acid buffering dissociates into CO_2 and H_2O. The CO_2 is eliminated by the lungs, leaving behind neutral water. Thus the lungs regulate H^+ of metabolic as well as respiratory origin.

Bicarbonate and Lactate Thresholds

Bicarbonate decrease approximates lactate increase, millimol for millimol, after the first minute of exercise [3, 9, 10]. Figure 4 shows the simultaneous arterial lactate and HCO_3^- concentrations as related to time, while cycling at three different work intensities [10]. Figure 5 shows that virtually all of the lactic acid buffering is by HCO_3^-, although the 1:1 relationship is displaced from the origin by about 0.5–1.0 millimol [9]. Beaver et al. showed that both the increase in lactate and decrease in bicarbonate have $\dot{V}_{O_2}$ thresholds [3]. HCO_3^- decrease is delayed relative to lactate increase by about 0.5 millimol [3]. This delay in HCO_3^- decrease relative to lactate increase was consistent in three studies in which the stoichiometry of the buffering was determined [3, 9, 10].

The buffer of the lactic acid accumulated during the first minute of exercise is also HCO_3^-. However, it is new bicarbonate formed during exercise with the alkalinization of muscle after the start of exercise [11]. It corresponds to the splitting of phosphocreatine. The phosphocreatine is an anion, which on splitting becomes

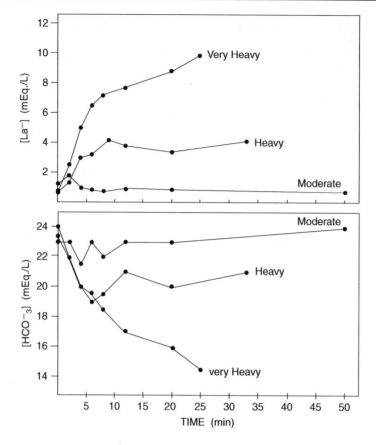

Anaerobic Threshold. Fig. 4 Arterial lactate increase and bicarbonate decrease with time for moderate, heavy, and very heavy exercise intensities for a normal subject. Bicarbonate changes in opposite direction to lactate and in a quantitatively similar manner. While the target exercise duration was 50 min for each work rate, the endurance time was reduced, the greater the lactate increase [5]

a neutral molecule (zwitter ion). This results in an excess of muscle cell cations (K^+), which is seen in the muscle venous blood as early as 5 s after the start of exercise (5 s sampling). The new anion balancing the K^+ is HCO_3^-, generated from aerobic metabolism. Within the first minute of exercise, K^+ and HCO_3^- appear to increase in the muscle venous blood, stoichiometrically [11] with a transient increase in pH. In summary, all of the buffering of the increased lactate concentration during exercise could be accounted for by HCO_3^- buffer, taking into account the HCO_3^- formed during exercise.

The Critical Capillary PO₂

In studies on normal male subjects in whom femoral vein (FV) lactate was measured simultaneous with FV PO_2, Stringer et al. [12] found that lactate did not increase until the end-capillary (FV) PO_2 of the exercising muscle reached a minimum value (approximately 20 mmHg).

The FV PO_2 remained constant, at its minimum value from the AT to peak $\dot{V}_{O_2}$, despite increasing work rate. While FV PO_2 did not decrease further above the lactate threshold, oxyhemoglobin saturation continued to decrease [12]. The decrease in oxyhemoglobin saturation, without a decrease in FV PO_2, could be accounted for by the rightward shift in the oxyhemoglobin dissociation curve caused by the acidification of the capillary blood (Bohr effect) [13].

Koike et al. [14] studied the critical capillary (femoral venous, FV) PO_2 during leg cycling exercise in ten patients with cardiovascular disease. Like the study of Stringer et al. on normal subjects, the FV lactate did not increase until the FV PO_2 decreased to its minimal value, i.e., the critical capillary PO_2. The gas exchange AT occurred soon after the critical capillary PO_2 was reached. Thereafter, the FV PO_2 during increasing work rate either remained constant (five patients) or reversed direction and increased (five

Heavy

Very Heavy

$$Y = .998\,(x) - 0.483$$
$$r = .904$$

$$Y = .951\,(x) - 0.989$$
$$r = .968$$

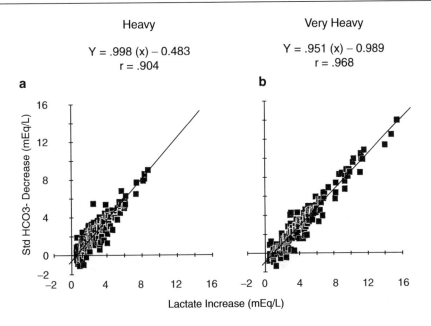

Anaerobic Threshold. Fig. 5 Arterial standard (Std) HCO_3^- decrease as function of lactate increase from resting values for heavy and very heavy work intensities. The decrease in Std HCO_3^- is delayed by about 1 min, allowing lactate to increase by about ½ to 1 millimol/l of arterial blood plasma before HCO_3^- decreases from rest (see regression equations in figure). Changes are approximately equal and opposite (heavy, n = 181: slope = 0.998 (CI 0.92–1.06), intercept = −0.48 (CI −0.71 to −0.26); very heavy, n = 141: slope = 0.951 (CI 0.92–0.98), intercept = −0.99 (CI −1.12 to −0.78)) [9]

patients). However, FV PO_2 did not decrease further, despite increasing work rate and FV lactate [14].

Does the Anaerobic Threshold Demarcate the O_2 Flow Insensitive and Sensitive Zones of Exercise Work Rate?

The mechanisms and patterns of lactate increase during exercise were studied in humans, particularly as related to the O_2 supply–O_2 demand relationships during exercise [15]. Altering O_2 transport was found to affect lactate increase and the AT [16]. Koike et al. [17] measured the effect of reducing blood O_2 content without changing arterial PO_2, by adding low concentrations of carbon monoxide to the inspired air. In this study, carboxyhemoglobin was increased to the 10% and 20% levels in each subject. Peak $\dot{V}O_2$ and AT decreased by approximately the same percent as the reduced O_2 content of the blood. Additionally, $\dot{V}O_2$ was not affected below the subjects measured AT, demonstrating its insensitivity to blood O_2 content. In contrast, the $\dot{V}O_2$ progressively decreased as work rate increased above the AT. The more reduced the arterial blood O_2 content, the greater the reduction in $\dot{V}O_2$. Thus $\dot{V}O_2$ is sensitive to O_2 transport above the AT.

Clinical Use/Application

Gas Exchange Methods for Measuring the Anaerobic (Lactate) Threshold

The use of gas exchange to measure the AT evolved over the past 45 years, as added factors affecting exercise gas exchange were learned. Today and for the past 25 years, we rely primarily on the V-slope method for measuring the AT [2]. The lactic acid increase above the AT is immediately buffered by HCO_3^-, releasing quantitatively, 22.3 ml of CO_2 for every millimol of lactic acid accumulating (Avogadro's number) [18]. The following is a brief overview of how gas exchange measurements evolved to measure the AT (lactate or ▶ lactic acidosis threshold) by gas exchange.

The Increase in Respiratory Exchange Ratio (R)

The 1964 approach was to detect the increase in CO_2 output ($\dot{V}_{CO_2}$) from HCO_3^- buffering of accumulating lactic acid [4]. This was attempted by measuring the increase in the ratio $\dot{V}_{CO_2}/\dot{V}_{O_2}$ or respiratory exchange ratio (R), breath by breath [4]. The hypothesis was that the rate of CO_2 output would increase by 22.3 ml, quantitatively, for each millimol of lactate accumulating. This approach proved insensitive because the R generally increased during exercise without a lactic acidosis. The increase in R below the *AT* resulted from muscle substrate being heavily in favor of carbohydrate (glycogen) [19] compared to the energy substrate used by the body as a whole. Therefore, R usually increased during exercise even without developing a lactic acidosis.

The Ventilatory Equivalent Method

This approach, described in 1973, took advantage of the disparity between the proportional increase in $\dot{V}E$ relative to $\dot{V}_{CO_2}$, at the onset of the buffering of the exercise lactic acidosis and the faster increase in $\dot{V}E$ relative to $\dot{V}_{O_2}$ [20]. At the AT, $\dot{V}E/\dot{V}_{O_2}$ increased due to the stimulus of the extra CO_2 released during HCO_3^- buffering, while $\dot{V}E/\dot{V}_{CO_2}$ remained constant,($\dot{V}E$ increasing proportionally to $\dot{V}_{CO_2}$). Thus $P_{ET}O_2$ increased at the *AT* while $P_{ET}CO_2$ remained constant for several minutes before it decreased in response to the acid drive [20]. The delay between the increase in $\dot{V}E/\dot{V}_{CO_2}$ relative to the increase in $\dot{V}E/\dot{V}_{O_2}$ is referred to as the isocapnic buffering period, because $PaCO_2$ and $P_{ET}CO_2$ remained constant during this interval. While this method was an improvement over the detection of an increase in R, particularly in normal subjects, it had limitations in some patient groups. It depended on the absence of physiological constraints on breathing, such as that due to severe airflow limitation or chest wall restriction (e.g., obesity).

The V-Slope Method for Measuring the Anaerobic Threshold

Recognizing the shortcomings of the earlier methods, Beaver et al. [2] developed a method for detecting the *AT* that depended only on the detection of the onset of the buffering of the lactic acidosis. This is an obligatory physical-chemical reaction that does not depend on the sensitivity of ventilatory chemoreceptors and the ventilatory response to the acid drive. Thus, it overcame the shortcomings of the prior methods. This method is called the V-slope method because it measures the volume of muscle CO_2 produced as a function of the simultaneous volume of muscle O_2 consumed on equal axes [2]. During exercise below the *AT*, $\dot{V}_{CO_2}$ increases at about the same rate as, or slightly less than, the increase in $\dot{V}_{O_2}$ because the muscle substrate is almost totally carbohydrate (respiratory quotient = 1.0). However, as soon as HCO_3^- in the cell starts to buffer the increase in lactic acid, $\dot{V}_{CO_2}$ increases relative to $\dot{V}_{O_2}$. The rate of $\dot{V}_{CO_2}$ increase must be 22.3 ml/mmol lactate buffered by HCO_3^-. This causes the slope of $\dot{V}_{CO_2}$ versus $\dot{V}_{O_2}$ to abruptly increase and

become >1.0. The rate of buffer CO_2 produced depends on the rate of lactate accumulating, not the lactate concentration itself. Thus the increase in work rate should be sufficiently rapid to easily visualize the steepening of the $\dot{V}_{CO_2}$ versus $\dot{V}_{O_2}$ slope (about 12 min or less from rest to peak $\dot{V}_{O_2}$). The $\dot{V}_{O_2}$ at the intercept of the two slopes (below and above the steepening of CO_2 output is the *AT*) correlates with the lactate and HCO_3^- thresholds [2, 3].

The Shortcut for Measuring the *AT* by the V-Slope Method

Measuring the AT by the V-slope principle does not require complex calculations. A clear plastic 45° right triangle suffices to line up on the points of $\dot{V}_{CO_2}$ vs $\dot{V}_{O_2}$ below the *AT*. The points falling, systematically, along the edge or slightly below the 45° slope of the triangle indicate the rate of CO_2 molecules produced relative to the number of O_2 molecules consumed. (Hyperventilation with respect to CO_2 does not occur until later, if it occurs.) At some point on this plot, the slope abruptly steepens, becoming >1.0 (>45°). The $\dot{V}_{O_2}$ at the intercept of the two slopes can be read from a perpendicular line to the X-axis. This is the *AT*. The V-slope method depends only on the physical chemistry of buffering.

The development of the V-slope method makes it possible to measure the *AT* in all normal subjects and almost all patients, regardless of the pathophysiology. The exceptions might be in patients with severe physical limitations, preventing the patient from reaching their *AT*, and patients with severe peripheral arterial disease so that the AT cannot be visualized by V-slope. However, this clinical problem can be quantified by other gas exchange methods during exercise.

Physiological Significance and Clinical Applications of the *AT*

A number of important physiological responses to exercise are altered above the *AT* [21]. Many of these have been described [5]. Among them are accelerated conversion of muscle glycogen to lactate, metabolic acidosis, increased ventilatory compensation for the metabolic acidosis, reduced exercise endurance, slowed $\dot{V}_{O_2}$ kinetics during step increase in work rate, increased CO_2 output relative to $\dot{V}_{O_2}$, hemoconcentration above the *AT*, and facilitation of oxyhemoglobin dissociation by the blood acidification (Bohr effect). Some of these are detrimental and some are beneficial in the performance of exercise. In the case of the latter, the maximal O_2 extraction and peak $\dot{V}_{O_2}$ would be reduced without the lactic acidosis [12].

Clinically, the *AT* is reduced when there is impaired O_2 delivery to the muscles during exercise. The *AT* correlates with peak $\dot{V}o_2$ in heart failure patients [22]. In applications in which a reliable peak $\dot{V}o_2$ cannot be obtained, the *AT* might replace it [23]. The *AT* measurement has proven to be of great value in defining the pathophysiology of exercise intolerance and its application in the differential diagnosis of physiological impairments that reduce exercise tolerance [24]. In addition, since it can be measured, noninvasively, the extent of its application has yet to be defined.

References

1. Wasserman K (1994) Coupling of external to cellular respiration during exercise: the wisdom of the body revisited. Am J Physiol 266:E519–E539
2. Beaver WL, Wasserman K, Whipp BJ (1986) A new method for detecting the anaerobic threshold by gas exchange. J Appl Physiol 60:2020–2027
3. Beaver WL, Wasserman K, Whipp BJ (1986) Bicarbonate buffering of lactic acid generated during exercise. J Appl Physiol 60:472–478
4. Wasserman K, McIlroy MB (1964) Detecting the threshold of anaerobic metabolism in cardiac patients during exercise. Am J Cardiol 14:844–852
5. Wasserman K, Hansen J, Sue DY, Stringer WW, Whipp BJ (2005) - Chapter 2. Physiology of exercise. In: Wasserman K et al (eds) Principles of exercise testing and interpretation. 4th edn. Lippincott, Williams and Wilkins, Philadelphia
6. McGilvery RW (1983) The oxidation of glucose. In: McGilvery RW (ed) Biochemistry: a functional approach. Saunders, Philadelphia
7. Wasserman K, Beaver WL, Davis JA, Pu J-Z, Heber D, Whipp BJ (1985) Lactate, pyruvate, and lactate-to-pyruvate ratio during exercise and recovery. J Appl Physiol 59:935–940
8. Wasserman K, Beaver WL, Whipp BJ (1990) Gas exchange theory and the lactic acidosis (anaerobic) threshold. Circulation 81(Suppl II): II-14–II-30
9. Stringer W, Casaburi R, Wasserman K (1992) Acid-base regulation during exercise and recovery in man. J Appl Physiol 72:954–961
10. Wasserman K, VanKessel A, Burton GB (1967) Interaction of physiological mechanisms during exercise. J Appl Physiol 22:71–85
11. Wasserman K, Stringer W, Casaburi R, Zhang YY (1997) Mechanism of the exercise hyperkalemia: an alternate hypothesis. J Appl Physiol 83:631–643
12. Stringer W, Wasserman K, Casaburi R, Porszasz J, Maehara K, French W (1994) Lactic acidosis as a facilitator of oxyhemoglobin dissociation during exercise. J Appl Physiol 76:1462–1467
13. Wasserman K (1999) Critical capillary PO2 and the role of lactate production in oxyhemoglobin dissociation during exercise. Adv Exp Med Biol 471:321–333
14. Koike A, Wasserman K, Taniguichi K, Hiroe M, Marumo F (1994) Critical capillary oxygen partial pressure and lactate threshold in patients with cardiovascular disease. J Am Coll Cardiol 23:1644–1650
15. Wasserman K, Beaver WL, Whipp BJ (1986) Mechanisms and patterns of blood lactate increase during exercise in man. Med Sci Sports Exerc 18(3):344–352
16. Wasserman K, Koike A (1992) Is the anaerobic threshold truly anaerobic? Chest 101:211–218
17. Koike A, Weiler-Ravell D, McKenzie DK, Zanconato S, Wasserman K (1990) Evidence that the metabolic acidosis threshold is the anaerobic threshold. J Appl Physiol 68:2521–2526
18. Zhang YY, Sietsema KE, Sullivan S, Wasserman K (1994) A method for estimating bicarbonate buffering of lactic acid during constant work rate exercise. Eur J Appl Physiol 69:309–315
19. Beaver WL, Wasserman K (1991) Muscle RQ and lactate accumulation from analysis of the VCO2-VO2 relationship during exercise. Clin J Sport Med 1(2):27–34
20. Wasserman K, Whipp BJ, Koyal S, Beaver WL (1973) Anaerobic threshold and respiratory gas exchange during exercise. J Appl Physiol 35:236–243
21. Wasserman K (1987) Determinants and detection of anaerobic threshold and consequences of exercise above it. Circulation 81(Suppl VI):VI-29–VI-39
22. Wasserman K, Sun X-G, Hansen J (2007) Effect of biventricular pacing on the exercise pathophysiology of heart failure. Chest 132:250–261
23. Older P, Hall A, Hader R (1999) Cardiopulmonary exercise testing as a screening test for perioperative management of major surgery in the elderly. Chest 116:355–362
24. Wasserman K (1997) Diagnosing cardiovascular and lung pathophysiology from exercise gas exchange. Chest 112:1091–1101

Androgen

A class of hormone that stimulates or controls the development and maintenance of male characteristics and associated with anabolic activity.

Cross-References

▶ Anabolic Steroids

Angiogenesis

THOMAS GUSTAFSSON, ERIC RULLMAN, ANNA STRÖMBERG
Department of Laboratory medicine, Karolinska Institutet, Stockholm, Sweden

Synonyms

Capillarization; Neovascularization; Vessel growth

Definition

Postnatal vessel growth naturally occurs in the female reproductive system, in wound healing, and in skeletal muscle in response to exercise. Postnatal vessel growth has been assumed to occur as a functional modification of existing arteries such as the growth of preexisting vessels into functional collateral arteries (arteriogenesis) or the formation of new capillaries from an already established capillary network (angiogenesis) [5] (Fig. 1). Arteriogenesis in response to increased muscle activity has been reported in animal

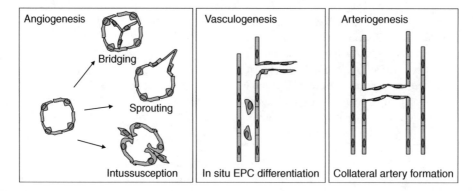

Angiogenesis. Fig. 1 A summary of the different mechanisms of vessel formation. Angiogenesis – proliferation of existing endothelial cells to form new capillary networks. Vasculogenesis – in situ differentiation of endothelial progenitor cells to form new endothelial cells. Arteriogenesis – remodeling of arterioles into collateral arteries

models, but only a few reports of arteriogenesis in response to exercise exist from healthy humans. Until recently, any increase in capillarity in human or animal skeletal muscle in response to exercise was assumed to reflect vessel growth due to angiogenesis [1, 4]. However, in 1997 the Isner laboratory reported that human peripheral blood contained CD34+/VEGFR2+ cells that contributed to angiogenesis in vivo, and questioned the view that blood vessel formation in adults depended solely on angiogenesis [6] (Fig. 1). These cells were termed EPCs (endothelial progenitor cells), and after this original publication lot of research has been performed to characterize these cells and explore their functionality in various experimental models. Their mode of action is to circulate the blood stream and migrate into tissues of active vessel growth where they mature in situ to endothelial cells, a process termed vasculogenesis, similar to how the vascular network is formed in embryos.

Basic Mechanisms

The British surgeon John Hunter used the term "angiogenesis" in 1787 to describe blood vessels growing in the reindeer antler, and in 1935, Arthur Tremain Hertig described angiogenesis in the placenta of pregnant monkeys. It is now accepted that there are at least two different types of angiogenesis: true sprouting of capillaries from preexisting vessels, and nonsprouting angiogenesis or intussusceptive growth [5]. True sprouting angiogenesis, the major type of growth, is a complex process involving many cell types, signaling pathways, growth factors, and receptors. It is initiated by the activation of endothelial cells and vasodilatation of the parent vessel, followed by an increase in vascular permeability. The basement membrane and the extracellular matrix are degraded, releasing numerous growth factors and allowing endothelial cells to migrate to sites where new capillaries are needed. Nonsprouting angiogenesis is also observed in skeletal muscle and is called luminal division, longitudinal splitting or bridging. An important advantage of intussusceptive capillary growth is that it permits rapid expansion of the capillary network and thus enlarges the endothelial surface for metabolic exchange.

Folkman's 1971 hypothesis that tumor growth is dependent on angiogenesis [5] stimulated intensive research on the basic mechanisms underlying angiogenesis. Regardless of the type of angiogenesis, it is now believed that the process is mediated by diffusible angiogenic factors through an increased synthesis or release from intracellular or extracellular storage pools. In 1996, Hanahan and Folkman introduced the term "angiogenic switch" to describe how this occurs. Angiogenesis may be induced by an increase in angiogenic regulators or a decrease in angiostatic regulators [5]. The development of in vivo bioassays, in vitro analytic techniques, and murine transgenic models has allowed the identification and characterization of more than 30 angiogenic and inhibitory factors that directly or indirectly affect angiogenesis. Of these, vascular endothelial growth factor-A (VEGF-A) is one of the major regulators of angiogenesis [5]. Angiogenesis is a multistep process that includes integration of different signaling pathways such as VEGF-A and the angiopoietins Ang-1 and Ang-2. [3]. Conditions that increase the expression of Ang-2 or the levels of VEGF-A enhance the angiogenic process through Ang-2-induced endothelial destabilization. This in turn facilitates the effects of VEGF-A on endothelial activation [3]. Other mechanisms are needed to complete the complex multistep angiogenic process. Remodeling the extracellular matrix, inflammation, and coagulation all clearly influence vascular growth in adults [4, 5].

Regarding vasculogenesis, the number of EPCs in the circulation is normally low but is increased when there is enhanced neovascularization and vessel repair. VEGF-A and stromal cell derived factor -1 (SDF-1) are important in guiding EPCs to regions of vessel growth (homing), and their expression is increased in tissues that have activated vessel formation. To enter the tissue from the circulation the EPCs need to traverse the endothelium, which is performed through binding to endothelial adhesion molecules. SDF-1 and VEGF induce the activation of Akt, which in turn enhances the expression of intercellular adhesion molecule 1 (ICAM-1) on endothelial cells. Other adhesion molecules important for EPC homing are the E- and P-selectins and vascular adhesion molecule 1 (VCAM-1) [6].

Exercise Intervention

Historical Review

Vanotti and Magiday (1934) first described increased capillarity following muscle activity alone, and with voluntary endurance exercise training in rat and guinea pig muscles. More recent studies confirm that electrical muscle stimulation and exercise training induce increased capillarity in skeletal muscle in various animal species. The first human studies demonstrating an increase in capillarity in response to increased physical activity were published in the mid-1970s, and by the early 1980s, the cessation of exercise training was shown to induce a rapid regression in capillarity [1].

Biological Significance

Increasing the number of capillaries in skeletal muscle improves oxygen uptake and utilization by increasing the surface area available for diffusion, decreasing the diffusion distance, and increasing the transit time for the exchange of oxygen, substrates, and waste products. Many of the metabolic pathways linked to levels of risk factors such as glucose and fatty acids, and lipoprotein turnover in humans, are controlled by the surface membranes of vascular endothelial cells in skeletal muscle [1]. Recent findings suggest that capillary formation, including utilization of EPCs, is crucial for the skeletal remodeling process.

Regulatory Mechanisms

Both animal and human experiments have contributed to the understanding of exercise-induced changes in angiogenic growth factors, with ex vivo studies adding to the analysis of the underlying mechanisms [1, 4]. The increase in VEGF-A expression observed in exercised skeletal muscle together with the inhibition of exercise-induced angiogenesis by gene deletion, VEGF-receptor inhibition, and trap models suggests that VEGF-A has a dominant role. However, the first characterized angiogenic factor, FGF-2, has consistently been shown to remain unchanged with exercise. The observations that VEGF-A mRNA levels increase transiently following acute exercise, whereas basal VEGF-A protein levels increase over a 5-week training program, suggest that protein translation must occur during the VEGF mRNA peak associated with each bout of exercise [2]. The angiopoietins are modulated during repetitive exercise bouts, producing a higher Ang-2/Ang-1 ratio that exerts a permissive effect on angiogenesis in both humans and rats [2]. In subjects in whom skeletal muscle has adapted to exercise training, the change in the Ang-2/Ang-1 ratio is reversed. This suggests that increased Ang-1 reflects a maturation of the capillary system during a later phase of the adaptation process [2].

Hypoxia, metabolic stress, and mechanical stretch appear to lead to sprouting angiogenesis, whereas shear stress appears to cause nonsprouting angiogenesis. A common feature in such situations is an increased expression of VEGF-A. Therefore, VEGF-A is crucial in both sprouting and nonsprouting angiogenesis [1, 4]. The regulation of VEGF-A by shear stress is clearly associated with nitric oxide production and the upregulation of endothelial nitric oxide synthase activity in endothelial cells. Several components of the hypoxia inducible factor 1 (HIF-1, the major transcription factor of hypoxic activation of cellular VEGF-A transcription) pathway are activated in response to a single bout of exercise in healthy human skeletal muscle. However, the mechanism responsible for the increase in VEGF-A in skeletal muscle fibers must be more complex than simply the activation of HIF-1. Numerous other factors and signaling pathways stimulated by exercise are known to activate the VEGF-A gene transcriptionally, for example 5'AMP-activated protein kinase (AMPK), adenosine, and peroxisome proliferator-activated receptor-coactivator (PGC-1) [1, 4]. In addition to the exercise-induced changes in gene expression, more rapid changes that may participate in the angiogenic response occur. For example, microdialysate obtained from skeletal muscle immediately following exercise stimulates endothelial cell proliferation and contains VEGF-A protein. During the initial phase of exercise, release of VEGF-A from the muscle is also observed. These changes occur long before any changes in gene transcription could result in protein synthesis and therefore support a release of VEGF-A from preexistent pools. Proteolysis of the extracellular membrane by proteases is a key event in sprouting angiogenesis and in addition to the degradation of membrane barriers, these enzymes can release bound growth factors through degradation of extra cellular matrix or binding proteins [4]. Another mechanism involved in the increase in available biofactors during bouts of exercise may thus be the activation of extracellular proteases in skeletal muscle tissue. Exercise-induced capillary growth probably results from the integrated activation of multiple systems and involves both nonsprouting and sprouting angiogenesis as well as vasculogenesis.

The levels of EPCs and recruiting stimulatory factors for circulating EPCs increase following exercise, and in animal models factors involved in homing and maturation processes increase in areas of neovascularization [6]. Thus, it is not possible to exclude vasculogenesis from this process. However, more information is required to establish whether homing and maturation processes are activated in the muscles of healthy individuals during exercise, although the processes that have been suggested to be involved in homing of EPCs to peripheral tissues are similar to those demonstrated to be of importance for rolling and homing of leukocytes. Since these mechanisms have been demonstrated to become activated by exercise, it indirectly proves the involvement of vasculogenesis in exercise-induced capillary growth.

Summary

Exercise-induced angiogenesis results from the integrated responses of multiple systems and involves both nonsprouting and sprouting angiogenesis. VEGF-A increases in exercising muscle and appears to be a key factor in exercise-induced capillary growth. More studies are needed before vasculogenesis can be added as a mechanism of exercise-induced capillary growth.

References

1. Gustafsson T, Kraus WE (2001) Exercise-induced angiogenesis-related growth and transcription factors in skeletal muscle, and their modification in muscle pathology. Front Biosci 6:D75–D89
2. Gustafsson T, Rundqvist H, Norrbom J, Rullman E, Jansson E, Sundberg CJ (2007) The influence of physical training on the angiopoietin and VEGF-A systems in human skeletal muscle. J Appl Physiol 103:1012–1020
3. Holash J, Maisonpierre PC, Compton D, Boland P, Alexander CR, Zagzag D, Yancopoulos GD, and Wiegand SJ (1999) Vessel cooption, regression, and growth in tumors mediated by angiopoietins and VEGF. Science 284:1994–1998
4. Prior BM, Yang HT, Terjung RL (2004) What makes vessels grow with exercise training? J Appl Physiol 97:1119–1128
5. Risau W (1997) Mechanisms of angiogenesis. Nature 386:671–674
6. Wahl P, Bloch W, Schmidt A (2007) Exercise has a positive effect on endothelial progenitor cells, which could be necessary for vascular adaptation processes. Int J Sports Med 28:374–380

Angiotensin Converting Enzyme

Angiotensin converting enzyme (ACE) converts angiotensin I into angiotensin II. The angiotensin-converting enzyme inactivates bradykinin, a powerful vasodilator.

Angiotensin I

A decapeptide with no biological activity, cleaved from precursor angiotensinogen by renin. It is converted by ACE into angiotensin II, a potent vasoconstrictor, after the removal of two amino acids at the C-terminal.

Angiotensin II

An octapeptide produced from angiotensin I after the removal of two amino acids at the C-terminal by ACE. Angiotensin II causes contraction of the arteriolar and renal vascular smooth muscle. In addition, angiotensin II stimulates the release of aldosterone from the adrenal zona glomerulosa, which in turn increases salt and water retention.

Angiotensinogen

An α2-globulin produced by the liver and secreted into blood circulation. Angiotensinogen is the inactive precursor of angiotensin I and II.

Anion

An ion which carries a negative ($-$) charge and migrates toward electrodes with a positive polarity (anode) when a current is applied.

Ankle/Brachial Index

The ratio of the ankle systolic blood pressure to the brachial systolic blood pressure.

▶ Peripheral Arterial Disease

Anoxia

▶ Hypoxia, Focus Hypoxic Hypoxia

Antigen

Usually a molecule foreign to the body but can be any molecule capable of being recognized by an antibody or T cell receptor.

Antihypertensive Effects of Exercise

▶ Hypertension

Antihypertensive Medications

Drugs taken to lower blood pressure that include α and β blockers, angiotensin converting enzyme inhibitors, calcium channel blockers, diuretics, and vasodilators among others.

Anti-inflammatory Activation

Anti-inflammatory activation is a macrophage inflammatory state characterized by the decrease of the secretion of many effectors and the release of high amount of IL-10. It can be triggered in vitro by IL-10 and/or glucocorticoids. Anti-inflammatory macrophages are associated with the resolution of inflammation and tissue repair.

Antioxidant Enzymes

Enzymes that are powerful scavengers of free radicals and other oxidants. In general, the oxidant is the substrate of the enzyme. In some cases, the presence of co-substrates (such as GSH) is essential for the activity of the enzyme.

Antioxidants

Any substance that can inhibit the oxidation of other compounds. There are enzymatic antioxidants (e.g., superoxide dismutate, catalase) and non-enzymatic antioxidans (e.g., glutathione). There are also a variety of dietary antioxidants and these include vitamin E and vitamin C and lipoic acid and lycopene.

Antiretroviral Medication

Drugs used to treat retroviral infections (e.g., HIV) by interfering with specific steps in the life cycle of the virus.

Anxiolytic

Exercise may have an anxiolytic effect – the anxiety level is reduced.

Cross-References
▶ Depression
▶ Psychiatric/Psychological Disorders

Aortic Coarctation

A stenosis of the proximal descending aorta usually at, or beyond, the site of the duct, which may vary in anatomy, physiology, and clinical presentation. It may present with discrete or long-segment stenosis, sometimes associated with hypoplasia of the aortic arch and bicuspid aortic valve.

AP-1

Activator protein-1 (AP-1) is usually a heterodimer composed of proteins belonging to the c-Fos, c-Jun, ATF, and JDP families. As a transcription factor, it regulates gene expression in response to a variety of stimuli, including inflammation via cytokines, growth factors, stress, and bacterial and viral infections. AP-1 in turn controls a number of cellular processes including differentiation, proliferation, and apoptosis.

Apelin

Apelin is a recently identified adipokine that has been reported to have a host of salutary effects on skeletal muscle and systemic carbohydrate and lipid metabolism. Apelin deficiency is associated with glucose intolerance, whereas the restoration of apelin concentrations reverses this condition. These effects may be caused in part by apelin's ability to increase muscle mitochondrial content and improve fat oxidation.

Apnea–Hypopnea Index

The primary measure of sleep-disordered breathing severity calculated as the number of apneas and hypopneas per hour of sleep; commonly abbreviated AHI.

Apoproteins

Are specific proteins that populate and dictate the action and function of lipoproteins. Examples include apoprotein A1, B100, B48, C1-3, E, a, and others.

Apoptosis

Amie J. Dirks-Naylor
School of Pharmacy, Wingate University, Wingate, NC, USA

Synonyms
Cell suicide; Programmed cell death

Definition

Apoptosis, programmed cell death, is a form of cell death that has an essential role in development, health, and disease [1]. Apoptosis plays a fundamental role in regulating cell number during developmental and post-developmental stages of the mammalian lifespan. For example, in the development of the central nervous system (CNS) half of the neurons produced during neurogenesis die via apoptosis before CNS maturation. In the mature adult, apoptosis is responsible for the death and shedding of cells in the epidermis and gastrointestinal tract. Apoptosis is also responsible for ridding the body of damaged or infected cells that may be harmful to the organism. Cells containing damaged DNA or dysfunctional mitochondria or cells infected with bacteria or viruses may die via apoptosis. Inadequate or excessive apoptosis contributes to pathophysiological conditions. For example, inadequate apoptosis is a vital mechanism of cancer development and progression. Excessive apoptosis has been implicated in the progression of many age-related diseases such as Alzheimer's, Parkinson's, and cardiovascular disease (e.g., atherosclerosis and diabetes mellitus). Furthermore, apoptosis has been implicated as an important mechanism in the loss of skeletal muscle mass and function with age. Exercise training has been shown to cause adaptations in apoptotic signaling making skeletal muscle more resistant to apoptotic stimuli [1]. Apoptotic signaling and the adaptations exerted by exercise training will be discussed.

Basic Mechanisms

Apoptosis is executed via specific signaling pathways that lead to distinct morphologic characteristics such as cell shrinkage, membrane blebbing, nuclear condensation, DNA fragmentation into ▶ mono- and oligo-nucleosomes, and phosphatidylserine translocation to the outer leaflet of the plasma membrane. Apoptosis is mediated by activation of a variety of cysteine proteases, known as caspases. Inactivated caspases, called ▶ procaspases, become activated by proteolytic cleavage. Initiation of apoptosis involves activation of a ▶ caspase cascade in which initiator caspases (e.g., caspase-8, caspase-9) first become activated and then cleave and activate effector caspases (e.g., caspase-3, caspase-7). The effector caspases carry out the proteolytic events that result in cellular breakdown and demise. There are 14 known mammalian caspases (i.e., caspase-1 through caspase-14), in which most participate in the apoptotic process depending on the stimulus and respective signaling pathway activated. The two major pathways extensively described include the intrinsic and extrinsic apoptotic signaling pathways (see Fig. 1).

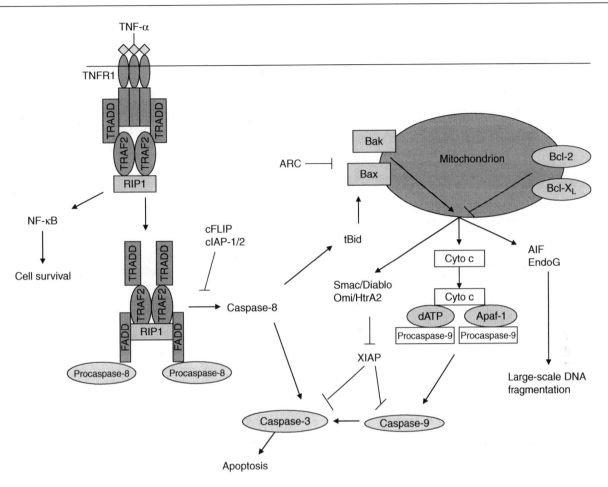

Apoptosis. Fig. 1 Simplified scheme of intrinsic and extrinsic apoptotic signaling pathways. *Arrows* indicate a stimulatory effect while blunt lines indicate an inhibitory effect

Mitochondria play a central role in the induction of apoptosis via the intrinsic pathway [2, 3]. Upon apoptotic stimulation, mitochondria can release cytochrome c into the cytosol, which forms a complex, the ▶ apoptosome, with procaspase-9, apoptotic protease activating factor 1 (Apaf-1), and dATP. Once the apoptosome is formed, procaspase-9 molecules can cleave and activate each other. Caspase-9 can then cleave and activate effector caspases such as procaspase-3, which leads to the typical morphological features of apoptosis. This process is highly regulated [2, 3]. First, cytochrome c release from the mitochondria is regulated. The B-cell lymphoma/leukemia-2 (Bcl-2) family of proteins was the first described to affect the release of cytochrome c. This family consists of a number of proteins, some of which are anti-apoptotic and others are pro-apoptotic. For example, Bcl-2 and Bcl-2 related gene, long isoform (Bcl-X_L) protect against cytochrome c release and are therefore anti-apoptotic, while

Bcl-2 associated x protein (Bax), Bcl-2 antagonist killer 1 (Bak), and Bcl-2 interacting domain death agonist (Bid) favor cytochrome c release and are therefore pro-apoptotic. The ratio and interaction of the Bcl-2 family of anti-apoptotic and pro-apoptotic proteins determines the fate of cytochrome c release from mitochondria. Often the Bcl-2/Bax ratio is used as an indicator of apoptotic potential where a high ratio protects against apoptosis and a low ratio favors apoptosis. Apoptosis repressor with caspase-associated recruitment domain (ARC) is another protein that regulates cytochrome c release. Upon stimulation, ARC translocates from the cytosol to the mitochondrial membrane and prevents cytochrome c release. Recent data show that ARC may prevent apoptosis by binding to Bax and interfering with its activation, which would ultimately protect against cytochrome c release. Another level of regulation involves the inhibition of caspase-9 and caspase-3 by the inhibitor of apoptosis protein (IAP) family member X-linked IAP (XIAP). XIAP binds the activated caspases and inhibits the enzyme activity. Mitochondria can release additional proteins, along with cytochrome c, to relieve the inhibition exerted by the XIAP allowing apoptosis to occur. These proteins include Smac/Diablo and Omi/HtrA2. Mitochondria can also release apoptosis inducing factor (AIF) and endonuclease G (EndoG), which translocate to the nucleus to induce chromatin condensation and large-scale DNA fragmentation in a caspase-independent manner.

The extrinsic pathway is mediated via the activation of membrane receptors, such as tumor necrosis factor receptor 1 (TNFR1) [4]. When activated by its ligand, tumor necrosis factor-alpha (TNF-α), TNFR1 can actually activate an apoptotic or an anti-apoptotic signal depending on the conditions. TNF-α binding leads to the formation of a complex on the cytosolic domain of TNFR1, which includes TNF receptor associated death domain (TRADD), TNF receptor associated factor-2 (TRAF2), and receptor interacting protein-1 (RIP1). Formation of this complex can lead to the activation of nuclear factor-kappa B (NF-κB) resulting in an anti-apoptotic response. However, under conditions where NF-κB is suppressed, the TRADD-TRAF2-RIP1 complex translocates to the cytosol and recruits fas-associated death domain (FADD) and procaspase-8 [4]. Once caspase-8 is activated, it can then activate caspase-3. Caspase-8 can also cleave Bid forming the truncated Bid (tBid), which leads to the activation of the mitochondrial-mediated signaling pathway via the activation of Bax and/or Bak. Activation of the mitochondrial-mediated pathway may be a mechanism for amplification of the apoptotic signal or it may actually be a required event for the induction of receptor-mediated apoptosis. The latter is true in cell types that require the release of Smac/Diablo and/or Omi/HtrA2 from the mitochondria in order to relieve the inhibition of caspase-3 by the XIAP. Cellular FADD-like interleukin-1 beta converting enzyme inhibitory protein (cFLIP) and cellular IAP1 and IAP2 (cIAP1/2) has been shown to inhibit activation of caspase-8.

In summary, apoptosis has an essential role in health and homeostasis as well as contributing to the pathogenesis of a variety of diseases. Apoptosis is mediated via intrinsic and/or extrinsic signaling pathways, which are both highly regulated. The intrinsic pathway involves release of cytochrome c from the mitochondria, formation of the apoptosome, and activation of procaspase-9. The extrinsic pathway involves activation of membrane receptors, such as TNFR1, which often leads to the activation of procaspase-8. Caspase-9 and caspase-8 can both activate procaspase-3, which results in cellular demise and the associated morphological characteristics such as cell shrinkage, DNA fragmentation into mono- and oligo-nucleosomes, membrane blebbing, and formation of apoptotic bodies.

Exercise Intervention

Exercise training results in many beneficial adaptations, including adaptations in apoptotic signaling leading to a potentially greater resistance to apoptosis [1]. Several studies have shown that the rate of apoptosis decreases in response to exercise training or chronic electrical stimulation (CES). For example, mono- and oligo-nucleosomal DNA fragmentation, a common marker of apoptosis, has been observed to slightly decrease in soleus muscle of young animals as a result of exercise training. Further, in apoptotic prone white gastrocnemius and extensor digitorum longus aged animals, exercise training can return DNA fragmentation to that matching youthful levels. During muscle disuse DNA fragmentation significantly increases. Yet, a brief 5–10 min bout of exercise three times per day substantially attenuates disuse atrophy-induced DNA fragmentation. Exercise training can modulate apoptosis in skeletal muscle, perhaps to a greater degree in skeletal muscle predisposed to apoptosis (i.e., aged and disused skeletal muscle), by altering mitochondrial-mediated and/or receptor-mediated apoptotic signaling.

Exercise training and/or CES appears to cause several adaptations in the intrinsic signaling pathway involving mitochondria [1]. First, exercise training causes adaptations in the Bcl-2 family proteins that may resemble an increase in the Bcl-2/Bax ratio, which would likely increase the resistance for cytochrome c release and formation of the apoptosome. For example, exercise training has been found to significantly increase Bcl-2 mRNA and protein and significantly decrease Bax mRNA in rat soleus muscle. The potential of exercise training to modulate Bcl-2 and Bax may not be as profound in young skeletal muscle as in old. Indeed, while 3 months of exercise training had no effect on Bcl-2 or Bax protein levels in young rat white gastrocnemius and rat soleus, the same stimulus restored Bcl-2 and Bax protein levels in aged rat white gastrocnemius and soleus to young expression levels. These data suggest that exercise training has the potential to reinstate a youthful anti-apoptotic potential in both fast and slow skeletal muscle. Secondly, in addition to potentially improving the Bcl-2/Bax ratio in apoptotic prone skeletal muscle, exercise training modulates ARC. ARC protein expression in the rat soleus is increased by exercise training or daily electrical stimulation of the rat tibialis anterior. By modulating the Bcl-2/Bax ratio and/or increasing ARC expression exercise training and/or CES limits mitochondrial cytochrome c release. For example, mitochondrial cytochrome c release has been shown to decrease in response to electrical stimulation. Intermyofibrillar mitochondria isolated from rat tibialis anterior muscle electrically stimulated daily results in a decrease in cytochrome c release under basal conditions and an attenuated release when subjected to a maximal reactive oxygen stimulus. Thirdly, Apaf-1 expression has been shown to be affected by exercise training. It was shown that 2 months of exercise training decreased Apaf-1 protein expression.

Furthermore, exercise training can increase the resistance to mitochondrion-mediated apoptosis by increasing the expression of XIAP thus, limiting the activity of caspase-3 and -9 [1]. One month of treadmill training increases XIAP protein expression in young rat soleus muscle, producing a negative correlation between XIAP protein expression and apoptotic DNA fragmentation. This correlative relationship suggests an important mechanism for the anti-apoptotic benefit of exercise training.

Lastly, adaptations may occur in apoptosis involving AIF and EndoG [1]. As previously discussed, mitochondrial release of AIF and EndoG induce chromatin condensation and large-scale DNA fragmentation in a caspase-independent manner. Daily exercise training does not alter cytosolic levels of AIF or EndoG in the rat extensor digitorum longus or soleus or human skeletal muscle. However, intermyofibrillar mitochondria isolated from rat tibialis anterior following daily electrical stimulation decreases AIF release under basal conditions and attenuates AIF release when subjected to a maximal reactive oxygen stimulus. These observations suggest that AIF and EndoG adaptations to exercise training may be muscle specific or exercise training and electrical stimulation produce differential adaptations.

In summary, exercise training and/or CES appears to cause adaptations in mitochondrial-mediated signaling that increase the resistance to apoptosis. Adaptations may include an increase in the Bcl-2/Bax ratio, increased expression of ARC and XIAP, and decreased expression of Apaf-1.

Exercise training also appears to modulate aspects of the extrinsic pathway involving TNFR1; however, very few studies have been published [1]. Aging and disease states such as chronic heart failure are associated with elevated plasma levels of TNF-α. Exercise training has been utilized as a possible means of altering plasma TNF-α levels. Acutely, plasma levels of TNF-α can dramatically rise and subsequently return to baseline in response to strenuous exercise. However, exercise training has been observed to significantly lower plasma TNF-α levels in many patients with heart failure. Further, individuals self-reporting a high level of physical activity have lower plasma TNF-α levels than sedentary individuals. Thus, basal plasma TNF-α levels vary with age, disease state, and chronic physical activity levels, perhaps predisposing individuals with high plasma TNF-α levels to apoptosis.

Skeletal muscle TNFR1 expression levels and plasma levels of soluble TNFR1 (sTNFR1) are altered by age and exercise [1]. Aging increases TNFR1 in old rat extensor digitorum longus but not rat soleus. The increased TNFR1 expression in aged rat extensor digitorum longus may result in the preferential sarcopenia of this fast muscle compared to the slow rat soleus. Exercise training restores TNFR1 expression to youthful levels in the aged rat extensor digitorum longus. sTNFR1 may function as a TNF-α inhibitor or carrier, the plasma level of which is considered to be an important marker of TNF-α. Indeed, 4 months of combined strength and endurance exercise training can significantly decrease the plasma level of sTNFR1 in patients with heart failure. While strength training alone does not alter plasma sTNFR1 levels in old subjects, a significant negative correlation exists between strength gain and pretraining levels of sTNFR1 suggesting that subjects with low sTNFR1 levels may experience greater strength gains. Thus, sTNFR1 levels are modifiable by exercise and may predict how beneficial exercise training will be.

The effects of chronic exercise training on the expression of adaptor molecules involved in TNFR1 signaling, such as TRADD, TRAF2, RIP1, and FADD have not been studied. However, exercise training has been shown to affect caspase-8 and -3 activation [1]. In the aged rat fast muscle, extensor digitorum longus, cleaved caspase-8 and -3 levels are elevated but not in the slow rat soleus muscle. However, increasing the activity level of old rat extensor digitorum longus restores cleaved caspase-8 and -3 levels to levels found in young rat extensor digitorum longus.

In summary, exercise training has a plethora of beneficial effects in skeletal muscle including the ability to enhance resistance against apoptosis. It appears that exercise training induces protective adaptations in regulatory proteins in both the mitochondrial- and receptor-mediated signaling pathways. Exercise training may lead to an increase in the Bcl-2/Bax ratio and ARC expression, which may explain the decrease in cytochrome c release in exercise-trained muscle. Expression of Apaf-1 decreases and XIAP expression increases with exercise training, both adaptations afford skeletal muscle protection from apoptosis. Exercise training also may lead to a decrease in expression of TNFR1 and plasma levels of TNF-α. The content of activated caspase-8 and -3 are also decreased.

Collectively, the data indicate that exercise training leads to a multitude of adaptations within skeletal muscle that decrease the apoptotic potential making skeletal muscle more resistant to cell death.

References

1. Dirks-Naylor AJ, Shanely RA (2009) Apoptosis in aging muscle and modulation by exercise, caloric restriction, and muscle disuse. In: Magalhães J, Ascensão A (eds) Muscle plasticity – advances in physiological and biochemical research. The Research Signpost, Kerala
2. Green DR (2000) Apoptotic pathways: paper wraps stone blunts scissors. Cell 102:1–4
3. Kroemer G, Galluzzi L, Brenner C (2007) Mitochondrial membrane permeabilization in cell death. Physiol Rev 87:99–163
4. Micheau O, Tschopp J (2003) Induction of TNF receptor 1-mediated apoptosis via two sequential signaling complexes. Cell 114:181–190

Apoptosome

A multi-protein complex comprised of cytochrome c, Apaf-1, dATP/ATP, and procaspase-9.

Arranged in Parallel

This is a mechanical term indicating the arrangement for which it is true that forces exerted by two or more element must be added to obtain the total force. Note that if the elements can change in length the displacements can*not* be added to obtain the total displacement (example, sarcomeres in parallel within a muscle fiber).

Arranged in Series

This is a mechanical term indicating that forces exerted on or by one element must also be borne by other element(s) with which it is arranged in series (equal force). If the elements can change in length, the displacements can be added to obtain the total displacement (example, sarcomeres in series within a muscle fiber).

Arterial Blood Gases

▶ Gas Exchange, Alveolar

Arterial Hypertension

Some clinical studies clearly have demonstrated that intervention affecting known atherosclerotic risk factor, especially arterial hypertension, improves endothelial function and reduces atherosclerotic risk. In particular, the united Kingdome Prospective Diabetes Study (UKPDS) demonstrated that a 12% reduction in cardiovascular events can be expected from a 10 mmHg reduction in systolic blood pressure. In total a tight control of blood pressure reduced both diabetes-related morbidity and mortality with a reduction of macrovascular and microvascular complications. Of note, the Hypertension Optimal Treatment (HOT) trial, demonstrated a 67% risk reduction in cardiovascular mortality during a period of 4 years, only when the diastolic blood pressure was reduced to <80 mmHg in patients with diabetes. It is also important to consider the result of the Heart Outcomes Prevention Evaluation (HOPE) Study, which demonstrated that despite almost equivalent levels of blood pressure, patients with diabetes treated with an angiotensin-converting enzyme inhibitor had a significant reduction in the combined primary outcome (MI, stroke, cardiovascular death, total mortality, and revascularization) by 25–30%. In patients with diabetes mellitus type 1 and type 2, administration of ACE-inhibitors has been shown to enhance NO-mediated endothelial function immediately after application, with further improvement evident after 4 weeks of therapy. Intensive treatment of hypertension in patients with newly diagnosed diabetes during an 8-year period, which decreased systolic and diastolic blood pressure by 10 and 5 mmHg, respectively, significantly reduced both the absolute risk of stroke and the combined end point of diabetes-related death, death from vascular causes, and death from renal causes by 5%. The HOT, which treated elevations in diastolic blood pressure for an average of 3.7 years, reported similar reductions in the risk of composite end points for macrovascular disease in subgroup analyses of patients with type 2 diabetes.

Cross-References

▶ Hypertension, Training

Arterial PCO$_2$

▶ Gas Exchange, Alveolar

Arterial PO$_2$

▶ Gas Exchange, Alveolar

Arteriosclerosis

RALF KINSCHERF
Head of the Department of Anatomy and Cell Biology,
Philipps-University of Marburg, Marburg, Germany

Synonyms
Atherosclerosis

Definition
Arteriosclerosis (from the Greek *arterio*, i.e., *artery*, and *sclerosis*, i.e., *hardening*) refers to an acampsia of arteries. Therefore, the term arteriosclerosis describes any hardening, calcification, or loss of elasticity of middle or large arteries caused by subendothelial lipid deposits and immigration of leukocytes, especially ▶ monocytes, ▶ macrophages (MΦ), and lymphocytes, as well as a proliferation of smooth muscle cells.

Basic Mechanisms
Arteriosclerosis is a systemic, arterial, inflammatory disease [1], which starts with the childhood and increases with age. Hallmark of the disease is a chronic, proceeding degeneration of the arteries, including progressive alterations of the vessel wall, especially the intima.

In symptomatical situations, arteriosclerosis can be obvious like coronary heart disease, myocardial infarction, peripheral arterial occlusion disease, or stroke. The clinical consequences of arteriosclerosis, especially cardiovascular diseases, are still the main cause of morbidity and mortality in the Western world. Several risk factors for the development of arteriosclerotic lesions are known like age, gender, diabetes, dyslipidemia, hypertension, hyperhomocysteinemia, overweight, sedentary lifestyle, smoking, and/or stress. Additionally, arteriosclerosis is characterized by a complex multifactorial pathophysiology, including several pro-arteriosclerotic factors and cells, like adhesion molecules, cholesterol, cytokines, fat, growth factors, collagen, lipoproteins, endothelial cells, monocytes, MΦ, smooth muscle cells, and thrombocytes. This makes it hard to define a simple hypothesis for the complex pathogenetic processes of arteriosclerosis. However, inflammation in the vessel wall is suggested to play a major role in the initiation, development, progression and the final steps of arteriosclerosis, i.e., plaque/lesion destabilization and eventually plaque rupture and stroke. During the growth of an arteriosclerotic plaque, inflammatory cells (i.e., monocyte-derived MΦ, T-lymphocytes) are localized in the vessel wall, which is mainly preceded by a dysfunction of endothelial cells, producing adhesion molecules that interact with inflammatory cells. MΦ secrete various cytokines, chemokines and growth factors that activate the proliferation of smooth muscle cells and induce the plaque progression, and finally the development of clinically relevant vulnerable plaques. Clinical cardiologists actually realize that coronary arteriosclerosis consists of two pathophysiological different syndromes, meaning stable and unstable plaques/lesions.

The initiation, development, and progression of arteriosclerotic plaques are multifactorial, complex processes, which progress over a long period of time and in which several factors are mainly involved. About five major steps seem to be of significant relevance.

Initial Step: Endothelial Dysfunction, Attachment, and Rolling of Leukocytes on the Endothelium
Figure 1a shows a "normal" artery under physiological conditions, which does not have any arteriosclerotic plaques, i.e., the lumen (Lu) has no signs of stenosis. These arteries consist of an endothelium (E; endothelial cells), media (M; smooth muscle cells and more or less elastic fibers), and adventitia (Ad; connective tissue with vasa vasorum). Increased production of reactive oxygen species [partly due to enhanced activity of NAD(P)H oxidases] named oxidative stress, but also infection, genetic factors, high blood pressure, poor diet, and/or smoking are suggested to be responsible for the dysfunction of the endothelium, which leads to deposition of native ▶ low-density lipoproteins (LDL) or oxidatively/enzymatically modified LDL (mLDL), inducing an increased expression of adhesion molecules. In this context, the selectin family of adhesion molecules are accountable for attachment and rolling of leukocytes (mainly monocytes), because of facilitated interactions between the sialylated carbohydrate portion of E- and P-selectin, which are expressed on endothelial cells and the carbohydrate structures on leukocytes.

Step 2: Firm Adhesion and the Transmigration of Leukocytes [Monocytes, T-Cells] into the Subendothelial Space
During this step, (inflammatory), leukocytes are directly in contact with/adhere to endothelial cells, mediated by adhesion molecules like intercellular adhesion molecule-1

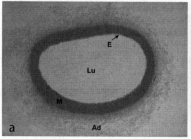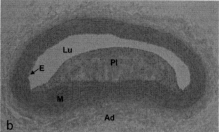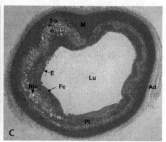

Arteriosclerosis. Fig. 1 (**a**) "Normal" artery (thoracic aorta) of a rabbit fed with standard chow (under physiological conditions); (**b**) arteriosclerotic artery (thoracic aorta) with an intermediate plaque of a cholesterol-fed rabbit; (**c**) arteriosclerotic artery (thoracic aorta) with a fibrous plaque of a cholesterol-fed rabbit: *Ad* adventitia, *E* endothelium, *Fc* fibrous cap, *Fo* foam cells, *M* media, *Lu* lumen, *Nc* necrotic core, *Pl* plaque

(ICAM-1) and vascular adhesion molecule-1 (VCAM-1), increasing the exposure to chemokines like interleukins (IL), e.g., IL-1, IL-6, and IL-18. These are essential for activation of integrins on the cell surface of leukocytes, which induce their transendothelial migration into the subendothelial space. Several studies have demonstrated an association between circulating pro-inflammatory molecules like IL-1, IL-6, tumor necrosis factor-α, C-reactive protein (CRP) or soluble adhesion molecules (sICAM-1, sVCAM-1), and future cardiovascular events in patients with coronary heart disease, but also in healthy individuals.

Step 3: From Fatty Streak to Intermediate Lesion

After transendothelial migration, leukocytes/MΦ (or even smooth muscle cells of the media) may modify deposited LDL to yield mLDL. Additionally, mLDL from the bloodstream may be localized in the subendothelial space. mLDL and transmigrated MΦ (e.g., by the secretion of chemokines) attract more and more MΦ, which results in the development of "fatty streak" consisting of a few MΦ, which may re-migrate to the bloodstream meaning that "fatty streaks" seem to be reversible up to a distinct degree. However, if "fatty streaks" do not disappear, they grow up to intermediated lesions due to the attraction of numerous leukocytes, which transmigrate into the subendothelial space. Figure 1b depicts an arteriosclerotic, intermediate lesion of the thoracic aorta of a cholesterol-fed rabbit. This arteriosclerotic plaque/lesion mainly consists of more or less lipid laden MΦ.

Step 4: From Intermediate Lesion to Atheroma and Fibrous Plaque

MΦ, which are localized in the subendothelial space, internalize mLDL by scavenger receptors, which are not downregulated. This leads to an intracellular accumulation of cholesterol and to the creation of "▶ foam cells," which finally may result in cell death (apoptosis/necrosis) of the foam cells. When foam cells die, their contents are released. This attracts the next MΦ from the bloodstream and generates a necrotic lipid core in the depth of an arteriosclerotic plaque. Additionally, smooth muscle cells migrate from the media overgrowing the foam cells to build a ▶ fibrous cap. Figure 1c shows an arteriosclerotic, atheromatous/fibrous lesion of the thoracic aorta of a cholesterol-fed rabbit. This lesion is characterized by foam cells (Fo; lipid laden MΦ), a fibrous cap (Fc; consisting of fibrous connective tissue and migrated smooth muscle cells from the media) and a necrotic lipid core (Nlc). Proliferation and apoptosis of MΦ are important events controlling destabilization, inflammatory response, and plaque vulnerability. Rupture-prone plaques are called "vulnerable plaques." A plaque destabilization by activation of matrix-metalloproteinases affecting the fibrous cap thickness may convert a chronic process into an acute disorder with clinical complication like acute coronary syndrome, coronary heart disease, myocardial infarction, or stroke.

Step 5: From a Fibrous Plaque to a Complicated Lesion/Rupture

Increased accumulation of foam cells, extracellular debris, necrotic lipid core in addition with a decrease in fibrous cap thickness by activation of matrix metalloproteinases enhances the risk for plaque rupture and thrombus formation. Plaque rupture with atheromatous debris and distal embolization is the major pathogenetic mechanism responsible for myocardial infarction and stroke. However, it is suggested that the plaque composition rather than lesion burden seems to be the determinant factor producing rupture and subsequent thrombosis.

An infarct prognosis concerning cardiovascular risk can be individually calculated online according to the

PROCAM (Prospective Cardiovascular Münster) study [2], the ESC Euro SCORE [3] or the Framingham study [4]. Additionally, an individual risk calculation for stroke can be performed according to the Framingham study by the d'Agostini-Score [5].

Exercise Intervention

Regular, long-term aerobic exercise even with low/moderate intensity (e.g., walking) has substantial inhibitory impact on development and progression of arteriosclerotic lesions and, thus, reduces the mortality from cardiovascular disease, but also all-cause mortality. In this context, it has been shown that men who participated in some form of regular moderate physical activity revealed direct vasoprotective effects, i.e., they had about 30% lower risk of mortality and a significantly diminished incidence of stroke. Long-term physical activity decreases the pro-arteriosclerotic activity of endothelial as well as peripheral blood mononuclear cells. The exercise-induced vasoprotective action seems to be due to a significant improvement of endothelial function (e.g., by enhancing NO bioavailability) and diminishing oxidative stress. However, regular aerobic exercise has beneficial (vasoprotective) effects such as induced suppression of inflammatory cytokines like interleukins or tumor-necrosis factor-alpha (TNF-alpha) and thereby offers protection against TNF-alpha-induced insulin resistance. Thus, regular physical activity results in increased insulin sensitivity, decreased fat content/obesity, as well as an attenuation of hyperlipidemia, but also enhances longevity by mechanisms independent of these risk factors.

Vasoprotective, aerobic physical exercise sport is suggested, like:

- Walking (>20 min/day)
- Cycling, ball games, jogging, skating, swimming, team sport, etc.
- Gym (low weight and many repeats [$n = 20$; $3 \times n$])

References

1. Ross R (1999) Atherosclerosis - an inflammatory disease. New Engl J Med 340:115–126
2. PROCAM (Prospective Cardiovascular Münster)-Study (2002) http://www.medical-tribune.ch/deutsch/fortbildung/kardiologie/procam.php. Accessed 12 Sep 2011
3. Kardiovaskuläre Risikoberechnung nach dem ESC Euro SCORE (2003) http://www.bnk.de/transfer/euro.htm. Accessed 12 Sep 2011
4. Kardiovaskuläre Risikoberechnung nach der Framingham-Studie (2004) http://www.bnk.de/transfer/framingham.htm. Accessed 12 Sep 2011
5. Risikoberechnung für Schlanganfall nach der Framingham-Studie (d'Agostini-Score) (2004) http://www.bnk.de/transfer/stroke.htm. Accessed 12 Sep 2011

Arteriovenous Oxygen Difference

The difference between the oxygen content of the arterial and mixed venous blood.

Arthritis

David L. Scott
Department of Rheumatology, King's College Hospital, Kings College London School of Medicine Weston Education Centre, London, UK

Synonyms

Arthrosis; Arthropathy; Inflammatory joint disease; Synovitis

Definition

Arthritis means inflammation of the joints. It spans a number of disorders. The commonest form of arthritis is osteoarthritis, which is primarily an example of joint failure. Its prevalence increases with age, and it is an inevitable consequence of longevity. Most other forms of arthritis have a more inflammatory drive. Classically, this is immune-driven inflammation; the best example of such inflammation is rheumatoid arthritis. It can also be due to crystal deposition; the best example of this is gout. Some forms of inflammatory arthritis involve only one or two joints; a good example of this is psoriatic arthritis. Connective tissue disorders that range from systemic lupus erythematosus to myositis are often accompanied by arthritis, though this is not usually their most prominent feature.

Characteristics

Arthritis results in joint inflammation. This is characterized by pain, swelling, tenderness, and stiffness. Acute arthritis can be associated with redness of the joints and may also give systemic features of inflammation with marked fatigue.

The features of arthritis vary depending on the cause. Osteoarthritis mainly causes pain and bony swelling of the joints; the stiffness of osteoarthritis is most marked after exercise. Rheumatoid arthritis more often results in joint swelling, which is symmetrical and involves the small joints of the hands. The stiffness of rheumatoid arthritis is most marked in the morning.

The distribution of arthritis is typical for the different types. Osteoarthritis involves large joints such as the knee

Arthritis. Table 1 Summary of main forms of arthritis

Type	Subgroup	Comment
Osteoarthritis	Generalized	Common, occurs in later life, generalized form shows female preponderance
	Individual joints (e.g., knee)	
Rheumatoid arthritis		Common, occurs at all ages, female preponderance
Seronegative arthritis	Psoriatic arthritis	Uncommon, occurs at all ages, some forms like ankylosing spondylitis show male preponderance
	Ankylosing spondylitis	
	Reactive arthritis	
	Colitic arthritis	
Crystal arthritis	Gout	Common, occurs at all ages, gout shows male preponderance, pyrophosphate disease linked to osteoarthritis
	Pyrophosphate crystal deposition disease	
Connective tissue diseases	Systemic lupus erythematosus	Uncommon, arthritis usually minor component, female preponderance
	Vasculitis	
	Scleroderma	
	Myositis	
Infections	Viral arthritis	Relatively uncommon, viral arthritis usually mild, septic arthritis usually severe and seen in immunocompromised patients
	Septic arthritis	

or hip together with the base of the thumb and the distal interphalangeal joints. Rheumatoid arthritis involves the small joints of the hands and feet in a symmetrical distribution. Gout involves one or two joints – classically the first metatarsal joint (base of the big toe) and is severe and short lived if correctly treated. The main forms of arthritis are shown in the table (Table 1).

Clinical Relevance

Arthritis results in pain and reduced function. Inflammation also results in pain and disability. As a consequence, inflammatory arthritis is more disabling than osteoarthritis. Persisting inflammatory arthritis also results in joint damage. As a consequence of pain and inflammation, and in the later stages of disease as a result of joint damage, mobility is lost and fitness declines.

Arthritis is common. Some degree of osteoarthritis is inevitable in the elderly and up to 30% of the over 65 have clinically relevant osteoarthritis. Inflammatory arthritis, which is mainly rheumatoid arthritis, is less common – involving up to 1% of adults – but it causes more disability. Gout is also common. Other forms of arthritis, such as psoriatic arthritis, are seen less frequently.

Arthritis has a complex relationship to sport and activity. Joint damage is linked to the development of osteoarthritis in later life. Therefore some sports increase the eventual likelihood of developing osteoarthritis. A good example is football; the knees are prone to be damaged while playing, and there is an increased risk of developing osteoarthritis. On the other hand, exercise also prevents obesity, and maintaining musculoskeletal fitness and avoiding obesity both reduce the chance of developing arthritis. As a consequence, overall, the benefits of sport and exercise outweigh the risks of developing osteoarthritis. Inflammatory arthritis such as rheumatoid arthritis has no specific relationship to sport and exercise.

Therapeutical Consequences

Drug Therapy
The treatment of arthritis involves extensive medical care, based on optimizing drug treatment. The treatments span using analgesics to reduce pain, anti-inflammatory drugs to reduce the symptoms of joint inflammation, disease-modifying drugs (DMARDs) to suppress immune-mediated inflammation, biologic treatment to suppress immune-mediated inflammation, and a number of specific treatments such as allopurinol for gout.

Although dietary modification is popular with patients, there is limited evidence that it is effective.

Glucosamine is widely used as a dietary supplement to treat osteoarthritis but is not usually considered to be effective. There is some evidence that certain dietary supplements can occasionally be useful in rheumatic diseases. An example is the use of creatine supplements in patients with myositis, which is one of the connective tissue diseases; when used in conjunction with physical exercise, these improve muscle power.

Drugs in arthritis are involved in a range of different metabolic pathways. The main ones are as follows:

- Analgesics: These mainly act through central receptors for opiates. Examples are codeine-based analgesics. Paracetamol, which is the dominant mild analgesic, has a different mechanism of action, and most probably affects central cyclooxygenase pathways.
- Anti-inflammatory drugs: These mainly act through inhibiting cyclooxygenase pathways, though there are multiple other metabolic effects. They affect both central and peripheral cyclooxygenase metabolism and so reduce both pain and inflammation.
- Steroids: these bind to cell receptors and reduce inflammation and also change glucose metabolism.
- DMARDs: There is a wide range of DMARDs, and they act in many different ways. They are considered as a group because they suppress joint inflammation, but otherwise they are a diverse group of unrelated drugs.
- Biologics: New molecular approaches have greatly changed the treatment of arthritis. Different biologics target specific molecules involved in inflammation. The most widely used group, inhibitors of tumor necrosis factor, specifically inhibit this cytokine and therefore reduce inflammation.
- Allopurinol: This is an enzyme inhibitor that stops the synthesis of uric acid, and therefore means that uric acid crystals, the basis of gout, cannot be deposited.

Almost all patients with arthritis need to take drug therapy from time to time. Most patients benefit from analgesics to treat pain. Anti-inflammatory drugs also reduce pain and they are widely used; caution is needed to balance their side effects with any benefits. They are best used for short periods rather than giving them for long periods.

Patients with rheumatoid arthritis and other forms of inflammatory arthritis usually need not only analgesics and anti-inflammatory drugs but also take DMARDs and biologics. The aim is to suppress joint inflammation. There has been a marked change in the last few years with more intensive treatment used to suppress inflammation, often involving combinations of DMARDs and early use of biologics.

Gout is treated using anti-inflammatory drugs in the acute phase. Persisting gout needs treating with allopurinol.

Steroids are also effective and widely used to treat arthritis. They can be given by local injection; for example, they can be injected into an inflamed knee. They can also be given by intramuscular injection or by mouth. They should only be used for short periods of time.

Although patients need to take effective drugs, all the treatments used have significant risks of adverse effects. Anti-inflammatory drugs are linked to gastric ulcers and cardiac infarctions. DMARDs can result in bone marrow depression, and biologics increase the risk of infections. Steroids are particularly prone to cause side effects such as osteoporosis, diabetes, and cardiac disease. All these treatments therefore need to be used with caution.

Exercise Intervention

Historically, patients with arthritis were encouraged to rest; bed rest decreased the pain and inflammation of active arthritis. The Spa approach characterized the historical treatment of arthritis with a focus on rest. As a consequence of rest, patients became deconditioned and unfit and their arthritis was in the long-term worsened.

The situation has now changed and patients with arthritis are encouraged to exercise and keep fit. The balance of evidence now strongly favors recommending exercise for all people with arthritis [1–4].

Two forms of exercise are used in arthritis. The first, and probably the most important, is general exercises to increase fitness. An example is to encourage patients to walk regularly. The second is specific exercises to improve strength; a good example is quadriceps strengthening in patients with osteoarthritis of the knee. Both of these approaches are effective and improve symptoms and reduce disability. The evidence to prefer one over the other is incomplete. However, not all patients are able to undertake aerobic exercise and vice versa. Therefore in clinical practice, it is important to have a choice of effective options available. Exercise in water, which has its historical background in hydrotherapy, is particularly effective in arthritis as the water provides support for active joints while allowing exercise to uninvolved areas.

Strength training has been studied in detail in knee osteoarthritis [1], and it improves a wide range of attributes. These include pain, disability, strength, and walking abilities. A summary of recent trials is shown in the figure (Fig. 1).

There is equally compelling evidence in rheumatoid arthritis [2]. A number of research studies have shown that exercise therapy, including aerobic or strengthening exercises, when used in conjunction with conventional drug

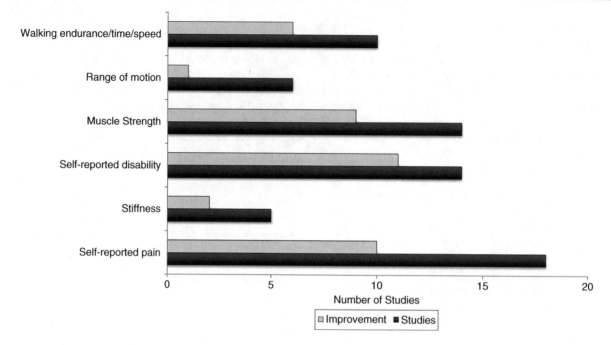

Arthritis. Fig. 1 Main outcomes in trials of exercise in arthritis. Numbers of studies and those reporting positive results are shown for different outcomes [1]

therapy, reduces pain and improves the quality of life in patients with rheumatoid arthritis. A key question is whether exercise worsens joint pain and inflammation in rheumatoid arthritis; the balance of evidence from many studies is that it does not do so.

Given the extent of the information in favor of exercise helping patients with arthritis, it is unfortunate that there remains significant resistance from patients and clinicians in implementing exercise programs. There are a number of limitations. These include lack of interest from patients, a relative unwillingness of specialists to recommend exercise for patients, and difficulties in meeting the costs of the programs for both patients and clinical staff undertaking these programs.

Measurements

There are many different assessments of muscle function and the impact of exercise in arthritis. One important measurement is quadriceps motor function; this can be assessed clinically or by more rigorous approaches such as using a strain gauge system. It is possible to calculate maximum voluntary contractions using such an approach.

A related issue is proprioceptive acuity, which indicates the patient's joint position sense. Measurement tools such as electrogoniometer are useful in this context.

As muscle function should improve performance, it is important to gain some understanding of patients' relative performance over time. One approach to this is the objective measure of the "aggregate functional performance time," which records the time taken to undertake four common activities of daily living. These comprise walking 50 ft on level ground, rising from a chair and walking 50 ft, and ascending and descending a flight of stairs. Shorter performance times indicate improved function.

The end result of muscle weakness can be captured by assessing disability. Conventionally patient-reported disability is measured. The most widely used method is the Health Assessment Questionnaire (HAQ), which records disability over a 0–3 scale. Higher HAQ scores indicate greater disability.

A number of more technical approaches are sometimes used. One example is measuring high-energy phosphate metabolites including ATP in the muscles before and after exercise; this can be achieved using phosphate magnetic resonance imaging. It is a highly specialized research method. Another example is the use of gait analysis to understand the mechanical issues underlying problems with performance in patients with arthritis; this tends to focus more on foot problems, but is useful to understand how patients are functioning.

References

1. Lange AK, Vanwanseele B, Fiatarone Singh MA (2008) Strength training for treatment of osteoarthritis of the knee: a systematic review. Arthritis Rheum 59:1488–1494
2. Oldfield V, Felson DT (2008) Exercise therapy and orthotic devices in rheumatoid arthritis: evidence-based review. Curr Opin Rheumatol 20:353–359
3. van den Berg MH, van der Giesen FJ, van Zeben D, van Groenendael JH, Seys PE, Vliet Vlieland TP (2008) Implementation of a physical activity intervention for people with rheumatoid arthritis: a case study. Musculoskeletal Care 6:69–85
4. Bearne LM, Scott DL, Hurley MV (2002) Exercise can reverse quadriceps sensorimotor dysfunction that is associated with rheumatoid arthritis without exacerbating disease activity. Rheumatology 41:157–166

Arthropathy

▶ Arthritis

Arthrosis

▶ Arthritis

Asthma Bronchiale

ANDRÉ MOREIRA, LUÍS DELGADO
Department of Immunology, and Immuno-allergology division, Faculty of Medicine, Hospital São João, E.P.E., University of Porto, Porto, Portugal

Synonyms

Asthma; Bronchial asthma; Exercise-induced asthma

Definition

▶ Asthma has a significant genetic component, but since its pathogenesis is not clear, much of its definition is descriptive: "...*a chronic inflammatory disorder of the airways in which many cells and cellular elements play a role. The chronic inflammation is associated with airway hyperresponsiveness that leads to recurrent episodes of wheezing, breathlessness, chest tightness, and coughing, particularly at night or in the early morning. These episodes are usually associated with widespread, but variable, airflow obstruction within the lung* that is often reversible either spontaneously or with treatment...*" in the Global Initiative for Asthma (GINA) Workshop Report 2009 available at: www.ginasthma.org. The pattern of inflammation in allergic asthma is characterized by T helper (Th) 2 inflammatory phenotype with a predominance of Th2 cytokines – such as interleukin-4 (IL-4), IL-5, IL-9, and IL-13. The allergic inflammation is characterized by increased IgE concentrations, mast-cell degranulation, and eosinophil-mediated inflammation.

In 2008, the PRACTALL initiative endorsed by the European Academy of Allergy and Clinical Immunology and the American Academy of Allergy, Asthma and Immunology, defined ▶ exercise-induced asthma (EIA) as lower airway obstruction and symptoms of cough, wheezing, or dyspnea induced by exercise in patients with underlying asthma [1]. The same clinical presentation in individuals without asthma was defined as ▶ exercise-induced bronchoconstriction. These definitions are however limited by the heterogeneity in asthma expression. In fact, multiple asthma phenotypes exhibiting differences in clinical response to treatment exist and assessment should be multidimensional, including variability in clinical, physiologic, and pathologic parameters. Two different clinical endotypes of asthma in athletes, reflecting different underlying mechanisms, have been recently suggested by Tari Haahtela *et al.* The pattern of "classical asthma" characterized by early onset childhood asthma, methacholine responsiveness, atopy and signs of eosinophilic airway inflammation; and another distinct phenotype with onset of symptoms during sports career, bronchial responsiveness to eucapnic hyperventilation test, and a variable association with atopic markers and eosinophilic airway inflammation [2, 3].

From the clinical point of view, the main physiological feature of asthma is intermittent and reversible airway obstruction, while the dominant pathological feature is airway inflammation sometimes associated with airway structural changes. Airway responsiveness is the tendency for airways to constrict under the influence of nonsensitizing physical stimuli such as cold air and exercise, chemical substances such as methacholine, or sensitizing agents such as allergens. Airway hyperresponsiveness can be defined as an abnormal increase in the degree to which the airways constrict upon exposure to these stimuli.

Pathogenesis

A consistent body of evidence has shown that Olympic level athletes have an increased risk for asthma and allergy, especially those who take part in endurance sports, such as swimming or running, and in winter sports.

The pathogenesis of EI-bronchoconstriction is likely multifactorial and is not completely understood. Classical postulated mechanisms behind exercise-induced asthma include the osmotic, or airway-drying, hypothesis [4]. As water is evaporated from the airway surface liquid, it becomes hyperosmolar and provides an osmotic stimulus for water to move from any cell nearby, resulting in cell shrinkage and release of inflammatory mediators that cause airway smooth muscle contraction. However, a proof of concept of this hypothesis would require that all athletes would develop bronchoconstriction at a certain point. This does not happen, suggesting the EIB explanatory model in athletes will probably include the interplay between environmental training factors including allergens and ambient conditions such as temperature, humidity, and air quality; and athlete's personal risk factors such as genetic and neuroimmunoendocrine determinants.

Genetic susceptibility to exercise-induced bronchoespasm has been linked with the gene for the aqueous water channel aquaporin. Airway hydration during exercise is mainly dependent on the water movement, following the osmotic force generated by sodium and chloride, through aquaporin channels expressed within the apical membrane of epithelial cells. It has been suggested that functional polymorphisms of the aquaporin gene may contribute to a phenotype where hyperhidrosis, sialorrhea, and excessive tearing are traits that may predict resistance of airways to nonspecific stimulus. However, it is also possible that mechanisms affecting both water and ion movement are commonly affected by nervous system dysfunction.

Intensive training can have effects on autonomic regulation promoting the vagal predominance, thus regulating contractions and relaxations of the airway smooth muscle. The increased parasympathetic activity could act as a compensatory response to the sympathetic stimulation associated with frequent and intense training. This could induce not only the resting bradycardia typical of athletes, but also an increase in bronchomotor tone and, in turn, an increased susceptibility to the development of asthma. A dysfunctional neuroendocrine–immune interface may then play a role in the pathogenesis of exercise-induced bronchoconstriction, mainly due to release and action of neuropeptides from primary sensory nerve terminals, in the so-called neurogenic inflammation pathway. This is also clinically supported by a positive effect of inhaled anticholinergic drugs in some athletes.

Exercise Response

Exercise is a powerful trigger of bronchoconstriction and symptoms in asthmatic patients and may result in avoidance of physical activity resulting in detrimental consequences to their physical and social well-being. Diagnosis demands the synthesis of medical history with respiratory symptoms, physical examination, and appropriate laboratory or field tests. Methods and thresholds to document exercise-induced bronchoconstriction may be different for recreational or competitive athletes, particularly in regulated sports. For recreational exercisers, free running for children or a simple 10 min jog for adults may be adequate to document exercise-induced bronchoconstriction ($\geq$10% drop in lung function measured by forced expiratory volume in the first second of forced vital capacity -FEV1). For others, the exercise challenge should elicit 90% of maximal heart rate or 40–60% of maximal ventilation during 6–8 min of exercise on a treadmill or stationary bicycle. For competitive athletes, precise criteria for diagnosing asthma have been set (Table 1).

Drugs effective in the treatment of asthma are likely to be effective in the treatment of EI-asthma or EI-bronchoconstriction. Inhaled β2-adrenoceptor agonists are most

Asthma Bronchiale. Table 1 Criteria set by the World Anti-Doping Agency to document asthma in athletes in 2011. www.wada-ama.org/.../WADA_Medical_info_Asthma_V3_EN.0.pdf

A rise in FEV1 to bronchodilator $\geq$12% of the baseline or predicted FEV1 and exceeds 200 ml
A fall in FEV1 $\geq$ 10% from baseline in response to exercise or eucapnic voluntary hyperpnea
A fall in FEV1 $\geq$ 15% from baseline after inhaling 22.5 ml of 4.5 g% NaCl or $\leq$635 mg of mannitol
A fall in FEV1 $\geq$ 20% from baseline in response to methacholine PC20 $\leq$ 4 mg/ml, or PD20 $\leq$ 400 µg (cumulative dose) or $\leq$200 µg (noncumulative dose) in those not taking inhaled corticosteroids (ICS), and PC20 $\leq$ 16 mg/ml or PD20 $\leq$ 1,600 µg (cumulative dose) or $\leq$800 µg (noncumulative dose) in those taking ICS for at least 1 month

Note: In the case of an athlete with known but well-controlled asthma, recording a negative result to the bronchial provocation test(s), but still seeking approval for the use of inhaled β2-agonist(s), the following documentation must be included in the submitted medical file: consultations with their physician for treatment of asthma, hospital emergency department visits, or admissions for acute exacerbations of asthma or treatment with oral corticosteroids. Additional information that may assist includes: the age of onset of asthma; detailed description of the asthma symptoms, both day and night; trigger factors; medication use; past history of atopic disorders and/or childhood asthma; and physical examination, together with results of skin prick tests or RASTs to document the presence of allergic hypersensitivity. Negative bronchial provocation and allergy test results also must be included with the submission to the National Anti-Doping Agency

effective in reversing EI-asthma/bronchoconstriction and are also used for prevention. The effectiveness of inhaled short-acting β-agonists such as salbutamol or terbutaline against EI-asthma/bronchoconstriction is optimal 20 min after inhalation and wane within a few hours. Long-acting β2-agonists, such as formoterol and salmeterol, protect for up to 12 h after a single inhalation. However, only formoterol acts as fast as quick-acting beta agonists; therefore, formoterol but not salmeterol, should be chosen to reverse EI-asthma/bronchoconstriction. Inhaled β2-agonists may mask worsening airway inflammation, and should never be used regularly without an inhaled glucocorticoid.

Regular treatments with inhaled ▶ glucocorticoids and/or ▶ leukotriene pathway antagonists control underlying asthma and reduce EI-asthma/bronchoconstriction. Zileuton is a leukotriene synthesis inhibitor, and montelukast, zafirlukast, and pranlukast are cysLT receptor-1 antagonists. H1-antihistamines have minimal effects on EI-asthma/bronchoconstriction, whereas cromones administered before exercise mildly reduce EI-bronchoconstriction. In difficult to control EI-asthma/bronchoconstriction, combining inhaled glucocorticoids, oral leukotriene antagonists, and/or inhaled β2-agonists may be beneficial.

Optimal control of underlying asthma minimizes airway narrowing during exercise. Worsening EI-asthma may be a sign of inadequate control of underlying asthma, and "step up" therapy should be considered. On the other hand, allergic rhinitis is also a very common disease among athletes, and may negatively impact athletic performance; its early recognition, diagnosis, and treatment are crucial for improving nasal function and reduce the risk of asthma during exercise and competition. Certain medications for athletes with asthma and rhinitis who participate in regulated competitions are not allowed and physicians, athletes, and coaches should be aware of the updated regulatory aspects of asthma treatment (Table 2).

A few notes should be taken on the effects of exercise as a non-pharmacological treatment of asthmatic patients. At the current knowledge, evidence-based prescription of physical activity in asthma seems to be restricted to improvements in the physical fitness of the subjects. It is recommended that children and adolescents participate in at least 60 min of moderate intensity physical activity most days of the week and preferably daily (Report of the Dietary Guidelines Advisory Committee Dietary Guidelines for Americans, 2010). Engagement in physical activity promotes the child normal psychosocial development, neuromuscular coordination, and self-esteem. Changing from sedentary behaviors such as television viewing and

Asthma Bronchiale. Table 2 Drugs regulated for asthma treatment during training and competition by the World Anti-Doping Agency in 2011

Beta agonists
All beta-2 agonists are prohibited except salbutamol (maximum 1,600 µg over 24 h) and salmeterol when taken by inhalation in accordance with the manufacturers' recommended therapeutic regime. Formoterol and terbutaline require a Therapeutic Use Exemption (TUE) with medical evidence of asthma. Reason why use of salbutamol and salmeterol is not suitable must be provided
The presence of salbutamol in urine in excess of 1,000 ng/ml is presumed not to be an intended therapeutic use of the substance and will be considered as an *Adverse Analytical Finding* unless the *Athlete* proves, through a controlled pharmacokinetic study, that the abnormal result was the consequence of the use of a therapeutic dose (maximum 1,600 µg over 24 h) of inhaled salbutamol
Glucocorticorticosteroid
Inhaled glucocorticosteroids (GCS) are permitted. All glucocorticosteroids are prohibited when administered by oral, intravenous, intramuscular, or rectal routes

computer games to moderate intensity physical activity has been associated with enhanced overall health and prevention of chronic diseases. In asthmatics, exercise training may reduce the perception of breathlessness through strengthening of respiratory muscle and decrease the likelihood of exercise-induced symptoms by lowering the ventilation rate during exercise.

Currently, the GINA Guidelines do not include recommendations for exercise as part of the treatment for patients with asthma. Exercise is a powerful trigger for asthma symptoms. For this reason, caretakers may be reluctant to allow their asthmatic children to engage in sports practice, fearing an exacerbation of the disease. Every child with asthma should be questioned about exercise performance, tolerance, and symptoms, but there is no reason to discourage asthmatic children with a controlled disease to exercise [5].

References

1. Schwartz LB et al (2008) Exercise-induced hypersensitivity syndromes in recreational and competitive athletes: a PRACTALL consensus report (what the general practitioner should know about sports and allergy). Allergy 63(8):953–961
2. Haahtela T, Malmberg P, Moreira A (2008) Mechanisms of asthma in Olympic athletes–practical implications. Allergy 63(6):685–694
3. Lotvall J et al (2011) Asthma endotypes: a new approach to classification of disease entities within the asthma syndrome. J Allergy Clin Immunol 127(2):355–360

4. Carlsen KH et al (2008) Exercise-induced asthma, respiratory and allergic disorders in elite athletes: epidemiology, mechanisms and diagnosis: part I of the report from the Joint Task Force of the European Respiratory Society (ERS) and the European Academy of Allergy and Clinical Immunology (EAACI) in cooperation with GA2LEN. Allergy 63(4):387–403

5. Moreira A et al (2008) Physical training does not increase allergic inflammation in asthmatic children. Eur Respir J 32(6):1570–1575

Atherosclerosis

▶ Arteriosclerosis
▶ Coronary Heart Disease

Athlete

One who participates in an organized team or individual sport that requires regular competition against others as a central component, places a high premium on excellence and achievement, and requires some form of systematic (and usually intense) training.

Athlete's Diet

RICHARD B. KREIDER, Y. PETER JUNG
Exercise & Sport Nutrition Lab, Department of Health and Kinesiology, Texas A & M University, College Station, TX, USA

Synonyms

Food regimes for active individuals; Macronutrient and micronutrient needs of athletes; Major nutrient requirements of sportsperson; Training table

Definition

The *athlete's diet* is a well-designed diet that meets energy intake, macronutrient, and micronutrient needs and incorporates proper timing of nutrients in order to optimize performance, recovery, and/or training adaptations [1–3]. The athlete's diet is the foundation upon which a sound performance enhancement training program can be developed. Research has clearly shown that not ingesting a sufficient amount of calories and/or enough of the right type of macronutrients may impede an athlete's training adaptations while athletes who consume a balanced diet that meets energy needs can augment physiological training adaptations. Moreover, maintaining an energy-deficient diet during training may lead to loss of muscle mass and strength, increased susceptibility to illness, and increased prevalence of ▶ overreaching and/or ▶ overtraining. Incorporating good dietary practices as part of a training program is one way to help optimize training adaptations and prevent overtraining.

Description

Energy Demands. Athletes need to consume enough calories to offset daily energy demands [1]. Individuals who participate in a general fitness program (e.g., exercising 30–40 min per day, three times per week) can typically meet nutritional needs following a normal diet (e.g., 1,800–2,400 kcals/day or about 25–35 kcals/kg/day for a 50–80 kg individual) because their caloric demands from exercise are not too great (e.g., 200–400 kcals/session). However, athletes involved in moderate levels of intense training (e.g., 2–3 h per day of intense exercise performed 5–6 times per week) or high volume intense training (e.g., 3–6 h per day of intense training in 1–2 workouts for 5–6 days per week) may expend 600–1,200 kcals or more per hour during exercise. For this reason, their caloric needs may approach 50–80 kcals/kg/day (2,500–8,000 kcals/day for a 50–100 kg athlete). For elite athletes, energy expenditure during heavy training and/or competition may reach as high as 12,000 kcals/day (150–200 kcals/kg/day for a 60–80 kg athlete). Additionally, caloric needs for large athletes (i.e., 100–150 kg) may range between 6,000–12,000 kcals/day depending on the volume and intensity of different training phases.

Although some argue that athletes can meet caloric needs simply by consuming a well-balanced diet, it is often very difficult for larger athletes and/or athletes engaged in high volume/intense training to be able to eat enough food in order to meet caloric needs. Maintaining an energy-deficient diet during training often leads to significant weight loss (including muscle mass), illness, onset of physical and psychological symptoms of overtraining, and reductions in performance [1, 4]. Nutritional analyses of athlete's diets have revealed that many are susceptible to maintaining negative energy intakes during training. Consequently, it is important for professionals working with athletes to ensure that athletes are well fed and consume enough calories to offset the increased energy demands of training, and maintain body weight. Although this sounds relatively simple, intense training often suppresses appetite and/or alters hunger patterns so that many athletes do not feel like eating. Further, travel and training schedules may limit food availability and/or the types of food athletes are accustomed to eating. This means that care should be taken to plan meal times in concert with training, as well as to make sure athletes have sufficient availability of nutrient-dense foods throughout the day for snacking between meals (e.g., drinks, fruit, carbohydrate/protein energy bars, etc.) [4].

Carbohydrate. In addition to meeting energy needs, athletes need to consume the proper amounts of carbohydrate (CHO), protein (PRO), and fat in their diet [1, 2]. Individuals engaged in a general fitness program can typically meet macronutrient needs by consuming a normal diet (i.e., 45–55% CHO [3–5 g/kg/day], 10–15% PRO [0.8–1.0 g/kg/day], and 25–35% fat [0.5–1.5 g/kg/day]) [1]. However, athletes involved in moderate and high volume training need greater amounts of carbohydrate and protein in their diet to meet macronutrient needs. In terms of carbohydrate needs, athletes involved in moderate amounts of intense training (e.g., 2–3 h per day of intense exercise performed 5–6 times per week) typically need to consume a diet consisting of 55–65% carbohydrate (i.e., 5–8 g/kg/day or 250–1,200 g/day for 50–150 kg athletes) in order to maintain liver and muscle glycogen stores. However, resistance-trained or power athletes may only need about 40–45% carbohydrate in their diet in order to maintain a sufficient amount of muscle and liver glycogen during training [1, 2]. Athletes involved in high volume intense training (e.g., 3–6 h per day of intense training in 1–2 workouts for 5–6 days per week) may need to consume 8–10 g/day of carbohydrate (i.e., 400–1,500 g/day for 50–150 kg athletes) in order to maintain muscle glycogen levels. Preferably, the majority of dietary carbohydrate should come from complex carbohydrates with a low to moderate glycemic index (e.g., whole grains, vegetables, fruit, etc.).

Protein. For people involved in a general fitness program, protein needs can generally be met by ingesting 0.8–1.0 g/kg/day of protein. Older individuals may benefit from a higher protein intake (e.g., 1.0–1.2 g/kg/day of protein) in order to help prevent ▶ sarcopenia. It is recommended that athletes involved in moderate amounts of intense training consume 1–1.5 g/kg/day of protein (50–225 g/day for a 50–150 kg athlete) while athletes involved in high volume intense training consume 1.5–2.0 g/kg/day of protein (75–300 g/day for a 50–150 kg athlete) [2]. Protein needs when living or training at altitude may be as high as 2.2 g/kg/day [2]. Although smaller athletes typically can ingest this amount of protein in their normal diet, larger athletes often have difficulty consuming this much dietary protein. Additionally, a number of athletic populations have been reported to

be susceptible to protein malnutrition (e.g., runners, cyclists, swimmers, triathletes, gymnasts, dancers, skaters, wrestlers, boxers, etc.). Therefore, care should be taken to ensure that athletes consume a sufficient amount of quality protein in their diet in order to maintain nitrogen balance (e.g., 1.5–2 g/kg/day).

Fat. The dietary recommendations of fat intake for athletes are similar to or slightly greater than those recommended for nonathletes in order to promote health. Generally, it is recommended that athletes consume a moderate amount of fat (approximately 30% of their daily caloric intake). For athletes attempting to decrease body fat, however, it has been recommended that they consume 0.5–1 g/kg/day of fat. Strategies to help athletes manage dietary fat intake include teaching them which foods contain various types of fat so that they can make better food choices and how to count fat grams.

Vitamins. Vitamins are essential organic compounds that serve to regulate metabolic processes, energy synthesis, neurological processes, and prevent destruction of cells. Although research has demonstrated that specific vitamins may possess some health benefit (e.g., Vitamin E, niacin, folic acid, vitamin C, etc.), few have been reported to directly provide ergogenic value for athletes. However, some vitamins may help athletes tolerate training to a greater degree by reducing oxidative damage (Vitamin E, C) and/or help to maintain a healthy immune system during heavy training (Vitamin C). Since dietary analyses of athletes have found deficiencies in caloric and vitamin intake, sports nutritionists' often recommend that athletes consume a low-dose daily multivitamin and/or a vitamin enriched post-workout carbohydrate/protein supplement during periods of heavy training [1].

Minerals. Minerals are essential inorganic elements necessary for a host of metabolic processes. Minerals serve as structure for tissue, important components of enzymes and hormones, and regulators of metabolic and neural control. Some athletes have been found to have deficiencies in some mineral intakes. Dietary supplementation of minerals in deficient athletes has generally been found to improve exercise capacity. Calcium supplementation with Vitamin D has been recommended for athletes susceptible to premature osteoporosis. Iron supplementation in athletes prone to iron deficiencies and/or anemia has been reported to improve exercise capacity. Sodium phosphate loading has been reported to increase maximal oxygen uptake, anaerobic threshold, and improve endurance exercise capacity by 8–10%. Increasing dietary availability of salt (sodium chloride) during the initial days of exercise training in hot and humid environments has also been reported to help maintain fluid balance and prevent dehydration. Finally, zinc supplementation during training has been reported to decrease exercise-induced changes in immune function. Consequently, in contrast to vitamins, there appear to be several minerals that may enhance exercise capacity and/or training adaptations for athletes under certain conditions [1].

Water. Water remains one of the most important nutrients for athletes. Exercise performance can be significantly impaired when 2% or more of body weight is lost through sweat. Weight loss of more than 4% of body weight during exercise may lead to heat illness, heat exhaustion, heat stroke, and possibly death. For this reason, it is critical that athletes consume a sufficient amount of water and/or glucose-electrolyte solution (GES) during exercise in order to maintain hydration status. Generally, athletes need to ingest 0.5–1 L/h of fluid per hour of exercise in order to prevent dehydration. This requires frequent ingestion of 6–8 oz of cold water and/or a GES sports drink every 5–15 min during exercise.

Nutrient Timing. In addition to these general nutritional guidelines, ▶ nutrient timing has also been reported to play a role in optimizing performance and training adaptations [3]. Pre-exercise meals should be consumed about 4–6 h before exercise. It is also advisable to ingest a carbohydrate and protein snack 30–60 min prior to exercise (e.g., 30–50 g of carbohydrate and 5–10 g protein). This serves to increase carbohydrate availability toward the end of an intense exercise bout and provide amino acids to help decrease exercise-induced catabolism of protein. When exercise lasts more than 1 h, athletes should ingest GES sport drinks in order to maintain blood glucose levels, help prevent dehydration, and reduce the immunosuppressive effects of intense exercise. Following intense exercise, athletes should consume carbohydrate and protein (e.g., 1 g/kg of carbohydrate and 0.5 g/kg of protein) within 30 min after exercise as well as consume a high carbohydrate meal within 2 h following exercise. This nutritional strategy has been found to accelerate glycogen resynthesis as well as promote a more anabolic hormonal profile that may hasten recovery. Finally, for 2–3 days prior to competition, athletes should taper training by 30–50% and consume 200–300 g/day of extra carbohydrate in their diet. This ▶ carbohydrate loading technique has been shown to supersaturate carbohydrate stores prior to competition and improve endurance exercise capacity.

Clinical Use/Application

Athletes engaged in intense training need to consume enough calories, macronutrients, and micronutrients to meet energy needs. Athletes who maintain energy-deficient diets and/or do not consume enough carbohydrate, protein, vitamins, and/or minerals to meet nutritional needs may experience a lack of positive training adaptations and poor performance leading to overtraining.

References

1. Kreider RB et al (2010) ISSN exercise and sport nutrition review: research and recommendations. J Int Soc Sports Nutr 7:7
2. Campbell B et al (2007) International Society of Sports Nutrition position stand: protein and exercise. J Int Soc Sports Nutr 4:8
3. Kerksick C et al (2008) International Society of Sports Nutrition position stand: nutrient timing. J Int Soc Sports Nutr 5:17
4. Kreider RB (2001) Nutritional considerations of overtraining. In: Stout JR, Antonio J (eds) Sport supplements: a complete guide to physique and athletic enhancement. Lippincott, Williams and Wilkins, Baltimore, pp 199–208

Athlete's Heart

WILFRIED KINDERMANN
Institute of Sports and Preventive Medicine, University of Saarland, Saarbrücken, Germany

Synonyms

Athletic heart syndrome; Marathoners' heart

Definition

The Finish physician Henschen described enlarged hearts in cross-country skiers in 1899 by means of percussion. He concluded that prolonged exercise training causes both dilatation and hypertrophy of the heart. Henschen referred to this enlargement induced by endurance training as athlete's heart. The nature of the athlete's heart has been controversially discussed for many decades. According to the Frank–Starling Law, it was assumed that the enlargement of the heart reflected a pathological state. Based on electrocardiographic and X-ray examinations in a number of highly trained athletes, Reindell from Freiburg, however, realized as early as in the first half of the twentieth century that the enlarged heart caused by sports reflects a physiological hypertrophy. Numerous detailed studies of elite athletes, using newer methods, confirmed that the athlete's heart is a physiological adaptation to chronic endurance exercise. The muscle mass of the heart increases and all heart cavities are enlarged, resulting in an eccentric hypertrophy. These changes have, since then, been well known as physiological cardiac remodeling [1, 4].

Mechanisms

Endurance exercise requires an increased cardiac output for extended periods of time. The resulting volume load is the

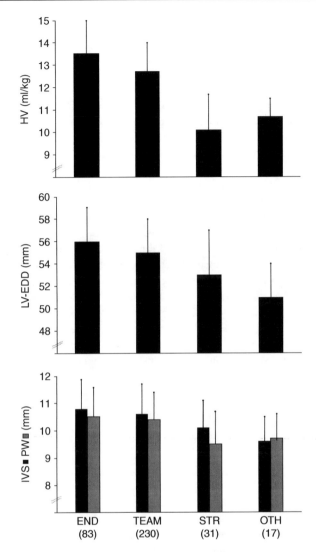

Athlete's Heart. Fig. 1 Mean values and standard deviation of heart volume (HV), left ventricular end-diastolic diameter (LV-EDD) and wall thicknesses (*IVS* interventricular septum, *PW* posterior wall) in endurance athletes (END), team sports (TEAM), strength athletes (STR), and other types of sports (OTH, e.g., bowling, dancing, golf, shooting)

crucial mechanism for the development of eccentric hypertrophy. This is similar to pathological volume-overloaded hearts such as aortic regurgitation although only the left ventricle is primarily enlarged in this case. By contrast, the athlete's heart is a balanced enlarged heart. Provided that duration and intensity of exercise are adequate, endurance training results in similar changes of left and right ventricle with regard to mass, volume, and function [4]. In particular, dimensions of heart cavities as well as wall thicknesses increase. The concomitant increase in wall thickness

maintains normal myocardial wall stress. Otherwise, the only increase in end-diastolic dimension would raise the wall stress according to the Law of Laplace. Furthermore, systolic and diastolic functions of left ventricle are not affected. Because of the heightened vagal tone, the ejection fraction may be in the lower normal range in some athletes, but will always return to normal during exercise. Several, but not all studies, evaluating transmitral flow by Doppler echocardiography, even demonstrated supranormal diastolic function of the athlete's heart. Finally, the enlarged heart of endurance athletes shows normal left ventricular filling pressures at rest and during exercise.

The increased blood pressure, especially during static exercise, is discussed as a further mechanism to develop changes of the heart. Concentric left ventricular hypertrophy, resembling the pattern of pathological pressure-overloaded hearts, was described in strength-trained athletes. It is assumed that the clearly increased afterload during mainly static exercise results in increased wall thickness without changes in end-diastolic ventricular dimensions. This type of an athlete's heart, however, is not generally accepted. Methodological pitfalls and in particular the influence of drugs such as anabolic steroids possibly misused have to be taken into account. Anabolic steroids can develop concentric hypertrophy of the left ventricle and are mostly, but not always, associated with an impaired diastolic function. If comparing the influence of different sports on left ventricle, the ratio between end-diastolic wall thickness and internal ventricular diameter was only significantly increased in body builders using anabolic steroids. All other athletes including anabolic-free strength-trained showed no concentric hypertrophy (Fig. 1). As a result of existing data, a specific influence of strength training is rather unlikely [5].

Exercise Response

An enlargement of the heart following sport is less common than generally assumed. Regular and intensive endurance training over the years for example, at least 5 h per week, is necessary. On the other hand, there are considerable individual differences with respect to a sports-related enlargement of the heart which are probably caused genetically. Even a running training of 100 km or more per week does not necessarily induce an enlarged heart. Accordingly, there is only a loose relationship between heart size or various echocardiographic parameters (e.g., left ventricular muscle mass, left ventricular end-diastolic diameter) and performance. Therefore, in the diagnosis of endurance performance, the knowledge of heart size cannot replace other physiological measures such as maximal oxygen uptake [1].

The heart size in athletes can be determined by echocardiography. The end-diastolic left ventricular volume, obtained from the modified Simpson rule, highly correlates with the radiologically determined total heart volume, which is usually expressed relative to body weight. The normal values in untrained healthy males and females are 10–12 (gray zone to 13) and 9–11 (gray zone to 12) ml/kg. There are no gender differences with regard to the percentage enlargement of the heart through training. The largest body weight-related heart volumes amount to approximately 20 (males) and 19 (females) ml/kg and are found in long-distance runners [1]. If expressed in absolute terms, however, the most enlarged athlete's hearts were found in endurance-trained or combined endurance- and strength-trained athletes with high body weight, e.g., rowing, cycling, swimming, and triathlon. Values of about 1,300 ml or more are possible. Accordingly, left ventricular end-diastolic diameter and wall thickness are also the greatest in endurance-trained athletes [3]. In team sports, especially soccer players, athletes may have slightly enlarged heart dimensions. Athletes hardly performing endurance training have no enlarged hearts, for example, types of sports such as athletics (sprinting, jumping, throwing, decathlon), gymnastics, alpine skiing, and weight lifting (Fig. 1). Children and adolescents are also likely to develop the same cardiocirculatory adaptations to endurance training, including moderate heart enlargement. Furthermore, if older persons perform regular dynamic training of a certain duration and intensity, they can also develop enlarged hearts.

From a technical point of view, the athlete's heart works with a larger swept volume and a reduced frequency. The dimensional changes lead to a significant increase in stroke volume and decrease in heart rate at rest and during exercise. Since the maximal heart rate remains largely unchanged, a high maximal cardiac output is achieved. The submaximal cardiac output, however, shows no relevant difference between trained and untrained heart [1].

The left ventricular hypertrophy can already decrease after a short period of detraining [3]. After long-term deconditioning, the regression of athlete's heart can be complete. The left ventricular dilatation, however, is frequently only partially reversible [1]. In some cases, the dimensions remain markedly enlarged (end-diastolic diameter ≥60 mm). In contrast, the wall thickness shows complete normalization. In addition to genetic influences, remaining physical activity and a usually increased body weight have to be considered causally. A relatively low training volume after the end of sporting career seems to be sufficient for a persistent moderate enlargement. There

is no evidence that former elite athletes with athlete's heart die prematurely. On the contrary, it was shown that the life expectancy of former endurance athletes is even higher than those of inactive subjects.

Athlete's heart is commonly associated with electrocardiographic (ECG) alterations [1, 3]. The most common changes are rhythm and conduction abnormalities (except intraventricular), increased QRS voltages, incomplete right bundle branch block, early repolarization patterns, and deep Q-waves. These alterations are mostly physiological and due to lower intrinsic heart rate, increased vagal tone, and cardiac remodeling. The ECG changes in female athletes are rarer. Rhythm and conduction abnormalities disappear during physical exercise because of decreased parasympathetic and increased sympathetic activity. Arrhythmias like frequent premature beats and nonsustained ventricular tachycardias may be part of the athletic heart syndrome. Nevertheless, pathological causes should be excluded. T-wave inversion, reported between 2% and 4% and mostly located in precordial leads, may be training related; however, further cardiac diagnosis is required. ECG abnormalities including T-wave inversions are more commonly present in black compared with white athletes.

Diagnostics

The differential diagnosis between physiological athlete's heart and pathological conditions may be difficult in some athletes. Cardiovascular diseases such as hypertrophic cardiomyopathy, dilated cardiomyopathy, arrhythmogenic right ventricular cardiomyopathy, hypertension, and valvular heart diseases induce changes mimicking certain morphological adaptations of the athlete's heart [2]. The knowledge of upper limits of cardiac dimensions helps to exclude pathological changes (Table 1). The diastolic dimensions of the left ventricle characterizing the

Athlete's Heart. Table 1 Upper limits of echocardiographic criteria of the athlete's heart (exceptional individual values in brackets)

	Men	Women
Heart volume (ml/kg)	20	19
Heart weight (g/kg)	7.5	7
LV muscle mass (g/m)	170	135
LV-EDD (mm)	63 (67)	60 (63)
Wall thickness (mm)	13 (15)	12
Left atrial dimension (mm)	45 (50)	43 (46)

LV left ventricular, *EDD* end-diastolic diameter

hypertrophy may be substantially increased in some athletes. Approximately 15% have an end-diastolic diameter of 60 mm or greater, and 2% show wall thicknesses of between 13 and 15 mm [3]. Combined strength- and endurance-trained athletes with great body dimensions like rowers or canoeists commonly show greater morphological adaptations than others because of isotonic and isometric training of both the arms and legs. Values of up to 67 mm for end-diastolic diameter and up to 15 mm for wall thickness are from such athletes [3]. Black athletes exhibit a greater left ventricular wall thickness and more frequently exceed the normal limit of 12 mm than white athletes.

The left atrium is enlarged in about 20% of the athletes and is part of the physiological remodeling. Two percent show a marked dilatation of 45 mm or greater (Table 1). There is a close association between the enlargement of the left ventricle and the size of the left atrium. Despite left atrial enlargement, atrial fibrillation is not more common in young athletes than in the general population.

Left ventricular wall thicknesses of 13 mm or more are suspect for pathological hypertrophy if the size of the left ventricle is normal or even rather small. The most important differential diagnosis is the presence of hypertrophic cardiomyopathy, the most common cause for sudden cardiac death in young athletes [2]. In contrast to athlete's heart, the diastolic function is mostly restricted, the left atrium can be marked enlarged, the wall thickness does not decrease after cessation of training, and the ECG often shows distinct changes.

A further clinical scenario is the differentiation between athlete's heart and dilated cardiomyopathy [2]. Diagnostic doubtful cases are athletes with an end-diastolic diameter of $\geq$60 mm and low-normal systolic function, e.g., ejection fraction of 50–55%. The systolic left ventricular function of the athlete's heart, however, is always normalized during exercise. Moreover, the ergometric performance is always increased in physiologically enlarged hearts.

Endurance training in athletes with aortic or mitral regurgitation can induce marked enlargement of left ventricle. Due to the combined volume load by training and valvular regurgitation, it is often difficult to evaluate the severity of regurgitation based on left ventricle dimensions. Mild valvular regurgitation per se does not influence the ventricle size. Therefore, if the left ventricular end-diastolic diameter of highly trained athletes with known valvular regurgitation is $\geq$60 mm, a significant regurgitation should be taken into account. In this case, consequences would result for the eligibility in competitive sports [2].

Cross-References

▶ Cardiac Hypertrophy, Physiological

References

1. Kindermann W (2007) Physiologische Anpassungen des Herz-Kreilauf-Systems an körperliche Belastung. In: Kindermann W, Dickhuth HH, Nieß A, Röcker K, Urhausen A (eds) Sportkardiologie. Steinkopff, Darmstadt, pp S1–S20
2. Maron BJ, Zipes DP (2005) 36th Bethesda conference: eligibility recommendations for competitive athletes with cardiovascular abnormalities. J Am Coll Cardiol 45:2–64
3. Pelliccia A, Maron BJ, Spataro A, Proschan MA, Spirito P (1991) The upper limit of physiologic cardiac hypertrophy in highly trained elite athletes. N Engl J Med 324:295–301
4. Scharhag J, Schneider G, Urhausen A, Rochette V, Kramann B, Kindermann W (2002) Right and left ventricular mass and function in male endurance athletes and untrained individuals determined by magnetic resonance imaging. J Am Coll Cardiol 40:1856–1863
5. Urhausen A, Kindermann W (1999) Sports-specific adaptations and differentiation of the athlete's heart. Sports Med 28:237–244

Athletic Amenorrhea

MARY JANE DE SOUZA, REBECCA J. TOOMBS
Women's Health and Exercise Laboratory, Noll Laboratory, Department of Kinesiology, Penn State University, University Park, PA, USA

Synonyms

Amenorrhea; Exercise-associated functional hypothalamic amenorrhea; Exercise-associated menstrual disorder; Female athlete triad-associated amenorrhea

Definition

Amenorrhea is the most serious menstrual disturbance observed in physically active women and athletes [1]. There are two classifications of amenorrhea, primary and secondary. ▶ Primary amenorrhea is defined as the failure to achieve menarche by age 15 in the presence of normal development of secondary sex characteristics [1]. The definition of ▶ secondary amenorrhea in the exercise literature has varied but should be defined conservatively as no menses for 90 days or 3 months, or less than five menses in 12 months. It is important to define amenorrhea conservatively (no menses for 90 days) versus liberally (no menses for 12 months) since serious clinical sequelae result from the presence of this disorder, particularly, low bone mass.

In athletes, the amenorrhea is termed as functional hypothalamic amenorrhea since the origin of the disorder

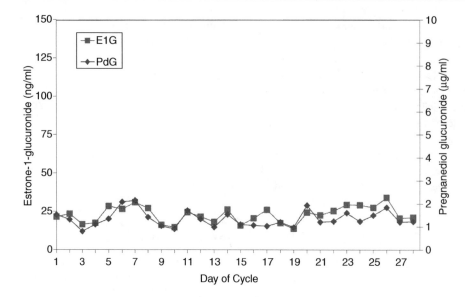

Athletic Amenorrhea. Fig. 1 Representative profile of estrogen and progesterone excretion in urine samples collected daily for 28 days in an amenorrheic athlete. *E1G* Estrone-1-glucuronide, *PdG* Pregnanediol glucuronide

resides in the hypothalamus [2, 3]. ▶ Functional hypothalamic amenorrhea in athletes is classically characterized by decreased gonadotropin-releasing hormone pulsatility and decreased pulsatility of the gonadotropins, particularly luteinizing hormone, in the face of chronic hypoestrogenism. The pituitary gland exhibits normal or exaggerated responsiveness to perturbation by gonadotropin-releasing hormone. Amenorrhea, whether primary or secondary, is associated with chronically suppressed levels of the ovarian steroids, estrogen and progesterone [2]. Figure 1 provides an example of a profile of estrogen and progesterone excretion in urine samples (urinary estrone and pregnanediol glucuronides) collected daily for 28 days in an amenorrheic athlete.

Mechanisms

In 1980, Dr. Michelle Warren first published the hypothesis that a long-term "energy drain" was associated with the reproductive suppression and amenorrhea observed in exercising women. Since then, this concept has been refined and the etiology of amenorrhea is predominately thought to be secondary to low energy availability [3]. ▶ Low energy availability means that the volume of energy an exercising woman has available is not enough to adequately support all of her physiological functions and results in her body making metabolic shifts to preserve the most important functions that are needed to sustain life and, as such, suppresses other less essential functions to conserve fuel, like reproductive function [2, 3]. Thus, in exercising women, the amenorrhea is attributable to low

energy availability where inadequate caloric intake combined with high energy expenditure causes an overall energy deficit. The energy deficit, in turn, stimulates compensatory metabolic shifts that cause weight loss and energy conservation, translating effects that result in hypothalamic suppression of ovarian function and amenorrhea [2, 3]. Mechanistically, when energy intake is inadequate to meet energetic demands, the body repartitions energy away from reproduction and growth and toward other more essential energy-consuming processes such as thermoregulation, cell maintenance, and locomotion. The primary metabolic shifts that are associated with energy conservation in amenorrheic athletes include a decrease in resting energy expenditure (REE), and suppression of triiodothyronine (TT_3), insulin-like growth factor-1 (IGF-1), and leptin concentrations and elevated ghrelin and cortisol concentrations [4]. Short-term and prospective training studies have provided convincing evidence of the effects of low energy availability on metabolic hormones and luteinizing hormone (LH) pulsatility [5–7]. Short-term manipulations of both dietary intake and energy expenditure at energy availability levels of mild, moderate, and severe levels of energy restriction (10, 20, or 30 kcal/kg LBM/d, respectively) for 4–5 days have consistently demonstrated suppressed peripheral concentrations of metabolic hormones, including TT_3, IGF-1, insulin, leptin, and decreased LH pulsatility [5]. Interestingly, the effects observed occurred in a dose–response manner with the most dramatic effects noted at the severe level of energy restriction.

Cause and effect relationships of low energy availability to actual menstrual function have been provided by the prospective training studies in monkeys [6, 7]. In these exercise training studies, amenorrhea was induced in monkeys during exercise training for a few months in an environment of inadequate energy availability, and the onset of the amenorrhea was directly related to the volume of calories restricted during the exercise training. Refeeding the amenorrheic monkeys by increasing their food intake without any moderation of their daily exercise training was associated with resumption of menses in the previously amenorrheic monkeys [6, 7]. It is of great interest that there was a dose-dependent relationship of the volume of energy intake and the resumption of ovulatory cycles in the amenorrheic monkeys such that the monkeys that ate the most calories recovered ovulatory function in the shortest period of time. Commensurate with the resumption of menses, total TT_3, a key marker of metabolic status, was significantly related to both the induction and reversal of amenorrhea. The short-term and prospective studies provide evidence that the suppression of reproductive function is linked with low energy availability when there is inadequate caloric intake in the face of increased exercise energy expenditure.

Exercise Response/Consequences

In the United States, the passage of Title IX in 1972 during the Richard Nixon administration dramatically increased opportunities for girls and women to engage in physical activity and sport. Research during the subsequent 3–4 decades has focused on the unique effects of many aspects of exercise on girls and women's health, particularly the impact of exercise on the menstrual cycle. One of the earliest reports of menstrual disorders in athletic women was published in 1962. In that report, a high prevalence of menstrual disorders was observed in athletes compared to nonathletes. Since that report, a plethora of studies have been published that confirm a high prevalence of the most serious menstrual disturbance, amenorrhea, in a wide variety of athletes, particularly those athletes involved in lean build sports like gymnastics, ballet, cross-country running, and figure skating [2, 3]. However, amenorrhea has been observed in virtually all sporting women, including women who participate in recreational physical activity [2, 3].

Amenorrhea is one of the most serious clinical problems observed in physically active women and athletes since amenorrhea plays a causative role in low bone mass observed in many female athletes [3, 8]. Inadequate energy intake precedes the clinical sequelae of amenorrhea and low bone mass. Inadequate energy intake in physically active women and athletes is typically associated with internal and external pressures to maintain a low body weight, and translates into disordered eating behaviors that include a high drive for thinness and dietary cognitive restraint [3, 4]. A syndrome of disordered eating, amenorrhea, and low bone mass was defined in 1997 by the American College of Sports Medicine as the Female Athlete Triad [3]. Helpful information for athletes, coaches, and parents is available from the Female Athlete Triad Coalition at http://www.femaleathletetriad.org.

Amenorrhea in athletes is associated with several bone health problems including stress fractures, loss of bone mass, the failure to achieve peak bone mass, and ▶ osteoporosis [3, 8]. Typically, bone mineral density (BMD) in amenorrheic athletes is 2–6% lower at the spine, hip, and total body when compared to athletes that are regularly menstruating [8]. Moreover, amenorrheic athletes have significantly lower lumbar spine and hip BMD Z-scores than age-matched sedentary women. In amenorrheic athletes, the prevalence of ▶ osteopenia is estimated to range from 1.4% to 50%, and the prevalence of osteoporosis is lower. Stress fractures are also 2–4 times more common in athletes with amenorrhea than athletes who are menstruating [3]. Three-dimensional imaging of bone in amenorrheic athletes also reveals a more definitive picture of the bone health of athletes. Indeed, trabecular BMD and bone strength are lower among athletes with amenorrhea-associated bone loss.

Guidelines published for premenopausal women by the International Society for Clinical Densitometry are used as the reference criterion to diagnose low BMD or osteoporosis in athletes. These criteria utilize a Z-score of −2.0 or lower to diagnose low BMD, and when a secondary risk factor is also present, such as hypogonadism or nutritional deficiency, a diagnosis of osteoporosis may be applied.

Chronic hypoestrogenism has typically been assumed to be the primary cause of bone loss in amenorrheic athletes. However, the effects of food restriction and energy deficiency on BMD represent an estrogen-independent mechanism for bone loss secondary to metabolic-related hormonal perturbations which include suppressed IGF-1 and leptin [8]. IGF-1 and leptin are important metabolic hormones that play a key role in optimizing bone formation. Figure 2 displays the mechanism by which high energy expenditure coupled with low energy intake result in bone loss among exercising, amenorrheic women.

Thus, the mechanism underlying low bone mass in amenorrheic athletes is twofold, and includes both hormonal and nutritional components [8]. Bone is an active

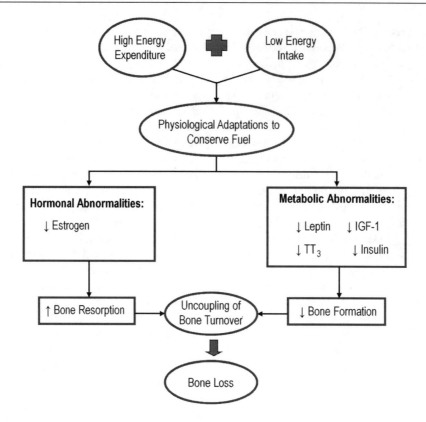

Athletic Amenorrhea. Fig. 2 Mechanism by which bone loss occurs in exercising, amenorrheic women. High energy expenditure coupled with low energy intake results in hormonal and metabolic alterations that contribute to the uncoupling of bone turnover and subsequent bone loss. TT_3 Triiodothyronine, *IGF-1* Insulin-like growth factor-1 (From [9] Reproduced with permission)

tissue, undergoing cycles of resorption and formation. In the face of both an estrogen and energy deficiency, an uncoupling of bone turnover occurs, creating an unfavorable environment of increased bone resorption and decreased bone formation, ultimately resulting in low bone mass [8]. The nutritional etiology of amenorrhea warrants emphasis, and treatment strategies should be focused on improving nutritional status in these physically active women and athletes. The best treatment approach is increased food intake and weight restoration, which are likely the best strategies for both resumption of menses and improved bone health [2, 3, 8].

Diagnostics

Due to the multiple causes of amenorrhea and its presence in many disease states, the diagnosis of functional hypothalamic amenorrhea is one of exclusion [1, 3]. The diagnosis of amenorrhea in athletes requires a thorough physical exam, review of the patient's medical history, and appropriate laboratory tests to rule out other underlying pathologies. Risk factors associated with functional hypothalamic amenorrhea include psychological stress, weight loss, and excessive exercise when coupled with inadequate nutrition [3]. In light of these risk factors, information regarding dietary habits, weight fluctuations, regular exercise regimen, and possible social or work-related stressors should be obtained during the physical exam [3]. When diagnosing amenorrhea, a pregnancy test should first be performed to exclude pregnancy as a cause. Subsequently, diagnostic tests of prolactin, thyroid hormones, follicle-stimulating hormone, and luteinizing hormone should be conducted to determine if the menstrual dysfunction is a result of endocrine pathologies such as (1) pituitary tumors, (2) adrenal diseases, (3) thyroid dysfunction, (4) polycystic ovarian syndrome (PCOS), (5) ovarian tumors, (6) gonadotropin mutations, (7) premature ovarian failure, and (8) hypothalamic causes [1, 9]. Hyperprolactinemia, as evidenced by high levels of prolactin, may indicate the presence of a prolactinoma in the pituitary, and abnormal levels of thyroid-stimulating hormone or thyroxine may indicate thyroid diseases such as hyper- or hypothyroidism. Elevated follicle-stimulating hormone (FSH) levels are indicative of premature ovarian failure; whereas, an abnormally high LH/FSH ratio is often observed among women with PCOS [1, 3]. If physical symptoms of hyperandrogenism (hirsutism, acne, androgenic alopecia) are observed during the physical exam, serum androgens should also be assessed [9]. In the case of functional hypothalamic amenorrhea, prolactin, thyroid hormones, and androgens will be in the normal range; however, gonadotropins (LH and FSH) may be low or normal [1]. Low levels of estradiol may also be used to corroborate hypothalamic causes of amenorrhea [3]. For a detailed algorithm describing the steps involved in identifying the cause and diagnosing amenorrhea, please refer to the following book chapter referenced here [9].

References

1. ASRM Practice Committee (2008) Current evaluation of amenorrhea. Fertil Steril 90(Suppl 1):S219–S225
2. De Souza MJ, Williams NI (2004) Physiological aspects and clinical sequelae of energy deficiency and hypoestrogenism in exercising women. Hum Reprod Update 10(5):433–448
3. Nattiv A et al (2007) American College of Sports Medicine position stand. The female athlete triad. Med Sci Sports Exerc 39(10):1867–1882
4. De Souza MJ et al (2007) Severity of energy-related menstrual disturbances increases in proportion to indices of energy conservation in exercising women. Fertil Steril 88(4):971–975
5. Loucks AB, Thuma JR (2003) Luteinizing hormone pulsatility is disrupted at a threshold of energy availability in regularly menstruating women. J Clin Endocrinol Metab 88(1):297–311
6. Williams NI et al (2001) Longitudinal changes in reproductive hormones and menstrual cyclicity in cynomolgus monkeys during strenuous exercise training: abrupt transition to exercise-induced amenorrhea. Endocrinology 142(6):2381–2389
7. Williams NI et al (2001) Evidence for a causal role of low energy availability in the induction of menstrual cycle disturbances during strenuous exercise training. J Clin Endocrinol Metab 86(11):5184–5193
8. De Souza MJ, Williams NI (2005) Beyond hypoestrogenism in amenorrheic athletes: energy deficiency as a contributing factor for bone loss. Curr Sports Med Rep 4(1):38–44
9. De Souza MJ, Toombs RJ (2010) Amenorrhea associated with the female athlete triad: etiology, diagnosis and treatment. In: Santoro NF, Neal-Perry G (eds) Amenorrhea: a case-based, clinical guide. Springer, New York, pp 101–125

Athletic Heart Syndrome

▶ Athlete's Heart

[Atot]

The total concentration of weak acid (and bases) in solution.

ATP

Major energy and signaling molecule in living cells.

Cross-References

▶ Adenosine Triphosphate

Atrial fibrillation

It's an irregular and often rapid heart rate that commonly causes poor blood flow to the body. During atrial fibrillation the heart's upper chambers (the atria) fibrillate, to be more precise they beat chaotically and irregularly, out of coordination with the two lower chambers of the heart (the ventricles). The blood is not pumped efficiently to the rest of the body which may cause shortness of breath, weakness and heart palpitation.

Atrioventricular Node

A localized area of the heart electrically connecting the atria to the ventricles which serves to delay the electrical signal to allow the cardiac atria to contract before the ventricles. The atria act as a primer pump for the larger ventricles.

Atrophy

The decrease in the size of an organ (e.g., muscle). This decrease is achieved by a decrease in the size of the cells by decreasing (i.e., cross sectional area) the components (e.g., contractile proteins) of the cell. In reference to skeletal muscle, a reduction in muscle or wasting of skeletal muscle which can result from disuse, aging, malnutrition, or disease such as muscular dystrophy.

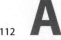

Automatic Implantable Cardioverter Defibrillator (AICD)

▶ Implantable Cardioverter Defibrillator

Autophagy

A process where damaged cellular constituents, including organelles, are targeted for elimination through an energy-dependent process.

Axon

The axon is an anatomical component of the neuron that transmits an action potential to other neurons, or to muscle fibers.

B

β-Endorphin

▶ Opioid Peptides, Endogenous

Balance

Keith Hill
Musculoskeletal Research Centre, La Trobe University and
Northern Health, Bundoora, VIC, Australia

Synonyms

Equilibrium; Postural control; Postural stability

Definition

▶ Balance is a complex and multidimensional phenomenon. It is defined as "the ability of an individual to successfully maintain the position of their body, or more specifically, the centre of gravity, within specific boundaries of space" [1]. Mancini and Horak [2] define the functional goals of the balance system as:

– "maintenance of a specific postural alignment, such as sitting or standing;
– Facilitation of voluntary movement, such as the movement transitions between postures; and
– Reactions that recover equilibrium to external disturbances, such as a trip, slip or push."

For healthy young people, balance is not stressed during routine activities, but may be challenged during higher level tasks including sports, or sensory challenged conditions or environments. For older people, effective balance is essential for safe, independent living, and maintaining an active lifestyle. Balance impairment is a strong, independent risk factor for falls among older people [3]. One in three people aged over 65 years fall each year. However, people with some health conditions such as stroke, Parkinson's disease, and lower limb arthritis have substantially higher risk of falling.

Focus of This Entry

While balance impairments can affect people of all ages, this entry will focus on assessment of balance performance, and training of balance impairment in older people (aged >65 years). This entry will also focus on balance in standing. The principles described can be applied at all ages [4] and all levels of balance abilities/dysfunction, and to other positions (e.g., sitting), although the specific measures and training approaches need to be tailored to meet individual needs.

Description

Balance performance for older people can vary across a continuum, from very poor balance (e.g., unable to stand unsupported) through to high-level balance (e.g., performing in a seniors acrobatic group). While balance performance on all performance-based tests does decline with increasing age, the decline solely due to the effect of age alone is relatively small. Healthy older people have sufficient balance abilities to maintain stability while undertaking an active lifestyle. Rather, it is the impact of health problems affecting the various components of the balance system that are the major contributors to decline in balance performance of older people.

Effective balance performance requires efficient sensory input (visual, vestibular, and somatosensory), central integration of this information, and effective and rapid motor responses (quick reaction time, generation of sufficient muscle force, sufficient joint flexibility, and good coordination) when balance is sensed as being challenged. When any component of this system is impaired through disease (e.g., cataracts, peripheral neuropathy, arthritis affecting lower limb joint flexibility and muscle strength), balance performance is reduced, and risk of falls increases.

Balance is ▶ multidimensional, therefore is unable to be fully reflected in a single test score. Factor analysis of performance of various groups of older people, including those with moderate balance impairment and falls risk, has identified a number of sub-domains that should be considered in assessment and treatment. One commonly used sub-domain is ▶ static balance (measuring postural sway, or timing ability to maintain stance) in a range of increasingly challenging stance positions (feet apart, feet

Frank C. Mooren (ed.), *Encyclopedia of Exercise Medicine in Health and Disease*, DOI 10.1007/978-3-540-29807-6,
© Springer-Verlag Berlin Heidelberg 2012

together, step stance, tandem stance, single leg stance), and ▶ dynamic balance. It is also important to utilize balance measures that challenge balance in a manner similar to the circumstances when balance dysfunction (i.e., falls) occur. Most common circumstances of falls include stepping, reaching and turning. Measures such as the four square step test, functional reach, step test, and timed up and go provide quick and simple measures of performance related to these [5]. There are several combinations of these dynamic balance tests (e.g., the BOOMER [6] and the BESTest [2]) that can provide a global balance score, as well as composite tests incorporating a range of balance destabilizing maneuvers, for example the Berg Balance Scale and the Tinetti Problem Oriented Mobility Assessment (POMA) [1, 2] (Table 1).

An additional challenge to the balance system during static or dynamic tasks is when sensory systems are compromised or not available. Comprehensive balance assessment can include assessment of any of the static or dynamic tasks described above, under conditions of sensory challenge. The most common approach to this is use of the Clinical Test of Sensory Integration for Balance (CTSIB) in which static balance is assessed with eyes open, eyes closed, and with a sensory conflict dome on a firm surface, then these three conditions are repeated standing on high-density foam (compromising somatosensory input) [2].

In real life, balance is often not performed as a single task, but often as a ▶ dual task. While balancing during activities, older people are often also performing a secondary cognitive task (e.g., talking while walking) or a secondary motor task (e.g., reaching into a handbag to take out a purse, while walking). There is limited but growing evidence that adding dual tasks to balance assessment may provide added value above single task assessment [7]. Tests such as the timed up and go tests have been reported under single and dual task (cognitive or motor dual task) [2]. To adequately assess and train balance, it is important that performance under dual task conditions is also considered. Reducing visual fixation (e.g., balancing while turning the head side to side or up and down) also produces an additional challenge to the balance system.

Identification of balance impairment serves a number of purposes. These include (1) to alert the patient about their impairment, and consider modifying related activities to reduce risk of falls; (2) to quantify the type of balance impairments and magnitude of impairment; (3) to use to guide specific balance exercise prescription; and (4) to use as an objective outcome measure to compare post intervention.

Balance. Table 1 Key standing balance domains and examples of assessments

Domain of balance	Assessment tool	Equipment required
Static balance	Clinical Test of Sensory Integration for Balance (CTSIB)	High density foam, sensory conflict dome, stopwatch
Dynamic balance – self-generated tasks		
1. Stepping	– Step test	– 7.5 cm block, stopwatch
	– Four square step test	– 4×walking sticks, stopwatch
2. Reaching	– Functional reach test	– Tape measure
3. Turning	– Timed up and go test	– Chair, marked out 3 meters, stopwatch
Dynamic balance– externally generated tasks	Pastors/Marsden's test	– nil
Combination tests	– Balance outcome measure for elder rehabilitation (BOOMER)	– Items for step test, timed up and go, and functional reach
	– BESTest	– Stopwatch, measuring tape mounted on wall, block of medium density foam, 10-degree incline ramp (at least 60 cm×60 cm) to stand on, step (height 15 cm) for alternate stair tap, two stacked shoe boxes as obstacle for gait, 2.5 kg weight for rapid arm raise, chair with arms, 3 and 6 m walkway, masking tape
	– Berg balance scale	– Stopwatch, chair with arms, table, object to pick up from floor, step stool, and a tape measure

It is also important to consider balance impairment as part of a comprehensive falls risk screen or assessment, as people with balance impairment may have a number of other falls risk factors that need to be identified and addressed optimally to minimize the risk of falls, in addition to addressing balance impairment. Ideally, this should include consideration of ▶ intrinsic falls risk factors (e.g., vision problems, polypharmacy, cognitive impairment, muscle weakness) as well as ▶ extrinsic falls risk factors (e.g., environmental hazards).

Clinical Use/Application

Assessment
In selecting the best mix of balance tests for a specific patient or clinical setting, factors to consider include:

- Reliability and validity of the test/s with the specific clinical group.
- The level of balance impairment. If the patient has mild balance dysfunction, tests that do not have ceiling effects should be used. Tests that have been reported as having ceiling effects include the Berg Balance Scale, the Tinetti POMA, and the timed up and go [2].
- Common circumstances when the patient's balance is threatened, or when falls have occurred.
- Be practical, easy to use, and low cost [2].

An example of a mix of simple clinical balance measures that covers the key domains of balance, includes reliable and valid measures, requires little equipment, can be completed quickly, and is suitable for patients presenting with mild to moderate severity balance impairment include (1) static balance – CTSIB; (2) dynamic balance – functional reach, step test, timed up and go (single task); and (3) dual task – timed up and go (with cognitive and/or motor dual task).

Training
Balance can be improved through specific exercise training no matter how poor initial performance is. A recent meta-analysis concluded that exercise training that includes balance, gait training, coordination, functional training, and muscle strengthening exercises, or combinations of these individual approaches, is effective in improving balance in older people [8]. However, to achieve the added benefit of reducing falls, meta-analysis recommendations are that exercise programs should (1) include balance exercises specifically (i.e., exercise programs that do not challenge the balance system are unlikely to reduce falls); and (2) that programs needed to include at least 50 h of exercise to be likely to be effective in reducing falls [9]. ▶ Multicomponent exercise approaches (that include two

or more of balance, strength, fitness, and flexibility exercises) are more likely to reduce falls risk [10]. ▶ Individualized home exercise programs (prescribed by a physiotherapist or other health professional trained in exercise prescription), group exercise programs, and tai chi have been shown to reduce falls in older people [10].

While there is good evidence that exercise programs, particularly those with a balance focus, can improve balance performance and reduce falls risk, some care needs to be used in prescribing these types of exercise programs, particularly for older people with moderate balance impairment or increased falls risk. To optimize outcomes, balance exercise needs to stress the system to be effective, but to do this safely. This requires tailoring of exercise selection, and choice of exercise mode (home exercise versus group exercise) and other safety considerations. Prior to undertaking a new exercise program, particularly one that aims to challenge balance ability, older people who have a history of falls, near falls, or unsteadiness should have a detailed balance assessment to determine suitability of a specific exercise program for the individual client. Those with increased risk may benefit initially from supervised exercise intervention (e.g., by a physiotherapist) to ensure safety and appropriate level of exercise is selected.

Conclusion
People presenting to health professionals complaining of unsteadiness, near falls, or actual falls should have a multidimensional assessment of their balance performance, as well as exploration of other factors that may increase their risk of falling. If balance impairment is identified, specific causes should be addressed, together with prescription of an appropriate and safe balance exercise program.

References
1. Matsumura BA, Ambrose AF (2006) Balance in the elderly. Clin Geriatr Med 22(2):395–412
2. Mancini M, Horak FB (2010) The relevance of clinical balance assessment tools to differentiate balance deficits. Eur J Phys Rehabil Med 46(2):239–248
3. Muir SW, Berg K, Chesworth B, Klar N, Speechley M (2010) Quantifying the magnitude of risk for balance impairment on falls in community-dwelling older adults: a systematic review and meta-analysis. J Clin Epidemiol 63(4):389–406
4. Zech A, Hübscher M, Vogt L, Banzer W, Hänsel F, Pfeifer K (2010) Balance training for neuromuscular control and performance enhancement: a systematic review. J Athl Train 45(4):392–403, 45
5. Bernhardt J, Hill K (2005) We only treat what it occurs to us to assess: the importance of knowledge based assessment. In: Refshauge K, Ada L, Ellis E (eds) Science based rehabilitation: theories into practice. Elsevier, Oxford
6. Haines T, Kuys SS, Morrison G, Clarke J, Bew P, McPhail S (2007) Development and validation of the balance outcome measure for elder rehabilitation. Arch Phys Med Rehabil 88(12):1614–1621

7. Zijlstra A, Ufkes T, Skelton DA, Lundin-Olsson L, Zijlstra W (2008) Do dual tasks have an added value over single tasks for balance assessment in fall prevention programs? A mini-review. Gerontology 54(1):40–49
8. Howe TE, Rochester L, Jackson A, Banks PMH, Blair VA (2007) Exercise for improving balance in older people. Cochrane database of systematic reviews 2007, Issue 4. Article No.: CD004963. doi:10.1002/14651858.CD004963.pub2
9. Sherrington C, Whitney JC, Lord SR, Herbert RD, Cumming RG, Close JC (2008) Effective exercise for the prevention of falls: a systematic review and meta-analysis. J Am Geriatr Soc 56(12):2234–2243
10. Gillespie LD, Robertson MC, Gillespie WJ, Lamb SE, Gates S, Cumming RG, Rowe BH (2009) Interventions for preventing falls in older people living in the community. Cochrane database of systematic reviews 2009, Issue 2. Article No.: CD007146. doi:10.1002/14651858.CD007146.pub2

Baroreflex

A negative feedback system that regulates blood pressure. Baroreceptors are mechanoreceptors found in the carotid bodies and aortic arch, and are sensitive to changes in stretch. If blood pressure increases, this is sensed by the baroreceptors, which send a signal to the brain, causing a reflex decrease in heart rate and vasodilation to the peripheral circulation to bring blood pressure back down to its set point. Conversely, if blood pressure decreases, this is sensed by the baroreceptors, which send a signal to the brain, causing a reflex increase in heart rate and vasoconstriction.

Basal Lamina

Next to the sarcolemma (on its extracellular side) a light zone is seen (sometimes called the lamina lucida). It contains molecules that connect trans-sarcolemmal molecules in muscle (called merosin) to a dense layer (lamina densa) seen at a certain distance (made up of a collagen IV network). Yet, other molecules connect this network to the endomysium to complete the myofascial link between the cytoskeleton and the continuous connective tissues of the extracellular matrix.

Basal Metabolic Rate

A clinical definition for metabolism measured under strictly standardized conditions.

Base

A single unit of the DNA sequence. There are four bases: adenine (A), guanine (G), thymine (T), and cytosine (C).

Basic Helix-Loop-Helix (bHLH) proteins

Basic Helix-Loop-Helix (bHLH) proteins are a family of transcription factors with a structurally conserved region consisting of two alpha helices joined by a loop domain (in a hair-pin like structure). The smaller of the helices contained basic amino acids, which enable dimerisation between two bHLH proteins, while the larger helix interacts with DNA to facilitate transcription of specific genes. The DNA sequence to which bHLH proteins bind is referred to as an Enhancer-box (E-box) domain with a consensus binging sequence of: CANNTG. In skeletal muscle myoD is a bHLH transcription factor which prescribes myogenic commitment. It can homo-dimerise with other myoD molecules or heterodimerise with myogenin (a bHLH protein belonging to the same myogenic regulatory factor (MRF) family as myoD) to promote skeletal muscle differentiation following enhanced expression of e.g., creatine kinase or the cell cycle inhibitor, p21. Alternatively, myoD can bind to id, which lacks the functional DNA binding domain and hence prevent skeletal muscle differenctation. These bHLH transcription factors are not limited to muscle transcription factors and include other members such as: Hypoxia-inducible factor-1 and c-myc, to name just two.

BDNF

Brain-derived neurotrophic factor is a protein produced and secreted from neurons that plays critical roles in learning and memory, and promotes the survival of neurons.

Behavior Change

TOM BARANOWSKI
Children's Nutrition Research Center, Department of Pediatrics, Baylor College of Medicine, Houston, TX, USA

Synonyms
Lifestyle change; Regimen adherence; Regimen compliance

Definition

Behavior Change is the outcome or the process of an intervention to promote a change in what a person does. The words ▶ regimen ▶ compliance and regimen ▶ adherence are used when changes are attempted in response to a medical prescription, often from a physician or other health professional. The word lifestyle change is used to refer to any of a variety of behavior changes.

Description

The ▶ Mediating-Moderating Variable Model (MMVM) provides a conceptual framework for a current understanding of behavior change [1]. Figure 1 provides the simple single mediator-single moderator version of the MMVM to explicate the principles. According to the MMVM, an intervention employs a behavior change procedure to induce change in a ▶ mediating variable, change in the mediating variable induces change in behavior, and a change in behavior induces change in a health outcome.

To maximize the likelihood of improvement in the targeted health outcome, a behavior must be selected and targeted that is causally and strongly related to the health outcome (e.g., daily long duration bouts of moderate to vigorous physical activity to adiposity), a mediating variable must be selected and targeted that is causally and strongly related to the targeted behavior (e.g., intrinsic motivation to perform daily long duration bouts of moderate to vigorous physical activity), and an intervention procedure (e.g., offering choice of fun sports activities done in a competitive fashion) must be selected and employed frequently and intensively enough to change the targeted mediating variable enough to change the targeted behavior enough to change the targeted health outcome.

Simple Mediating-Moderating Variable Model
as a Conceptual Framework

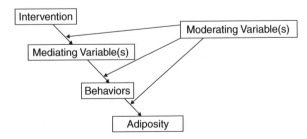

Behavior Change. Fig. 1 This model demonstrates the simple pathway of effects from an intervention to health outcomes, allowing for differences of effects across demographics or other moderating variables

The intervention is usually employed with diverse people in diverse contexts. If the intervention works differently with some people (but not others), or in some contexts (but not others), the characteristic of people or context for which the behavior change is different is a ▶ moderating variable. For example, gender is a common moderator, e.g., the intensive sport intervention is most likely to have the desired behavior change effects with boys, but not girls.

In the real world, an intervention will often have multiple intervention procedures targeting multiple mediating variables related to multiple behaviors (e.g., physical activity and diet) to influence the targeted health outcome. This complexity imposes complications in selecting appropriate behaviors, mediators and change procedures, and constraints in how to accommodate and effectively interdigitate all the selected procedures in one intervention, and prioritize measures of all the possible pathways in the evaluation.

Application

Since the variables and pathways in the MMVM in regard to physical activity have not been clearly delineated for many health outcomes with different participants in diverse settings, professionals interested in behavior change often select a promising theory of behavior which has provided ample evidence that variables within that theory are strongly and causally related (preferably from longitudinal research) to the behavior of interest [2]. Similarly, these professionals would select for their intervention procedures those which have been demonstrated (preferably in experimental research) to change the targeted mediators enough to change the behaviors enough to influence the health outcomes in the desired direction. At this time, the research on these issues is not sufficiently detailed to provide practitioners ample and easy choices. Often the interventions which have been evaluated have attained no changes in health outcomes [3], little or no changes in health behaviors [4], and needed statistical mediating variable analyses have not been done (often because statistical power is too low to have confidence in the results) [4, 5].

References

1. Baranowski T, Baranowski J, Cullen K, Hingle M, Hughes S, Jago R, Ledoux T, Mendoza J, Nguyen T, O'Connor T, Thompson D, Watson K (2010) Problems and possible solutions for interventions among children and adolescents. In: O'Dea J, Eriksen M (eds) Childhood obesity prevention - International research, controversies and interventions. Oxford University Press, NY, pp 408–421
2. Baranowski T, Cullen K, Nicklas T, Thompson D, Baranowski J (2003) Are current health behavior change models helpful in guiding prevention of weight gain efforts? Obes Res 11(Suppl 1):23S–43S

3. Brown T, Kelly S, Summerbell C (Mar 2007) Prevention of obesity: a review of interventions. Obes Rev 8(Suppl 1):127–130
4. van Stralen MM, Yildirim M, Velde ST, Brug J, van Mechelen W, Chinapaw MJ (2011) What works in school-based energy balance behaviour interventions and what does not? A systematic review of mediating mechanisms. Int J Obes (Lond)
5. Cerin E, Barnett A, Baranowski T (2009) Testing theories of dietary behavior change in young using the mediating variable model with intervention programs. J Nutr Educ Behav 41(5):309–318

Beta 2-Adrenoceptor Agonists

These drugs act as bronchodilators, stimulating the airways to open wider, allowing more air to pass. Bronchodilatation is kept for various lengths of time, depending on the beta-2 agonist used. As for 2011, the World Anti-Doping Agency allows the use of selected beta-2 agonists (salbutamol, salmeterol, terbutaline, and formoterol) in athletic competition only by asthmatic athletics, to prevent or treat exercise-induced asthma or bronchial constriction, and only used by inhalation. Oral and injected forms of beta-2 agonists are illegal.

Beta-Adrenergic Receptors

One of the three major subfamilies of adrenergic receptor, divided into beta1-, beta2-, and beta3-adrenoceptors.

Cross-References

▶ Adrenergic Receptors

Beta-Blockers

Antagonist drugs that block the actions of catecholamines at beta-adrenoceptors. Actions of beta-blockers include slowing of the heart, narrowing the airways, and reducing tremor. The latter action explains why they are banned by WADA in competition for sports such as shooting and snooker.

Bicarbonate Threshold

The O_2 uptake at which arterial bicarbonate starts to decrease due to its buffering action during exercise.

Bicycle

Pedal-driven, human-powered, single-track vehicle.

Bicycling

▶ Cycling

Biking

▶ Cycling

Bioactive Substances in Intercellular Signal Transduction

▶ Cytokines

Bioavailability

Is the fraction of an administered drug dosage which reaches the systemic circulation. Therefore, the bioavailability of intravenously administered drugs amounts to 100%. Bioavailability of orally administered drugs depends on the interaction with other food compounds and the intestinal uptake routes. It can therefore be affected by malabsorptive diseases as well as the competition of food compounds for the same intestinal transport mechanism. On the other hand, bioavailability can be selectively enhanced.

Bioenergetics

▶ Energy Metabolism

Biomarker

A biomarker, or biological marker, is in general a substance used as an indicator of a biological state. It is a characteristic that can be objectively measured and evaluated as an indicator of normal biological processes, pathogenic processes, or pharmacologic responses to a therapeutic intervention. A biomarker may serve as a surrogate clinical endpoint when it is appropriately qualified to substitute as a marker of how a patient feels, functions, or survives.

Biomechanics

Science dedicated to the study of the structures and functions of biological systems using mechanical principles.

Biosynthesis

The formation of chemical compounds by a living organism.

Bipolar disorder

When abnormally elevated mood (manic episodes) is followed by abnormally lowered mood (depressive episodes). Also referred to as manic-depressive disorder.

Cross-References
▶ Psychiatric/Psychological Disorders

Block Periodization Concept (BPC)

The block periodization concept utilizes sequenced mesocycles where training is focused on a small number of athlete skills and capacities.

Blood

Walter Schmidt, Nicole Prommer
Department of Sports Medicine, University of Bayreuth, Bayreuth, Germany

Definition
Blood is a suspension consisting of fluid (plasma) and cells or cell fragments which are classified in erythrocytes, leucocytes and lymphocytes, as well as thrombocytes (platelets). Blood is the transport medium within the cardiovascular system and supplies the tissues with nutrients and oxygen. It also transports metabolites like CO_2, lactic acid, and urea to the excretory and metabolizing organs and is essential for the regulation of the body's temperature, acid-base, as well as electrolyte and water status. Its immune cells, antibodies and its coagulatory function protect the body.

The role blood plays in sports and vice versa is multifarious. Especially the red cells are the target of training measures and manipulations as they are the main predictor of endurance performance. The immune system and the coagulatory systems which are often impaired due to a sedentary lifestyle are positively affected by prolonged submaximal training whereas vigorous exercise may acutely exert the contradictory effect. In the following, the performance enhancing effects of erythrocytes and blood volume will be emphasized.

Mechanisms
▶ VO_{2max} is the key parameter of endurance performance and directly depends on quantitative and qualitative characteristics of the blood. According to Fick's law, VO_{2max} is the product of cardiac output (CO) and the arteriovenous oxygen difference ($avDO_2$). Prerequisites for a high CO are (1) an enlarged heart size (athlete's heart) allowing a high stroke volume and (2) a high blood volume facilitating venous return and herewith improving the filling volume of the heart. $avDO_2$ is determined by the ▶ hemoglobin concentration, which is the key factor for blood oxygen transport capacity, and the tissue oxygen extraction. This oxygen extraction itself depends on (1) the oxygen demand, (2) the aerobic metabolic capacity of the muscle cell, and (3) the capability of the hemoglobin molecule to unload oxygen, i.e., the hemoglobin-oxygen affinity. The hemoglobin molecule, therefore, may influence performance (Fig. 1) in a triple way [7]:

1. It contributes to the blood volume via the red cell volume and thereby increases CO (Figs. 2 and 3).
2. It determines the hemoglobin concentration and thereby the oxygen transport capacity in dependency on the absolute ▶ hemoglobin mass of the body and the plasma volume (Fig. 2).
3. It influences the tissue oxygen supply by the quality of O_2 binding, i.e., by changing the hemoglobin O_2-affinity during the passage through the body: A left-shifted oxygen dissociation curve ensures a nearly complete O_2-saturation of the hemoglobin in the lung, while a right shift during the muscle

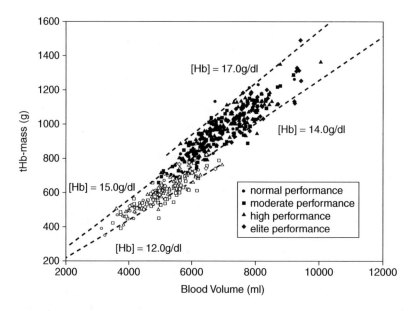

Blood. Fig. 1 Relationship between absolute maximal oxygen uptake and absolute total hemoglobin mass (Data derive from boys aged 9–14 years, fit untrained subjects, leisure sports athletes, elite runners, and elite rowers [6])

Blood. Fig. 2 Total hemoglobin mass vs total blood volume. Presented are data of 490 differently trained subjects (male subjects n=314, female subjects n=176). The *dashed lines* indicate the hemoglobin concentration ([Hb]) as a function of blood volume and hemoglobin mass [6]

passage facilitate the O_2-unloading from the blood to the muscle cell due to an increased blood temperature and due to allosteric influences of the metabolites CO_2 and lactic acid (▶ Bohr-effect).

During maximum exercise, the whole blood volume circulates approximately four times per minute through the body [6], i.e., it is four times saturated in the lungs and four times desaturated in the muscle tissue (see Fig. 3).

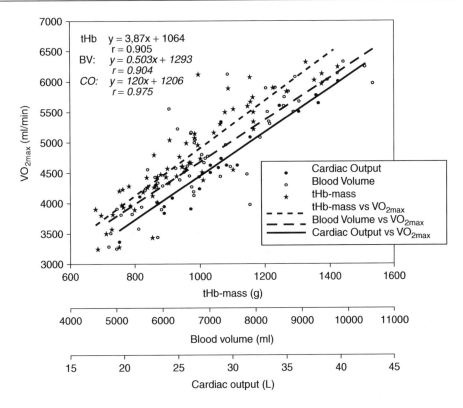

Blood. Fig. 3 Relationship between maximal oxygen uptake (VO$_{2max}$) and total hemoglobin mass (tHb-mass), blood volume (BV), and cardiac output (CO) [6]

Since 1 g of hemoglobin binds ~1.39 ml of oxygen (Huefner's number) and since at maximum exercise the hemoglobin molecules release ~80% of the ligated oxygen 1 g of hemoglobin contributes up to 4 ml/min to VO$_{2max}$. This relationship is described in cross-sectional and also in longitudinal studies when changes in hemoglobin mass due to phlebotomy or to manipulative erythrocyte expansion are associated with changes in VO$_{2max}$ [6].

In untrained subjects, the impact of hemoglobin mass on VO$_{2max}$ is less since the muscle tissue is unable to utilize all the oxygen offered by the circulating blood. In endurance athletes, however, the metabolic capacity of the muscles exceeds the oxygen transport capacity of the cardiocirculatory system. This is the reason why blood is the probably most important limiting factor for VO$_{2max}$ in elite athletes [8].

Endurance athletes posses ~50% more blood and hemoglobin than sedentary subjects [1]. Most reasonably, but not yet proven, the genetic predisposition is the main cause. However, several years of training may also contribute to the athlete's erythrocyte expansion. Since the relationship between hemoglobin mass and performance is that apparent, many athletes try to improve their

performance by increasing hemoglobin mass by altitude training or by blood manipulations.

Exercise Response/Consequences

During acute exercise, plasma volume decreases as a function of intensity and duration. Increased blood pressure combined with high muscle perfusion augments the fluid efflux from the vascular space. This effect is present already at moderate exercise and it tremendously increases during high intensity exercise when the rising osmotic pressure within the muscle cells due to accumulating metabolites augments the fluid drag from the vascular space. Furthermore, during long-lasting bouts of exercise especially in hot environments the fluid loss via sweat considerably contributes to the decrease in plasma volume. The effect of these regulations on the amount of plasma volume is between ~3% at moderate exercise and may exceed 20% at exhaustion; i.e., ~1 l in elite athletes [3].

Within 24 h after intensive exercise, plasma volume may be overcompensated by 5–10% which is the first step of a rapid increase of plasma and blood volume. The reasons are acute hormonal changes (increases in ADH and aldosterone, decrease in ANP and urodilatin) during and after exercise leading to elevated renal sodium and water retention. These acute responses are stabilized by increased intravascular protein content and a weakened vascular baroreceptor response. Interestingly, all these mechanisms can still be observed in highly trained endurance athletes: During stage races (e.g., Tour de France) plasma volume increases by approximately 1 l reducing the hemoglobin concentration by >1.0 g/dl since hemoglobin mass remains constant. On the other hand, an abrupt stop of endurance training induces a rapid reduction in plasma volume which is reflected by increased hemoglobin concentration.

Red cell mass is normally only slightly affected by acute exercise. When untrained subjects start a training program a small destruction occurs (~2% of red cell mass within a week), but also in some trained athletes the so-called foot strike hemolysis can be observed.

In contrast to the pO_2 in the muscle tissue, the renal pO_2 seems not to be affected during exercise resulting in a stable plasma erythropoietin concentration during and after exercise. However, a small reticulocytosis can be observed in sedentary subjects when starting a training program while endurance athletes show relatively low ▶ reticulocyte numbers. Training programs lasting 4–6 weeks are too short to increase hemoglobin and red cell mass. At the earliest 3 months after intensive endurance training, an effective increase in red cell mass by 3.5% and after 9 months by 6% can be observed [5]. The genetic contribution to the high red cell mass of endurance athletes has not been completely clarified. However, the fact that sedentary subjects who do not practice any sports but show ~50% elevated VO_{2max} and hemoglobin mass values compared to the normal sedentary population indicates a considerable genetic contribution.

Although red cell and hemoglobin mass is considerably higher in endurance athletes than in sedentary subjects their hemoglobin concentration is similar or even decreased which can be referred to the plasma volume expansion. In non-manipulating athletes, hemoglobin concentration is, therefore, not related to aerobic performance and high hemoglobin concentration and hematocrit values may hint to non-physiological situations like ▶ blood manipulation.

In professional endurance athletes, the individual oscillation of red cell mass during a training year is low and training influences on total hemoglobin mass are below 3% [2]. Most pronounced effects on the athlete's red cell and hemoglobin mass are altitude and illness or injury, respectively. At altitudes above 1,600 m the lower ambient pO_2 induces an elevated erythropoiesis and yields

to increases in red cell mass of ~12% at 2,500 m and of up to 50% during life-long adaptation to 5,000 m. Athletes living and training at altitude benefit from both, the altitude and the training effects, and show highest red cell volumes. Therefore, also athletes from lowlands try to increase their red cell mass by altitude or by hypoxic training. During 3 weeks lasting traditional altitude training camps at ~2,300 m the gain in hemoglobin mass is 3–7%. But also the training concept "▶ live high – train low" yields similar results when the daily hypoxic exposure exceeds 12 h [5]. No effect on red cell mass, however, occurs after hypoxic training or hypoxic exposure for only some hours per day.

Illness and injury reduce red cell mass due to the lacking training stimulus. Additionally, the inhibition of the erythropoietic activity by pro-inflammatory cytokines contributes to a fast reduction of the athlete's red cell mass. Another major factor disturbing an adequate red cell mass is iron deficiency which can occur due to, e.g., low alimentary iron uptake, low iron absorption, lacking cofactors as vitamin B-12 or folic acid, or blood loss. Controlling the iron status and providing the optimal iron availability is, therefore, a prerequisite for a sufficient erythropoiesis and for the optimal individual red cell mass.

During the recent years, many endurance athletes manipulated their blood with erythropoietic-stimulating substances like recombinant erythropoietin and by homologous or autologous blood transfusions. The effects of these measures on red cell mass and endurance performance exceed by far the effects of training at sea level and even of training at altitude. Non-manipulating athletes, therefore, have no winning chance when competing against doped colleagues.

Diagnostics

Until some years ago, hemoglobin concentration and hematocrit were the only blood parameters, which were used to estimate blood volumes and hemoglobin content. Due to dilution or concentration mechanisms, however, this information only scarcely provided reliable quantitative data on hemoglobin and blood volume. Methods using radioactive labeling to determine the absolute volumes were also not suitable for routine measurements in sports medicine. Since 2005, the optimized CO-re-breathing method now facilitates an accurate and noninvasive measurement of total hemoglobin mass which can frequently be applied to an individual subject [4]. The method is based on the inhalation of a small bolus of carbon monoxide for 2 min and on the measurement of CO-labeled hemoglobin before and some minutes after the inhalation period. It is characterized by a small error of measurement (typical error $\sim 1.5\%$), very short experimental time (10 min), and absolute harmlessness (maximum COHb-increases $\sim 5\%$). The application of the method is recommended to monitor the stimulating effects of training at sea level and altitude and the disturbing effects of, e.g., inflammation, iron deficiency, and injury. In some sports physiological research centers, the method is also used for talent identification. The World Anti-Doping-Agency (WADA) considers the method to monitor the athlete's hemoglobin profile to detect possible blood manipulations.

References

Literature

1. Heinicke K, Wolfahrt B, Winchenbach P, Biermann B, Schmid A, Huber G, Friedmann B, Schmidt W (2001) Blood volume and hemoglobin mass in elite athletes of different disciplines. Int J Sports Med 22:504–512
2. Prommer N, Sottas PE, Schoch C, Schumacher YO, Schmidt W (2008) Total hemoglobin mass - a new parameter to detect blood doping? Med Sci Sports Exerc 40:2112–2118
3. Sawka MN, Convertino VA, Eichner ER, Schnieder SM, Young AJ (2000) Blood volume: importance and adaptions to exercise training, environmental stresses, and trauma/sickness. Med Sci Sports Exerc 32:332–348
4. Schmidt W, Prommer N (2005) The optimised CO-rebreathing method: a new tool to determine total haemoglobin mass routinely. Eur J Appl Physiol 95:486–495
5. Schmidt W, Prommer N (2008) Effects of various training modalities on blood volume. Scand J Med Sci Sports 18:57–69
6. Schmidt W, Prommer N (2010) Impact of alterations in total hemoglobin mass on VO_{2max}. Exerc Sport Sci Rev 38:68–75
7. Schmidt WFJ, Böning D, Maassen N (2005) Erythrocytes. In: Mooren FC, Völker K (eds) Molecular and cellular exercise physiology. Human Kinetics, Champaign, pp S.309–S.319
8. Wagner PD (2000) New ideas on limitations to VO_{2max}. Exerc Sport Sci Rev 28:10–14

Blood Boosting

▶ Blood Doping

Blood Doping

MICHEL AUDRAN
Biophysics & Bio-Analysis Laboratory, Montpellier, France

Synonyms

Blood boosting; Oxygen delivery in sports

Definition

The Word Antidoping Agency (WADA) defines blood doping as "the misuse of certain techniques and/or substances to increase one's red blood cell mass which allows the body to transport more oxygen to muscles and therefore increase stamina and performance." But this definition could be extended to any method or substance which allows to increase oxygen transport by blood without necessary increase in the red blood cell mass (blood boosting).

Energy for the muscular contraction is provided by adenosine triphosphate (ATP) conversion into adenosine diphosphate (ADP) and inorganic phosphate. As ATP is not stored in the body, it must be synthesized continuously. For endurance sports that require prolonged energy expenditure, ATP is produced by the aerobic system. Theoretically, the more oxygen you can use during high-level exercise, the more ATP you can produce. This maximum amount of oxygen (O_2) that an individual can utilize during maximal exercise is called ▶ VO_2max and is generally considered to be a good indicator of aerobic endurance. VO_2max is a distributed property, dependent on the interaction of oxygen transport and mitochondrial oxygen uptake. It is mainly limited by the maximal cardiac output multiplied by the oxygen content of the arterial blood. It was speculated that an increase in the oxygen transport of arterial blood could increase the VO_2max and thereby increases performance in endurance sports.

The ergogenic effects of blood doping are known since 1947. But widespread use among endurance athletes started after the 1968 Olympic Games in Mexico City. The International Olympic Committee (IOC) forbade blood doping for the 1988 Olympics. At this time, the ▶ recombinant human erythropoietin (rHu-Epo) became available and the increase of red blood cell mass could be much easier achieved. In addition to the rHu-EPO the first "blood substitutes," perfluorocarbons (PFCs) and hemoglobin oxygen carriers (HBOCs) which were designed to enhance the oxygen-carrying capacity of blood, and which have been in clinical development since a quarter of century, were in phase III clinical trials or available. So a large battery of methods and substances has become available for the manipulators and blood doping is also named blood boosting. In a very near future new ▶ erythropoiesis-stimulating agents (ESAs) and gene therapy may further enlarge this battery of techniques (Fig. 1).

Mechanism of Action

Erythropoiesis and Oxygen Transport

Erythropoiesis, a complex physiologic process to maintain O_2 homeostasis in the body, is primarily regulated by

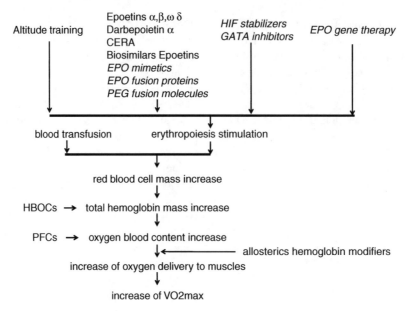

Blood Doping. Fig. 1 Main methods to increase oxygen delivery to muscles

▶ erythropoietin (EPO) a 30-kDa glycoprotein hormone. Its plasma half-life varies between 2 and 13 h and serum concentrations range from 6 to 32 U/l. In the presence of EPO, bone marrow erythoid precursor cells proliferate and differentiate into red blood cells (RBCs). EPO is mainly synthesized in renal peritubular intersticial cells (90%) and is production is regulated at the level of its gene by tissue oxygenation. A lower partial pressure of Oxygen in blood (pO_2) is sensed by cellular oxygen sensors particularly the members of the hypoxia inducible factors (HIF) family. It takes 3–5 days between the EPO secretion and the appearance of the reticulocytes (immature RBCs) in the blood and extra 2–3 days for mature RBCs.

Increase in HGB and VO$_2$max

By the 1970s it was clear that maneuvres that increased total body ▶ hemoglobin also increased VO$_2$max. As Hb is inside the RBC (a small amount is dissolved in the plasma but is physiologically insignificant) such maneuvres consisted in increasing the RBC number. Therefore, the primary determinant of VO$_2$max was assumed to be total body Hb or t-Hb mass, and it is now well established that increase the t-Hb mass increases both VO$_2$max and endurance performance in sports. Each fully saturated gram of Hb carries 1.34 ml of O_2; a 20 g/l increase in Hb will raise the O_2 carrying capacity of 1 l of blood by 25 ml. A number of studies have confirmed the positive impact of increased t-Hb mass on performance. These studies showed that VO$_2$max per gram increased for about 20 ml per gram of

Hb administered and this increase was the same whether the subject's normal baseline Hb concentration ([Hb]) was 130 or 170 g/l. However, the intraindividual variation in the change of VO$_2$max was great.

Physiological Methods to Increase Blood Oxygen Content

Altitude which lowers blood pO_2, is a stimulus for endogenous EPO synthesis and thus affects blood oxygen content. However the first phenomenon to occur is a decrease in plasma volume, beginning hours after arrival at high altitude (>2,000 m). Thus, altitude exposure provokes an increase in Hb concentration due to decreases of the blood volume giving the false impression of rapid RBC volume expansion. If altitude exposure continues beyond some weeks, then total Hb increases at a rate of about 1% per week with a maximal effect requiring as much as 80 days (or less in higher altitudes). Moreover, training is harder at altitude as less O_2 is available to the tissues. One solution is the "live high-train low" (LHTL). Athletes living (18 h/day) at moderately high altitude (≈ 2,500 m) and training at lower altitude (≈ 1,000 m) exhibit a t-Hb mass expansion (5.3%) and approximately a 5% improvement in VO$_2$max after 3–4 weeks. An alternative method is to use "altitude houses" which are normobaric hypoxic units that create an artificial hypoxic environment via nitrogen dilution or hypoxic sleeping devices that stimulates altitude up to about 4,500 m. The effects on the increase in t-Hb mass and performance are limited and depend of the length of time spent at low pO_2. Improved performance requires at least 12–16 h, but 50% of competitive athletes have been identified as "nonresponder." The mechanisms underlying the wide variability in erythrocyte and performance responsiveness are unknown.

Illegal Methods to Improve Blood Oxygen Content

Increasing Erythrocyte Volume

Erythrocyte volume and thus t-Hb mass can be artificially increased by infusing erythrocytes or administering human recombinant EPO (rHuEPO) and related pharmacological products called erythropoiesis-stimulating agents (ESA).

Blood transfusions are of two types: either from a matching donor (hetero transfusion) or a donor of the same ABO and rhesus D blood group (homo transfusion) or by reinfusion of RBCs of the athlete himself (autologous transfusion). In the latter case, 450–1,800 ml (1–4 units) of blood are withdrawn and then centrifuged. The plasma components are generally immediately reinfused. The phlebotomy is performed several weeks earlier so that the athlete has returned to a normal blood count prior to infusion. RBCs can be stored either the usual way in a refrigerator (4°C) or in a frozen state in glycerol solutions. In the first case, the blood must be reinfused within 4–8 weeks, due to RBC hemolysis which is roughly 1% per day. In the second case, the interval between blood withdrawal and reinfusion can extend up to several years, but, before reinfusion, the cell must be thawed and washed to remove the glycerol and suspended in a saline solution.

Blood transfusion increases t-Hb mass immediately and the improvement in performance is striking and rapid though at least one unit of packed RBCs (450 ml) seems to be necessary. In well-designed double-blind studies, reinfusion of 900–1,350 ml of blood increased VO_2max by 4–11% but the elevated erythrocyte level lasts only a few weeks. The introduction of rHuEPO therapy late of 1980s provided a far easier, though lower acting, alternative to blood transfusion. In 2001 however, direct detection of rHuEPO was introduced and blood doping practices regained interest among cheating athletes.

The human EPO gene was cloned in 1983, allowing development of rHuEPO. Early studies in patients with renal failure or severe anemia showed that this hormone and the associated increase in whole body Hb and packed cell volume had profound effects on their exercise tolerance. Studies in trained subjects and athletes showed the expected increase in VO_2max. The maximal rate of erythrocyte expansion from EPO stimulation is about

50 ml/week or 3 g/l of Hb per week, and this increase will be sustained if treatment continues.

By the early 1990s, rHuEPO had become the "drug of choice" for unscrupulous athletes seeking to increase their endurance performance and the International Olympic Committee placed it on the forbidden substances list in 1990. From a technical viewpoint, rHuEPO has several advantages. It could be administered by subcutaneous or intravenous route two or three times per week and require no complex logistically difficult manipulations such as blood withdrawal, storage, and reinfusion. Moreover, with no blood withdrawal, there is no reduction in training or competition performance. From the late 1980s to 2001, rHuEPO was widely used notably by cross-country skiers and cyclists, in triathlon and marathon athletes. This is unsurprising as it was undetectable. rHuEPO with the same amino acid sequence as human EPO are called epoetins: epoetin alpha, the first rHuEPO, has been commercially produced since 1989 and is worldwide available and marketed under different names: Epogen, Procrit, Eprex, Erypo, and Espo. Other epoetins exist: Epoetin beta, available only outside the USA under the name of Neorecormon or Epogin, EPO omega (Epomax), Epoetin delta (now discontinued). Attempts to improve rHuEPOs to meet the demands of patients and caregivers led to additional ESAs with increased serum half life: Darbepoetin α (Aranesp, Nespo), whose serum half-life is three- or fourfold longer than that of epoetin alpha or beta and continuous erythropoietin receptor activator (CERA), sold as Mircera, a methoxy-polyethylene glycol epoetin beta whose serum half-live is about 5, 5 days.

With the expiration of patents many epoetin, called Biosimilar epoetins, are being produced today at lower cost throughout Asia, Africa, and Latin America as well in Europe. These are mostly erythropoietins of the epoetin alpha, beta, or omega type.

Other ESAs are currently in preclinical or clinical trials and can be classified in three categories: (1) substances that activate the erythropoietin receptor (EPOR): protein-based EPO derivatives and large (CTNO 528) and small (Hematide®,SEStide) molecule ESAs, (2) substances that stimulate endogenous EPO production by activating the EPO gene:HIF stabilizers and GATA inhibitors, and (3) EPO gene therapy.

EPO gene therapy which may be able to generate lower and continuous levels of EPO is a potentially attractive area of research. Following a single intramuscular injection of a vector containing the EPO gene under control of a rapamycin-sensitive promoter, regulated, inducible expression of EPO was obtained in macaques for a period of 7 years. In 2002, OxforBiomedica developed

Repoxygen, a viral gene delivery vector carrying the murine EPO gene under the control of a "hypoxia control element" ("HRE") designed to be delivered to muscles by injection and therefore to induce EPO synthesis in the muscle tissue. Animal experiments have shown that it is possible to obtain oxygen-dependent feedback regulation of the transgene similar to that of the endogenous EPO gene.

Red blood cell mass can also, but to lesser extent, be increased by the use of several hormones, prostanoids, thyroid hormone, angiotensin II, growth hormone corticosteroids and anabolic-androgenic steroids (SAA). Theses substances either may stimulate the endogenous EPO production or stimulate the proliferation of erythrocytic progenitors in the bone marrow or, as it is the case with SAA, both of them.

Artificial Oxygen Carriers (Blood Substitutes) and Allosteric Hemoglobin Modifiers

ESAs and blood transfusion work by enhancing the body's normal O_2 delivery mechanisms. The WADA list bans other compounds that artificially enhance the oxygen transport or delivery. The attempt to develop a viable blood substitute spans more than seven decades. For many years, two approaches were envisaged: perfluorocarbon emulsions (PFCs), first presented to the world in movie "The Abyss," and modified hemoglobins known as hemoglobin-based oxygen carriers (HBOCs). But most attempts to synthesize blood substitutes have failed because of significant adverse effects. Today only Hemopure (OPK Biotech), a polymerized form of bovine hemoglobin, is sold (since 2001) in South Africa. Hemospan (Sangart Inc.), PEG-conjugated human hemoglobin is in advanced-phase clinical trials and Oxycyte, (Oxygen Biotherapeutics), a PFC emulsion, is in phase II clinical trials. Although the US Food and Drug Administration and the European Medicines Agency have approved no oxygen-carrying blood substitutes for human use, some athletes have tried to use them. Later, all gave up because of the side effects.

The synthetic ▶ allosteric Hb modifier, Efaproxiral (Efaproxyn™, RSR13) has been discontinued. It decreases Hb-O_2 binding affinity and was designed to enhance oxygenation of hypoxic tumors to increase the effectiveness of radiotherapy.

Clinical Use

Blood transfusions can be life saving in some situations, such as massive blood loss due to trauma, or can be used to replace blood lost during surgery. Blood transfusions may also be used to treat a severe anemia or thrombocytopenia caused by a blood disease. People suffering from hemophilia or sickle-cell disease may require frequent blood transfusions.

ESAs are effective treatment of anemia and avoidance of the blood transfusion risks.

Side Effects of Blood Doping

Blood transfusions, independent of type, and ESA treatment increase total RBC mass leading to increased Hb concentration, hematocrit (Hct), and blood viscosity and they may cause iron overloading. In the general population and in patients with primary polycythemia, there is an exponential increase in the risk of cardiovascular mortality with elevated [Hb] and/or Hct. Besides the risk of thrombosis, homologous transfusions carry significant risks of contraction of infectious diseases and life-threatening immune reactions.

rhuEpo use has a greater thrombotic potential than blood transfusion due to increased platelet reactivity and increased systolic blood pressure particularly at submaximal exercise. In the early 1990s, 18 Europeans cyclists died and EPO was a key suspect in many of these deaths. Far more threatening is the risk of red cell aplasia characterized by an arrest in RBC production.

HBOCs have a number of problems with toxicity related to their radical reactivity: Outside the RBC, Hb scavenges nitric oxide which causes vasoconstriction and it is able to initiate free-radical-mediated lipid peroxidation via peroxidative heme reaction.

PFC toxicity is associated with its immunogenicity.

Diagnostics

Blood Doping Detection

Blood doping detection strategies include direct and indirect approaches. Markers of enhanced or reduced erythropoiesis are used as well as direct detection of the various molecules, but until 2001 no direct test was available. Some sports federations (International Cycling Union, International Skiing Federation) adopted a strategy based on arbitrary thresholds for hemoglobin and/or hematocrit and reticulocyte values. Athletes exceeding the threshold limits were suspended from competition for rather arguable reasons of health. Nevertheless, this action prevented heavy EPO use.

Direct Testing

A method for detecting rHuEPO in human urine was published in 2000 and adopted for antidoping control in 2001. This method is based on isoelectric focalization in polyacrylamide slab gels. Due to differences in the composition of carbohydrate chains, EPO exhibits microheterogenicity. Isoelectric focalization (separation according to the overall electrical charge of the molecule in a pH gradient) shows a variety of isoforms (Fig. 2). Due to a slightly different sugar composition, rHuEPO exhibits more basic isoforms (more acidic for Aranesp) than natural EPO. First, second, and third generations of rHuEPO can thus be separated from endogenous EPO in urine as in plasma or serum. However, in some cases the SDS-PAGE method which separates proteins according to their apparent molecular mass is needed to interpret of the results particularly for epoetin delta which contains a slightly higher quantity of "endogenous" isoforms. The detection window, from several days to only 12 h, depends on the half-life of molecule, the dose, and the administration route. This method differentiates transgenic EPO and physiological EPO, at least in the macaques. Other methods (membrane-assisted isoform immunoassay and liquid chromatography-tandem mass spectrometry) are currently being tested.

The principles for detecting of homologous blood transfusions by fluorescence-based flow cytometry were established in 2002. The detection method was adopted in 2005. This method is based on the quantification of antigenically distinct donor and recipient RBCs. Individual's erythrocytes are characterized by the genetically defined combination of at least 45 independents antigens. The test uses up to 12 antibodies. Unfortunately, this test does not detect autologous blood transfusion.

Oxygen carriers are not eliminated in urine but are easy to detect by chromatography-mass spectrometry in blood and also in breathing air for the PFCs.

Indirect Testing

Indirect methods were the first to detect rHuEPO and relied on the variations of blood and serum parameters. The first indirect test (2000) consisted of two models: the "ON" model based on reticulocyte hematocrit, serum EPO, soluble transferin receptor, hematocrit, and % of macrocytes to reveal administration of EPO and the "OFF" model based on reticulocyte hematocrit, serum EPO, and hematocrit for the washout phase. This test was subsequently improved (second generation of ON and OFF models). The new "OFF" model, known as the stimulation index, is based on [Hb] and % of reticulocytes (RET%), and is a means to detect athletes who have stopped EPO administrations a week or more early or who have received a blood transfusion. More sophisticated statistical approaches have been developed and have led to the concept of the "hematological passport." In the third-generation model, Hb values and "OFF" scores were compared with the athlete's entire historical baseline rather with a population threshold. This approach heightened the capacity to detect blood doping by removing within subject variability. But this model relied on the use of a unique value of non-inter-individual, variation presupposing that this value is the same for every athlete. The most recent improvement was contributed by the Swiss Laboratory of Doping Analyses which proposed the "Athlete's Biological Passport" (ABP). Three distinct modules can be distinguished in ABP: the hematological, steroidal, and endocrinological modules. The hematological module of ABP aims to detect any form of blood doping. It includes a longitudinal follow-up of Hb, "OFF" score, RET%, and the "Abnormal Profile Score" (ABPS), a multiparametric marker that responds to modifications

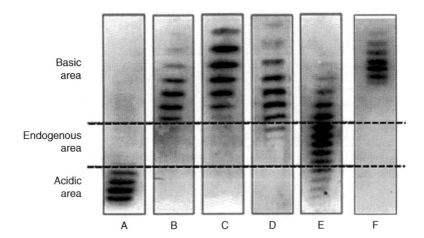

Blood Doping. Fig. 2 Isofocalization profiles of different epoetin and human EPO. Aranesp (A), epoetin α and β (B), epoetin ω (C), epoetin δ (D), human EPO (E), Myrcera (F)

in seven different indirect markers (erythrocyte count, Hb, Hct, RET%, mean corpuscular volume, mean corpuscular Hb, mean corpuscular Hb concentration) that may result from either rHuEPO administration or blood transfusion. This method, adopted by IUC since 2008 but now adopted by some other international federations, is the only indirect method used today as evidence of doping.

References

1. Bassett DR Jr, Howley ET (2000) Limiting factors for maximum oxygen uptake and determinants of endurance performance. Med Sci Sports Exerc 32(1):70–84, Review
2. Cooper CE, Beneke R (eds) (2008) Essays in biochemistry: drugs and ergogenic aids to improve sport performance. Portland Press, London
3. Ekblom BT (2000) Blood boosting in sport. Baillere's Clin Endocrinol Metab 14(1):89–98
4. Fourcroy JL (ed) (2009) Pharmacology, doping and sports. Routledge, London
5. Thieme D, Hemmerscbach P (2010) Doping in sports. In: Handbook of experimental pharmacology, vol 195. Springer, Berlin/Heidelberg

Blood Fats

▶ Lipoproteins

Blood Flow

Movement of blood through the circulatory system.

Blood Lactate

Lactate (lactic acid) produced within resting and working skeletal muscle that appears within the blood stream.

Cross-References

▶ Lactate Metabolism

Blood Manipulation

Artificial increase in hemoglobin mass mostly due to the use of erythropoietic stimulating agents (ESA) or blood transfusions. Today, approximately 100 ESAs exist which cannot all be detected.

Blood Rheology

Philippe Connes
Laboratoire ACTES (EA 3596), Département de Physiologie, Université des Antilles et de la Guyane, Pointe-à-Pitre, Guadeloupe, French West Indies

Synonyms

Hemorheology; Red blood cell rheological properties

Definition

Blood rheology is the scientific field working on the biophysical properties and flow properties of blood. One of the well-known hemorheological parameter is blood viscosity. Blood viscosity depends on plasma viscosity, hematocrit, and the ability of red blood cell to deform and aggregate under specific hemodynamic conditions. The French physician Poiseuille [1] was the first to study the principles of fluid flow in order to understand blood circulation. He formulated the relationship between pressure gradient and flow in a cylindrical tube as follows:

$$Q = \frac{\Delta P \cdot \pi \cdot r^4}{8 \cdot L \cdot \eta}$$

where Q is the volumetric flow rate through a tube of radius r under a pressure difference ΔP over the vessel length L and η is the viscosity of the flowing fluid.

According to the law derived from this work, vascular geometry is the most important factor of blood flow resistance and, consequently, the impact of blood viscosity and the other hemorheological factors have often been ignored. Poiseuille's law has been used extensively in scientific and medical research, and critical elements of blood rheology in cardiovascular physiology continue to be studied.

Basic Mechanisms

Today, it seems that the use of Poiseuille law has some limits to study integrative cardiovascular function. Poiseuille law does not consider the fact that blood interacts directly with ▶ endothelium, and that hemorheological properties may be strong modulators of vascular function and geometry. For example, it was demonstrated that a rise in plasma viscosity may cause a counterintuitive and surprising decrease in vascular resistance [2]. The increase in viscosity causes a greater ▶ shear stress applied at the endothelium level, which stimulates the production of nitric oxide by the endothelial nitric oxide synthase (e-NOs) and results in compensatory vasodilatation. In addition, Baskurt et al. [3] recently reported an effect of red blood cell (RBC) aggregation on the vasodilatory function of muscular microcirculation. They described depressed e-NOs activity and decreased NO-mediated relaxation of arterioles when red blood cell (RBC) aggregation was increased. This effect was explained by the enhanced axial migration of cellular elements of blood, which reduced the frictional forces on the endothelial cells and downregulated NO synthesis.

In the microcirculation, Poiseuille law cannot be applied easily to understand how blood flows. Blood flow and adequate oxygen delivery to tissue are mainly dependent on RBC deformability. Parthasarathi and Lipowsky [4] studied the effect of reduced RBC deformability on microvessel recruitment attendant to a reduction in tissue oxygen pressure (PO_2) in rat cremaster muscle. These authors found that impaired RBC deformability may adversely affect capillary recruitment and the physiological mechanisms that ensure adequate delivery of oxygen to tissue. Studies on the rheological behavior of RBCs in the capillary network clearly demonstrated that capillary flux and velocity are strongly dependent on the ability of RBCs to deform in the capillaries. A decrease in RBC deformability adversely affects capillary perfusion. Baskurt et al. [5] demonstrated that a 15–17% reduction in RBC deformability can cause a 75% rise in flow resistance in isolated-perfused rat hind limbs when vasoactivity is intact and more than 250% when vasoactivity is inhibited.

These data demonstrate that, although Poiseuille law is useful to grossly understand cardiovascular regulations, integrative cardiovascular approaches should keep in mind that blood rheology and vascular function are related to each other.

Blood Viscosity (ηb)
Rheology is the study of flow and deformation. Hemorheology specifically deals with the flow properties of blood. Fluidity of blood is strongly influenced by flow conditions. More specifically, ηb depends on ▶ shear rate, decreasing with increased shear rate. This property is known as shear-thinning and is characteristic of a non-Newtonian fluid. Therefore, blood fluidity cannot be described with a single value of viscosity, but it should be expressed as a function of shear rate.

This specific flow behavior of blood is mainly determined by its structure. Blood is a two-phase liquid and its rheological properties are determined by the flow properties of both phases and the relative contribution of these phases to the total volume of blood. The two phases are plasma and cellular components and their relative contribution is represented by hematocrit (Hct) value. Therefore, Hct value is the major determinant of ηb. Plasma viscosity (ηp) contributes to high shear ηb significantly. Plasma is a Newtonian fluid, with its viscosity being independent of shear rate.

Shear thinning properties of blood are mainly determined by the mechanical properties of cellular components of blood, more specifically by the properties of RBCs, which constitutes 99% of cellular components.

RBC Deformability and Aggregation
RBCs possess two special mechanical properties that determine the non-Newtonian behavior of whole blood. At high shear rates (characterized with higher shear forces), RBCs exhibit an extensive shape change, which leads to an efficient orientation of them to laminar flow streamlines, decreasing their distortion and reducing internal resistance of fluid to flow [5]. This means a reduction in viscosity. Therefore, high shear rate viscosity is mainly determined by this ability of RBC to deform under shear, which is called "deformability." RBC deformability is determined by the geometric properties, cytoplasmic composition, and viscosity and membrane properties of RBC [5].

RBCs return to biconcave discoid shape as shear forces become smaller (being related to lower shear rates) and orientation to flow streamlines become less effective, resulting in increased ηb [5]. Additionally, RBCs tend to form aggregates under conditions of low shear rates, further increasing viscosity, due to increased distortion of flow streamlines. RBC aggregation is a physiological process dominating under low shear or stasis conditions, characterized by the formation of regular structures where RBCs form face-to-face contacts resulting in structures looking like stacks of coins. This special way of clumping of RBC depends on the presence of fibrous macromolecules with molecular weights above a certain size [5]. Fibrinogen is the physiological aggregating macromolecule for RBC. RBC aggregation is determined by both plasma composition and cellular properties [5]. The third factor determining the extent of RBC aggregation is the magnitude of effective shear forces, as aggregate formation is a reversible process.

Exercise Intervention

Blood Rheology and Aerobic Performance

Significant correlations have been reported between baseline blood fluidity and indices of physical fitness such as time of endurance until exhaustion, aerobic working capacity at 170W (W170) or maximal oxygen consumption (VO_{2max}) [6]. Brun et al. [7] proposed that decreased resting ηb could improve O_2 delivery to muscle during exercise in trained individuals.

However, recent data support that the relationships between blood rheology and aerobic performance/fitness could be a little bit more complex. And none of these previous studies investigated the relationships between the hemorheological changes induced by exercise and the aerobic fitness. Connes et al. [8] recently studied the relationships between the changes in ηb, vascular resistance, NO production and oxygen consumption induced by a submaximal exercise. The authors observed: (1) a positive correlation between the increase in ηb and the increase in NO production during exercise; (2) a negative correlation between the increase in NO production and the decrease in vascular hindrance; (3) a negative correlation between the increase in ηb and the decrease in systemic vascular resistance. These findings suggest that a marked rise in ηb during exercise could be necessary for NO production and adequate vasodilation, to reach the highest aerobic performance. Having decreased resting ηb could be a way to obtain the largest rise in ηb in response to exercise; that could explain why decreased baseline ηb is also related to improved aerobic fitness. It must be kept in mind that these data have been observed in healthy subjects with healthy endothelium and that these conclusions are not necessary applicable to other populations.

Blood Rheology and Acute Exercise

As mentioned above, acute exercise usually leads to a rise in ηb. This rise is related to change in Hct, ηp, RBC deformability, and RBC aggregation [6].

The increase in Hct with exercise can be explained by several mechanisms including fluid shift, water loss, release of sequestered RBCs from spleen, and water trapping in muscle [6].

Exercise also increases ηp. This increment has been attributed to a rise in plasma protein content, such as fibrinogen, a1-globulins, a2-globulins, b-globulins and g-globulins, and probably to plasma volume loss, at least in part [6].

The effects of exercise on RBC deformability have been examined in several studies, with most reporting a decrease [6]. This decrease has been attributed to the effects of lactic acid and oxidative stress on the membrane of RBCs [6]. However, few studies also observed a surprising improvement of RBC deformability during exercise [9]. This increase in RBC deformability is not well understood but it has been shown that a rise in lactate concentration was able to cause RBC rigidification in sedentary people whereas it resulted in RBC deformability improvement in endurance-trained athletes [10]. It seems that RBC from endurance sportsmen could better cope with lactate than RBC from sedentary subjects. Another molecular agent, which may positively influence RBC deformability, is NO [11]; but very few studies investigated the effects of NO on RBC deformability during exercise.

Few studies have investigated RBC aggregation in response to exercise and the results are not in agreement: some studies describe no change, an increase or a delayed decrease of RBC aggregation [6]. The reasons for these various results are unclear, but may be related to: (1) the population tested; (2) the exercise performed; and (3) the technique used to measure aggregation (backscattered technique vs light transmission technique).

Blood Rheology and Exercise Training

Most of the studies investigating the effects of exercise training on blood rheology focused on patients with cardiovascular disease.

Epidemiological, case control, and clinical studies have reported relationship between cardiovascular risk factors (elevated low density lipoprotein cholesterol, decreased high density lipoprotein cholesterol, elevated arterial blood pressure, smoking) and ηb and ηp. Impaired hemorheology has been demonstrated in ischemic heart disease, peripheral arterial disease, arterial hypertension, and in venous disorders. Whatever the causes of hemorheological impairment, these alterations are widely thought to contribute to cardiovascular diseases/complications.

For Brun et al. [7], exercise must be considered as a "hemorheological therapy" in cardiovascular diseases. For example, Church et al. [12] reported blood rheology improvement in patients with coronary heart disease after a phase II cardiac rehabilitation and exercise training. Blood viscosity at corrected Hct (0.45) and ηp were significantly reduced and RBC transport efficiency was enhanced after training [12]. Several other studies have suggested that regular exercise could improve ηb in healthy persons too [7] and therefore, decrease the risks for the development of cardiovascular diseases.

References

1. Poiseuille JLM (1835) Recherches sur les causes du mouvement du sang dans les vaisseaux capillaires. CR Acad Sci Paris 1:554–560
2. Tsai AG, Acero C, Nance PR, Cabrales P, Frangos JA, Buerk DG, Intaglietta M (2005) Elevated plasma viscosity in extreme hemodilution increases perivascular nitric oxide concentration and microvascular perfusion. Am J Physiol Heart Circ Physiol 288:H1730–H1739
3. Baskurt OK, Yalcin O, Ozdem S, Armstrong JK, Meiselman HJ (2004) Modulation of endothelial nitric oxide synthase expression by red blood cell aggregation. Am J Physiol Heart Circ Physiol 286:H222–H229
4. Parthasarathi K, Lipowsky HH (1999) Capillary recruitment in response to tissue hypoxia and its dependence on red blood cell deformability. Am J Physiol 277:H2145–H2157
5. Baskurt OK, Meiselman HJ (2007) In vivo hemorheology. In: Baskurt OK, Hardeman PR, Rampling MW, Meiselman HJ (eds) Handbook of hemorheology and hemodynamics. IOS Press, Netherlands, pp 322–338
6. Connes P, Brun JF, Baskurt OK (2010) Blood rheology and exercise. In: Connes P, Hue O, Perrey S (eds) Exercise physiology: from a cellular to an integrative approach. IOS Press, Netherlands, pp 213–229
7. Brun JF, Varlet-Marie E, Connes P, Aloulou I (2010) Hemorheological alterations related to training and overtraining. Biorheology 47:95–115
8. Connes P, Pichon A, Hardy-Dessources MD, Waltz X, Lamarre Y, Simmonds MJ, Tripette J. Blood viscosity and hemodynamics at exercise. Clin Hemorheol Microcirc (in press)
9. Connes P, Tripette J, Mukisi-Mukaza M, Baskurt OK, Toth K, Meiselman HJ, Hue O, Antoine-Jonville S (2009) Relationships between hemodynamic, hemorheological and metabolic responses during exercise. Biorheology 46:133–143
10. Connes P, Bouix D, Py G, Prefaut C, Mercier J, Brun JF, Caillaud C (2004) Opposite effects of in vitro lactate on erythrocyte deformability in athletes and untrained subjects. Clin Hemorheol Microcirc 31:311–318
11. Bor-Kucukatay M, Wenby RB, Meiselman HJ, Baskurt OK (2003) Effects of nitric oxide on red blood cell deformability. Am J Physiol Heart Circ Physiol 284:H1577–H1584
12. Church TS, Lavie CJ, Milani RV, Kirby GS (2002) Improvements in blood rheology after cardiac rehabilitation and exercise training in patients with coronary heart disease. Am Heart J 143:349–355

Blood Substitutes

Are solutions which injected in blood increase oxygen transport and delivery but do not replace all compound and functions of blood (coagulation factors, white blood cells, etc.).

Cross-References

▶ Blood doping

Blood-Borne Infections

Ramiro L. Gutiérrez, Catherine F. Decker
Division of Infectious Diseases, National Naval Medical Center, Uniformed Services University of the Health Sciences, Bethesda, MD, USA

Synonyms

Hepatitis B; Hepatitis C; HIV

Definition

Blood-borne infections are acute and chronic infections which may be transmitted from person-to-person by way of contact with blood and/or other secretions. Although several pathogens may be transmitted in this fashion, the three main pathogens of concern are all viruses; the human immunodeficiency virus (▶ HIV), ▶ hepatitis C virus, and ▶ hepatitis B virus. Transmission of these infections during sports has been rare and risk varies depending on virus type and degree physicality and risk of injury associated with different sports. Available evidence suggests that much of the risk for acquisition of these diseases among athletes, stems not from participation in sports themselves, but rather from risky off-field behaviors such as unsafe sexual practices and the sharing needles in the setting of blood doping and use of illicit recreational and performance-enhancing drugs.

Characteristics

Hepatitis B virus, hepatitis C virus, and HIV are all able to cause chronic infectious state where the individual remains contagious despite being asymptomatic. After acute HIV infection, and almost invariably, individuals enter a chronic state of infection. Acute HBV and HCV infections may be spontaneously cleared in some cases, but a variable number of individuals go on to develop chronic infection and remain infectious to others. All three viruses may be found to varying degrees in the blood and other bodily fluids of acute and chronically infected individuals. Those chronically infected will often be asymptomatic for long periods and conceivably are able to participate in athletic activities. Generally, blood exposures with hepatitis B are most contagious, followed by hepatitis C coming second, while HIV is the least transmissible of the three.

Transmission of hepatitis B during athletic activity has been reported in high-prevalence regions in the world. During an outbreak among sumo wrestlers in Japan, transmission was attributed to a single chronically infected individual who participated while he had an uncovered wound [4]. Also in Japan, five cases of acute hepatitis B infection in a college football team were associated with exposure to a teammate who was a chronic carrier and again, contact with an open uncovered wound was the likely source [5].

There have been no documented reports of hepatitis C acquisition as a result of exposure during sports related activities, but cases of athletes acquiring hepatitis C due to the use of injectable steroids and other performance enhancing drugs have been published. In a study of 208 former professional and amateur soccer and basketball players in Brazil, the study population had a higher prevalence of hepatitis C infection (7.2%) than the general population. In that study, previous use of injectable performance enhancing drugs was the only risk factor to have a significant association with infection rates and suggests that such behavior patterns may pose a significant and modifiable risk for infection among athletes [6].

HIV transmission during athletic activity has been difficult to document but the risk appears to be low. In 1990, the only known case of possible transmission of HIV between athletes was published, the report described two soccer players in Italy who collided during play and sustained significant soft tissue injuries and mucocutaneous blood exposure. Seroconversion of the HIV-negative player occurred over the next month and no other significant risk factors for acquisition were elucidated [7]. Early data from healthcare workers exposed to HIV infected patients suggests that such mucocutaneous exposure is less efficient as a means of transmission and risk of acquisition may be 0.1% per exposure [8].

Some have tried to quantify the possible risk of transmission of HIV during contact sports. In one study in the United States, National Football League teams were observed during regular season games and the frequency of bleeding injuries was calculated in order to obtain an estimate of risk of mucocutaneous exposure to blood-borne pathogens during routine play. Based on conservative calculations the authors concluded that the risk for transmission of HIV during play was low and in the range of less than 1 in 85 million contacts [9].

Clinical Relevance

In 2009 the American Academy of Pediatrics (AAP) updated their 1999 recommendations on the prevention of blood-borne diseases in the athletic setting [10]. These guidelines have been widely adopted by youth, collegiate,

amateur, and professional athletic programs. The guidelines recommend against mandatory testing and against disclosure or removal of participants based on blood-borne pathogen infected status. Instead, they recommend: (1) adherence to Universal Precautions by trainers and coaches when managing bleeding injuries, (2) the provision of hepatitis B vaccination for athletes and support staff that may come in contact with injured athletes, (3) the education of athletes regarding the risks of acquisition of blood-borne pathogens on and off the athletic field, and (4) suggest that United States Occupational Safety and Health Administration (OSHA) standards (Standard 29 CFR 1910.1030 is available at: http://osha. gov) be followed for the prevention of blood-borne pathogen transmission even when not required by the State.

Many professional and international athletic groups have established their own guidelines for prevention of blood-borne pathogen transmission and these have largely been similar to AAP guidelines. In the United States, the National Football League, National Basketball Association, and Major League Baseball, as well as the NCAA, generally abide by AAP and OSHA guidelines and do not mandate testing or exclusion of participants. With regards to hepatitis B, the NCAA Sports Medicine Handbook (available at: http://www.NCAA.org/health-safety) does recommend that programs consider removal of athletes with acute hepatitis B from participation in close contact sports, such as wrestling, until they become negative for hepatitis B surface antigen (HBsAg). They go on to suggest that if the athlete does not become negative for hepatitis B surface antigen (HBsAg); that is, does not develop hepatitis B surface antibody and clear the infection, and goes on to develop chronic hepatitis B, they should be removed from close contact sports. In March 2009, the International Olympic Committee (IOM) published guidelines for the execution of the pre-participation physical exam for athletes and although it recommends that a history of blood-borne pathogen infection be obtained, testing is left to the discretion of the examiner. The IOM does not recommend the barring of athletes based on blood-borne pathogen infected status [11]. Similarly, the International Federation of Sports Medicine has issued position statements on AIDS and hepatitis and sports which are available at http: www.fims.org.

Although there have been no reports of HIV transmission in the setting of boxing or other combative sports, in the United States, mandatory testing for HIV and other blood-borne pathogens is required by most states in order to obtain a professional boxing, or combat sport license.

The AAP guidelines specifically comment that boxing is not a recommended sport for youth but agree that such sports may pose a higher-risk of exposure to blood-borne infection [10].

The risk of transmission of blood-borne pathogens during athletic activity appears to be quite low. Reports of possible instances of transmission have been rare. Hepatitis B may pose the greatest risk, whereas HIV poses the least risk. Similarly, sports with close contact, and high likelihood of bleeding injuries, such as martial arts, wrestling, and boxing, may pose a greater risk of exposure but there have been no documented cases of such transmission. Athletes and trainers, in addition to being educated on Universal Precautions and their possible exposure risk to blood-borne pathogens, should be offered hepatitis B vaccination. Blood-borne pathogen prevention programs for athletes must emphasize modification of traditional risk factors and risky off- the- field behaviors which may pose the greatest risk of acquisition of these pathogens.

Disclaimer: The views expressed in this article [lecture, etc.] are those of the author and do not necessarily reflect the official policy or position of the Department of the Navy, Army, Department of Defense, nor the U.S. Government. I/We certify that all individuals who qualify as authors have been listed; each has participated in the conception and design of this work, the analysis of data (when applicable), the writing of the document, and the approval of the submission of this version; that the document represents valid work; that if we used information derived from another source, we obtained all necessary approvals to use it and made appropriate acknowledgements in the document; and that each takes public responsibility for it. Nothing in the presentation implies any Federal/DOD/DON endorsement (when applicable).

Copyright Statement: I am a military service member (or employee of the U.S. Government). This work was prepared as part of my official duties. Title 17 U.S.C. §105 provides that 'Copyright protection under this title is not available for any work of the United States Government.' Title 17 U.S.C. §101 defines a U.S. Government work as a work prepared by a military service member or employee of the U.S. Government as part of that person's official duties.

References

1. Koziel MJ, Thio CL (2009) Hepatitis B virus and hepatitis delta virus. In: Mandell GL, Bennett JE, Dolin R (eds) Principles and practice of infectious diseases, 7th edn. Churchill Livingstone Elsevier, Philadelphia, pp 2059–2081
2. Ray SC, Thomas DL (2009) Hepatitis C. In: Mandell GL, Bennett JE, Dolin R (eds) Principles and practice of infectious diseases, 7th edn. Churchill Livingstone Elsevier, Philadelphia, pp 2057–2086
3. International Olympic Committee (2005) Together for HIV and AIDS prevention: a toolkit for the sports community. Available at: http://www.olympic.org. Accessed 20 Feb 2010
4. Kashiwagi S, Hayashi J, Ikematsu H, Nishigori S, Ishihara K, Kaji M (1982) An outbreak of hepatitis B in members of a high school sumo wrestling club. J Am Med Assoc 248:213–214
5. Tobe K, Matsuura K, Ogura T, Tso Y, Iwasaki Y, Mizuno M, Yamamoto K, Higashi T, Tsuji T (2000) Horizontal transmission of hepatitis B virus among players of an American football team. Arch Intern Med 160:2541–2545
6. Costa-Passos AD, de Castro-Figueiredo JF, Candolo-Martinelli A, Villanova M, Nascimento MM Passeri do, Secaf M (2008) Hepatitis C among former athletes; association with the use of injectable stimulants in the past. Mem Inst Oswaldo Cruz, Rio de Janeiro 103(8):809–812
7. Torre D, Sampietro C, Ferraro G, Zeroli C, Speranza F (1990) Transmission of HIV-1 infection via sports injury. Lancet 335:1105
8. Gelberding JL (1995) Management of occupational exposures to blood-borne viruses. N Engl J Med 332(7):444–451
9. Brown LS, Drotman DP, Chu A, Brown CL, Knowlan D (1995) Bleeding injuries in professional football: estimating the risk of HIV transmission. Ann Intern Med 122(4):273–274
10. Committee on Sports Medicine and Fitness, American Academy of Pediatrics (1999) Human immunodeficiency virus and other blood-borne viral pathogens in the athletic setting. Pediatrics 104:1400–1403
11. International Olympic Committee (2009) The International Olympic Committee (IOC) consensus statement on periodic health evaluation of elite athletes. J Athletic Training 44(5):538–557

BMD

▶ Bone Mineral Density

BMI

▶ Body Mass Index

Body Builder Training

Training for muscular hypertrophy. Typically 10–12 dynamic repetitions in 5–7 series to complete exhaustion in slow movements.

Body Composition

GUY PLASQUI, KLAAS R. WESTERTERP
Department of Human Biology, NUTRIM School for
Nutrition, Toxicology & Metabolism, Maastricht
University Medical Centre +, Maastricht, The Netherlands

Synonyms
Composition of the human body

Definition
The relative amounts of various components in the body, such as the percentage body fat.

Description
In vivo, body composition can only be measured indirectly. There are nowadays a great variety of methods available with different assumptions and limitations. All these assumptions stem from the chemical analysis of a limited number of cadavers with a normal body condition until death, the only direct method to assess human body composition.

The most commonly used outcome measure from human body composition analysis is the percentage body fat or percent fat mass (%FM). Excess body fat is a risk factor for metabolic complications, such as insulin resistance, cardiovascular disease, and type 2 diabetes, which makes it an important outcome measure in health related and clinical research. Body composition however comprises more than just the %FM. The human body can be subdivided into multiple components, fat mass (FM) being just one of those. A variety of techniques is available to assess these components, each technique having its limitations and assumptions. Below, an overview is given of the different models used in body composition assessment as well as the techniques commonly used.

Multiple Compartment Models
The two-compartment (2C) model is the most commonly used model to assess the composition of the human body. Basically, the body is divided into fat mass (FM) and all other tissues, referred to as ▶ fat-free mass (FFM). The assessment of ▶ body density, using hydrodensitometry or air-displacement plethysmography, or total ▶ body water (TBW) using isotope dilution techniques, are examples of 2C-models. Each method has an uncertainty of the order of magnitude of at least 1.5 kg FM and FFM. A combination of independent measurements can reduce this measurement bias, adopting a three- or four-compartment model. An example of a 3C-model is when

▶ body volume is assessed using hydrodensitometry and TBW is assessed using deuterium dilution. This provides some more insight into the composition of the FFM, as the three compartments being calculated are FM, TBW, and remaining solids. This approach would enhance the accuracy to about 1.0 kg for FM and 0.7 kg for FFM. In some clinical situations, such as significant depletion of bone mineral mass, the composition of the "remaining solids" may also be altered. In that case, further improvement in accuracy can be achieved with a 4C-model, including a measure of total bone mineral content from dual-energy X-ray absorptiometry (DEXA).

As the number of techniques combined increases, fewer assumptions are made about the composition of FFM and as a consequence the accuracy to estimate FM and FFM will improve. Therefore, the 4C-model is currently considered the "gold" standard to assess body composition.

"Classical 2C-Models"

Densitometry
Densitometry requires the measurement of ▶ body weight and body volume from which body density can be calculated. It assumes a constant chemical composition of FM and FFM resulting in a density of 0.90 and 1.10, respectively. Body volume can be assessed in water (underwater weighing) or air (air-displacement plethysmography).

Underwater weighing is based on Archimedes' principle, stating that: "Any object, wholly or partially immersed in a fluid, is buoyed up by a force equal to the weight of the fluid displaced by the object." This means that when a subject is first weighed in air and then when completely submerged under water, the difference in weight equals the weight of the amount of water displaced by the person's body. As the volume of water displaced equals the volume of the subject, and when the density of the water at a specific temperature of the water is known, body volume can be calculated.

Body volume has to be corrected for lung volume, ideally by measuring simultaneously residual lung volume during submersion. Densitometry has gained widespread use and was until recently the "gold standard" for body composition measurement with other techniques.

The theoretical error of densitometry for predicting FM and FFM is 3–4%, associated with the uncertainty in the density and chemical composition of FFM. The main variables are water content and bone density. In practice additional error sources are variability in gastrointestinal gas volume and residual lung volume, the latter when lung volume is not measured during but before or after submersion. An error of 0.1 L in lung volume is roughly equivalent to a 1% error in FM and FFM. Usually errors are not additive and the overall accuracy of densitometry for body composition is 1–2%.

Body volume measurement by submersion in water is not always applicable in adult subjects, e.g., patients or the elderly. A recent development is to measure body volume in air instead of water [1]. The advantage of air-displacement plethysmography using the Bod Pod® (Life measurement, Inc. Concord, CA, USA), is the applicability and the required time for an observation. Underwater weighing in a trained subject takes about half an hour while measuring body volume in air is done in 5–10 min. Several studies have compared the Bod Pod with underwater weighing and found mean differences in %FM varying between −4.0% and +2.0% and individual-level differences in the order of ±6–8%.

Body fat can be calculated from body weight and body volume with the two equations: body weight = FFM + FM; volume = FFV + FV, where FFV = fat-free volume and FV = fat volume. With the assumed density for FFM of 1.1 and for FM of 0.9, body volume = FFM/1.1 + FM/0.9. Solving the two equations with two unknowns we get the Siri equation (5):

$$\%FM = (4.95/D_b - 4.50)100$$

where

D_b – body density = (body weight)/(body volume)

Isotope Dilution Techniques

Isotope dilution can be used to assess total body water. From TBW, FFM can be calculated by assuming a constant hydration fraction of FFM. In adults, the hydration fraction is usually 73% whereas in children it is higher, depending on the age [2]. From body mass (BM) and TBW, FFM can be calculated as TBW/0.73 and FM as BM minus FFM.

TBW is measured with dilution of isotopes of water, i.e., isotopes of hydrogen and oxygen: ^3H, ^2H, or ^{18}O. The underlying assumption is that these have the same distribution volume as water. A subject gets an accurately measured oral or intravenous dose of labeled water, followed by an equilibration period of at least 2 h and subsequent sampling of the body fluid [3]. Dose, equilibration time, and sampling medium depend on the isotope, the dosing route, and the facilities for sample analysis. Tritium or ^3H is a radioisotope, which is measured with liquid scintillation counting. Deuterium or ^2H and ^{18}O are both stable isotopes, ^2H can be measured in higher concentrations with infrared absorption and both isotopes are measured in low concentrations with isotope ratio mass spectrometry (IRMS). Body fluids for

sampling are saliva, blood, and urine. The length of the equilibration period is minimally 2 h with intravenous dosing and taking blood as a sampling medium. Using the less invasive oral route of dosing and sampling urine needs a minimal equilibration time of 4–6 h. The calculation of TBW is based on the relationship:

$$C_d \times V_d = (C_1 - C_0) \times TBW$$

where

C_d – concentration of the tracer
V_d – volume of the dose
C_0 – basal concentrations of the tracer
C_1 – concentrations of the tracer after dose consumption

In practice, using a noninvasive method with stable isotopes at low concentrations, subjects get a dose of labeled water in the post-absorptive state after collecting a background sample, i.e., saliva or urine. Background levels for ^2H and ^{18}O are around 150 and 2,000 ppm, respectively. The minimal excess enrichment to be reached is around 100 ppm. After equilibration, lasting 4–6 h, a final saliva or urine sample is collected. For urine this should be a sample from at least a second voiding after dosing the labeled water. The use of ^{18}O as a tracer is preferred over ^3H and ^2H as the dilution space of ^{18}O is very close to TBW. The dilution space for the hydrogen isotopes is on average 4% larger and the dilution space for ^{18}O is on average 1% larger than TBW, due to the exchange of the label with nonaqueous substances in the body. On the other hand the cost of ^{18}O is 100 times higher than the other labels.

Imaging Techniques

Dual-Energy X-ray Absorptiometry (DEXA)

DEXA is an imaging technique that has gained much popularity, especially in clinical settings. It was primarily designed to assess total bone mineral mass and mineral density but is also widely applied to assess %FM. An advantage is that it also provides some information about regional distribution of FM, e.g., upper or lower body. It is a technique that allows rapid acquisition with minimal radiation dose, which is applicable to a wide variety of subjects, including patients.

DEXA will differentiate between bone and soft tissue. A second differentiation within the soft tissue needs to be made between FM and FFM. A limitation inherent of this technique, which limits the accuracy, is that soft tissue behind or in front of bone cannot be assessed. Therefore, the assumption needs to be made that the distribution of

FM versus FFM is the same behind or in front of the bone as it is next to the bone.

The consequence is that the accuracy is lower than that of underwater weighing or deuterium dilution and DEXA can certainly not be regarded as a criterion method [4].

Magnetic Resonance Imaging (MRI)

MRI is an imaging technique that is rapidly gaining popularity, also in the assessment of body composition. A major advantage compared to the "classical" techniques is that it can provide detailed information about regional body composition, e.g., subcutaneous versus visceral fat and can further differentiate within the FFM compartment, e.g., differentiate muscle from organs and bone. The disadvantage is that the analysis of the images is prone to some error, i.e., which part of the image is actually fat mass (or other tissue) and which is not. Measuring total muscle mass, for example, would require to acquire several transversal images (covering the entire body) and to calculate the surface of muscle tissue within each image. This could be done with appropriate software or manually, but in either case accuracy will depend on the ability to determine the actual surface and volume of the tissue of interest. As the resolution of MRI machines is rapidly increasing, the ability to accurately assess different tissues is also increasing.

It is not a technique to replace underwater weighing or deuterium dilution when it comes to assessing total %FM and FFM, but for specific regional interests or more detailed assessment of a specific organ, it has great potential.

"Field" Techniques to Measure Body Composition

Anthropometry

The quickest and cheapest method to measure body composition is from skin fold thickness. The assumptions forming the basis for the method are:

- The thickness of the subcutaneous FM reflects a constant proportion of the total FM.
- The average thickness of skin folds at selected sites reflects the subcutaneous FM.

Skin folds are usually measured at four sites: triceps, biceps, sub scapula, and iliac crest. The sites are measured at least three times and the sum of the separate measurements is averaged. Equations to predict body fat from the sum of skin folds use a logarithmic transformation of skin fold thickness, as body fat is not linearly related to skin fold thickness, age, and gender of the subject.

The measurement is made with a caliper, with the skin grasped between thumb and forefinger, gently shaken to exclude underlying muscle, and pulled away to allow the jaws of the caliper to take over. The caliper is calibrated to exert a constant pressure. The measurement requires the skill to grasp the skin in the right way at the right site. Other sources of variation are interindividual differences in compressibility of the subcutaneous tissue. Some people have firm subcutaneous tissue and in others it is very flabby and easily deformable. The method is not applicable in extremely fat subjects where the subcutaneous fat layer gets too large to allow the proper grasping of a skin fold.

The errors estimating FM and FFM from BM and skin fold thickness are reported between 3% and 9%, highly depending on the experience of the observer and generally higher than the methods mentioned earlier. On the other hand, it sometimes is one of the few possibilities to obtain information on body composition.

Bio-electrical Impedance Analysis (BIA)

A BIA instrument creates a current through the body and measures impedance with contact electrodes positioned on the hands and feet. The technique seems attractive, especially in a clinical setting, because it is safe, quick, noninvasive, and easy to use. Therefore, BIA instruments have been widely used and validated in different populations. From these validation studies it can be concluded that the accuracy is poor. On a group level, BIA may provide a %FM within 2% of the gold standard 4C-model, but 95% limits of agreement may be as large as ±9% [5]. The same accuracy can be achieved by population-specific prediction formulas based on body mass, height, gender, and age.

Clinical Use/Application

As indicated in previous paragraphs, some techniques are more suitable for clinical application than others. It should be obvious that underwater weighing is not suitable to apply in a clinical setting. Air-displacement plethysmography may be a good alternative, when the assumptions of densitometry are not violated. Indeed, aging, starvation, and disease may violate the general assumptions of the two compartment models as adopted with the densitometry and the total body water measurement. In addition, as with densitometry, isotope dilution techniques are generally not readily available in a clinical setting.

As a consequence, DEXA and some "field" techniques have gained widespread popularity in the clinic. DEXA provides reasonably accurate results and is because of its applicability the most clinically used technique to assess body composition. Accuracy of skin folds highly depends on the experience of the observer. BIA is easy to use, but accuracy is too low to allow proper measurement of body composition on the individual basis.

In conclusion, all techniques, except for carcass analysis, are indirect. For the assessment of total body fat mass and fat-free mass, hydrodensitometry and isotope dilution are indirect techniques, whose assumptions are based on the direct analysis of a limited number of cadavers with a normal body condition until death. When these assumptions are violated, accuracy can be improved by combining several techniques into a three- or four-compartment model. DEXA is less accurate but suitable in a clinical setting. Imaging techniques such as MRI offer great perspective for assessing regional and more detailed body composition measurements. The so-called field techniques such as skin folds or BIA are basically double indirect methods. For example, skin fold measurements are first translated to body density which is then translated to %FM, based on the assumptions that also apply for densitometry.

Interestingly, when it comes to estimating a %FM in a large group of healthy subjects, prediction formulas based on body mass, height, age, and gender will provide you with the correct answer on the group level. Thus the essential starting point of any measurement of body composition and changes in body composition is an accurate measurement of BM using properly calibrated weighing scales. For comparative studies subjects should be measured with minimal clothing, minimal gut contents (post-absorptive), and with an empty bladder.

References

1. Dempster P, Aitkens S (1995) A new air displacement method for the determination of human body composition. Med Sci Sports Exerc 27(12):1692–1697
2. Lohman TG (1989) Assessment of body composition in children. Pediatr Exerc Sci 1:19–30
3. van Marken Lichtenbelt WD, Westerterp KR, Wouters L (1994) Deuterium dilution as a method for determining total body water: effect of test protocol and sampling time. Br J Nutr 72(4):491–497
4. Schoeller DA et al (2005) QDR 4500A dual-energy X-ray absorptiometer underestimates fat mass in comparison with criterion methods in adults. Am J Clin Nutr 81(5):1018–1025
5. Jebb SA et al (2000) Evaluation of the novel Tanita body-fat analyser to measure body composition by comparison with a four-compartment model. Br J Nutr 83(2):115–122

Body Composition in Youths

▶ Obesity in Children

Body Density

Body weight divided by body volume and expressed in kilograms per liter.

Cross-References

▶ Body Composition

Body Mass Index

The body mass index (BMI) is a number calculated from a person's weight and height. It is used as a reliable indicator of body fatness for most people and is used to screen for weight categories. Body mass index is defined as the individual's body weight divided by the square of the height. The unit of measure is kg/m2. The following BMI categories have been defined: Underweight = <18.5, Normal weight = $18.5-24.9$, Overweight = $25-29.9$, Obesity = BMI of 30 or greater.

Body Movement

▶ Physical Activity

Body Temperature

Refers to the thermal state of the internal organs, known as core temperature (T_{core}). It may be measured at various sites including esophageal, tympanic, rectal, or insulated intra-aural temperature. Oral and axillary temperatures are less reliable and intestinal or gut temperature is acceptable, recorded by means of an ingestible radio-sensitive pill. There is a gradient from core to skin of about $4°C$ that facilitates transfer of heat for peripheral cooling and normally a further gradient between skin surface and ambient air. These flows of heat can be depicted using infrared thermography. Skin temperatures can be recorded at various sites using thermistors or thermocouples and a weighted average incorporating various skin sites and core temperature used to indicate mean skin temperature.

Body Temperature Control

▶ Thermoregulation

Body Volume

The volume of an organism's body, measured in liters.

Body Water

The total amount of water in the body, including intracellular water and extracellular water.

Body Weight

The mass of an organism's body, measured in kilograms. Standard measurement conditions: without any items on, minimal gut contents (post absorptive) and with an empty bladder.

Bohr Effect

A rightward shift in the O_2-hemoglobin dissociation curve which facilitates off-loading of O_2 at the tissue level. Extremely pronounced in contracting muscle(s) during heavy/severe exercise.

Bone Density

▶ Bone Mineral Density

Bone Mass

▶ Bone Mineral Density

Bone Mineral Density

PHIL CHILIBECK
College of Kinesiology, University of Saskatchewan, Saskatoon, SK, Canada

Synonyms
BMD; Bone density; Bone mass

Definition
Bone mineral density is defined clinically as the amount of bone mineral (grams) in a given area of bone (cm^2). Technically, density refers to the mass of a material in a given volume; therefore, when bone mineral density is expressed as g/cm^2, it is often referred to as "areal" bone mineral density. Most studies on exercise examine the effect of exercise on areal bone mineral density, but in the last 10–15 years, more researchers are using novel measurement techniques to assess true volumetric bone mineral density (expressed as g/cm^3). Bone mineral density is a significant determinant of bone strength and low bone mineral density increases susceptibility to fracture [1, 2].

Mechanisms
The mechanisms by which bone mineral density is increased with exercise training are complex. Bone has four different types of cells. Osteoblasts are cells involved in bone formation and are activated by exercise. Osteoclasts are involved in bone resorption (bone breakdown) which is important in the process of repair of damaged bone and for keeping blood calcium levels stable (which in turn is important for other physiological functions such as maintaining excitability of muscle and nervous tissue). Osteocytes are cells embedded in the bone matrix and are important for detection of loads on bone induced by exercise and for transmitting signals from these loads to osteoblasts to stimulate bone formation. The fourth type of bone cell is bone-lining cells, derived from inactivated osteoblasts, which reside on the surface of bone [1, 2].

The process that initiates signals for increased bone formation as a result from exercise loading is thought to involve the induction of fluid flow through bone. Exercise loading of bone stimulates fluid flow through small canals in the bone surface, called canaliculi [2]. These canaliculi span the bone matrix and connect the different bone cell types. Increased fluid flow caused by an exercise stimulus increases delivery of nutrients to bone cells. The fluid flow also stimulates osteoblasts or osteocytes by disturbing integrins, which are glycoproteins that extend from the cell, spanning its membrane and connecting to an internal cellular actin cytoskeleton which is connected to the nucleus of the cell. Disturbing of the osteoblast's or osteocyte's cytoskeleton may activate transcription within the cell's nucleus to initiate the process of synthesis of important collagenous proteins that, when secreted, form the organic matrix of bone. This results in formation of immature bone, referred to as osteoid. Hydroxyapatite crystals (calcium and phosphate) are then incorporated into osteoid to form mature, mineralized bone. The movement of integrins by fluid flow past osteoblasts and the resulting disruption of the osteoblast cytoskeleton may also open calcium channels in the cell's membrane or activate calcium release from intracellular stores. Calcium is involved in the activation of enzymes involved in production of prostaglandins, a hormone-like molecule, which when released, may activate osteoblasts to increase production of collagenous protein [2].

Exercise may increase bone mineral density by inhibiting bone resorption in addition to stimulating bone formation. Formation is usually coupled to resorption in a "bone remodeling cycle," the purpose of which is to break down and repair damaged bone and to keep blood calcium levels constant. Osteoblasts release a compound called "receptor activator of nuclear factor kappa beta ligand" (RANKL) which activates osteoclasts (and bone resorption) by binding to its receptor (RANK) on the osteoclast membrane. Stimulation of osteoblasts through exercise loading increases production of a protein called osteoprotegerin from osteoblasts, which acts as a decoy receptor for RANKL. This prevents binding of RANKL to RANK on osteoclasts, preventing osteoclast activation and bone resorption [3]. In this way, activation of osteoblasts by exercise loading may result in inhibition of bone resorption in addition to stimulation of bone formation.

Exercise Responses/Consequences

The optimum loading characteristics for inducing bone formation and increasing bone mineral density are derived mainly from animal or cellular studies [4]. Static loading of bone does not appear to be effective because it does not induce the pulsatile fluid flow through bone that is important for stimulation of bone formation. Isometric exercise, although imparting large loads on muscle and bone, may therefore not be effective for stimulating bone formation. Loading at high frequencies is effective for inducing bone formation and this has led to the promotion of exercise on vibration platforms. High magnitude loads are effective for inducing bone formation; therefore, exercises such as gymnastics or

heavy resistance training (weight lifting) are effective. Loads that induce high strain rates are effective; therefore, exercises such as jumping increase bone mineral density. Loads are most effective if they induce novel strain distributions on bone; therefore, unaccustomed exercise may be most effective. Examples would be gymnastics or weight lifting that incorporates the training principle of variety. On the other hand, exercises that we are accustomed to (i.e., walking) are not as effective for inducing bone formation. Ironically, walking is probably the most prescribed exercise for older people at risk for bone loss and osteoporosis. Walking has many health benefits (i.e., cardiovascular and metabolic benefits) but its effectiveness for increasing bone mineral density is minimal. One final characteristic of bone to consider is that once a load is applied, bone quickly loses its sensitivity to the load [4]. This means that a load may be effective for stimulating bone formation, but the effectiveness dissipates the longer the load is applied. Long distance running, therefore, might be effective for stimulating bone formation at the beginning of an exercise session, but not continuously throughout the exercise session. It may be best therefore to break exercise sessions up into shorter, more frequent sessions, rather than a lower number of sessions of long duration.

While dynamic exercise that induces strains of high magnitude, frequency, stain rate and abnormal distribution are important for inducing bone formation, an important point to consider is that excessive exercise may be detrimental to bone. Excessive exercise reduces estrogen secretion in young females, leading to the condition of athletic amenorrhea (i.e., where menstrual cycles are halted). Estrogen is an important hormone for maintaining bone mineral density; therefore, reduction in estrogen caused by excessive exercise, or inadequate dietary compensation to offset the increased caloric expenditure of exercise, can result in decreased bone mineral density [1, 2]. There is also evidence that excessive exercise in males may reduce testosterone levels and reduction in this anabolic hormone may also lead to reductions in bone mineral density [1].

Exercise loading is beneficial for building bone as we grow, and important for maintaining bone mineral density as we age; however, certain exercise loads may induce fracture in people with very brittle bones. There is evidence that exercises that involve trunk forward flexion or twisting of the trunk at high velocities may increase susceptibility to fractures of spinal vertebrae [2]. People at high risk of fracture should therefore avoid exercise such as sit-ups or crunches or exercises that involve bending at the waist (i.e., to pick up weights).

Diagnostics

Clinically, bone mineral density (g/cm^2) is assessed by dual energy X-ray absorptiometry. Bone mineral density is usually assessed at the lumbar spine, the hip (i.e., proximal femur), and the distal forearm (radius) because these sites are susceptible to bone loss and development of osteoporosis. Bone is made up of hard cortical bone, and softer trabecular bone, which has a higher turnover. These skeletal sites are more susceptible to fracture because of their higher amount of trabecular, relative to cortical bone, and in the case of the hip and distal forearm, these absorb impact if someone has a fall. Bone mineral density as assessed by dual energy X-ray absorptiometry is compared against the young adult mean (i.e., 30 years of age and of the same sex). A t-score for bone mineral density measurements refers to the standard deviation units from the young adult mean. A t-score higher than -1.0 is considered normal. A t-score between -1.0 and -2.4 is considered "oteopenic" where an individual is at increased risk of fracture and a t-score of -2.5 or less is considered "osteoporotic" where one is at a high risk of fracture. A t-score of -1.0 means that you have a bone mineral density which is lower than approximately 85% of young individuals (i.e., aged 30 years); whereas a t-score of -2.5 means you have a bone mineral density lower than approximately 99.4% of young individuals. A one standard deviation decrease in your t-score increases fracture risk at the lumbar spine, hip, or radius two to three times [2].

T-scores are good for predicting fracture risk at the population level; however, it is now recognized that two individuals with the same t-score can have very different levels of fracture risk. New guidelines have therefore recently been developed to take other factors into consideration when interpreting t-scores and fracture risk. These additional factors include age, past fragility fracture, and use of systemic corticosteroids [5].

While areal bone mineral density (g/cm^2) is used for diagnosing osteoporosis, measurements of volumetric bone mineral density (i.e., g/cm^3) may be more sensitive to the effects of exercise. Peripheral quantitative computed tomography (pQCT) is a technique which allows assessment of volumetric cortical and trabecular bone mineral density in long bones (mainly the proximal and distal parts of the radius and tibia). There is evidence that changes in trabecular or cortical volumetric bone mineral density in response to exercise training as detected by pQCT might not be reflected in changes in areal bone mineral density measured by dual energy X-ray absorptiometry [2]. Peripheral quantitative computed tomography also more easily allows measurement of geometric changes in bone (i.e., cross-sectional area), an important

predictor of bone strength. Geometric properties of bone may change to a greater extent with exercise training, than traditionally measured areal bone mineral density [2].

References

1. Chilibeck PD, Sale DG, Webber CE (1995) Exercise and bone mineral density. Sports Med 19:103–122
2. Khan K, McKay H, Kannus P, Bailey D, Wark J, Bennell K (2001) Physical activity and bone health, 1st edn. Human Kinetics, Champaign
3. You L, Temiyasathit S, Lee P, Kim CH, Tummala P, Yao W, Kingery W, Malone AM, Kwon RY, Jacobs CR (2008) Osteocytes as mechanosensors in the inhibition of bone resorption due to mechanical loading. Bone 42:172–179
4. Turner CH, Robling AG (2003) Designing exercise regimens to increase bone strength. Exerc Sport Sci Rev 31:45–50
5. Papaioannou A, Morin S, Cheung AM, Atkinson S, Brown JP, Feldman S, Hanley DA, Hodsman A, Jamal SA, Kaiser SM, Kvern B, Siminoski K, Leslie WD (2010) 2010 clinical practice guidelines for the diangnosis and management of osteoporosis in Canada: summary. Can Med Assoc J 182:1864–1873

Bone Modeling

Is the process by which bone shape is formed and maintained throughout growth through the independent function of bone formation and resorption.

Bone Remodeling

Christopher L. Newman, Matthew R. Allen
Department of Anatomy & Cell Biology, Indiana University School of Medicine, Indianapolis, IN, USA

Synonyms

Bone renewal; Bone turnover

Definition

Despite its caricature as a static and inactive system, the skeleton is in a constant state of renewal. Bone remodeling is the physiological mechanism by which the replacement of bone matrix occurs. It is a spatially and temporally coordinated process in which bone matrix is removed by ▶ osteoclasts and subsequently formed by ▶ osteoblasts [1]. The integration of these two cellular functions distinguishes it from ▶ bone modeling in which resorption and formation occur in spatially isolated locations. Remodeling is triggered by local cellular signals (activation) that stimulate the degradation of bone (resorption) and initiate the successive production of new tissue (formation) [2]. Perturbations in bone remodeling are a hallmark of many metabolic bone disorders [3, 4].

Characteristics

Bone matrix is a composite material consisting of ▶ hydroxyapatite crystals embedded in a highly organized meshwork of collagen fibers. Structurally, it is classified as either cortical (compact) or cancellous (trabecular). Remodeling occurs in both types of bone. Remodeling can occur upon three different types of surfaces: the periosteal, the endosteal/cancellous, and intracortical (or Haversian) surfaces. During intracortical remodeling, teams of osteoclasts and osteoblasts burrow through the matrix (Fig. 1). This group of cells, and its associated blood vessels, is called a bone remodeling unit or basic multicellular unit (BMU). The final product of remodeling within the cortex is an osteon, a structure composed of concentric layers of bone enclosed by a cement line with a central (Haversian) canal containing blood vessels and nerves. BMUs can arise from the bone marrow, the periosteum, or the vasculature within an existing osteon. On endocortical/cancellous and periosteal surfaces, bone remodeling does not include the incorporation of a blood vessel, and its resulting structure is called a hemiosteon (Fig. 1). Bone remodeling on endosteal/cancellous surfaces is common during growth and development as well as in adulthood, while remodeling on the periosteal surface is a far less frequent phenomenon.

The majority of bone surfaces at any given time are quiescent meaning that there is no cellular activity. Quiescent bone surfaces are covered by a single layer of inactive osteoblasts known as bone lining cells.

The first step in bone remodeling is activation, the process by which osteoclasts are recruited to a specific skeletal site for resorptive activity. Several activation signals have been identified including ▶ microdamage formation and ▶ osteocyte apoptosis. The specific signal for recruiting osteoclasts to a given spatial region is unclear but is thought to arise from the osteocytes either as an active signal for resorption or the cessation of an inhibitory signal that normally suppresses osteoclast recruitment.

Following activation, bone lining cells withdraw from the surface of the bone to expose the mineralized matrix to osteoclasts, commencing the resorptive phase of bone remodeling. During this process the mineral is dissolved and the collagen fragments liberated. These fragments can be measured in the blood and urine, providing useful biomarkers for the assessment of bone remodeling.

The reversal phase is characterized by the cessation of osteoclast resorption and the initiation of bone formation. The signal for reversal within BMUs is unknown, though numerous molecules have been implicated [2]. Once osteoclasts are finished resorbing bone, the exposed surface is cleaned by specialized bone lining cells that degrade any remaining collagen fragments. They also are thought to deposit a thin layer of new bone matrix (the cement/reversal line), a clear histological feature that delineates the boundaries of osteons and hemiosteons from the surrounding, older matrix.

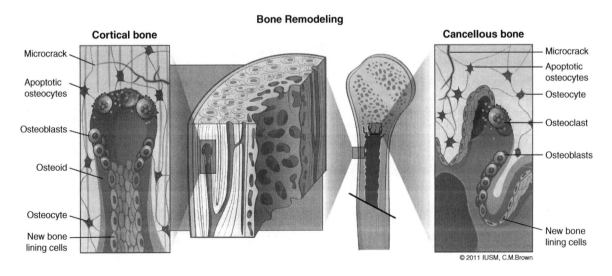

Bone Remodeling

Cortical bone — Cancellous bone

Microcrack, Apoptotic osteocytes, Osteoblasts, Osteoid, Osteocyte, New bone lining cells

Microcrack, Apoptotic osteocytes, Osteocyte, Osteoclast, Osteoblasts, New bone lining cells

© 2011 IUSM, C.M.Brown

Bone Remodeling. Fig. 1 Bone remodeling in cortical and cancellous bone

During bone formation osteoblasts lay down an unmineralized organic matrix called osteoid, which is primarily composed of type I collagen fibers and serves as a template for inorganic hydroxyapatite crystals. Osteoid mineralization occurs in two distinct phases. Primary mineralization, the initial incorporation of calcium and phosphate ions into the collagen matrix, occurs rapidly over 7-21 days and accounts for roughly 70% of the final mineral content. Secondary mineralization, the final addition and maturation of mineral crystals, occurs over a much longer timeframe (up to a year or more).

The osteoblasts participating in new bone formation undergo one of three fates. The majority of them die through apoptosis. The remaining osteoblasts are either incorporated into the osteoid matrix and become osteocytes or remain present until the end of the formation event to become bone lining cells. Osteocytes play a crucial role in mineral metabolism and in the physiological response to mechanical stresses placed upon bones.

Clinical Relevance

In a healthy individual, slightly less bone is formed by osteoblasts than is resorbed by osteoclasts, leading to a negative bone balance at each site of remodeling. In cortical bone, this is necessary to accommodate blood vessels within the central (Haversian) canal. The purpose of a negative bone balance on cancellous and endocortical surfaces, however, is not clear. Yet its significance is illustrated by the fact that individuals with metabolic bone disease often have an increased negative bone balance, resulting in an accelerated rate of bone loss.

Altered bone remodeling is the primary mechanism underlying numerous bone diseases, including osteoporosis. In postmenopausal osteoporosis, this increased remodeling rate results from declining estrogen levels. The combination of negative bone balance at each remodeling site and an increase in the total number of these sites leads to an accelerated rate of bone loss. Several other metabolic diseases (e.g., hyperparathyroidism) cause increased bone remodeling rates as well.

Substantial decreases in bone remodeling can also have adverse consequences. An extreme case is osteopetrosis, a genetic disease disrupting normal osteoclast function. Individuals with osteopetrosis often have very high bone mineral density but routinely experience bone fracture because the lack of resorption leads to low quality (highly mineralized) skeletal tissue.

Pharmaceutical agents aimed at reducing fracture risk in persons with metabolic bone disease are primarily focused on the suppression of bone remodeling [5].

Anti-remodeling (or anti-resorptive) medications accomplish this by reducing the number of newly initiated remodeling sites. However, they do not affect bone balance at a given remodeling site. In the months following the initiation of anti-remodeling therapy, the refilling of active remodeling sites with new bone matrix and the formation of fewer remodeling sites combine to produce an initial gain in bone mass. Since any site that initiates remodeling will still have a negative bone balance, patients will eventually begin to lose bone mass, but they will do so at a much slower rate than an untreated individual.

Anti-resorptives include bisphosphonates, estrogen, ▶ selective estrogen receptor modulators (SERMs), calcitonin, and denosumab. All of these different classes of drugs slow bone loss, and therefore fracture risk, by reducing bone remodeling. Bisphosphonates physically bind to the bone matrix and lead to either osteoclast apoptosis or inactivity during the resorptive phase of remodeling. Estrogen and SERMs act through estrogen receptors on osteoclasts to reduce their activity. Calcitonin is a hormone crucial for calcium ion metabolism that acts to reduce serum calcium levels. It achieves this indirectly by reducing osteoclast development and activity. Denosumab is an antibody that inhibits ▶ RANK ligand, an integral membrane protein necessary for osteoclast maturation, thereby preventing bone resorption. There is considerable variation in the efficacy of these agents in the prevention of fractures. Bisphosphonates and denosumab exert far more significant inhibition of remodeling than estrogen, SERMs, or calcitonin. Even within the general class of bisphosphonates, each of the specific compounds differs in the magnitude of remodeling inhibition. These medications impacting the level of bone remodeling have played an important role in addressing human bone disease.

References

1. Parfitt AM (2008) Skeletal heterogeneity and the purposes of bone remodeling: implications for the understanding of osteoporosis. In: Marcus R, Feldman D, Nelson D, Rosen C (eds) Osteoporosis, 3rd edn. Elsevier, San Diego
2. Henricksen K, Neutzsky-Wulff AV, Bonewald LF, Karsdal MA (2009) Local communication on and within bone controls bone remodeling. Bone 44:1026–1033
3. Eriksen EF (1986) Normal and pathological remodeling of human trabecular bone: three dimensional reconstruction of the remodeling sequence in normals and in metabolic bone disease. Endocr Rev 7:379–408
4. Seeman E, Delmas PD (2006) Bone quality – The material and structural basis of bone strength and fragility. N Engl J Med 354:2250–2261
5. Kawai M, Modder UI, Khosla S, Rosen CJ (2011) Emerging therapeutic opportunities for skeletal restoration. Nat Rev Drug Discov 10:141–156

Bone Renewal

▶ Bone Remodeling

Bone Turnover

▶ Bone Remodeling

Bradyarrhythmias

Any disturbance of cardiac rhythm in which the mean heart rate is < than 60 beats per minute.

Brain Hemisphere

One of the paired structures forming the bulk of the human brain, which together comprise the cerebral cortex, centrum semiovale, basal ganglia, and rhinencephalon, and contain the lateral ventricles.

Bronchial Asthma

▶ Asthma Bronchiale

Bronchial Hyperresponsiveness

▶ Pulmonary System, Training Adaptation

Bronchiectasis

The end result of the inexorable cycle of airway infection, injury and mucus plugging, and obstruction characteristic of the latter stages of cystic fibrosis. Bronchiectatic airways are abnormally dilated, do not allow normal mucus transport, and are particularly prone to recurrent infection with organisms such as *Pseudomonas aeruginosa* and *Staphylococcus aureus*. Treatment approaches include airway clearance methods (chest physical therapy), often in conjunction with an exercise program, cycling oral and/or inhaled antibiotics, and inhaled medications geared at promoting altering the abnormal mucus observed in CF, including recombinant human DNase and hypertonic saline.

Cross-References
▶ Chronic Obstructive Pulmonary Disease
▶ Cystic Fibrosis

Brown Adipose Tissue (BAT)

A particular form of adipose tissue with selected distribution. Its color is brownish, depending on its content of cytochromes and of fat which is distributed in multiple droplets and also on its dense vascularization. Its heat-generating capacity relates to the rate of fatty acid oxidation which is not constrained by cellular ATP catabolism. BAT appears to be restricted to mammalian species, especially of smaller body size, but is also present in newborns of larger species including humans. BAT activity has been recently shown also in adult humans.

Buffer Capacity

The amount of acid or base needed to change pH one unit.

Buffering of Acid

Restricting a shift of acid–base status of an aqueous solution, by reacting with a buffer salt with properties of a weak acid and strong base.

C

γH2AX Foci Analysis

Histon H2AX is phosporylated rapidly in response to DNA double-strand breaks (DSB), leading to the formation of nuclear foci visualized by immunocytochemical detection of γH2AX. γH2AX analysis is an exquisitely sensitive technique to monitor DSB repair, amenable for use with very low doses.

2-(Carbamimidoyl-Methyl-Amino) Acetic Acid

▶ Creatine

Ca²⁺ Release Channels

▶ Excitation–Contraction Coupling
▶ Ryanodine Receptors

Ca²⁺-Induced Ca²⁺ Release (CICR)

Ca^{2+}-induced Ca^{2+} release (CICR) in myocytes is mediated via opening of ryanodine receptors on the SR. Ryanodine receptors are activated by adjacent L-type voltage-operated Ca^{2+} channels, which are in turn activated by depolarized plasma membranes. CICR subsequently leads to significant elevation of Ca^{2+} levels intracellularly, allowing Ca^{2+} to bind to myofilament proteins and initiate contraction of myocytes.

Caffeine

JAYNE M. KALMAR
Wilfrid Laurier University, Waterloo, ON, Canada

Synonyms

3,7-dihydro-1,3,7-trimethyl-1 H-purine-2,6-dione; 1,3,7-trimethylxanthine; 1,3,7-trimethyl-2,6-dioxopurine

Definition

Caffeine (1,3,7-trimethylxanthine) is a plant ▶ alkaloid with a purine structure. Its chemical formula is $C_8H_{10}N_4O_2$ and it has a molecular weight of 194.19 g. Pharmacologically, caffeine is most frequently defined as a central nervous system stimulant, although it is also a weak diuretic and smooth muscle relaxant [1].

Description

Caffeine is an alkaloid that can be extracted from plants such as tea leaves, cacao seeds, cola nuts, and coffee beans or synthesized from uric acid. Once purified, caffeine is a white crystalline substance that is somewhat soluble in water (as caffeine citrate) and many organic solvents. Caffeine has a number of dimethylated metabolites including ▶ paraxanthine, ▶ theobromine, and ▶ theophylline that differ with respect to the number and location of methyl groups on their purine heterocyclic ring structure (Fig. 1). Paraxanthine is the primary metabolite of caffeine that acts as a central nervous system stimulant with potency similar to caffeine. The metabolites theobromine and theophylline are also naturally occurring plant alkaloids. As indicated by its chemical name (1,3,7-trimethylxanthine), caffeine has three methyl groups positioned on N1, N3, and N7 of the purine ring structure [1].

Pharmacologically, caffeine is best known for its actions as a central nervous system stimulant; however,

Frank C. Mooren (ed.), *Encyclopedia of Exercise Medicine in Health and Disease*, DOI 10.1007/978-3-540-29807-6,
© Springer-Verlag Berlin Heidelberg 2012

Caffeine. Fig. 1 Caffeine is a trimethylated xanthine that is metabolized to three dimethylated xanthines including theobromine, theophylline, and paraxanthine. Caffeine, theobromine, and theophylline are plant alkaloids widely consumed in a variety of foods and beverages such as coffee, tea, and chocolate, while the primary metabolite, paraxanthine, is only found endogenously. Due to its structural similarity to adenosine, caffeine acts as a competitive adenosine receptor antagonist. This is the primary mechanism for caffeine's effects as a central nervous system stimulant

the drug is sufficiently small and hydrophobic to cross the blood-brain barrier and other cell membranes and therefore has the capacity to affect many tissues depending on its concentration. Caffeine and other methylxanthines are used therapeutically to prevent drowsiness, to treat mild to moderate headaches in combination with analgesics, and to treat apnea and arrhythmias in preterm infants [1]. Caffeine is approved by the US Food and Drug Administration as a safe and effective stimulant and is available over the counter. Three mechanisms of caffeine's actions have been observed in vitro: (1) intracellular calcium mobilization via direct interaction with calcium channels in the sarcoplasmic reticulum, (2) phosphodiesterase inhibition, and (3) adenosine receptor antagonism [2]. The first two of these three mechanisms require millimolar concentrations of caffeine that would be toxic in humans. Nonetheless, it has been suggested that endogenous modulators such as ATP may potentiate caffeine and paraxanthine's effects on the ▶ ryanodine receptor to increase intracellular calcium concentration in intact skeletal muscle preparations. If this is the case, caffeine may alter muscle function in vivo at concentrations much lower than predicted by in vitro studies. In contrast, caffeine functions as an adenosine receptor antagonist at caffeine concentrations in the micromolar range associated with plasma and brain levels following low to moderate oral doses of the drug. Accordingly, the widespread effects of caffeine on human tissues are largely attributed to antagonism of adenosine receptors [2].

Application

Caffeine is well known for its effects on wakefulness and mental alertness. In 1958, Axelsson and Thesleff reported that caffeine could generate muscle contractions in the absence of neural or electrical activation, suggesting that this legal, widely available, and socially acceptable drug may improve both physical and mental performance. Several decades of research have since clearly established that caffeine is indeed ergogenic, enhancing performance in many types of sports and exercise. It is now clear, however, that the primary mechanism for these ergogenic effects is via adenosine receptor antagonism rather than direct effects on muscle.

Caffeine's effects on human performance are most evident in endurance sports such as running and cycling. In these sports, dosages ranging from 3 to 9 mg/kg body weight have been found to increase time to exhaustion or time trial performance in placebo-controlled studies [4].

The effects of caffeine on high-intensity exercise are not as clear. There are some reports that caffeine improves performance on tests of anaerobic power, such as the Wingate test, and other studies that report no effect of caffeine or a decline in anaerobic performance in the caffeine trail compared to placebo. In tests of anaerobic performance, it appears that caffeine is more likely to enhance the performance of trained athletes than untrained individuals [3]. Although caffeine is a weak diuretic, it does not appear to alter sweat rate and total body water loss to an extent that would impair performance or pose any risk to the athlete [3].

Because caffeine is distributed to all body compartments, it is difficult to isolate the biological mechanisms responsible for its ergogenic effects. Previously, caffeine was thought to enhance endurance performance through enhanced lipolysis and glycogen sparing secondary to phosphodiesterase inhibition and increased catecholamine release. However, caffeine does not inhibit phosphodiesterase activity at physiological doses and while caffeine is associated with elevated plasma epinephrine levels, there is very little evidence to suggest that caffeine enhances fat oxidation [4]. Consequently, it is now generally accepted that the ergogenic effects of caffeine are not of a metabolic origin and focus has shifted to alternative theories.

One possibility is that caffeine enhances skeletal muscle contractile force, although there is some question as to whether physiological levels of caffeine would be sufficient to elicit the increase in intracellular calcium observed in vitro. Most human studies report no effect of caffeine on twitch amplitude, twitch half relaxation time, or maximal instantaneous rate of twitch relaxation in either unfatigued or fatigued human muscle [5]. However, caffeine does offset the decline in tetanic force observed during low-frequency electrical stimulation of muscle. Because ▶ low-frequency fatigue has been attributed to a reduction in calcium release by the ryanodine receptor, it is possible that caffeine improves contractile output of fatigued muscle under some conditions.

Placebo-controlled studies report increased muscle activation and endurance times following caffeine administration that could not be attributed to changes in neuromuscular transmission or muscle contractile function. This suggests that caffeine may also enhance human performance via central mechanisms [5]. ▶ Adenosine is an endogenous neuromodulator that exerts a tonic inhibitory influence in the central nervous system by decreasing excitatory neurotransmitter release and the firing rates of central neurons. Due to its structural similarity to adenosine, caffeine functions as an adenosine receptor antagonist and reverses many of the inhibitory effects of adenosine at microMolar concentrations [2]. Caffeine has been found to increase neurotransmitter release and firing rates via A_1 receptor antagonism, increase dopaminergic transmission, and increase spontaneous motor activity and treadmill running time of rats [5]. In human studies of corticomotor excitability, caffeine potentiates cortically evoked potentials and reduces the duration of the ▶ cortical silent period. It also increases the amplitude of the ▶ Hoffman reflex and self-sustained firing of motor units which suggests that the drug may also act on the neuromuscular system at a spinal level. Finally, caffeine is associated with reductions in pain and force sensation which may contribute to enhanced endurance performance [5].

Restricting or banning a substance consumed in foods and beverages by many people on a daily basis poses a challenge to anti-doping agencies. In the past, the International Olympic Committee (IOC) restricted the use of caffeine by athletes, allowing a maximal urine level of 12 µg/ml. Over 95% of ingested caffeine, however, is excreted as paraxanthine-derived urinary metabolites rather than caffeine. As such, athletes would have to consume approximately 9 mg of caffeine per kg body weight to reach the IOC urinary caffeine limit whereas ergogenic effects have been demonstrated following oral caffeine dosages as low as 3 mg/kg body weight. Although caffeine use is not prohibited by the World Anti-Doping Agency (WADA), it is monitored for use in competition via the WADA Monitoring Program for the purposes of detecting patterns of misuse of this stimulant in sport. Use of caffeine out of competition is not monitored.

References

1. Brunton LB, Lazo JS, Parker KL (eds) (2005) Goodman & Gilman's the pharmacological basis of therapeutics, 11th edn. McGraw-Hill, New York
2. Fredholm BB (1995) Astra award lecture. Adenosine, adenosine receptors and the actions of caffeine. Pharmacol Toxicol 76:93–101
3. Goldstein ER, Ziegenfuss T, Kalman D, Kreider R, Campbell B, Wilborn C, Taylor L, Willoughby D, Stout J, Graves BS, Wildman R, Ivy JL, Spano M, Smith AE, Antonio J (2010) International society of sports nutrition position stand: caffeine and performance. J Int Soc Sports Nutr 7:5
4. Graham TE (2001) Caffeine and exercise: metabolism, endurance and performance. Sports Med 31:785–807
5. Kalmar JM (2005) The influence of caffeine on voluntary muscle activation. Med Sci Sports Exerc 37:2113–2119

Calcium

Calcium is a chemical element belonging to the group of alkaline earth metals. It has the atomic number 20 and an atomic mass of 40.078 Da. Ca is named as a macroelement as the Ca content of humans amounts to about 1 kg, which is used predominantly for mineralization of bones. Important food sources include milk and milk products, nuts, and vegetables such as broccoli, beans, and collard greens. Serum Ca is under hormonal control, e.g., calcitriol, calcitonin, and parathyroid hormone, and its typical concentration range is between 2.1 and 2.6 mmol/L. There exists a steep concentration gradient for calcium across the plasma membrane as the intracellular levels are around 100–200 nmmol/L. This gradient is an important prerequisite for calcium's role as an important intracellular signaling factor thereby activating many cellular processes such as myofilament contraction, gating of ion channels, derangement of cytoskeletal and organelle structures, and gene expression.

Cross-References

▶ Intracellular Signaling

Calmodulin

Calmodulin (CaM) is an abbreviation for *cal*cium-*modul*ated prote*in*, which is an important calcium-binding protein ubiquitously expressed in eukaryotic cells. It contains four so-called EF-hands motifs, which represent the calcium-binding unit. Upon Ca^{2+} binding, calmodulin becomes an important regulator of several intracellular targets which are involved in processes such as inflammation, immune response, metabolism, apoptosis, cell growth, etc.

Canaliculi

Small canals that run through the bone matrix. Fluid flows through these canals when strain is applied to bone. This fluid flow is thought to stimulate bone formation.

Cancer

Cancer is a group of diseases characterized by uncontrolled growth and spread of abnormal cells. If the spread is not controlled, it can result in death. Cancer is caused by both external (e.g., tobacco, chemicals, radiation, infectious organisms, etc.) and internal (e.g., inherited mutations,

hormones, immune conditions, metabolic conditions, etc.) factors. These casual factors may act together or in sequence to initiate or promote carcinogenesis.

Cancer Cachexia

A complex metabolic syndrome associated with underlying illness and characterized by skeletal muscle wasting with or without loss of fat mass. It is associated with muscle weakness and fatigue and accounts for more than 20% of all cancer-related deaths. Cancer cachexia is associated with reduced mobility, increased risk of complications in surgery, impaired response to chemo-/radiotherapy, and increased psychological distress, leading to an overall reduction in quality of life. "Cachectic" pertains to a state of poor health, malnutrition, and weight loss.

Cancer Survivorship

Term given to describe individuals who have been diagnosed with cancer from the point of diagnosis through end of life.

Cancer, Prevention

Brigid M. Lynch, Christine M. Friedenreich
Department of Population Health Research, Alberta Health Services – Cancer Care, Calgary, AB, Canada

Synonyms

Malignancy; Neoplasm; Tumor

Definition

▶ Cancer describes diseases that arise when normal regenerative processes are disrupted by uncontrolled cell growth or by cellular loss of the ability to undergo apoptosis. Abnormal cells continue dividing, forming tumors that can spread to other tissues via invasion or metastasis. Cancer can originate nearly anywhere in the body. The most common type of cancer, carcinoma, begins in the skin or in cells that line or cover internal organs, such as the lungs or colon. Other forms of cancer include sarcoma (arises in bone, cartilage, fat, muscle, or other connective tissue); myeloma (plasma cells); lymphoma (lymphatic system); and leukemia (white blood cells).

Each year, an estimated 13 million people are diagnosed with cancer, and there are approximately eight million cancer-related deaths [1]. Breast cancer is the leading cancer site amongst women (representing 23% of new diagnoses and 14% of deaths), whilst lung cancer is the most frequently diagnosed cancer in men (17% of new diagnoses and 23% of deaths) [1]. Cancer is the leading cause of death in developed countries, and the second most common cause of death in developing countries [1]. The developing world has cancer incidence rates approximately half those seen in the developed world; however, overall cancer mortality rates are similar. The poorer cancer survival rates in developing countries is likely due to the disease being diagnosed at a later stage and limited access to appropriate treatments [1].

The burden of disease is expected to increase globally: by 2030, the number of people with cancer is projected to double, to more than 20 million new cases [2]. This increase will be partly attributable to population growth and aging, but also because of increasing adoption of a "western" lifestyle amongst the developing world. Hence, a disproportionate increase in cancer incidence will occur within the developing world in years to come.

Pathogenesis

The etiological pathway leading to cancer is a complex one, involving a series of changes that likely occur over decades. Various models of carcinogenesis have been proposed, but generally there are four definable stages: initiation, promotion, progression, and malignant conversion. Initiation describes the point at which genetic errors occur spontaneously when cells divide or as a result of exposure to carcinogens. Cells have a number of mechanisms to repair damaged DNA, but if repair does not occur, the mutated cells may begin to replicate (promotion), eventually becoming a benign tumor. During progression, the tumor cells continue to replicate and additional mutations may occur in genes that regulate growth and cell function. These changes contribute to further growth until malignant conversion occurs.

Epidemiological studies have identified a wide range of environmental and genetic factors associated with increased cancer risk. Some environmental risk factors, such as tobacco smoking, alcohol consumption, exposure to UV radiation, dietary intake, and physical activity levels, are modifiable. Hence, a large proportion of common cancers are potentially preventable. Expert review has concluded that approximately one third of cancer cases are attributable to tobacco smoking or exposure, and another third of cases are due to a combination of poor diet, physical inactivity, and overweight/obesity [2].

Physical activity is thought to reduce cancer risk via a number of biological mechanisms [3]. These mechanisms may impact different stages of carcinogenesis: for an in-depth review, see [4]. Key biological mechanisms by which physical activity may reduce cancer risk include:

Adiposity

Physical activity may reduce body fat, which is associated with colon, postmenopausal breast, endometrial, ovarian, kidney and esophageal cancers, and cancer-related mortality. ▶ Adiposity is likely an independent contributor to cancer risk, and it may facilitate carcinogenesis through a number of pathways, including increased levels of ▶ sex hormones, ▶ insulin resistance, chronic ▶ inflammation, and altered secretion of adipokines.

Endogenous Sex Hormones

Physical activity decreases endogenous sex hormone levels and increases circulating sex hormone binding globulin (SHBG). Exposure to estrogens/androgens is a risk factor for breast, endometrial, ovarian, and prostate cancers. SHBG may affect cancer risk by binding to sex hormones, rendering them biologically inactive.

In premenopausal women, estrogens are predominantly produced by the ovaries. Very high levels of physical activity might lower estrogen exposure by delaying onset of menarche, causing menstrual irregularity or reducing the total number of menstrual cycles. For postmenopausal women, adipose tissue is the primary source of endogenous estrogens. Physical activity may decrease adiposity and thus production of estrogens. In men, the effect of physical activity on androgen levels is unclear, but dihydroxytesterone (a testosterone metabolite) may be increased.

Insulin Resistance

Physical activity improves insulin sensitivity by increasing the number and activity of glucose transporters in both muscle and adipose tissue. In addition, physical activity may indirectly reduce insulin resistance by promoting fat loss and preservation of lean body mass. Associations between insulin levels and colorectal, postmenopausal breast, pancreatic, and endometrial cancers have been demonstrated in epidemiological studies. Fasting glucose levels have been directly associated with pancreatic, kidney, liver, endometrial, biliary, and urinary tract cancers.

Neoplastic cells use glucose for proliferation; therefore, hyperglycemia may promote carcinogenesis by providing an amiable environment for tumor growth. High insulin levels increase bioavailable insulin-like growth factor-I, which is involved in cell differentiation, proliferation, and apoptosis. Decreasing blood insulin levels also results in increased hepatic synthesis of SHBG; hence, insulin indirectly increases bioavailability of endogenous sex hormones.

Inflammation

Physical activity may decrease levels of proinflammatory factors, namely adipokines (leptin, tumor necrosis factor-α, interleukin-6) and C-reactive protein, and increase anti-inflammatory factors (adiponectin). Chronic inflammation is acknowledged as a risk factor for most types of cancer.

Obesity represents a low-grade, systematic inflammatory state. It has been hypothesized that perpetual cell proliferation, microenvironmental changes, and oxidative stress associated with chronic inflammation could deregulate normal cell growth to promote malignancy.

Other Possible Mechanisms

Physical activity results in improved pulmonary function, which may promote expulsion of carcinogenic agents from the lungs. This mechanism is specific to physical activity and lung cancer.

Physical activity may increase circulating levels of 25-hydroxyvitamin D, possibly through increased ultraviolet radiation exposure as a result of time spent outdoors. In addition, ▶ vitamin D is fat soluble and is readily stored in adipose tissue. Hence, physical activity may also increase vitamin D levels by reducing adiposity. Vitamin D has been associated with colorectal, breast, and pancreatic cancer risk.

Regular, moderate physical activity may also modulate the immune system's ability to recognize and repair or eliminate damaged cells.

It is likely that these proposed mechanisms are interrelated, and that the relative contribution of each mechanism varies by cancer type. Further research is required to elicit a clearer understanding of the biological mechanisms involved in the pathways between physical activity and cancer [3].

Training/Exercise Response

The association between physical activity and cancer has been systematically reviewed by international agencies [2] and individual scientists [3, 5]. The level of epidemiological evidence varies by cancer site. There is convincing evidence that physical activity decreases the risk of developing colon cancer, probable evidence for an effect on breast and endometrial cancer, and possible evidence for a reduced risk of developing ovarian, prostate, and lung cancer [3, 5].

Epidemiological reviews estimate that physical activity reduces colon cancer risk by 20–25% amongst both men and women who report participation in the highest level of physical activity assessed, compared with men and women who report participating in the lowest level of physical activity. There is a 25% average breast risk reduction amongst most physically active women compared to least active women. A stronger physical activity-associated risk reduction exists amongst postmenopausal women. For endometrial cancer, reviews have concluded that physical activity reduces risk by 20–30%. There is consistent evidence for a dose–response effect for colon and breast cancer, whereas for endometrial cancer a dose–response effect has been found in approximately half of all studies.

Whilst the evidence is weaker for ovarian, prostate and lung cancers, epidemiological reviews estimate that risk reductions are modest (10–20%) for ovarian and prostate cancer. For lung cancer, there appears to be no effect of physical activity on risk amongst nonsmokers. However, there may be substantial risk reductions (20–40%) among smokers. The associations between physical activity and cancer risk for other sites are either null or there is insufficient evidence to draw any conclusions about the link.

It remains unclear what type and dose of physical activity are required to achieve significant cancer risk reductions. Randomized, controlled trials are required to provide answers about these areas of uncertainty. Nonetheless, there is strong and consistent epidemiological evidence that physical activity reduces the risk of several major cancers types. Public health guidelines for physical activity and cancer prevention recommend 30–60 min of moderate-to-vigorous-intensity physical activity per day [2].

References

1. Jemal A, Bray F, Center MM, Ferlay J, Ward E, Forman D (2011) Global cancer statistics. CA Cancer J Clin 61:69–90
2. World Cancer Research Fund, The American Institute for Cancer Research (2007) Food, nutrition, physical activity, and the prevention of cancer: a global perspective. American Institute for Cancer Research, Washington, DC
3. Friedenreich CM, Neilson HK, Lynch BM (2010) State of the epidemiological evidence on physical activity and cancer prevention. Eur J Cancer 46:2593–2604
4. Rundle A (2005) Molecular epidemiology of physical activity and cancer. Cancer Epidemiol Biomarkers Prev 14:227–236
5. Courneya KS, Friedenreich CM (eds) (2011) Recent results in cancer research: physical activity and cancer. Springer, Heidelberg

Cancer, Therapy

Lee W. Jones
Department of Surgery, Duke University Medical Center,
Duke Cancer Institute, Durham, NC, USA

Synonyms

Exercise and cancer-related side effects; Exercise and prognosis after cancer diagnosis

Definition

The benefits of physical activity to reduce the primary and secondary risk of cardiovascular-related diseases have been recognized since antiquity. The first formal investigation was not until the early 1950s when James Morris and colleagues reported that occupational exercise was associated with substantial reductions in coronary heart disease in the seminal London Busmen study [1]. This pioneering work led to extensive epidemiological investigation of the association between both occupational and leisure-time exercises and the risk of cardiovascular disease by numerous research groups. As a result of the burgeoning evidence, in 1995, the American College of Sports Medicine and Centers for Disease Control published the first prescription guidelines to encourage increased participation in exercise in Americans of all ages for health promotion and disease prevention [2]. Over the past 15 years, physical activity guidelines have been published for secondary prevention of numerous chronic conditions, including type II diabetes, chronic obstructive pulmonary disease, heart failure, and heart transplant recipients [3].

The putative relationship between exercise and ▶ cancer was not formally recognized until 2002 wherein the American Cancer Society recommended regular exercise to reduce the risk of breast, colon, and several other forms of cancer. In contrast, investigation of the role of exercise following a diagnosis of cancer has, until recently, received scant attention. The precise reasons for this are not known but likely reflect the prevailing dogma that a cancer diagnosis and associated therapeutic management preclude participation in and benefit from physical activity. The reversal of interest in exercise results from the alignment of several factors including recognition of ▶ cancer survivorship as a major public health concern, a stronger evidence base, and strong interest of cancer patients themselves in pursuing adjunct approaches to optimize recovery and longevity. In the past decade, however, exercise–oncology research has become increasingly

recognized as a legitimate and important field of research in cancer management [4]. This review will provide an overview of the putative evidence supporting the role of exercise across the cancer survivorship continuum (i.e., diagnosis to palliation).

Characteristics

The use of conventional and novel cytotoxic therapies is associated with a diverse range of debilitating physiological (e.g., deconditioning, skeletal muscle atrophy, cardiac and pulmonary dysfunction) and psychosocial (e.g., fatigue, nausea, depression, anxiety) toxicities that impair recovery and increase susceptibility to concomitant age-related conditions [5]. To address these concerns, in the mid- to late 1980s, researchers initiated the first studies to explore whether structured physical activity may be an appropriate intervention to mitigate ▶ chemotherapy- and radiation-induced fatigue and anticipated loss of functional capacity among women with early-stage breast cancer. Since this early work, ~80 studies have now examined the safety, feasibility, and preliminary efficacy of structured physical activity interventions on a broad range of physiological and psychosocial outcomes before, during, and/or following cancer therapy. Since this early seminal work, the number of publications has steadily increased over the past 20 years, with studies becoming progressively more sophisticated in scope, design, and size to address the major questions in the field. A chronological timeline of significant landmarks in "exercise–oncology" research is presented in Fig. 1.

Several excellent systematic reviews and meta-analyses have evaluated the pertinent literature [6]. Findings of these reviews indicate that structured exercise training is a safe and well-tolerated intervention associated with favorable improvements in cancer-related symptoms and functional outcomes both during and following the completion of adjuvant therapy. To summarize, the majority of studies were conducted in women with early breast cancer, with fewer studies in nonsmall-cell lung cancer (NSCLC), hematologic malignancies, or mixed cancer populations. Exercise modality consisted of aerobic training alone, resistance training alone, or the combination of aerobic and resistance training prescribed at a moderate–vigorous intensity (50–75% of baseline maximum heart rate or cardiorespiratory fitness), three sessions or more per week, for 10–60 min per exercise session. The length of the exercise training ranged from 2 to 24 weeks. Overall, exercise was associated with significant improvements in muscular strength, cardiorespiratory fitness, functional quality of life (QOL), fatigue, anxiety, and self-esteem. Few adverse events (AEs) were observed. It was concluded

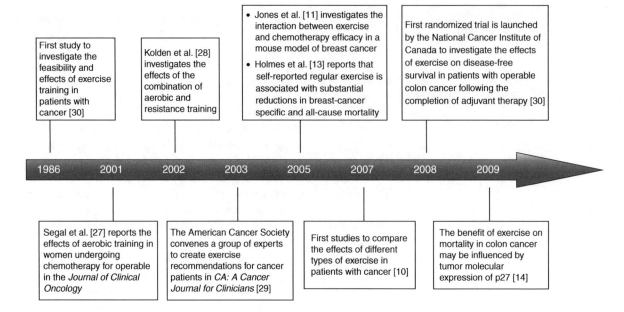

Cancer, Therapy. Fig. 1 Exercise–oncology research timeline

that exercise is a beneficial adjunct therapy both during and following the completion of adjuvant therapy in adult cancer patients, with low incidence of AEs [6].

To further clarify this issue, Jones et al. [7] conducted a meta-analysis to determine the effects of supervised exercise training on cardiorespiratory fitness, including only those studies employing a randomized controlled design and direct measurement of peak oxygen consumption (VO_{2peak}), the gold standard assessment of cardiorespiratory fitness. Cardiorespiratory fitness is determined by the integrative capacity of the cardiopulmonary system (i.e., pulmonary–cardiac–vascular–skeletal muscle axis) to deliver oxygen from the atmosphere to muscle mitochondria. Cardiorespiratory fitness is one of the most powerful predictors of cardiovascular and all-cause mortality in healthy adults as well as those with cardiovascular disease (CVD) even after controlling for traditional CVD risk factors.

Jones et al. [7] only identified a total of six studies that met eligibility criteria involving a total of 571 adult cancer patients ($n = 344$, exercise; $n = 227$, usual-care control). Pooled data indicated that exercise training was associated with a statistically significant increase in VO_{2peak} (WMD = 2.91 mL·kg^{-1}min^{-1}; 95% CI, 1.18–4.64) with minimal adverse events, although significant heterogeneity was evident in this estimate ($I^2 = 87\%$). It was concluded that the effect of exercise on VO_{2peak} is promising but the current evidence base is emergent with many fundamental questions (e.g., optimal prescription, timing,

and setting of exercise; effects of exercise on tumor biology; and therapeutic efficacy) remaining to be addressed.

In the following sections, we review the efficacy of exercise training in specific areas across the cancer survivorship continuum (i.e., presurgery, postsurgery during adjuvant therapy, survivorship (following the completion of primary adjuvant therapy), and palliation), with a view toward areas requiring future research.

Clinical Relevance

Exercise Therapy Prior to Surgical Resection

Surgery is the most common form of cancer therapy for patients with solid tumors. Pulmonary resection is the treatment of choice for a variety of disorders, including non-small cell lung cancer and selected cases of oligometastatic disease (sarcoma, colorectal cancer, melanoma, etc.), and involves removal of a substantial portion of lung parenchyma that can negatively impact VO_{2peak}. In addition, the majority of lung cancer patients also present with several significant concomitant comorbid diseases. The extent of surgery, together with comorbid disease, significantly complicates the treatment process, and perioperative and postoperative complications are common. In order to evaluate complication risk, cancer surgeons often assess VO_{2peak} to determine preoperative physiologic status of operable candidates. VO_{2peak} is strongly inversely associated with surgical complication rate in NSCLC patients. Given this, an important question is whether exercise training prior to surgical resection can improve VO_{2peak} and, in turn, lower surgical complications.

To date, two studies have addressed the initial feasibility, tolerability, and potential efficacy of presurgical exercise-based rehabilitation in patients diagnosed with NSCLC. In the first study, Jones et al. [8] examined the efficacy of presurgical aerobic training on VO_{2peak} among 20 patients with suspected NSCLC. Mean VO_{2peak} increased by 2.4 $mLkg^{-1}min^{-1}$ from baseline to presurgery. Exploratory analyses indicated that presurgical VO_{2peak} decreased postsurgery but did not decrease beyond baseline values. In the second study, Bobbio et al. [9] reported that short-term exercise-based pulmonary rehabilitation increased VO_{2peak} by 2.8 mL $kg^{-1}min^{-1}$ prior to pulmonary resection in 12 NSCLC patients with chronic obstructive disease. Larger randomized trials investigating the efficacy of exercise training on surgical complications and postsurgical recovery in cancer patients appear warranted.

Exercise Therapy During Adjuvant Therapy

The use of anticancer therapies is associated with unique and varying degrees of direct and indirect physiological injury that dramatically reduces patients' ability to tolerate exercise (i.e., low VO_{2peak}), predisposing them to morbidity, poor psychosocial functioning, and increase susceptibility to concomitant age-related conditions [5]. To address these concerns, in mid- to late 1980s, researchers explored whether structured exercise training may be an effective intervention to prevent and/or mitigate adjuvant therapy–associated toxicities and poor cardiorespiratory fitness among women with early-stage breast cancer. Since these early studies, approximately 40 studies have been conducted, investigating the safety, tolerability, and efficacy of structured exercise training on symptom control and other pertinent outcomes in patients undergoing cancer therapy. In summary, the current evidence base provides promising evidence that exercise training is a well-tolerated and safe adjunct therapy that can mitigate several common treatment-related side effects among patients undergoing different types of ▶ cytotoxic therapy, including chemotherapy, radiation, and androgen deprivation therapy (ADT).

In addition to examining symptom control, a question of significant importance is whether the effects of exercise are similar among those patients undergoing therapy as those who have completed therapy. The meta-analysis by Jones et al. [7] indicated that exercise training was associated with superior VO_{2peak} improvements following adjuvant therapy compared to during adjuvant therapy, although no study has formally investigated this question.

For example, Courneya et al. [10] found that ∼17 weeks of aerobic training did not improve VO_{2peak} among women receiving anthracycline-containing chemotherapy for early breast cancer. Similarly, Jones et al. reported that 14 weeks of aerobic training led to negligible improvements in VO_{2peak} among patients undergoing cisplatin-based adjuvant chemotherapy for early NSCLC. It is also important to stress that although exercise training caused minimal improvements in VO_{2peak}, these effects occurred against the background of declines in VO_{2peak} in patients assigned to the control condition; in the study by Courneya et al., VO_{2peak} declined ∼5% among women randomized to usual-care control. Intriguingly, several other studies have reported significant improvements in VO_{2peak} and other pertinent outcomes in patients receiving other types of conventional cytotoxic therapies, such as radiation and ADT. These findings suggest that exercise-induced adaptations in the cardiopulmonary system may be contingent on the type of cytotoxic therapy being administered.

Another question that has received less attention but is one of critical importance is whether exercise impacts the therapeutic efficacy of conventional or novel cytotoxic agents. Exercise is a potent multifactorial intervention that influences a wide spectrum of pathways that could potentially modulate the cytotoxicity of chemotherapeutic agents. Jones et al. [11] investigated the effects of 8 weeks of forced exercise (treadmill running) on the antitumor efficacy of ▶ doxorubicin in female mice bearing human breast cancer ▶ xenografts. Overall, there were no significant differences on tumor growth between groups receiving doxorubicin alone versus doxorubicin plus exercise training ($p = 0.33$), suggesting that exercise does not significantly modulate doxorubicin-induced breast cancer growth inhibition. However, further work by Jones et al. [12] found that although tumor growth was comparable between exercised and sedentary animals bearing ▶ orthotopically implanted breast cancer xenografts, tumors from exercising animals had significantly improved blood perfusion/vascularization relative to the sedentary control group, suggesting that aerobic exercise can significantly increase intratumoral vascularization, which may "normalize" the ▶ tumor microenvironment and, in turn, inhibit tumor cell ▶ metastatic dissemination and improve therapeutic efficacy. Future studies are required to test these intriguing questions.

Exercise Therapy Following the Completion of Adjuvant Therapy (Survivorship)

Improvements in early detection and surveillance together with more effective locoregional and systemic therapies have led to significant survival gains for individuals diagnosed with early-stage cancer. Indeed, ∼13 million Americans who have been diagnosed with cancer are alive today. However, it is becoming increasingly apparent that improved outcomes in patients with early stage disease may come at the price of therapy-induced late effects. As a result, there has been a significant paradigm shift toward long-term therapy-associated toxicity and its resultant effects on morbidity, premature noncancer, competing causes of mortality, and QOL.

Exercise has emerged as an intervention of central importance in cancer survivorship, with numerous research groups examining whether exercise performed following the completion of therapy can accelerate recovery from the rigors of adjuvant cytotoxic therapy [4]. Similar to during therapy, the current literature base suggests that exercise is a safe and well-tolerated therapy associated with significant improvements in certain physiological and psychosocial therapy late effects.

A major goal in exercise–oncology survivorship research is to determine the optimal exercise prescription in cancer survivors. The vast majority of studies to date have investigated the effects of either aerobic training alone, resistance training alone, or the combination of aerobic and resistance training following traditional exercise prescription guidelines (3–5 day week^{-1} at 50–75% of baseline VO$_{2peak}$ for 12–15 weeks) in cancer survivors. As the field progresses, it will be important to conduct adequately powered studies that identify the optimal type, intensity, duration, and frequency of exercise training to improve symptom control in cancer survivors. At least three ongoing trials are addressing different aspects of this question in NSCLC, breast, and prostate cancer survivors. Of particular interest is high-intensity exercise training. Several recent randomized trials have demonstrated that high-intensity aerobic training (i.e., ≥75% of baseline exercise capacity) causes superior improvements in VO$_{2peak}$ relative to low- or moderate-intensity exercise training in patients with or at risk of CVD. However, there is a dearth of data regarding effects of exercise intensity following a cancer diagnosis.

Arguably, one of the most important questions in exercise–oncology research is to determine whether the benefits of exercise extend beyond to impact prognosis following a cancer diagnosis [4, 6]. The extant literature indicates that, in general, regular physical activity is associated with 15–61% reduction in the risk of death from breast or colorectal cancer (Table 1). The association between physical activity and cancer-specific mortality is not uniform and appears to vary according to volume of physical activity and even cancer type. In breast cancer,

the amount of physical activity that was significantly inversely associated with cancer death ranged from ≥9 MET-h week^{-1} (brisk walking for 30 min, 5 day week^{-1}) to ≥21 MET-h week^{-1} (brisk walking for 75 min, 5 day week^{-1}); in colorectal cancer, the range was ≥18 MET-h week^{-1} (brisk walking for 60 min, 5 day week^{-1}) to ≥27 MET-h week^{-1} (brisk walking for 90 min, 5 day week^{-1}). In addition, exploratory analyses suggest that the effects of physical activity may also differ by histological subtype and tumor expression of certain molecular markers. For example, Holmes et al. [13] reported that ≥9 MET-h week^{-1} was associated with a relative risk reduction in mortality of only 9% in women with estrogen receptor (ER)–negative tumors relative to a mortality reduction of 50% in women with ER-positive tumors. Meyerhardt et al. [14] reported that the association between exercise and mortality in patients with stage I–III colon cancer may depend on p27 status. Specifically, in tumors with loss of p27, the HR for colon cancer mortality was 1.40 (95% CI, 0.41–4.72) for patients reporting ≥18 MET-h week^{-1} relative to those reporting <18 MET-h week^{-1}. Conversely, in tumors with expression of p27, the HR for colon cancer mortality was 0.33 (95% CI, 0.12–0.85). Molecular status of fatty acid synthase, K-ras, p53, p21, and PI3KCA did not modify the association between exercise and clinical outcome. More studies are required to further investigate the association between postdiagnosis physical activity and clinical outcomes in breast and colorectal cancer as well as other cancer populations.

Exercise Therapy in Advanced (Palliative) Disease

Median survival of patients with advanced (inoperable) disease is heterogeneous and varies dramatically, depending on cancer site, molecular subtype, and therapeutic response. Patients with advanced disease are treated with aggressive combination therapeutic regimens that cause a wide spectrum of toxicities that negatively impact physical functioning, leading to higher disease-related symptoms and impaired QOL.

Exercise–oncology research is a new field, and investigators have predominately focused on the role of exercise in patients with early-stage disease – patients, in general, with better physical functioning and prognosis and who are experiencing less treatment-related toxicities. The investigation of exercise interventions in patients with advanced disease represents a unique challenge. For instance, patients with advanced cancer, by definition, have systemic (metastatic) disease, have often been heavily pretreated for prior early-stage disease, and are likely

Cancer, Therapy. Table 1 Association between postdiagnosis physical activity and cancer-specific mortality and all-cause mortality following a cancer diagnosis

Cancer site/ author	N	Cohort/setting	Cancer-specific mortality			All-cause mortality		
			Risk reduction (HR)	Exercise dose	Dose response	Risk reduction (HR)	Exercise dose	Dose response
Breast cancer								
Holmes et al. [13]	2,987	Stages I–III; Nurses' health study	0.50[a]	9–14.9 METs-h week[b]	No	0.56[a]	15–23.9 METs[b]	No
Sternfeld et al. [16]	1,970	Stages I–IIIa; Life after cancer epidemiology	0.69[a]	3–<6 h week moderate exercise	No	0.66[a]	3–<6 h week moderate exercise[b]	No
Holick et al. [17]	4,482	Invasive disease free of recurrence 2 yr > after diagnosis	0.51[a]	≥21.0 METs-h week[b]	Yes	0.44[a]	≥21.0 METs-h week[b]	Yes
Irwin et al. [18]	933	Operable disease; health, eating, activity, and lifestyle	0.65[a]	≥9 METs-h week	Yes	0.33[a]	≥9 METs-h week[b]	Yes
Pierce et al. [19]	1,490	Stages I–IIIa; Women's health eating and living	0.58	≥1,320–6,420 METs-min week	Yes	–	–	–
Dal Maso et al. [20]	1,453	Invasive	0.85[a]	≥2 METs-h week	N/a	0.82[a]	≥2 METs-h week	N/a
Colon cancer								
Meyerhardt et al. [21]	832	Stage III	0.39[a]	≥18.0 METs-h week[b]	Yes	0.43[a]	≥18.0 METs-h week[b]	Yes
Colorectal cancer								
Meyerhardt et al. [22]	573	Women with stages I–III; Nurses' health study	0.51[a, c]	≥18.0 METs-h week[b]	No	0.37[a]	≥27.0 METs-h week[b]	Yes
Meyerhardt et al. [23]	668	Men with stages I–III; Nurses' health study	0.47[a]	≥27.0 METs-h week[b]	No	0.59[a]	≥27.0 METs-h week[b]	No
Prostate cancer								
Kenfield et al. [24]	2,705	Men from health professionals follow-up study	0.67[a]	≥9 METs-h week[b]	Yes	0.65[a]	≥9 METs-h week[b]	Yes
Ovarian								
Moorman et al. [25]	638	Invasive disease; NC ovarian cancer study	n/a	N/a	N/a	0.69[a]	≥2 METs h week[b]	No
Primary glioma								
Ruden et al. [26]	243	WHO grade III/IV recurrent glioma	n/a	N/a	N/a	0.64[a]	≥9 METs-h week[b]	N/a
Lung cancer								
Jones et al.	118	Stage IV, NSCLC	n/a	N/a	N/a	0.67	≥9 METs-h week[b]	N/a

[a]Multivariate-adjusted relative risk
[b]$p < 0.05$
[c]Cancer recurrence or death from any cause (disease-free survival);
HR hazard ratio, *METs* Metabolic equivalent, *n/a* not applicable, *WHO* World Health Organization, *NSCLC* nonsmall-cell lung cancer

receiving aggressive combination cytotoxic and supportive care therapies. As such, these patients are likely experiencing more disease-related and treatment-related toxicities that will modify the exercise response.

A recent systematic review by Lowe et al. [15] identified a total of six studies investigating the effect of exercise training on symptom control in patients with advanced cancer. In general, all studies reported positive findings, but overall, methodological quality was poor. There is currently insufficient evidence for definitive conclusions regarding the tolerability, safety, or efficacy of exercise in cancer patients with advanced disease. Given the poorer prognosis and elevated treatment toxicity in this setting, we stress the importance of rigorous AE and safety monitoring in planned exercise studies is comparable to that required for pharmaceutical intervention trials, in conjunction with appropriate correlative science components. Such an approach will ensure the optimal safety and efficacy of exercise in this unique setting.

Summary

Research, as well as clinical interest, in the role of exercise following a cancer diagnosis has increased dramatically and is likely to increase even further over the next decade with the emergence and increasing importance placed on cancer survivorship. The current evidence base provides strong but preliminary evidence that exercise training is a well-tolerated and safe adjunct therapy that can mitigate several common treatment-related side effects among patients receiving adjuvant therapy for early-stage disease. Results of these "first-generation" studies provide a solid platform to launch "second-generation" studies that will extend the scope and application of exercise–oncology research to address the major unanswered questions in this emerging field.

Acknowledgements

Dr. Jones is supported by NIH CA143254, CA142566, CA138634, CA133895, CA125458 and George and Susan Beischer.

References

1. Morris JN, Heady JA, Raffle PA et al (1953) Coronary heart disease and physical activity of work. Lancet 265:1111–20
2. Pate RR, Pratt M, Blair SN et al (1995) Physical activity and public health. A recommendation from the Centers for Disease Control and Prevention and the American College of Sports Medicine. J Am Med Assoc 273:402–407
3. Warburton DE, Nicol CW, Bredin SS (2006) Health benefits of physical activity: the evidence. Canadian Med Assoc J 174:801–809
4. Jones LW, Peppercorn J (2010) Exercise research: early promise warrants further investment. Lancet Oncol 11:408–410
5. Jones LW, Eves ND, Haykowsky M et al (2009) Exercise intolerance in cancer and the role of exercise therapy to reverse dysfunction. Lancet Oncol 10:598–605
6. Schmitz KH, Courneya KS, Matthews C et al (2010) American College of Sports Medicine roundtable on exercise guidelines for cancer survivors. Med Sci Sports Exerc 42:1409–1426
7. Jones LW, Liang Y, Pituskin EN et al (2011) Effect of exercise training on peak oxygen consumption in patients with cancer: a meta-analysis. Oncologist 16:112–120
8. Jones LW, Eves ND, Peddle CJ et al (2009) Effects of presurgical exercise training on systemic inflammatory markers among patients with malignant lung lesions. Appl Physiol Nutr Metab 34:197–202
9. Bobbio A, Chetta A, Ampollini L et al (2008) Preoperative pulmonary rehabilitation in patients undergoing lung resection for non-small cell lung cancer. Eur J Cardiothorac Surg 33:95–98
10. Courneya KS, Segal RJ, Mackey JR et al (2007) Effects of aerobic and resistance exercise in breast cancer patients receiving adjuvant chemotherapy: a multicenter randomized controlled trial. J Clin Oncol 25:4396–4404
11. Jones LW, Eves ND, Courneya KS et al (2005) Effects of exercise training on antitumor efficacy of doxorubicin in MDA-MB-231 breast cancer xenografts. Clin Cancer Res 11:6695–6698
12. Jones LW, Viglianti BL, Tashjian JA et al (2010) Effect of aerobic exercise on tumor physiology in an animal model of human breast cancer. J Appl Physiol 108:343–348
13. Holmes MD, Chen WY, Feskanich D et al (2005) Physical activity and survival after breast cancer diagnosis. J Am Med Assoc 293:2479–2486
14. Meyerhardt JA, Ogino S, Kirkner GJ et al (2009) Interaction of molecular markers and physical activity on mortality in patients with colon cancer. Clin Cancer Res 15:5931–5936
15. Lowe SS, Watanabe SM, Courneya KS (2009) Physical activity as a supportive care intervention in palliative cancer patients: a systematic review. J Support Oncol 7:27–34
16. Sternfeld B, Weltzien E, Quesenberry CP Jr et al (2009) Physical activity and risk of recurrence and mortality in breast cancer survivors: findings from the LACE study. Cancer Epidemiol Biomarkers Prev 18:87–95
17. Holick CN, Newcomb PA, Trentham-Dietz A et al (2008) Physical activity and survival after diagnosis of invasive breast cancer. Cancer Epidemiol Biomarkers Prev 17:379–386
18. Irwin ML, Smith AW, McTiernan A et al (2008) Influence of pre- and postdiagnosis physical activity on mortality in breast cancer survivors: the health, eating, activity, and lifestyle study. J Clin Oncol 26:3958–3964
19. Pierce JP, Stefanick ML, Flatt SW et al (2007) Greater survival after breast cancer in physically active women with high vegetable-fruit intake regardless of obesity. J Clin Oncol 25:2345–2351
20. Dal Maso L, Zucchetto A, Talamini R (2008) Effect of obesity and other lifestyle factors on mortality in women with breast cancer. Int J Cancer 123:2188–94
21. Meyerhardt JA, Heseltine D, Niedzwiecki D et al (2006) Impact of physical activity on cancer recurrence and survival in patients with stage III colon cancer: findings from CALGB 89803. J Clin Oncol 24:3535–3541
22. Meyerhardt JA, Giovannucci EL, Holmes MD et al (2006) Physical activity and survival after colorectal cancer diagnosis. J Clin Oncol 24:3527–3534
23. Meyerhardt JA, Giovannucci EL, Ogino S et al (2009) Physical activity and male colorectal cancer survival. Arch Intern Med 169:2102–2108
24. Kenfield SA, Stampfer MJ, Giovannucci E et al (2011) Physical activity and survival after prostate cancer diagnosis in the health professionals follow-up study. J Clin Oncol 29:726–732

25. Moorman PG, Jones LW, Akushevich L et al (2011) Recreational physical activity and ovarian cancer risk and survival. Ann Epidemiol 21:178–187
26. Ruden E, Reardon DA, Coan AD et al (2011) Exercise behavior, functional capacity, and survival in adults with malignant recurrent glioma. J Clin Oncol 29(2):2918–2923
27. Segal R, Evans W, Johnson D et al (2001) Structured exercise improves physical functioning in women with stages I and II breast cancer: results of a randomized controlled trial. J Clin Oncol 19:657–665
28. Kolden GG, Strauman TJ, Ward A et al (2002) A pilot study of group exercise training (GET) for women with primary breast cancer: feasibility and health benefits. Psycho Oncol 11:447–456
29. Brown JK, Byers T, Doyle C et al (2003) Nutrition and physical activity during and after cancer treatment: an American Cancer Society guide for informed choices. CA Cancer J Clin 53:268–291
30. Courneya KS, Booth CM, Gill S et al (2008) The colon health and life-long exercise change trial: a randomized trial of the national cancer institute of Canada clinical trials group. Curr Oncol 15:279–285

Capillarization

▶ Angiogenesis

Capillary Hematocrit

The ratio of red blood cells (RBCs) to plasma volume within the capillaries at any given time. The number of RBCs within the capillaries that lie adjacent to the myocytes determines, in part, the O_2 diffusion capacity (DO_2).

Carbohydrate

▶ Nutrition

Carbohydrate Loading

A. N. Bosch
Human Biology, University of Cape Town MRC Research Unit for Exercise Science and Sports Medicine, Sports Science Institute of South Africa, Newlands, South Africa

Synonyms

Glycogen loading; Glycogen super-compensation

Definition

Carbohydrate loading is the use of a dietary technique used primarily by endurance athletes before participation in prolonged events such as the marathon. It involves ingestion of high-carbohydrate foods or drinks for 1–3 days before competition to increase muscle glycogen stores.

Mechanism of Action

In 1967, the introduction of the needle biopsy technique for the sampling of muscle tissue in exercise physiology studies provided important new data on the relationships between diet, muscle glycogen concentration, and fatigue during prolonged exercise.

Muscle Glycogen Concentrations

Using the biopsy technique, initial studies determined that the concentration of glycogen in the leg muscles of untrained people eating a normal diet varies from approximately 80 to 120 mmol/kg of wet muscle (ww), whereas average muscle glycogen concentrations of athletes who ingest a diet high in carbohydrate and are in training are somewhat higher, around 130 mmol/kg ww [1]. Values as high as 140–200 mmol/kg ww are attained in trained athletes who have not exercised for 24–48 h and who have consumed a high-carbohydrate diet.

Muscle Glycogen Concentrations, Diet, and Exercise Performance

Diet can affect both muscle glycogen content and exercise performance. Possibly the best known studies that contributed to the development of the dietary practice that was to become known as "carbohydrate loading" are those of Ahlborg et al. [2] and Bergstrom et al. [3] in which muscle glycogen concentrations were manipulated through various combinations of diet and exercise. In these studies, muscle glycogen concentration was found to average 97 mmol/kg ww at the start of exercise. Subjects then cycled to exhaustion at 75% of VO_{2max} on a cycle ergometer, which averaged 114 min. Following this initial exercise bout, for the next 3 days a high fat-protein diet was ingested, after which muscle glycogen concentrations had decreased to 35 mmol/kg ww and average exercise time to exhaustion was reduced to 57 min. The dietary regimen was then changed to a high carbohydrate one for the next 7 days. With this regimen, mean muscle glycogen concentrations increased to 184 mmol/kg ww and exercise time increased to 167 min. Thus, it became apparent that initial glycogen concentration influenced exercise time to exhaustion, and that muscle glycogen concentration could be influenced by dietary manipulation. It was not long before this procedure of first depleting muscle glycogen stores by an exercise bout followed by 3 days of a diet low in carbohydrate (high fat-protein diet), followed subsequently by eating a large amount of carbohydrate (∼600 g of carbohydrate daily), was used by endurance athletes in an effort to enhance performance. This became known as the "carbohydrate loading" diet, although the period of high carbohydrate intake became reduced from 7 to 3 days when used by athletes.

Importantly, this original work was done using relatively untrained people in the experiments. Subsequently, it was demonstrated that the depletion phase of eating only protein and fat is unnecessary in well-trained athletes [4, 5]. Simply eating a high-carbohydrate diet for 3 days (500–600 g/day; 10 g/kg body weight/day), combined with a reduction in training, was found to result in similar amounts of glycogen being stored to that obtained when the original loading regimen was followed. This is because glycogen synthase, one of the enzymes involved in muscle glycogen synthesis, is activated by the carbohydrate and glycogen depletion regimen in untrained people; in trained individuals, however, glycogen synthase is already maximally activated as a result of daily training and no further activation occurs following a period of low carbohydrate intake.

More recently, it has been shown that in highly trained athletes even 3 days of carbohydrate loading is longer than needed to maximize muscle glycogen stores. By ingesting 10 g/kg body weight/day of carbohydrate, maximal muscle glycogen concentrations can be attained within 24 h [6, 7].

Carbohydrate loading with high glycemic index carbohydrate foods rather than low glycemic index foods has been found to have no effect on performance in a 10-km performance run, after an initial run for 1 h at 70% VO_{2max} [8]. Unfortunately, muscle glycogen concentration was not measured in this study, and the total exercise performed may not have been sufficient to deplete muscle glycogen stores, and therefore, it cannot be assumed that the high glycemic index foods did not result in higher initial muscle glycogen stores, based only there being no differences in performance in this particular study. The effect of glycemic index on the rate of muscle glycogen storage remains to be resolved. It should be noted, however, that in the study which showed that maximal muscle glycogen stores could be attained within 24 h, a high glycemic index carbohydrate was ingested to carbohydrate load.

Once a high muscle glycogen concentration has been attained by carbohydrate loading, it is possible for an athlete to maintain these high concentrations without continued loading. Specifically, the muscle glycogen concentration remains elevated for 3 [9] to 5 days [10], provided only moderate intensity exercise of approximately only 20 min duration is performed during that time.

Following the findings of Bergstrom et al. [3] of increased dietary carbohydrate resulting in increased muscle glycogen stores and an apparently related increase in exercise time to exhaustion, a number of papers were published which examined in greater detail the relationship between diet, muscle glycogen content, and the possibility of improved exercise performance. These studies showed that fatigue in endurance exercise appeared to consistently coincide with low muscle glycogen concentrations, and it was therefore concluded that exhaustion during prolonged exercise was due to muscle glycogen depletion. Therefore, starting exercise with raised muscle glycogen levels by prior carbohydrate loading was confirmed as being advantageous. In some respects, however, the coincidence between muscle glycogen depletion and exhaustion during prolonged exercise may be an over simplification, as in many of the studies that examined the effect of carbohydrate loading on performance, blood glucose concentration was either not measured or not carefully considered when results were analyzed. It appears that in some studies which attributed fatigue to depleted muscle glycogen stores, lowered blood glucose concentration could also have accounted for the fatigue experienced by the subjects. Nevertheless, the majority of studies have shown that starting exercise with high muscle glycogen concentration delays the onset of fatigue.

Although, in some cases, low blood glucose concentrations together with low muscle glycogen concentration make interpretation of the cause of fatigue difficult, the importance of muscle glycogen concentrations alone was demonstrated in a study in which subjects started exercise with either high or low muscle glycogen content as a result of ingesting a diet either low in carbohydrate or after having carbohydrate loaded for 4 days prior to the experiment. As expected, time to fatigue was longer in the athletes with high initial muscle glycogen content. At exhaustion, glucose was infused to restore plasma glucose to pre-exercise levels. Interestingly, although this eliminated symptoms of hypoglycemia, it did not improve performance time, suggesting that muscle glycogen depletion specifically, and not hypoglycemia was responsible for exhaustion in these subjects. In contrast, Coyle et al. [11] showed that exercise could be continued even when muscle glycogen content was low, provided that the blood glucose concentration remained high. Cyclists ingested either a glucose polymer solution or water placebo while cycling at 70% of VO_{2max}. Those subjects ingesting the carbohydrate solution were able to exercise for an hour longer than subjects ingesting the placebo, even though the muscle glycogen concentrations of the carbohydrate ingesting subjects during the final hour were as low as those of the subjects who could not continue and who were exhausted. Thus, it was concluded that it could not have been muscle glycogen depletion that stopped the subjects from continuing to exercise, but rather an inadequate supply of plasma glucose for oxidation. The final conclusion of the study was that as long as the muscle was provided with sufficient glucose to oxidize, exercise could be continued when normally this would not be possible because hypoglycemia terminated exercise prematurely. However, if the data are examined carefully, it becomes apparent that the muscle glycogen concentrations at exhaustion in this study did not reach the very low concentrations that are usually associated with exhaustion. Values were around 40 mmol/kg ww, whereas it has previously been reported that 17–28 mmol/kg ww is the concentration consistent with exhaustion [12]. Thus, it is likely that the ergogenic effect of the carbohydrate was mainly due to the maintenance of euglycemia, and therefore the concept of muscle glycogen being implicated in exhaustion remains.

One of the few field studies that have investigated the theory that glycogen depletion is an important element in the cause of fatigue is that of Karlsson and Saltin [12]. Using well-trained subjects, they found that after following a carbohydrate-loading regimen, subjects ran a faster time in a 30-km road race than when eating a normal diet. Of particular interest was the finding that loading did not result in a faster initial running speed. Rather, it allowed the athletes to maintain their initial speed for longer before slowing down. The time in the race at which the runners slowed down correlated with their starting muscle glycogen concentrations.

Although there have been many studies that have concentrated on the effect of high muscle glycogen concentration subsequent to carbohydrate loading on endurance exercise performance at moderate intensity (70% VO_{2max}), there have also been studies which have shown that even if exercise intensity is low, high muscle glycogen content at the start of exercise is important. For example, muscle glycogen depletion has been implicated in exhaustion in exercise performed as low as 43% of VO_{2max}. At the other extreme, it has also been shown that exercise at very high exercise intensities (greater than 80% VO_{2max}) may also be affected by muscle glycogen content at the start of exercise. Specifically, an increase in time to exhaustion after carbohydrate loading and decreased time to exhaustion after glycogen depletion compared to exercise which commenced with normal muscle glycogen levels, has been shown when exercise was performed at 100% of VO_{2max}. This was despite the short duration of exercise performed at such a high intensity.

Despite the majority of studies showing a positive effect on exercise performance as a result of starting exercise with high muscle glycogen content after carbohydrate loading, there have been some that have shown no effect. For example, in one study, there was no difference in running time to fatigue (77 min) at 75–80% of VO_{2max} between carbohydrate-loaded and non-loaded groups of well-trained runners. Glycogen concentrations at exhaustion, however, were too high in both groups to be considered a possible cause of fatigue (125 and 100 mmol/kg ww, respectively). Similarly, a field trial over a distance of 21 km showed no improvement in running performance as a result of prior carbohydrate loading. The failure to show an improvement over this distance is most likely due to muscle glycogen stores not becoming depleted before the end of the 21-km distance. Other studies, however, have shown an effect over a distance of 25 km. Thus, although there is some conflicting evidence, generally it appears that carbohydrate loading only becomes important when exercise duration is so long, or of such high intensity that muscle glycogen becomes depleted during the event. It is also important to remember that fatigue can occur due to factors other than muscle glycogen depletion or low blood glucose concentration. For example, Costill et al. [13] found that trained runners may became fatigued even though muscle glycogen concentrations at exhaustion were 63 mmol/kg ww in the vastus lateralis and 86 mmol/kg ww in the soleus.

In summary, carbohydrate loading increases muscle glycogen concentration, which has generally been shown to enhance endurance performance, and in some studies, to enhance shorter duration exercise performed at a higher intensity.

References

1. Sahlin K, Katz A, Broberg S (1990) Tricarboxylic acid cycle intermediates in human muscle during prolonged exercise. Am J Physiol 259(5 Pt 1):C834–C841
2. Ahlborg B, Bergstrom J, Brohult J et al (1967) Human muscle glycogen content and capacity for prolonged exercise after different diets. Forvarsmedicin 3:85–99
3. Bergstrom J, Hermansen L, Hultman E, Saltin B (1967) Diet, muscle glycogen and physical performance. Acta Physiol Scand 71(2): 140–150
4. Sherman WM, Costill DL, Fink WJ, Miller JM (1981) Effect of exercise-diet manipulation on muscle glycogen and its subsequent utilization during performance. Int J Sports Med 2(2):114–118

5. Costill DL, Sherman WM, Fink WJ et al (1981) The role of dietary carbohydrates in muscle glycogen resynthesis after strenuous running. Am J Clin Nutr 34(9):1831–1836
6. Bussau VA, Fairchild TJ, Rao A et al (2002) Carbohydrate loading in human muscle: an improved 1 day protocol. Eur J Appl Physiol 87(3):290–295
7. Fairchild TJ, Fletcher S, Steele P et al (2002) Rapid carbohydrate loading after a short bout of near maximal-intensity exercise. Med Sci Sports Exerc 34(6):980–986
8. Chen Y, Wong SH, Xu X et al (2008) Effect of CHO loading patterns on running performance. Int J Sports Med 29(7):598–606
9. Goforth HW Jr, Arnall DA, Bennett BL, Law PG (1997) Persistence of supercompensated muscle glycogen in trained subjects after carbohydrate loading. J Appl Physiol 82(1):342–347
10. Arnall DA, Nelson AG, Quigley J et al (2007) Supercompensated glycogen loads persist 5 days in resting trained cyclists. Eur J Appl Physiol 99(3):251–256
11. Coyle EF, Coggan AR, Hemmert MK, Ivy JL (1986) Muscle glycogen utilization during prolonged strenuous exercise when fed carbohydrate. J Appl Physiol 61(1):165–172
12. Karlsson J, Saltin B (1971) Diet, muscle glycogen, and endurance performance. J Appl Physiol 31(2):203–206
13. Costill DL, Sparks K, Gregor R, Turner C (1971) Muscle glycogen utilization during exhaustive running. J Appl Physiol 31(3):353–356

Carbon Dioxide Output

▶ Gas Exchange, Alveolar

Cardiac Arrhythmias

ALESSANDRO BLANDINO, ELISABETTA TOSO, FIORENZO GAITA
Cardiology Division, Department of Internal Medicine, San Giovanni Battista Hospital, University of Turin, Turin, Italy

Synonyms
Abnormal cardiac electrical activity; Disturbance of the heartbeat; Rhythm disorder

Definition
The term "arrhythmia" comes from the ancient Greek a-rhuthmos) and identifies a loss of normal heart activity. Cardiac arrhythmias can be classified into bradyarrhythmias (when heart rate is < than 60 beats for minute) or ▶ Tachyarrhythmias (when heart rate is > than 100 beat for minute), that may arise from supraventricular regions or ventricles. Bradyarrhythmias include sinus bradycardia, wandering pacemaker, sinus pause, and

atrioventricular blocks. Supraventricular tachyarrhythmias include premature ectopic beats, AV nodal reentrant tachycardia (AVNRT), orthodromic AV reentrant tachycardia (AVRT) due to an ▶ Accessory Pathway, ectopic atrial tachycardia, atrial fibrillation (AF), and atrial flutter (AF1). Ventricular tachyarrhythmias include premature ectopic beats, non-sustained ventricular tachycardia, idio-ventricular accelerated rhythm, benign idiopathic ventricular tachycardia, and malignant ventricular tachycardia, such as sustained ventricular tachycardia, polymorphic ventricular tachycardia, torsades de pointes, and ventricular fibrillation.

Characteristics and Eligibility for Sports Practice

Bradyarrhythmias
In the trained athlete, sinus bradycardia (defined as sinus heart rate < 60 beats per minute) and sinus pauses are frequent and are generally benign conditions, secondary to high vagal tone and reduced sympathetic tone (▶ Bradyarrhythmias). These conditions are generally asymptomatic and do not affect maximum heart rate attainment. Anyway, if symptomatic, 24-h Holter monitoring and exercise testing are recommended, plus echocardiography whether structural heart disease is suspected.

High vagal tone and reduced adrenergic tone are also responsible for the high prevalence of atrioventricular (AV) blocks in athletes. In AV block, atrial activation is conducted to the ventricles with a delay, or it is not conducted at all, during a period when the AV conduction pathway (AV node or His-Purkinje system) is not expected to be refractory. On the basis of the electrocardiographic criteria, AV block is classified as first, second, or third degree, and depending on the anatomical point at which the conduction of the activation wave front is impaired, it is described as supra-Hisian, intra-Hisian, or infra-Hisian.

In the athletes, the most common AV blocks seen are as follows: first-degree AV block (each atrial stimulus is conducted to the ventricles with a prolonged PR interval more than 200 ms) and second-degree AV block type I (Wenckebach or Mobitz I, defined as progressively increased PR interval until an atrial stimulus is not conducted to the ventricles). AV blocks typically occur during sleep or at rest and resolve during exercise, showing the supra-hisian nature of conduction impairment.

If asymptomatic, with no cardiac disease, and with resolution of block during exercise, the athlete is eligible for all sports. In case of severe bradycardia (heart rate <40 bpm), sinus pause >3 s, and when symptomatic, it is necessary to interrupt any sports activity and further diagnostic monitoring (24-h Holter monitoring and exercise testing) be recommended. At least after 3 months when the symptoms are absent, physical effort can be restarted with yearly clinical controls.

Tachyarrhythmias

As previously described, tachyarrhythmias are classified into supraventricular (when they originate from atria or AV junction) and ventricular (when they originate from myocardium under the AV junction).

Supraventicular Arrhythmias

Premature Supraventricular Complex

Supraventricular premature ectopic beats (PSVCs) are premature activation of the atria or AV junction arising from a site other than the sinus node. They are a common finding in many individuals, including athletes, and they may be asymptomatic or cause mild symptoms such as "skipping" sensation or palpitations; they are often single and isolated, but may be frequent or occur in a bigeminal pattern. In predisposed individuals, PSVCs may trigger supraventricular and, less commonly, ventricular arrhythmias. In the absence of structural heart disease, thyroid dysfunction, initiation of sustained arrhythmias and moderate/severe symptoms, no further evaluation or therapy is required. If the athlete is asymptomatic, with no cardiac disease, eligibility is for all sports, without further yearly clinical assessment.

Atrioventricular Nodal Reciprocating Tachycardia

Atrioventricular nodal reciprocating tachycardia (AVNRT) is the most common form of paroxysmal supraventricular tachycardia. It is more prevalent in females, is associated with palpitations, dizziness, and neck pulsations, and rarely is associated with structural heart disease.

Rates of tachycardia are often between 140 and 250 per minute. The reentrant circuit comprises the compact AV node and frequently a perinodal atrial tissue. AVNRT involves reciprocation between two functionally and anatomically distinct pathways (fast and slow pathways). The fast pathway appears to be located near the His bundle at the Koch's triangle apex, whereas the slow pathway extends infero-posterior to the compact AV-node tissue and stretches along the septal margin of the tricuspid annulus at the level of the coronary sinus.

During typical AVNRT, the fast pathway serves as the retrograde limb of the circuit, whereas the slow pathway is the anterograde limb (slow–fast AV-node reentry). After conduction through the slow pathway to the His bundle

and ventricle, brisk conduction back to the atrium over the fast pathway results in inscription of the shorter duration (40 ms) P wave during or close to the QRS complex (less than or equal to 70 ms) often with a pseudo-r in V1. Less commonly (approximately 5–10%), the tachycardia circuit is reversed such that conduction proceeds anterogradely over the fast pathway and retrogradely over the slow pathway (fast–slow AV-node reentry, or atypical AVNRT) producing a long R-P tachycardia. The P wave, negative in leads III and augmented vector foot (aVF), is inscribed prior to the QRS. Infrequently, both limbs of the tachycardia circuit are composed of slowly conducting tissue (slow–slow AV-node reentry), and the P wave is inscribed after the QRS, producing an RP interval more than 70 ms.

Adequate evaluation of the athlete with AVNRT includes history with emphasis on the characteristics of the arrhythmia onset and symptoms during tachycardia. When based on ECG documentation an AVNRT is suspected, an electrophysiological study aimed to define the reentry mechanism and to confirm the diagnosis is recommended. In order to be eligible for sports activity, the athlete must undergo ▶ Catheter Ablation. If the athlete refuses the procedure, eligibility can still be released only when a cardiac disease has been ruled out, paroxysmal palpitations occur rarely and the arrhythmia is well tolerated with no correlation with effort. Anyway, sports activity with increased risk (▶ Bradyarrhythmias) is forbidden.

Atrioventricular Reciprocating Tachycardia (Extra Nodal Accessory Pathways)

Accessory pathways (APs) are extra nodal pathways that connect the atrial myocardium to the ventricle across the AV groove. Pathways can be classified on the basis of conduction direction (anterograde, retrograde, both), location (along the mitral or tricuspid annulus), and mode of conduction (decremental or non-decremental). Typical APs usually exhibit rapid, non-decremental conduction, similar to that present in normal His-Purkinje tissue. APs that are capable of only retrograde conduction are referred to as "concealed," whereas those capable of anterograde conduction are "manifest," demonstrating delta wave on a standard ECG. Delta wave results from the contemporary activation of ventricles by two distinct wave fronts: the first across the accessory pathway, the second across the His-Purkinje system. The degree of pre-excitation is variable and strongly related to the relative conduction to the ventricle over the AV-node-His bundle versus the accessory pathway. In some patients, anterograde conduction is apparent only with pacing close to the atrial insertion site, as, for example, for left-lateral pathways. Manifest APs usually conduct in both anterograde and retrograde directions. Those that conduct in the anterograde direction only are uncommon, whereas those that conduct in the retrograde direction are common.

The diagnosis of Wolff–Parkinson–White (WPW) syndrome is reserved for patients who have both pre-excitation and tachyarrhythmias. Among patients with WPW syndrome, atrioventricular reciprocating tachycardia (AVRT) is the most common arrhythmia, followed by atrial fibrillation. AVRT may be orthodromic or antidromic. During orthodromic AVRT, the reentrant impulse conducts anterogradely over the AV node and the specialized conduction system from the atrium to the ventricle and utilizes the accessory pathway for retrograde conduction to the atrium. During antidromic AVRT, the circuit is traveled in the reverse direction, with anterograde conduction from the atrium to the ventricle occurring via the accessory pathway and retrograde conduction over the AV node or a second accessory pathway. However, antidromic conduction occurs in only 5–10% of AVRT. Atrial fibrillation is the second most frequent arrhythmia in WPW patients (about one third) and may be a potential life-threat: in fact, if the AP has a short anterograde refractory period, rapid repetitive conduction to the ventricles during AF can result in a rapid ventricular response with possible VF degeneration. In symptomatic WPW patients, ventricular fibrillation occurs rarely (0.15–0.4%) during pre-excitated atrial fibrillation, whereas in symptomatic WPW patients, the risk appears to be higher (2.2%). Evaluation of the athlete with ventricular pre-excitation includes history, physical examination, ECG, stress test, and echocardiography to exclude an associated structural heart disease such as Ebstein anomaly or hyperthrophic cardiomyopathy, if physical examination is doubtful. Assessment of the risk of sudden cardiac death (SCD) is mandatory and is based on delta wave intermittence on the ECG, sudden disappearance of delta wave while heart rate increases, presence of multiple accessory pathways, and easy induction of AF and short AP anterograde refractory period evaluated by the electrophysiological or the transesophageal study (currently used criteria are <240 ms at rest and <220 ms during effort or isoproterenol infusion).

Asymptomatic athletes with absence of both risk criteria and arrhythmia induction in the electrophysiological study can perform sports without undergoing catheter ablation. However, sports activity with increased risk (▶ Bradyarrhythmias) is forbidden. Instead, WPW athletes with risk criteria or symptoms or AF/AVRT induction in the electrophysiological study, in order to obtain sports eligibility, must undergo ablation procedure.

Ectopic Atrial Tachycardia

Ectopic atrial tachycardia (EAT) is characterized by a regular atrial activation originating from a localized atrial site with subsequent centrifugal spread. Atrial rate ranges between 100 and 250 bpm with isoelectric baselines between atrial deflections on the surface ECG. Neither the sinus node nor the AV node plays a role in the initiation and perpetuation of the tachycardia. The outlook of patients with focal AT is usually benign with the exception of incessant forms, which may lead to tachycardia-induced cardiomyopathy. EAT can occur in the absence of cardiac disease, but it is often secondary to underlying cardiac abnormalities (especially in children with congenital heart disease). Clinical management is similar to that applied in atrial fibrillation. ▶ Sports Eligibility may be released only when a cardiac disease, sick sinus syndrome, and substance abuse have been ruled out, paroxysmal palpitations occur rarely, and the arrhythmia is well tolerated with no correlation with effort. Anyway, sports activity with increased risk (▶ Bradyarrhythmias) is clearly forbidden.

Atrial Fibrillation

Atrial fibrillation (AF) [1] is the most frequent arrhythmia in general population, especially in the elderly and in patients with heart disease. However, although this arrhythmia is very rare in the young, recent data highlighted a relationship between long-term endurance sports and occurrence of AF. At surface ECG, AF is characterized by irregular RR intervals without distinct P waves but with an atrial cycle length (interval between two atrial activations), when visible, extremely high (>300 bpm). Clinically, it is reasonable to distinguish four types of AF based on the presentation and duration of the arrhythmia: paroxysmal, persistent, long-standing persistent, and permanent AF. Paroxysmal AF is typically self-terminating, anyway lasting less than 7 days. Persistent AF is present when an AF episode either lasts longer than 7 days or requires cardioversion for termination. Long-standing persistent when AF has lasted for ≥1 year but a rhythm control strategy has been adopted. AF becomes permanent when a rhythm control strategy has been definitively abandoned. In the general population, up to 80% of patients with AF show symptoms such as palpitations, fatigue, dyspnea, and reduced tolerance to physical effort, while the remaining 20% are asymptomatic and AF is occasionally diagnosed on the ECG. In the athletes' population, the percentage of asymptomatic forms is much higher than 20%. In 40% of athletes with AF, a possible substrate, such as WPW syndrome, cardiomyopathy, or silent myocarditis can be identified. Doping substances, such as anabolic steroids, are also a likely cause of AF in athletes. Evaluation of the athlete with AF includes clinical history, physical examination, ECG, echocardiography to exclude an underlying structural heart disease, stress test, and 24-h continuous ECG monitoring to confirm the diagnosis when paroxysmal and evaluate the mean ventricular rate while AF is persistent/long-standing persistent. In patients with paroxysmal AF, sports eligibility may be obtained when an underlying cardiac disease, sick sinus syndrome, and WPW syndrome have been ruled out and AF recurrences have not occurred 3 months before assessment. Furthermore AF must be well tolerated with no correlation between symptoms and effort. Patients with persistent/permanent AF are eligible for sports on individual basis after careful evaluation of heart rate control and exclusion of bradycardia-related ventricular arrhythmias. Clearly, the need for anticoagulation therapy excludes individuals from sports with a risk of bodily collision or trauma.

Atrial Flutter

Atrial flutter (AFl) is characterized by an organized atrial rhythm with a rate ranging from 250 to 350 bpm, without clear isoelectric baselines between atrial deflections on the surface ECG. AFl may be classified as typical and atypical. Typical AFl includes isthmus-dependent forms, in which the circuit is defined anteriorly by the tricuspid orifice, posteriorly by a combination of anatomical obstacles (orifices of superior and inferior vena cava and the Eustachian ridge), and functional barriers (the region of the crista terminalis). The critical isthmus is between the inferior vena cava orifice and the tricuspid annulus. In 90% of cases, impulse crosses the circuit counterclockwise ("common type"), while in the remaining 10% of cases the circuit is traveled clockwise ("uncommon type or reverse"). In counterclockwise atrial flutter, a characteristic ECG "sawtooth" pattern is present in leads II, III, aVF with a positive flutter deflection in lead V1 and a negative in lead V6. Clockwise isthmus-dependent flutter shows the opposite pattern, generally with no "sawtooth" aspect.

All the other atrial flutter not fitting the typical and reverse typical flutter patterns described above are considered atypical. Evaluation of the athlete includes ECG for a precise classification of the arrhythmia and a complete clinical assessment including clinical history, physical examination, and echocardiography to exclude an underlying structural heart disease. Furthermore stress test and 24-h continuous ECG monitoring are useful to confirm the diagnosis and evaluate the mean ventricular rate. Catheter ablation and at least 3-month follow-up freedom from AFl recurrences without antiarrhythmic drugs are the requirements for sports eligibility.

Ventricular Arrhythmias

Premature Ventricular Complex

Premature ectopic ventricular beats (PVCs) are premature ventricular contractions, frequently found in athletes as well as in the general population. The main predictor of a good prognosis is the absence of heart disease. In the absence of CV abnormalities, PVCs are not associated with an increased risk of malignant ventricular arrhythmias and convey a good outcome. However, PVCs may also be the initial and unique manifestation of clinically silent arrhythmogenic conditions such as Arrhythmogenic Right Ventricular Cardiomyopathy (ARVC), Hypertrophic Cardiomyopathy (HCM), and myocarditis. For this reason, athletes with PVCs require careful evaluation including clinical history (familial history of sudden death and symptoms, such as palpitations or syncope, particularly during exertion), physical examination, echocardiography, exercise testing, and 24-h Holter monitoring. In athletes with suspected heart disease, further invasive testing (such as gadolinium-enhancement MRI, coronary angiography, and endomyocardial biopsy) may be required in individual case in order to rule out cardiac disease and establish appropriate management. Sports eligibility is released as follows. The individual is asymptomatic, without cardiac disease and family history for SCD; there is no relationship among PVCs and efforts, and PVCs are monomorphic and not precocious with respect to the previous QRS and T complex.

Non-sustained Ventricular Tachycardia

Non-sustained ventricular tachycardia (NSVT) is defined as three or more consecutive beats of ventricular origin with a heart rate >100 bpm and lasting <30 s. It is an uncommon finding in healthy subjects and requires extensive clinical assessment, including exercise testing, 24-h Holter monitoring, and echocardiography (or other imaging techniques) to rule out underlying cardiac disease. The electrophysiological study should be reserved to selected patients. Sports eligibility is the same as for PVBs, with the need for further clinical assessment every 6 months.

Idio-Ventricular Accelerated Rhythm

It is a focal ventricular rhythm with a heart rate <100 bpm, due to increased ventricular automaticity, frequently secondary to bradycardia. It is generally asymptomatic, disappears during effort, and, in the absence of an underlying cardiac disease, it is not associated with an increased risk of fatal outcome. So, evaluation aims to rule out structural cardiac abnormalities and includes clinical history, physical examination, ECG, echocardiography, and exercise testing. A 24-h Holter monitoring may be useful to precisely define the idio-ventricular rhythm pattern and duration.

In the absence of structural heart disease, sports activity is not contraindicated.

Benign Idiopathic Ventricular Tachycardia

This group includes several different forms of VT of which right ventricle outflow tract tachycardia (RVOTT) and idiopathic left ventricular tachycardia (ILVT) are the most frequent in clinical practice. RVOTT is a cathecolamine-sensitive tachycardia arising from a focal region in the outflow tract of the right ventricle. On the ECG, it is characterized by left bundle branch block QRS morphology and inferior axis. ILVT is a verapamil-sensitive tachycardia often arising from a region along the posteroinferior left ventricular septum, near the left posterior fascicle. On the ECG it is characterized by right bundle branch block QRS morphology and left axis deviation. These two distinct entities are not usually associated with heart disease and are related with an excellent long-term prognosis. When present, the most frequent symptoms are palpitations, fatigue, and dyspnea. Both VTs are usually induced by adrenergic trigger and physical exercise. Considering that a certain degree of overlapping between idiopathic RVOTT and ARVC has been described, it is mandatory to evaluate carefully cardiac structure in order to rule out any underlying cardiac disease. To this regard, a complete clinical assessment including clinical history, physical examination, and echocardiography must be achieved. Furthermore, stress testing and 24-h Holter monitoring are very useful to well characterize the arrhythmic burden in terms of number, morphology, and complexity of VT. In selected cases, an electrophysiologic study may be necessary for the differential diagnosis among benign RVOTT in the context of ARVC and aberrant supraventricular tachycardia. Sports eligibility is quite similar to that used for PVBs, with the need for further clinical assessment every 6 months. Anyway, sports activity with increased risk is forbidden. Catheter ablation is a useful therapeutic option for these VTs. After a successfully transcatheter ablation (freedom from VTs recurrences without antiarrhythmic drugs at least after 3 months of follow-up), the athletes are newly eligible for sports practice.

Malignant Ventricular Tachycardia

Malignant ventricular tachycardias (VTs) include sustained monomorphic ventricular tachycardia, polymorphic ventricular tachycardia, torsades de pointes, and ventricular fibrillation. These VTs are usually associated with acute ischemia, structural heart disease, genetic cardiac abnormalities, severe electrolyte imbalance, and drug poisoning. They lead to hemodynamic deterioration with high risk of cardiac arrest. In young and "healthy" people, they are caused by different pathologic conditions, including hypertrophic cardiomyopathy, ARVC, and congenital coronary anomalies. Affected individuals need a thorough clinical assessment and therapeutic options for SCD prevention. In athletes with documented malignant VT, competitive sports are contraindicated. Exception is represented by ventricular arrhythmias secondary to acute and transient myocardial lesions, such as myocarditis, commotio cordis, acute electrolytic depletion, and drug abuse, when the cause has been completely resolved.

Arrhythmogenic Disorders and Sudden Death

Strenuous exercise in young individuals may precipitate fatal arrhythmias and sudden death, particularly in those with pre-existing structural heart diseases such as hypertrophic cardiomyopathy (HCM), congenital coronary abnormalities, arrhythmogenic right ventricular cardiomyopathy (ARVC), Wolff–Parkinson–White (WPW) syndrome and channelopathies (▶ Sudden Cardiac Death) [2–5].

Sudden death among young athletes is uncommon, ranging from 0.5 to 3 per 100,000 per year. The first cause of athlete deaths is HCM (responsible for approximately one third of the cases), followed by congenital coronary artery anomalies (particularly those characterized by a wrong aortic sinus origin). Channelopathies account for 3% of the global SCD burden in athletes (▶ Sudden Cardiac Death) and are represented by long and short QT, Brugada syndrome, and catecholaminergic ventricular tachycardia.

Long QT syndrome (LQTS) is a congenital disorder characterized by a prolongation of the QT interval on ECG and a propensity to ventricular tachyarrhythmias, which may lead to syncope, cardiac arrest, and sudden death. The QT interval on the ECG, measured from the beginning of the QRS complex to the end of the T wave, represents the duration of activation and recovery of the ventricular myocardium. Long QT interval is defined as heart rate–corrected QT interval (according to the Bazett's formula, QTc) measured in lead II exceeding 440 ms in males and 460 ms in females. On the other hand, considering that a longer QT interval has been reported in elite athletes, a new QTc cutoff $\geq$ 500 ms has been proposed as a modified diagnostic criterion in this cohort of people. Congenital long QT syndrome has been associated with genetically defective cardiac potassium and sodium channels which result in prolongation of ventricular repolarization and predispose to torsade de pointes and ventricular fibrillation. To exclude potential causes of acquired long QT interval, electrolyte depletion (hypokalemia) or chronic intake of drugs capable to prolong repolarization (antibiotics, antihistaminics, etc.) should be first investigated. Athletes with borderline QT lengthening should be evaluated with exercise testing and 24-h Holter monitoring. Genetic testing is mandatory for definitive diagnosis, genotype-related risk stratification, and therapy. Congenital long QT syndrome is a contraindication for any type of sports, even without documented major arrhythmic events.

Short QT syndrome (SQTS) is a congenital disorder characterized by a shortening of the QT interval on ECG and a propensity to ventricular fibrillation, syncope, and/or atrial fibrillation in young patients. Patients with short QT interval are characterized by rate-corrected QT interval < 320 ms. Congenital short QT syndrome has been associated with genetically defective cardiac potassium channels. The possible substrate for the development of ventricular tachyarrhythmias may be a significant trasmural dispersion of the repolarization due to a heterogeneous abbreviation of the action potential duration. Athletes with borderline short QT should be evaluated with exercise testing and 24-h Holter monitoring. Genetic testing is mandatory to achieve the definitive diagnosis. Congenital short QT syndrome is a contraindication for any type of sports, even without documented major arrhythmic events.

The Brugada syndrome is a genetic condition characterized by a peculiar ECG pattern in the anterior precordial leads V1–V3 (ST-segment elevation ≥ 2 mm, with "coved or saddle back type" and negative T wave in same derivation, either spontaneous or induced by pharmacological sodium channel blockade) in association with related arrhythmic events (syncope, cardiac arrest). This syndrome, associated to a sodium channel gene mutation (SCN5A) in 30% of cases, is correlated to a risk of SCD due to malignant ventricular arrhythmias (sustained VT, VF), which usually occur at rest and often at night, as a consequence of increased vagal stimulation and/or withdrawal of sympathetic activity. Increased vagal tone as a consequence of chronic athletic conditioning may eventually enhance the propensity of athletes with Brugada syndrome to die at rest, during sleep, or during the recovery after exercise. Therefore, although no relation between exercise and arrhythmias has been found, subjects with definite diagnosis of Brugada syndrome should be restricted from competitive sports. Whether healthy genetic carriers of the Brugada syndrome without phenotypic expression should be restricted from sports participation is at present uncertain.

Catecholaminergic ventricular tachycardia is a polymorphic ventricular tachycardia (most often with "bidirectional pattern") induced by exercise which can degenerate in ventricular fibrillation. This arrhythmia has been linked to mutations of the ryanodine receptor and calcequestrin genes leading to abnormal calcium release from the sarcoplasmic reticulum. Unlike long QT syndrome and Brugada syndrome, this condition is not associated with abnormalities of the basal ECG and remains unrecognized unless the athlete undergoes exercise testing. Clearly, this condition is a contraindication for any type of sport, even if major arrhythmic events have not been documented.

Clinical Relevance

Several previous data showed that a low-intensity regular physical activity is a healthy habit associated with a reduced burden of atherosclerotic risk factors, coronary artery disease, and mortality. For this reason, competitive athletes are believed to be the healthiest segment of the population. Instead, long-term exhaustive sports practice may lead to an increased risk of cardiovascular events, mainly represented by arrhythmias, with a clinical scenario ranging from mild palpitations to sudden cardiac death. In light of these considerations, when an athlete with symptoms suggestive for cardiac arrhythmias is evaluated, it is pivotal to identify precisely which arrhythmia occurred, to exclude the presence of an underlying heart disease, to evaluate the hemodynamic tolerance during exercise, to select which people are at increased risk of ventricular fibrillation and sudden death, always with a glance to specific type of sport and its intrinsic risk.

In this respect, the European Society of Cardiology [3] recommendations provide a classification of sports according to the physical effort intensity, dividing them into low, moderate, and high. This classification is intended to provide a schematic indication of the cardiovascular demand associated with different sports, with an additional notification of those disciplines associated with increased risk of bodily collision and those associated with an enhanced risk if syncope occurs (which should be avoided in certain cardiac patients).

The Basic Mechanism of Cardiac Arrhythmias in the Athletes

As previously described, arrhythmia occurrence, not only in athletes, depends on the interaction among substrate, trigger, and modulator factors: all these elements are strongly affected by physical training [4, 5]. In fact

Cardiac Arrhythmias. Table 1 Synopsis about cardiac arrythmias in athletes

Arrhythmias	Evaluation	Eligibility and Recommendations
Bradyarrhythmias		
1- Sinus Bradycardia and sinus pauses	History, 24-h Holter monitoring, exercise test, echocardiography	If asymptomatic, no cardiac disease, resolution of block during exercise: eligible for all sports
2- AV block first and second degree, type I		If severe bradycardia (heart rate <40 bpm), sinus pause >3 s and when symptomatic: interruption any sport activity and further diagnostic monitoring
Supraventricular Arrhythmias		
1- Supraventricular premature beats	History, ECG, thyroid function	Absence of structural heart disease, thyroid dysfunction, initiation of sustained arrhythmias, symptoms or therapy: eligibility for all sports
2- Atrioventricular Nodal Reciprocating Tachycardia	History, ECG, electrophysiological study	In order to be eligible for sport activity: catheter ablation
3- Atrioventricular Reciprocating Tachycardia (extra nodal accessory pathway)	History, ECG, stress test, echocardiography, electrophysiological study	In case of risk criteria, symptoms or tachyarrhythmias induction at electrophysiological study: catheter ablation
5- Ectopic atrial tachycardia, atrial fibrillation and atrial flutter	History, physical examination, ECG, echocardiography, stress test and 24-h Holter	Anticoagulation therapy: exclusion from sports. Catheter ablation is requirement for sports eligibility
Ventricular Arrhythmias		
1- Premature ectopic ventricular beats	History (familial history of SCD and symptoms), physical examination, echocardiography, exercise testing, 24-h Holter	If asymptomatic, no cardiac disease, no history of SCD, no relationship among PVBs and efforts, PVBs monomorphic and not precocious: eligible for all sports
2- Non-sustained ventricular tachycardia	History, physical examination, echocardiography, exercise testing, 24-h Holter	Sport eligibility is the same as for PVBs, with the need for further clinical assessment each 6 months
3- Idio-ventricular accelerated rhythm	History, physical examination, ECG, echocardiography, exercise testing, 24-h Holter	In the absence of structural heart disease, sport activity is not contraindicated
4- Benign idiopathic ventricular tachycardia	History, physical examination, echocardiography, exercise testing, 24-h Holter. In selected cases electrophysiologic study	Sport activity with increased risk is forbidden. Catheter ablation is a useful therapeutic option for these VTs
5- Malignant ventricular tachycardia	History, physical examination, echocardiography, exercise testing, 24-h Holter, electrophysiologic study according to underlying heart disease	Competitive sports are contraindicated (exception is represented by ventricular arrhythmias secondary to a cause completely resolved)
Arrhythmogenic disorders and sudden death		
1- Long QT syndrome	History, physical examination, echocardiography, exercise testing, 24-h Holter, genetic testing. In selected cases electrophysiologic study	These conditions are a contraindication for any type of sport
2- Short QT syndrome		
3- Brugada syndrome		
4- Catecholaminergic ventricular tachycardia		

Source : References [3] and [5].

during physical effort, the heart undergoes several structural changes. These physiologic adaptations, called "Athlete's Heart," include structural modifications such as left ventricular hypertrophy, diastolic dysfunction, atrial enlargement, and fibrosis that are associated with intense, long-standing endurance training and permit to satisfy the increased oxygen demand of skeletal muscle during rigorous activity. Intense sports practice typically also affects trigger: the increased incidence of precocious atrial ectopic beats originating from pulmonary veins, a well-known cause for paroxysmal supraventricular arrhythmias, is a common example. Finally, in athletes, a combination of sympathoexcitation, related to effort and competition stress, and high vagal tone at rest occurs, playing a determinant role as modulator factor. In fact, high vagal tone acts by shortening the effective refractory periods and increasing atrial and ventricular dispersion, while adrenergic stimulation can enhance automaticity, modify conduction, and cause afterdepolarization, by membrane potential oscillations as a result of increased Calcium current and Sodium–Calcium exchange.

Treatment

Bradyarrhythmias
These arrhythmias are usually benign, and evaluation may be limited to history, physical examination, and ECG. If asymptomatic and without structural heart disease, treatment is usually not necessary. Sometimes, a deconditioning period of 1–2 months may be useful to clarify the clinical significance of extreme ▶ Bradyarrhythmias. Pacemaker implant is usually reserved for few and selected cases.

Tachyarrhythmias
In the absence of underlying structural heart disease and once the tachyarrhythmia was documented, athlete may become eligible for sports practice after catheter ablation.

Catheter ablation of focal and reentry tachyarrhythmias has become an available and effective therapeutic strategy with high success rate (>95%) and minimum risk of side effects (≈1%).

Lethal complications are very uncommon (<1%) and usually occur when ablation is performed on the left-sided heart. The occurrence of AV blocks is rare (<1%), and limited to ablation of AV nodal reentry tachycardia, para-hisian accessory pathways, and ectopic atrial tachycardia involving the peri-AV nodal region. In athletes, indications for catheter ablation differ from those in the general population, because the procedure is not only aimed to eliminate disabling symptoms, but also to allow resumption of competitive sports activity. When

cardiac abnormalities (which are per se responsible for non-eligibility) are excluded, catheter ablation is recommended in athletes with the following conditions:

- WPW syndrome, either symptomatic or asymptomatic, with evidence of short anterograde refractoriness of the AV accessory pathway and AF/AVRT induction in the electrophysiological study
- Supraventricular reentry tachycardia, either paroxysmal (frequent and sustained episodes with heart rate faster than maximum heart rate by age) or incessant and iterative (with the exception of episodes with slow heart rate)
- Typical atrial flutter, either common or uncommon
- Symptomatic RV outflow ventricular tachycardia or fascicular ventricular tachycardia

Three months after successful catheter ablation, patients can resume competitive sports, after an ECG confirmation of the absence of ventricular pre-excitation in case of WPW syndrome and that they are asymptomatic and without recurrence of tachycardia. Repeated electrophysiologic assessments may be required in selected cases when the outcome of the procedure is considered uncertain.

References
1. Molina L, Mont L, Marrugat J et al (2008) Long-term endurance sport practice increases the incidence of lone atrial fibrillation in men: a follow-up study. Europace 10:618–623
2. Mont L (2010) Arrhythmias and sport practice. Heart 96:398–405
3. Pelliccia A, Fagard R, Bjornstad HH et al (2005) Recommendations for competitive sports participation in athletes with cardiovascular disease: a consensus document from the study group of sports cardiology of the working group of cardiac rehabilitation and exercise physiology and the working group of myocardial and pericardial diseases of the European Society of Cardiology. Eur Heart J 26:1422–1445
4. Pluim BM, Zwinderman AH, Van DerLaarse A et al (2002) The athlete's heart. A meta-analysis of cardiac structure and function. Circulation 105:944–949
5. Maron BJ et al (2007) Recommendations and considerations related to preparticipation screening for cardiovascular abnormalities in competitive athletes: 2007 update: a scientific statement from the American Heart Association Council on Nutrition, Physical Activity and Metabolism: endorsed by the American College of Cardiology Foundation. Circulation 115:1643

Cardiac Energy Metabolism

The processes that allow the transformation of chemical energy into work in the cardiomyocyte.

C

Cardiac Growth

▶ Cardiac Hypertrophy, Pathological
▶ Cardiac Hypertrophy, Physiological

Cardiac Hypertrophy, Pathological

RENÉE VENTURA-CLAPIER
Faculté de Pharmacie, U-769 Inserm,
Université Paris-Sud,
Châtenay-Malabry, France

Synonyms

Cardiac growth; Cardiomyocyte dysfunction; Cardiomyopathies; Failing cardiomyocyte; Heart failure; Maladaptive cardiac remodeling; Marathoners' Heart

Definition

▶ Cardiac hypertrophy can be defined as the growth of the heart due to the enlargement of myocardial cells and hyperplasia of nonmuscular cardiac components. Cardiac hypertrophy is generally a response to pressure and volume overload and sometimes to neurohumoral factors. Clinically, chronic systolic overload of the left ventricle (LV) most commonly results from regional loss of myocardial tissue (myocardial infarction) or elevated impedance to LV outflow (hypertension and aortic stenosis). It occurs in response to diverse pathophysiological stimuli such as hypertension, ischemic heart disease, valvular insufficiency, infectious agents, or mutations in sarcomeric and metabolic genes [1]. Hypertrophy is compensatory when the cardiac growth unables the heart to sustain the increased workload and to normalize LV wall stress. When the stress to the heart is prolonged and exceeds the adaptive capacity, chronic pressure or volume overload induces further remodeling, fibrosis increases, and cardiac hypertrophy becomes maladaptive and even pathological. Pathological ▶ cardiomyocyte growth is associated with an increase in cardiomyocyte death via apoptotic and necrotic pathways which plays a significant role in the transition between ▶ compensated hypertrophy to LV dilatation. This reduces cardiac output so that the heart is unable to pump blood adequately and contribute to the development of ▶ heart failure. Chronic pathological hypertrophy may be deleterious because it decreases the adaptive reserve. It is associated with increased risk for the development of heart failure (HF) and premature death. Heart failure is a clinical syndrome characterized by systemic perfusion inadequate to meet the body's metabolic demands as a result of impaired cardiac pump function.

Basic Mechanisms

In response to stress, the heart hypertrophies to bear the extra load and normalize the pressure. Because very early after birth, the cardiomyocytes cease to divide, cardiac hypertrophy is due to the enlargement of existing cardiomyocytes. In response to pressure overload, the parallel addition of sarcomeres (the contractile unit of the striated muscle) causes an increase in myocyte width, which in turn increases wall thickness. This remodeling results in concentric hypertrophy. On the other hand, volume overload engenders myocyte lengthening by sarcomere replication in series and an increase in ventricular volume. This pattern of eccentric hypertrophy is also initially compensatory, such that the heart can meet the demand to sustain a high stroke volume. In the pathological stages of response to stress, hypertrophy is accompanied by cardiomyocyte dysfunction.

Heart failure is associated with profound remodeling of the cardiomyocyte [2]. Complex changes in gene expression affect all cellular functions, including contractile apparatus composition and regulation, energy metabolism, components of hormonal pathways, and intracellular ion homeostasis. Although some of these switches are at first adaptive and promote a more favorable energetic economy, in the long-term, they may participate in the cardiomyocyte failure. Cellular abnormalities in excitation and contraction include changes at the level of the sarcolemma, sarcoplasmic reticulum, myofilaments, and mitochondria, all of which contribute to depressed contractile function and reserve. At the level of the cardiomyocyte, energy for contraction is mainly produced aerobically by the oxidation of lipids in the mitochondria, and sophisticated energy transfer systems ensure the close matching between energy production and utilization [3]. In response to physiological stimuli as well as during compensated hypertrophy, mitochondrial content increases in proportion to other cell components to maintain an optimal ratio between mitochondria and energy consuming organelles like myofilaments. During progression to heart failure, these adaptive mechanisms become insufficient to maintain oxidative metabolism and cardiac performances. In pathological uncompensated hypertrophy, mitochondrial dysfunction is associated with decreased energy production, increased production of reactive oxygen species, and increased mitochondrial permeability. Together with increased intracellular calcium, these events are key mediators of cardiomyocyte cell death. Decreased mitochondrial biogenesis and mitochondrial dysfunction appear as a hallmark of the failing heart. The energetic unbalance between cardiac work demand and energy production participates in altered calcium handling and contractile dysfunction.

Heart failure is characterized by an augmented energy demand due to the increased load, a decreased energetic efficiency, and diminished energy metabolism leading to energetic imbalance of the myocardium. It is worth mentioning that skeletal muscle is similarly but secondarily affected, explaining the early fatigue of HF patients and their reduced ability to perform aerobic exercise.

Deciphering the causative changes continues to be a challenge. Increases in the production of reactive oxygen species, altered calcium regulation, and impaired energy metabolism are characteristics of heart failure. ▶ Signaling pathways involved in cardiac remodeling depend on the hypertrophic stimuli. They can be classified in two main categories: mechanical (pressure and stretch) or hormonal (renin angiotensin aldosterone system (RAAS), estrogens, adrenergic drive, growth factors) stimuli. The combination of signals varies according to the origin of the cardiac overload. For example, exercise-induced hypertrophy involves stretch signals, growth hormones, and catecholamines will pressure overload-induced hypertrophy mainly activates RAAS, adrenergic and mechanical signals. It is generally accepted that pathological hypertrophy results from activation of calcium-dependent pathways while exercise-induced hypertrophy involves insulin-like growth factor 1 (IGF-1) [4]. Thus, according to the origin of the stress to the myocardium, combination of these different pathways leads to signal specific cardiac remodeling (Fig. 1).

Exercise Intervention

Regular exercise has well-documented benefits in most patients with stable cardiac diseases. It may improve survival, delays the onset of decompensated heart failure, reverses or attenuates pathological LV remodeling, and improves quality of life. Moderate exercise training was shown to improve diastolic function, heart rate variability,

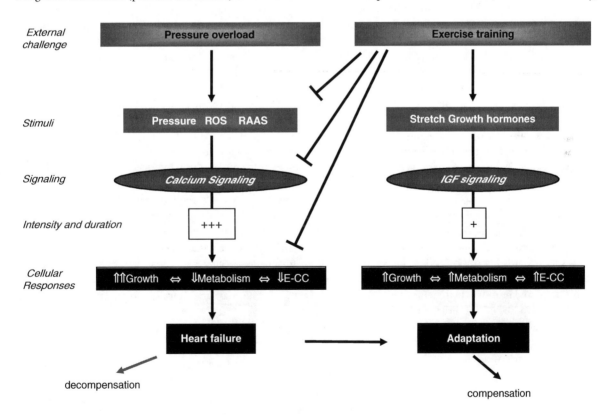

Cardiac Hypertrophy, Pathological. Fig. 1 Schematic representation of processes leading to heart failure and effects of endurance exercise training. *ROS* reactive oxygen species, *E-CC* excitation–contraction coupling, *RAAS* rennin-angiotensin aldosterone system

to decrease the incidence of arrhythmias, and to reduce blood pressure and fibrosis. It is noteworthy that even minimum guidelines for activity (30 min walk most of the days) are sufficient to reduce all-cause and cardiovascular mortality. The large randomized controlled multicentre clinical trial, HF-ACTION, recently demonstrated that a program of recommendation of regular exercise training at moderate intensity is safe, improves quality of life, and reduces the combined endpoint of all-cause death and hospitalization in patients with chronic heart failure [5]. However, the size of beneficial effects was modest compared to results published in smaller single studies and meta-analyses, emphasizing the difficulty in monitoring observance and the importance of compliance with a long-term exercise training program. However, in which patients and at which stages of the pathology regular exercise exerts beneficial effects is not completely established and may depend critically on the underlying cause of HF. Moreover, there are still controversies regarding the level and format of exercise that can yield optimal beneficial effects (resistance vs. aerobic, low vs. high intensity, interval vs. continuous exercise training) and the effects of long-term training remains to be investigated.

While adaptive responses of the skeletal muscle are well known, the adaptive response of the heart is less established. Skeletal muscles adapt to repeated prolonged exercise by marked quantitative and qualitative changes in mitochondria, increased capillary supply, and vasorelaxation. Exercise training is able to oppose the deleterious effects of heart failure on skeletal muscle energy metabolism, atrophy, and contractile dysfunction, although this is less clear for cardiac muscle [3].

If the beneficial effects of endurance training in CHF patients are well established in terms of exercise capacity, quality of life, and even morbi-mortality, there is increasing evidence that it is at least not harmful and may even be beneficial for the failing heart itself. Aerobic exercise in heart failure reduces the level of vasoactive compounds, increases myocardial perfusion and angiogenesis, normalizes sympathetic–parasympathetic balance, decreases oxidative stress, and improves peripheral arterial compliance. Adaptive responses of the heart to endurance training result in bradycardia, improved ventricular function and increased resistance of the heart to ischemic insult. Our knowledge of the molecular pathways involved is still under investigation and relies mainly on experimental studies. It has been shown that aerobic endurance training attenuates ventricular and cellular hypertrophy and consistently restores contractile function, intracellular Ca^{2+} handling, and Ca^{2+}-sensitivity in cardiomyocytes. Exercise training also reverses the abnormal metabolic status

and myocardial energetics of heart failure (Fig. 1). Improvement in energy metabolism involves increased oxidative capacity and fatty acid utilization, improved mitochondrial function, and restoration of energy transfer. This may serve to improve the abnormal Ca^{2+} cycling and inotropy. All these factors participate in the beneficial effects of exercise training on cardiac function mainly by reducing the load to the myocardium and improving perfusion and energy supply, thus re-equilibrating the energetic balance.

The signaling pathways involved in the beneficial effects of exercise in heart failure are currently under investigation. It seems at first paradoxical that exercise training which per se induces hypertrophy and increases cardiac work is able to reverse pathological hypertrophy. This can be tentatively explained by the fact that exercise training lowers adverse hormonal stimulation like RAAS and inflammatory factors while producing the release of growth factors. Indeed, exercise training reduces hormonal overdrive and induces deactivation of the pathological calcineurin/NFAT pathway leading to anti-remodeling effects in HF. This results from the fact that separate genetic and signaling networks may be responsible for the pathological development of the heart and the changes that occur in response to exercise training. This may also explain that the ability to respond to exercise training remains intact despite a pathological phenotype in HF.

In clinical setting, exercise training in heart failure is nowadays considered as a nonpharmacological, nonsurgical, and non-device management intervention that has well-documented benefits. Although beneficial effects of endurance training in heart failure are indubitable, further work is needed to delineate the pleiotropic effects of physical activity on cardiac and skeletal muscle functions. Further research examining the mechanisms of these beneficial effects at the whole organ and cellular levels will be of vital importance to identify potential advantageous effects of pharmacological and physical therapy. Adaptation of training programs to the specificity, seriousness, and duration of heart failure is also necessary.

References

1. Lorell BH, Carabello BA (2000) Left ventricular hypertrophy: pathogenesis, detection, and prognosis. Circulation 102:470–479
2. Katz AM, Konstam MA (2008) Heart failure: pathophysiology, molecular biology, and clinical management. Lippincott Williams & Wilkins, Philadelphia
3. Ventura-Clapier R, Mettauer B, Bigard X (2007) Beneficial effects of endurance training on cardiac and skeletal muscle energy metabolism in heart failure. Cardiovasc Res 73:10–18

4. Bernardo BC, Weeks KL, Pretorius L, McMullen JR (2010) Molecular distinction between physiological and pathological cardiac hypertrophy: experimental findings and therapeutic strategies. Pharmacol Ther 128:191–227

5. O'Connor CM, Whellan DJ, Lee KL, Keteyian SJ, Cooper LS, Ellis SJ, Leifer ES, Kraus WE, Kitzman DW, Blumenthal JA, Rendall DS, Miller NH, Fleg JL, Schulman KA, McKelvie RS, Zannad F, Pina IL (2009) Efficacy and safety of exercise training in patients with chronic heart failure: HF-ACTION randomized controlled trial. J Am Med Assoc 301:1439–1450

Cardiac Hypertrophy, Physiological

OLE JOHAN KEMI[1], ØYVIND ELLINGSEN[2]
[1]Institute of Cardiovascular and Medical Sciences, University of Glasgow, Glasgow, Scotland, UK
[2]Department of Circulation and Medical Imaging, Norwegian University of Science and Technology, Trondheim, Norway

Synonyms

Athlete's heart; Cardiac growth; Exercise training; Marathoners' Heart

Definition

Physiological hypertrophy or ▶ athlete's heart denotes enlargement of the myocardium (heart muscle) in response to exercise. The term physiological distinguishes normal adaptation to exercise from excessive growth associated with pathological conditions like hypertension, valve disease, and heart failure. Physiological hypertrophy typically entails a balanced increase in muscle mass and chamber volume of both ventricles, whereas pathological hypertrophy is either associated with the increase or reduction of ventricular wall thickness relative to chamber volume (concentric versus eccentric hypertrophy). In physiological hypertrophy, cardiac muscle function and pump capacity are increased, whereas pathological hypertrophy is associated with structural changes that eventually impair function (remodeling). Both types of hypertrophy result from increased mechanical loading of the heart muscle and (partially) reverse when the hypertrophic stimulus is removed (or reduced) by detraining or treatment of the pathological condition. In some cases, exercise training may reverse pathological hypertrophy associated with heart failure and significantly improve cardiac function. Physiologic growth of the heart also occurs in response to increased circulatory needs in pregnancy and in the normal stages of development and growth of the body from fetus and newborn through childhood and teenage toward a fully grown-up adult.

The main stimulus of ▶ physiological cardiac hypertrophy is systematic, long-term endurance exercise training. Such exercise training has traditionally been thought to induce eccentric hypertrophy, but involvement of concentric hypertrophy has also been observed in endurance athletes, as well as a higher than expected ratio between wall thickness and lumen diameter. Physiological hypertrophy associates with increased contractility and, as a result, increased pump function. The effect of this is an increased capacity for oxygen transport to skeletal muscles that therefore increases exercise capacity. In fact, the largest magnitude of physiological hypertrophy is generally observed in endurance athletes with a high maximal oxygen uptake (VO_{2max}). Simultaneous effects occurring in these athletes include improved excitation-contraction coupling, larger blood volume that increases central venous pressure, increased myocardial endothelial function and vascularity, and improved metabolic capacity of the myocardial and skeletal muscle. These changes also contribute toward improving pump function and exercise capacity. Also, a common finding of resting endurance athletes with physiological cardiac hypertrophy is bradycardia.

Resistance or strength training may induce concentric cardiac hypertrophy, which has a different induction. Resistance or strength training is characterized by short and powerful exercise bouts that raise blood pressure. During static isometric strength exercise, systolic blood pressure may exceed 220 mmHg, such that this effectively induces a hypertrophy response reminiscent of pressure-overload-induced cardiac hypertrophy, as observed in, for instance, hypertensive patients. Under these circumstances, the cardiac phenotype is characterized by increased ventricular wall thickening, with no changes or reduced lumen diameter.

The different growth responses of the heart in response to different stimuli are schematically shown in Fig. 1.

Mechanisms

For gaining a mechanistic understanding of physiological cardiac hypertrophy, experimental studies of exercising laboratory animals have proven inevitable. These studies have demonstrated that the increased heart-to-body weight ratio is mainly due to cellular changes and in particular, adaptation of the cardiac muscle cell (cardiomyocyte). In very young individuals, this may be caused by cellular hyperplasia, whereas in adult individuals with limited cardiac generative capacity, the evidence suggests that hypertrophy occurs secondary to individual

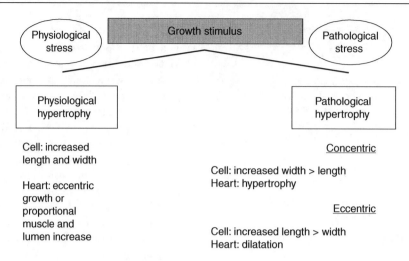

Cardiac Hypertrophy, Physiological. Fig. 1 Schematic of cardiac hypertrophy in response to different stimuli

cardiomyocyte hypertrophy, which involves a pattern of proportional length and width growth but no change in cell numbers [1].

Physiological hypertrophy of the cardiomyocyte in response to exercise training includes both transcription and translation mechanisms, though these may be temporally distinct. First, it has been convincingly and repeatedly demonstrated that both running and swimming exercise protocols activate the phosphoinositide-3-kinase (PI3K)/protein kinase B (Akt)/mammalian target of rapamycin (mTOR) intracellular pathway, an important inducer of physiological hypertrophy. Exercise causes both local and systemic releases of insulin-like growth factor-1 (IGF1), and this stimulates ribosomal protein synthesis by phosphorylation of the p70S6-kinase/ribosomal protein S6 and the eukaryotic translation initiation factor-4E binding protein-1 (4E-BP1) cascades, of which the latter allows eukaryotic translation initiation factor-4E and factor-4G (eIF4E and eIF4G) to combine. These factors increase ribosomal activity and hence stimulate translation of proteins from messenger ribonucleic acids (mRNA). Initiation and regulation of hypertrophy by this signal pathway may be particularly important since the same experiments found no chronic activation of either mitogen-activated protein kinase (MAPK) or fetal genes. In contrast, pressure-overload-induced pathological hypertrophy is characterized by inactivation of the PI3K/Akt/mTOR signal cascade [2], which thus seems to differentiate between physiological and pathological cardiac hypertrophies.

Although MAPK-associated signals may not be chronically activated by exercise training, it has been shown that members of this pathway, such as extracellular-signal-regulated kinases (ERKs), p38 isoforms, and c-Jun N-terminal kinases (JNKs), are transiently increased shortly after exercise training bouts in untrained, but not in trained, individuals. This transient activation may initiate nuclear transcription by the myocyte enhancer factor-2 (Mef2), a well-known regulator of genes that transcribe for cellular hypertrophy. Thus, MAPK activation may facilitate induction, but not maintenance, of physiological hypertrophy.

Several adjacent molecular pathways have been implicated in the control of physiological hypertrophy of the heart [1, 2]. Exercise acutely increases and chronically improves intracellular Ca^{2+} cycling as part of the excitation-contraction coupling, and this activates the Ca^{2+}/calmodulin-dependent kinase II (CaMKII), which subsequently inhibits class II histone deacetylases (HDAC). As HDAC suppresses Mef2, the exercise-induced increase in CaMKII activation will partially abort the Mef2 suppression, and this may chronically increase the transcription of genes that control cellular hypertrophy by coding for hypertrophy-associated proteins. In contrast, some studies suggest that exercise training may modulate gene transcription by reducing the activity of calcineurin and its target, nuclear factor of activated T-cell (NFAT) in the nucleus. Since NFAT activates Mef2, the result would be a reduced activation of Mef2-controlled genes.

The exact role of nuclear gene transcription to induction and maintenance of cardiomyocyte physiological hypertrophy remains therefore incompletely understood, although it is clear that it does contribute at least to some spatio-temporal aspect of cellular hypertrophy. The transcription factor Mef2 also exerts control over several micro-RNAs, which innately suppress mRNA translation by binding and cleaving complementary mRNA strands. This process targets the mRNA pools within the cell and inhibits translation. Exercise training downregulates micro-RNAs 1 and 133, such that mRNA translation may increase.

Mechanisms that maintain the translated proteome may also contribute to maintain cellular hypertrophy. This may include increased heat shock proteins (HSPs) that are activated by stress signals and act as cellular chaperones to protect downstream protein structures. Protease systems and apoptosis-inducing pathways may also be involved; for example, the ubiquitin-proteasome pathway (UPS) is reduced after exercise training.

An overview of signaling mechanisms causing or maintaining physiological cardiac hypertrophy in response to exercise training is provided in Fig. 2.

Exercise Response/Consequences

Although the cardiomyocyte responds by hypertrophy to dynamic endurance exercise, the magnitude of the response may differ according to the intensity and duration of the exercise training program as well as the duration and frequency of the individual exercise sessions. For instance, the response to a program of daily high-intensity exercise training at 85–90% of VO_{2max} is a proportional ~20% increase in the length and width of the cardiomyocyte, which is substantially greater than the response to lower-intensity exercise training. The hypertrophy becomes observable already after a few weeks of exercise training and reaches a plateau after ~2–3 months of daily high-intensity exercise training, although the possibility remains that further hypertrophy may be induced by manipulating the exercise training with respect to

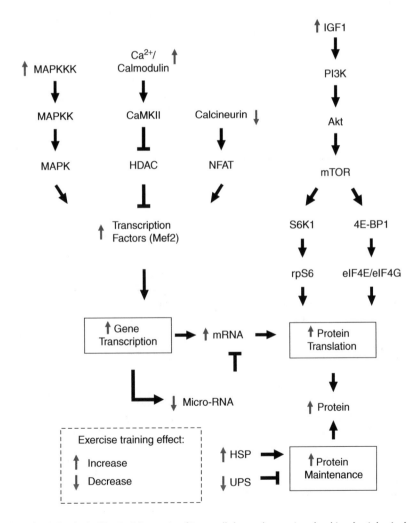

Cardiac Hypertrophy, Physiological. Fig. 2 Schematic of intracellular pathways involved in physiological cardiac hypertrophy; see text for details

intensity or duration. Moreover, in detraining (abortion of regular exercise training), the hypertrophic effect is reversed [2]. The cellular responses correspond closely with whole-heart measurement of organ hypertrophy and also with differential exercise effects on VO_{2max}, indicating that cellular hypertrophy precedes cardiac hypertrophy and that these adaptations contribute to improving exercise capacity.

The dose- and time-response relationships of exercise-induced cardiac hypertrophy as described above have been obtained by experimental animal studies. However, physiological cardiac hypertrophy has been confirmed also in humans by both cross-sectional and longitudinal studies using necropsy, radiography, echocardiography, electrocardiogram, and magnetic resonance imaging techniques [3, 4]. In general, cross-sectional studies of endurance athletes versus untrained control subjects have indicated that resting ventricular end-diastolic volume in male endurance athletes is usually ~150–200 mL, whereas in untrained subjects, the normal value is ~120 mL. Left ventricular muscle mass in the same athletes is generally ~200–280 g, whereas the equivalent in untrained subjects is ~130–180 g. Females present with smaller values but with intact differences between endurance-trained and untrained subjects. However, non-uniform body weights complicate direct comparisons between studies. Nonetheless, the difference between endurance athletes and untrained subjects is mainly attributed to the eccentric hypertrophy and can be explained by the cellular hypertrophy, including magnitude of the hypertrophy by numerically comparing the 10–20% cellular hypertrophy to the left ventricular muscle gain or the 10–20% increased wall thickness observed in athletes, though the increased central venous pressure also contributes. Stroke volume at rest is increased from ~80 to ~120 mL, but because of the bradycardia, cardiac output is normally not increased at rest. However, during maximal endurance exercise, cardiac output in endurance athletes may reach values of 30–40 L/min, well above untrained subjects. This is explained by the greater stroke volume in endurance athletes, as maximal heart rate does not change.

Serial assessments of cardiac size and dimension parameters before and after a program of exercise training also tend to report physiological hypertrophy, albeit the effect size rarely is of the same magnitude as cross-sectional comparisons between endurance athletes and untrained sex- and age-matched subjects. This is not surprising, as most longitudinal studies have limited follow-up periods, small sample sizes, and difficulties obtaining appropriate and therefore unbiased control volunteers.

Diagnostics

Some studies have suggested that exercise-training-induced physiological hypertrophy may transform to a more malignant form of hypertrophic cardiomyopathy, especially after deconditioning and detraining [4], although this remains controversial. Similarly, case reports of a possible association between physiological hypertrophy and sudden cardiac deaths also exist, although this has not been confirmed by more controlled trials. Some earlier reports suggested that physiological cardiac hypertrophy may associate with various disturbances to electrical conduction that may increase the risk of developing arrhythmias. However, such events may be linked to the increased vagal tone that associates with exercise training. Issues such as whether the causes of sudden cardiac deaths, conduction abnormalities, and electrical disturbances are directly or indirectly linked to cardiac hypertrophy, and which populations of athletes may be affected, remain unresolved.

Interventions to target pathological hypertrophy in heart disease have brought evidence that exercise training may have a therapeutic potential for reversing pathological hypertrophy and remodeling [5]. Several studies have demonstrated this possibility, and in a pilot study, 3 months of systematic high-intensity exercise training in NYHA class II–III post-infarct heart failure patients resulted in a reduction of the left ventricular dilatation and mass and an increase in ejection fraction, stroke volume, and systolic and diastolic motion parameters [5]. Albeit a small study, it demonstrates that if targeted to specific patient populations and if appropriately prescribed, exercise training may have the potential to reverse pathological hypertrophy. Experimental studies of rodents with similar post-myocardial infarction heart failure subject to similar exercise training programs have confirmed the ▶ reverse remodeling to a cellular level [2]. In both humans and rodents, natriuretic peptide levels correspond closely with the development and reversal of pathological hypertrophy.

References

1. Hunter JJ, Chien KR (1999) Signaling pathways for cardiac hypertrophy and failure. N Engl J Med 341:1276–1283
2. Kemi OJ, Wisloff U (2010) Mechanisms of exercise-induced improvements in the contractile apparatus of the mammalian myocardium. Acta Physiologica 199:425–439
3. Fagard R (2003) Athlete's heart. Heart 89:1455–1461
4. Maron BJ, Pelliccia A (2006) The heart of trained athletes – cardiac remodeling and the risks of sports, including sudden death. Circulation 114:1633–1644

5. Wisloff U, Stoylen A, Loennechen JP, Bruvold M, Rognmo O, Haram PM, Tjonna AE, Helgerud J, Slordahl SA, Lee SJ, Videm V, Bye A, Smith GL, Najjar SM, Ellingsen O, Skjaerpe T (2007) Superior cardiovascular effect of aerobic interval training versus moderate continuous training in heart failure patients – a randomized study. Circulation 115:3086–3094

Cardiac Output (Q)

The amount of blood pumped by the heart into the systemic circulation per unit of time, most frequently expressed as liters per minute. At rest the cardiac output is approximately 5 L min^{-1}. Maximal cardiac output in young, healthy people varies between 15 and 25 L min^{-1}. In elite endurance athletes maximal cardiac output can reach about 40 L min^{-1}.

Cardiac Preconditioning

▶ Ischemia-Reperfusion Injury, Exercise-Induced Cardioprotection

Cardiac Rehab

▶ Rehabilitation, Cardiac

Cardiac Rehabilitation

▶ Heart Failure, Training
▶ Rehabilitation, Cardiac

Cardiac Transplantation

▶ Transplantation, Heart

Cardioembolic Stroke

A type of ischemic stroke that is a result of a cardiac thrombus dislodging and occluding a vessel within the intracranial circulation.

Cardiomyocyte

The muscle cell of the heart.

Cardiomyocyte Dysfunction

▶ Cardiac Hypertrophy, Pathological

Cardiomyopathies

▶ Cardiac Hypertrophy, Pathological

Cardiopulmonary Exercise Test

An exercise test with the addition of ventilatory gas exchange equipment, often referred to as CPX.

Cross-Referencess
▶ Exercise Electrocardiogram

Cardiopulmonary Exercise Testing (CEPT)

Cardiopulmonary exercise testing is a dynamic, noninvasive, physiologic test which provides a global assessment of the integrative exercise responses involving the pulmonary, cardiovascular, skeletal muscle, hematopoietic, and neuropsychological system. The whole procedure gives the physician the opportunity to evaluate both submaximal and peak exercise responses, thus, providing important information for clinical decision making.

Cross-References
▶ Ergometry
▶ Exercise Testing

Cardiorespiratory Endurance Capacity

▶ Maximal Oxygen Uptake ($\dot{V}O_{2\ max}$)

Cardiorespiratory Fitness

▶ Aerobic Power, Tests of

Cardiovascular System

Body system consisting of the heart, blood vessels, and the circulating blood. It supplies oxygen to all parts of the body and removes waste materials.

Caspase

Cysteine proteases that play a central role in apoptosis, which cleaves its target substrates after aspartate residues (cysteine-dependent aspartate specific protease).

Catabolic

Metabolic reactions that break down molecules into smaller units and releases energy.

Catabolism

Subdivision of metabolism involving all degradative chemical reactions in the living cell.

Catecholamines

NIELS JUEL CHRISTENSEN
Endocrine Research Laboratory, Department of Medicine, Herlev Hospital, University of Copenhagen, Herlev, Denmark

Synonyms
Stress hormones

Definition
▶ Catecholamines are hormones (epinephrine) or neurotransmitters (epinephrine, dopamine, and norepinephrine).

They are derived from the amino acid tyrosine and are therefore relatively small molecules. Epinephrine (E) is primarily a hormone secreted from the adrenal medulla in response to stress like aerobic ▶ exercise. The release is controlled by the nervous system. E is important for mobilization of substrates to working muscles. NE is transmitter in the sympathetic nervous system, which is important for the regulation of blood pressure in response to gravitational stress in the upright position and vascular dilatation in working muscles during exercise.

NE activates ▶ receptors so-called α-adrenoceptors on the cell surface (Table 1). The receptors pass through the cell membrane and activation results in mobilization of Ca^{++} inside vascular smooth muscle cells. Vessels not involved in exercise activity will constrict. NE will also increase heart rate and contraction of the heart by activating β-adrenoceptors on heart muscle cells. Activation of β-adrenoceptors on the cell surface increases cAMP production inside cells.

E is released into the blood stream and it can therefore reach all receptors in the organism except for receptors in the brain due to the so-called blood-brain barrier. Neurotransmitters like NE in the sympathetic nervous system are released from nerve endings close to the receptors on smooth muscle cells. The nerve endings are not in direct contact with the cells and NE may leak into plasma.

E and the sympathetic nervous system are often designated as the sympathoadrenal system, which is functioning largely without control of the conscious mind.

In the brain, all three catecholamines are neurotransmitters. Dopamine in the brain is especially important for regulation of movements, for enjoyment and reinforcement mechanisms, and for regulation of the pituitary gland. Clearly, catecholamines are important for many aspects of exercise regulation.

To understand the relationship between catecholamines and exercise, it is important to know something about methods of measuring NE and E and sympathetic nervous activity (Table 2).

Basic Mechanisms
The increase in blood flow and oxygen delivery to working muscles during aerobic (dynamic) exercise is mediated by an increase and redistribution of cardiac output. NE and E in plasma increase with the intensity and duration of aerobic exercise and the size of the contracting muscle mass [1, 2]. There is a close correlation between the plasma NE concentration and the level of muscle sympathetic nerve activity as measured by microneurography. Several hormones increase during exercise but the relative increase is less than the increase in NE and E, which may

Catecholamines. Table 1 Adrenergic receptors

	α-adrenergic receptors		β-adrenergic receptors	
Subtypes	α_1	α_2	β_1	β_2
Agonists	NE > E	E ≥ NE	E = NE	E > NE
Antagonists	Phentolamine	Yohimbine	Atenolol	
Function	Smooth muscle contraction	Inhibitor of NE release and insulin secretion	Increase in heart rate and contraction	Vasodilatation, glycogenolysis
Second messenger	$Ca^{++} \uparrow$	$Ca^{++} \downarrow$ cAMP $\downarrow$	cAMP $\uparrow$	cAMP $\uparrow$

NE Norepinephrine, *E* Epinephrine, *cAMP* cyclic adenosine monophosphate

Catecholamines. Table 2 Methods of measuring NE and E and the activity in the sympathetic nervous system

1. Quantification of NE and E in plasma, tissue, and in spinal fluid. In specific tissues it is possible to measure amounts of catecholamines present (depots) or the release of NE by microdialysis or by isotope techniques
2. Recordings of muscle sympathetic nerve activity by microneurography (MSNA)
3. Recordings of cardiovascular responses and reflexes in combination with adrenoceptor blockade
4. Recording of specific responses to infusion of catecholamines or agonists in combination with various types of adrenoceptor antagonists
5. Studies of intracellular signaling systems after activation of adrenoceptors (Ca^{++}, c-cyclic AMP, proteins)
6. DNA sequencing to study genetic variants, which may influence exercise performance
7. Quantification of messenger RNA of specific proteins or noncoding RNA, which may influence exercise responses

increase more than 15-fold above basal levels. Furthermore, it is not possible to perform dynamic exercise without an intact sympathetic innervation due to the decrease in arterial blood pressure, when working muscles are dilated. Sympathetic nervous system activity during dynamic exercise is regulated by (1) central command and (2) afferent impulses from working muscles to the central nervous system. The increase in plasma NE during exercise is negatively correlated with the level of mixed venous oxygen saturation and the splanchnic blood flow. In the basal state sympathetic activity is inversely related to plasma volume and cardiac output, and the NE response to exercise may also be increased by volume depletion.

β-adrenoceptor blockade during exercise decreases cardiac output and heart rate and reduces physical performance. Isometric exercise may increase muscle sympathetic activity but to a minor degree and the level is controlled by chemical stimuli especially accumulation of hydrogen ions in working muscles. Increments in plasma E may be relatively high during isometric exercise.

Sympathoadrenal activity plays a major role in mobilization of substrate during exercise. NE decreases insulin secretion by an α-adrenergic mechanism. The decrease in insulin is important for mobilization of lipids especially free fatty acids from fat tissue by sympathetic nerves. This response is mediated by a β-adrenergic mechanism and may in part be regulated by the brain. Furthermore, the decrease in plasma insulin and the rise in plasma E and glucagon increase glucose production in the liver. Finally, E is important for the breakdown of glycogen to lactate in working muscles. Glucose in active muscles is taken up by the so-called alternatively pathway, because insulin levels in the blood are reduced.

Exercise influences ► immunology [3]. Both infusion of E and exercise increase the number of NK-cells in the blood. Severe exercise may, however, results in suppression of the immune system.

Plasma catecholamines especially E is increased by ► training. This is observed even if trained and untrained subjects are examined at the same relative workload. This is due to the development of the so-called sports adrenal medulla.

Exercise Intervention

Exercise and ► aging: We showed many years ago that resting plasma NE concentrations increased with age in normal subjects. This response is due to an increase in the sympathetic nerve activity and not due to a decrease in the degradation rate of NE. The increase may be due a decrease in the responsiveness in the elderly to NE released at nerve endings. NE responses during exercise are also greater in the elderly compared to young subjects. The increase in plasma NE in the basal state and in response to exercise is even greater in long-term smokers as compared with nonsmokers.

Exercise and ▶ mortality: We studied plasma E and NE in a group of 802 subjects 70 years of age with no overt disease and followed them for 7 years. The mortality rate was positively correlated with plasma NE concentrations and inversely correlated with plasma E. The latter mentioned relationship was probably explained by a positive correlation between E and physical working capacity. Furthermore, plasma NE was inversely related to forced vital capacity and to smoking.

Lifestyle interventions and exercise: Public health interventions should help people to remain physically active and abstain from smoking. Exercise is also recommended in weight management of obesity. The effect of exercise on weight reduction is, however, relatively small and should be combined with caloric restriction. In general, these interventions are not very successful probably due to lack of appropriate motivation factors and reinforcement mechanisms.

▶ Cognition performance and exercise: The relationship between exercise and cognition performance is of great interest. Some studies have indicated that exercise and exercise training are associated with improvements in attention and processing speed [4]. Exercise may increase dopamine levels in the brain as suggested in some experiments in animals.

Insulin-dependent diabetic patients and exercise: In these patients, insulin is released from skin depots, and the plasma insulin concentration cannot be reduced by an increase in sympathetic activity. If plasma insulin values are high at the start of the exercise period, mobilization of substrate to active muscles may be attenuated. Blood glucose concentrations decrease to low levels and the patient may develop hypoglycemia.

Exercise and ▶ cardiac arrhythmias: Exercise may induce cardiac arrhythmias due to structural diseases of the heart. Ventricular arrhythmias may be life threatening. Catecholaminergic polymorphic ventricular tachycardia is a genetic disease in subjects with no structural heart disease. It is due to abnormalities in specific genes, which results in cytosolic Ca^{++} overload and ventricular tachycardia. Many patients will respond to β-adrenoceptor blocker therapy [5].

Isometric exercise and shooting: β-adrenergic blockers may be useful during activities, which require accuracy and precision such as shooting. The blockers may reduce muscle tremor and improve performance.

Future experiments: We need to get more information about brain catecholamines and exercise. We also need to get more information about ▶ genetic polymorphism in genes, which are important for cardiovascular performance during exercise (a sports genetic profile) [6].

References

1. Christensen NJ, Galbo H (1983) Sympathetic nervous activity during exercise. Annu Rev Physiol 45:139–153
2. Seals DR, Victor RG (1991) Regulation of muscle sympathetic nerve activity during exercise in humans. Exerc Sport Sci Rev 19:313–349
3. Pedersen BK, Hoffman-Goetz L (2000) Exercise and the immune system: regulation, integration and adaptation. Physiol Rev 80:1055–1081
4. Smith PJ, Blumenthal JA, Hoffman BM, Cooper H, Strauman TA, Welsh-Bohmer K, Browndyke JN, Sherwood A (2010) Aerobic exercise and neurocognitive performance: a meta-analytic review of randomized controlled trials. Psychosom Med 72:239–252
5. Walker J, Calkins H, Nazarian S (2010) Evaluation of cardiac arrhythmia among athletes. Am J Med 123:1075–1081
6. Eisenach JH, Wittwer ED (2010) {beta}-Adrenoceptor gene variation and intermediate physiological traits: prediction of distant phenotype. Exp Physiol 95:757–764

Catheter Ablation

It's an electrophysiological invasive procedure directed to treat certain cardiac arrhythmias through the destruction of small localized areas of heart tissue. It involves the use of flexible catheters inserted into the patient's blood vessels and then advanced towards the heart where high-frequency electrical impulses are used first to induce the arrhythmia, and then to ablate (destroy) the abnormal tissue that is causing the heart rhythm disturbance.

Cation

An ion which carries a positive (+) charge and migrates toward electrodes with a negative polarity (cathode) when a current is applied.

Cell Suicide

▶ Apoptosis

Cell-to-Cell Lactate Shuttle

Proposed by George Brooks (University of California, Berkeley) in 1984, this is the process whereby lactate, which is continuously being formed as the end product of glycolysis, moves from one cell to adjacent cells or into the blood for transfer to other cells throughout the body. Lactate is produced by glycolysis even in the presence of ample O_2 for oxidative phosphorylation, and can move via monocarboxylate transporters (MCT1, MC2, and MCT4) from lactate-producing cells to lactate-consuming cells. The lactate can then be further metabolized as a fuel, or converted to glucose or glycogen depending on the metabolic characteristics of the cell that takes it up.

Cellular Oxidation

▶ Aerobic Metabolism

Cellular Plasticity

A form of plasticity that modifies the cellular stage, structure, and function.

Central Sleep Apnea

A type of sleep-disordered breathing in which the majority of the apneas are due to lack of respiratory drive; commonly abbreviated CSA.

Cerebral Autoregulation

A physiological mechanism by which the blood pressure to the brain is maintained within a relatively narrow range.

Cerebral Hemorrhage

▶ Stroke

Cerebral Infarct

▶ Stroke

Cerebral Palsy

Cerebral palsy is a condition which refers to damage to one or more areas of the brain. It can occur during fetal development, during the birthing process or shortly after birth. The condition is nonprogressive and can impair body movement and muscle coordination. The excessive muscle tone reduces metabolic efficiency during exercise which can result in premature fatigue.

Cerebral Plasticity

The term Cerebral plasticity depicts the ability of the brain to modify its function or structure according to the needs in response to injury or challenge. While neurogenesis (i.e., the formation of new neurons) also occurs in the adult brain, cerebral plasticity mainly is synaptic plasticity. Following Hebb's hypothesis (Donald O. Hebb) that synapses that fire together also wire together, research has shown that synapses that are active when the firing rate of the postsynaptic neuron is high will be strengthened. This will only occur, when many synapses are active at the same time. Otherwise, the change in postsynaptic membrane potential induced by the firing of the synapse will not be sufficient to alter the neurons own firing activity. Synapses that fire "out of tune" will therefore lose their link over time. Those processes are important for everyday learning as well as for reorganization of brain functions following injury.

Cross-References
▶ Neural Plasticity

Cerebrovascular Accident

▶ Stroke

CFTR

The cystic fibrosis transmembrane regulator protein that functions abnormally in cystic fibrosis patients, ultimately leading to the clinical manifestations of CF. The CFTR protein is a cAMP-regulated chloride channel present on the apical surface of different cell types. These include most importantly respiratory epithelial cells and cells lining the exocrine glands, including the pancreas. The CFTR protein also influences movement of sodium and water across respiratory epithelial cells.

Chain-Breaking Antioxidants

Some oxidative mechanisms, especially lipid peroxidation proceeds through propagation reactions depending on the generation of peroxyl radicals. These reactions are produced in lipophilic environments. The chain-breaking antioxidants, which are essentially nonpolar antioxidants, act inactivating the peroxyl radicals, preventing the propagation of the oxidation. Vitamin E is suggested to be the most powerful chain-breaking antioxidant.

Cross-References
▶ Redox Status

Chalone

A biological factor produced in the exact same amount by only one cell type in the body (i.e., liver or muscle cells). When enough of this factor circulates through the body, further growth of cells that produce the chalone is prevented. This is thought to explain why when a portion of the liver is removed the remaining liver grows back at exactly the same size as before the injury.

Change of Direction Speed

▶ Agility

Changes in Brain Capabilities

▶ Neural Plasticity

Channellopathy

Cardiac channellopathy is a type of primary electrical disorder, only recently recognized, which were caused by mutations of genes encoding for cardiac channel subunits that regulate ion currents. Such diseases include long and short QT syndrome, Brugada syndrome and catecholaminergic ventricular tachycardia.

Chemoattraction

The tendency of neuronal processes to grow and extend along a chemical gradient.

Chemokines

A group of chemotactic cytokines classified into four separate families. The main families are the CC group and CXC group, so named based on the position of their cysteine (C) residue, and they include cytokines such as IL-8 and MCP-1. Chemokines act on several transmembrane pass receptors and cause chemotaxis (increased directional migration of cells in response to concentration gradients of certain chemotactic factors) and cell activation of the target cells.

Cross-References
▶ Cytokines

Chemotherapy

Drugs (agents) used to kill tumor cells. These drugs are often used as a single agent (monotherapy) or more commonly in combination with other chemotherapies or cytotoxic agents over a prolonged period of time (3–12 months).

Children Competition Sport

▶ Children, in Competitive Sports

Children, in Competitive Sports

NICOLA MAFFULLI[1], UMILE GIUSEPPE LONGO[2], FILIPPO SPIEZIA[2], VINCENZO DENARO[2]
[1]Centre for Sports and Exercise Medicine, Barts and The London School of Medicine and Dentistry, Mile End Hospital, Queen Mary University of London, London, UK
[2]Department of Orthopaedic and Trauma Surgery, Campus Biomedico University, Rome, Italy

Synonyms

Children competition sport; High-intensity training young athletes

Definition

Children who practice competitive sports may perform intensive training to an intensity and duration similar to an adult athlete. Hence, the effects of the high work imposed to the body of a young athlete have to be known by coaches and medical personnel who deal with athletes of such age group. Cardiovascular, muscular, skeletal, and soft tissues responses to training in children are often discussed. However, concerns about physical and psychological injuries remain, and it is likely that the age of the child and the particular sport could influence the type and intensity of training. Young athletes are not just smaller athletes, and they should not become sacrificial lambs to a coach's or parent's ego. The "not too much and not too soon" rule should apply, although it must be admitted that it remains unclear as to how much is "too much" and how soon is "too soon."

Description

Competitive sport participation has become an established feature of Western society [1–3]. Intensive training and high level competition for several years in sports like gymnastics, swimming, or tennis [4]. The "Catch them young" philosophy is one of the factors which influences the early enlisting of children in competitive training activities.

Self-esteem, confidence, team play, fitness, agility, and strength may be increased in children practicing competitive sport [5]. Also, the age of starting organized sport is decreasing.

Participation in physical exercise at a young age should be encouraged, because of the health benefits it produces. Preventive programs may also decrease the incidence and severity of competitive sports injuries in young athletes, and may produce a long-term favorable economic impact in health care costs. Active prevention measures are the main weapon to decrease the (re)injury rate and to increase athletic performance [6].

Talking about competitive sport in young athlete should bring to mind some questions:

Should young children participate in intensive training and high level competition? Are children involved in intensive training at risk of injuries to their developing musculoskeletal system? Can psychological problems arise from intensive sports participation at a young age?

We will try to answer some of these questions in the present chapter. Physical, cardiovascular and muscular effects, increase in strength, and endurance are an established feature of growth and development and training. The effects of sport participation and training on young athletes have to be separated from those of normal puberty.

A certain amount of physical activity may be required for normal growth, but the minimum needed has not been identified, and the ill effects of intensive training have not been fully clarified. Menarche and menstrual disorders have been studied. The age of achieving menarche, and the incidence and duration of menstrual disturbances in young athletes engaged in intensive training, have been also studied. Menarche is delayed in female athletes engaged in intensive training, who may also experience menstrual irregularities, even though this issue has not been convincingly researched. Genetic influences or nutritional status may have an influence on time of menarche, but they have to be systematically studied [5]. Regular physical activity has no effects on the growth of young male athletes, based on the study of skeletal maturation of young male athletes engaged in cycling, rowing, and ice hockey from 12 to 15 years old.

Athletic potential is another question to be addressed. The response of a given athlete to a particular training regimen seems to derive from an inherited genotype [7]. Training accounts for only approximately 30% in the variance in maximal oxygen uptake (▶ VO_2 max) and maximal force and power of top class competitors, and those young athletes undergoing vigorous training were taller and had less body fat and higher VO_2 max than sedentary controls. In another study, boys engaged in competitive middle and long distance running were compared controls not undergoing intensive training and they had less body fat and lower resting heart rates, larger heart volumes, and a higher VO_2 max relative to body weight and respiratory capacity.

The effects of endurance and sprint training on the vastus lateralis muscles of boys aged 16 and 17 years have been evaluated in another work in which endurance training resulted in a significant increase to type I and HA fiber areas, together with increased activity of some of the enzymes of the Kreb's cycle. On the other hand, sprint-trained boys showed a significant increase in the activity of glycolytic enzymes. Muscular strength trainability in children is another interesting topic. Pre- and post-pubescent children of both sexes can significantly increase their muscular strength by resistance training. The natural increase in strength in boys reaches its maximum only approximately 1 year after the growth spurt, while in girls this occurs during the period of growth spurt itself.

Fatigue syndrome has been described in top class athletes. Hence, intensive training in young athletes may result in staleness. Evidences in this field are lacking. An increased predisposition to viral infections, fatigue from overtraining or combination of physical and psychological fatigue analogous to the "burn out syndrome" have been reported. Sports mediated immune response alterations may play a major role in determining increased susceptibility to infections.

Young athletes undergo increased stress and anxiety in competitions and workout time, and this may be increased by parents, potentially leading to a greater incidence of aggression in the young athletes. These concerns have led to the extreme position of calling for a complete ban on high level competition in preadolescence because of the possible long-term deleterious effects.

The physiological responses to training in children appear to be similar to those found in adults and, in the short term at least, seem beneficial. It should be clear to people dealing with young athletes that children are not just adults in miniature, and they should not be assumed to be able of the same amount and quality of exertion as adults. Adults dealing with highly athletic children must not exploit the youngsters, but maintain the state of health of the children under their care, while helping them to improve their athletic performance. Time is needed for growing children to incorporate their own body changes, and probably little room is left at this critical stage for developing speed, strength, and resistance.

Young Female Athletes

The differences observed in stature between athletes and nonathletes are mainly the result of nature rather than nurture. With regard to pubertal development, the evidence suggests that the tempo is slowed down in some sports, but it has not been yet possible to identify whether this is a result of athletic training. On average, young female athletes from most sports have statures that equal or exceed the median for the normal population. Female basketball players, volleyball players, tennis players, rowers, and swimmers have been shown to have mean

statures above the 50th centile of the reference populations from 10 years onward. However, gymnasts consistently present mean values below the 50th centile, with a secular trend for decreased stature: today's elite female gymnasts are, on average, shorter than girls training intensively in other sports. On average, young female athletes from most sports have statures that equal or exceed the median for the normal population.

Usually, female athletes tend to have body masses that equal or exceed the reference medians. Gymnasts, figure skaters, and ballet dancers consistently have lighter body mass. However, gymnasts and figure skaters have appropriate body mass for their height, whereas ballet dancers and distance runners have low body mass for their height. Although female athletes from a number of sports tend to be heavier than reference populations, they also, in general, have lower percentage body fat.

Successful early adolescent and adolescent athletes (about 12–18 years of age) tend to have, on average, somatotypes similar to adult athletes in their respective sports.

Physique may be of particular importance in aesthetic sports such as gymnastics, figure skating, and diving, where performance scores may be influenced by how the judges perceive the athlete's physique. Maturity differences among young female athletes are most apparent during the transition from childhood to adolescence, and particularly during the adolescent growth spurt. During childhood, the skeletal ages of gymnasts are average or on time for chronological age. As they enter adolescence, most are classified as average and late maturing, with few early maturing girls. In later adolescence, most gymnasts are classified as late maturing. Gymnasts and ballet dancers tend to attain menarche later than the normal population and girls in other sports. Early and average maturing girls are systematically represented less often among gymnasts as girls pass from childhood through adolescence, probably reflecting the selection criteria of the sport, and perhaps the performance advantage of later maturing girls in gymnastics activities. Ballet dancers and distance runners show a similar maturity gradient in adolescence. In contrast, young female swimmers tend to have skeletal ages that are average or advanced in childhood and adolescence.

The smaller size of elite gymnasts is evident long before any systematic training starts, and is in part familial. In our own studies, we have found that gymnasts have parents who are shorter than average. There is also a size difference between those who persist in the sport and those who drop out. Female athletes in volleyball, diving, distance running, and basketball show rates of growth in height that, on average, closely approximate rates observed in nonathletic children [3] which are well within the range of normally expected variation among youth.

There is no good evidence to suggest that training causes changes in anthropometric variables. Available data also indicate no effect of sport training on the age at peak height velocity or the growth rate of height during the adolescent spurt. There are no sufficient evidences that intensive training may delay the timing of the growth spurt and stunt the growth spurt in female gymnasts. Confounding factors should also be considered, such as the rigorous selection criteria for gymnastics, marginal diets, and short parents. Female gymnasts, as a group, show the growth and maturation characteristics of short, normal, slow maturing children with short parents. Even though is not clear whether training may compromise adult stature, studies suggest this association. A short-term longitudinal study in which the adult stature of gymnasts and swimmers was predicted concluded that gymnasts were failing to obtain full familial height. However, decreasing predicted adult height during puberty is a characteristic of slow or late maturation, confirmed by the late onset of menarche in these subjects. Longitudinal data for girls active in sport compared with nonathletic girls are limited, and indicate that there is no effect of training on the timing and progress of secondary sexual characteristics (development of breast and pubic hair). The interval between ages at peak height velocity and menarche (1.2–1.5 years) for girls active in sport and non-active girls also does not differ, and is similar to that of nonathletic girls.

Children' Injuries in Competitive Sports

There is no evidence that intensive training in young athletes may affect either positively or negatively growth and maturation, and the idea that competitive sports may cause growth inhibition effects is still under debate.

Up to 30–40% of all injuries in children and adolescents occur during sports, but the rate of injury is lower in children than in mature adolescents.

The growing musculoskeletal system has typical peculiarities in comparison with the musculoskeletal system of the adult. Tendons and ligaments are relatively stronger than the epiphyseal plate, and considerably more elastic. Hence, in severe trauma, the epiphyseal plate, being weaker than the ligaments, gives way. Growth plate damage is more common than ligamentous injury. Bones and muscles in children present increased elasticity and heal faster. Around the period of peak linear growth, adolescents are prone to injuries because of imbalance in strength and flexibility and changes in the biomechanical

properties of bone. As bone stiffness increases and resistance to impact diminishes, sudden overload may cause bones to bow or buckle. High-intensity training can inhibit bone growth; however, low-intensity training can stimulate it. Up to puberty, muscular strength is similar in girls and boys, and adaptive changes to sport activity have been reported. Growth plate disturbances may result in limb length discrepancy, angular deformity or altered joint mechanics, and marked long-term disability. Also, children produce more heat relative to body mass, have a low sweating capacity, and also tend not to drink enough compared with adults. This may produce heat exhaustion more promptly than in adults, especially if the sport activity is performed in hot climates. This may also result in an increased number of injuries.

After growth spurt, the decrease in flexibility from the relative lengthening of the bone may predispose to injury if stretching exercises before the sport activity are not performed. Evidences show that, in adults, stretching before exercise does not reduce the incidence of injury: it is not clear whether this holds true also in children. Inadequate training devices such as improper footwear may cause an injury. Cross training and gradual change in training schedules is good practice. Players should be matched for body size, athletic ability and biological maturity, and play with appropriate body protection and supervision. Nutrition also plays an important role for success of amenorrhoeic anorexic females. Given their reduced bone mineral density, these subjects are at higher risk of injury. High-resistance training may also predispose children to an increased risk of injury [6].

The epiphysis is located at the end of a long bone. The epiphyseal growth plate is usually called physis in the long bones, and it is a pressure growth plate. The apophysis, on the other hand, is a traction physis, is located at the site of attachment of major muscle tendons to bone, and is subjected primarily to tensile forces. The apophyses contribute to bone shape but not to longitudinal growth. Although a sport injury may involve the apophyseal growth plates, it will not produce disruption of longitudinal bone growth.

Epiphyseal growth plates are mainly subjected to compressive and, at times, shearing forces. The process of endochondral ossification depends on the growth plate health. Growth disturbance can be a consequence of injuries to the epiphyses and their associated growth plates. These are weaker areas, and therefore predisposed to injury.

Young gymnasts and divers are exposed to overuse and acute spinal injuries. The damaging effects repetitive microtrauma and/or acute macrotrauma may be revealed at plain radiography. Damage to the pars interarticularis resulting in spondylolysis or spondylolisthesis, discal pathology, and abnormalities of the vertebral endplates and vertebral ring apophyses of the thoracolumbar spine are example of young athletes injuries.

Spondylolysis or spondylolisthesis are associated with certain types of sport (example in gymnastics and ballet, weight-lifting, wrestling, football, swimming and some light athletics) characterized by extreme hyperextension and rotation of the lumbar spine.

A possible relationship has been hypothesized between back pain and the spinal abnormalities in young athletes. However, there is no evidence about the effects of the long-term effects of spinal trauma in athletes.

There is no definitive evidence about the relationship between acute knee injuries during adolescence and osteoarthritis developed in adulthood and maturity. In a long-term follow-up of young athletes with meniscus surgery, more than 50% of subjects presented knee osteoarthritis.

Anterior cruciate ligament (ACL) injury is common in young athletes, but little is known about the effect of age as a risk factor for ACL injury because of lack of age-related exposure studies. Regardless of management, athletes who suffered an ACL injury usually retire from active sports at a higher rate than athletes without this injury.

Long-term follow-up studies showed that, 12–20 years after knee injury (meniscus or ACL), more than 50% of those injured will experience knee osteoarthritis compared with 5% in the uninjured population. Hence, it is reasonable that proper management of knee injuries in childhood or adolescence may reduce future impairments in sport career of young athletes.

Dislocations in adolescents are typically traumatic. Glenohumeral dislocations are uncommon prior to closure of the growth plate. Recurrence is highly likely given the age of the young athlete and the traumatic nature of injury. Soft tissue injuries are commonly associated with shoulder dislocation, especially affecting the rotator cuff and biceps tendon. An excessive throwing action in sports such as baseball may damage the glenoid labrum. Elbow dislocation is common in gymnastics and football, and can be associated with fractures of the medial epicondyle of the humerus. Also, fractures of the neck of the radius or injury to the median or ulnar nerve may happen.

In young athlete, shoulder dislocations are usually posterior or posterolateral. Emergency reduction is required at all ages, and active rehabilitation encouraged. The return to sport activities is reasonable when the child will have regained full range of movement, likely after 8–12 weeks. A twisting injury of the knee is a common cause of patellar subluxation or dislocation. The typical

mechanism of injury is that the femur is twisted medially with the foot planted on the ground. A direct trauma may also cause dislocation. Patella alta predisposes to patellar instability, and may be accompanied by chronic low-grade knee pain from patellofemoral stress syndrome.

Muscle injuries may occur from a direct blow, sudden explosive action or occasionally from a more trivial action. Quadriceps contusions may cause local muscle bleeds associated with injury. Chronic compartment syndrome may also occur, even in young athletes, typically in runners. Tendinopathy of the lower extremity are common in young athletes. Achilles tendinopathy can be caused by excessive eccentric weight bearing, and tibialis anterior tendinopathy may result from direct pressure in skates or ski boots. Ankle sprains are more common in patients suffering from weak and deconditioned peroneal muscles and cavovarus deformity of the foot. As ligaments in youth are considerably more elastic than in adults, this kind of injuries are well tolerated in lax individuals.

Economical interests in international sports are present even in children. In high level sports, the demand for better performances is constantly increasing, and the diffusion of ► doping even in young athletes is a major problem. Athletes of all ages and levels of competition may use doping to increase their performances. However, adolescents are more likely to be persuaded that drug-taking is necessary to achieve success in sport. Ergogenic aids are now commonly used not only by professional athletes but also by physically active individuals in the normal tasks of daily life. Obviously, the effort to control this dangerous behavior is probably inadequate. Obtaining precise data in this field is difficult. The anti-doping strategy has to be focused and enhanced to eradicate doping in elite athlete through repression measures, and, in parallel, fighting the commercial diffusion of drugs. More research is necessary to devise systems to discover the presence of the always better hidden doping in athletes. Education should focus against the concept that high level sport is made possible only by high sophisticated drugs. The culture of doping in young competitors does not come from the children themselves, but may have its own origin in parents craving for success of their children, and also in their frustrated sport aspirations. Furthermore, some parents unreasonably challenge other parents in a foolish hunger for their own children superiority among their young companions. These "bursting" motivations should come from the children's love for the sport and their natural competition spirit. The motivational role of coaches it is paramount for children involved in competitive sport. Coaches, not pharmacological substances, should be able to nurture the better qualities of the children, rightly directing in the different abilities of youngsters. No "chemical doping" may compete with such a "motivational doping": the history of modern sport is full of such examples.

References

1. Maffulli N, Longo UG, Spiezia F, Denaro V (2011) Aetiology and prevention of injuries in elite young athletes. Med Sport Sci 56:187–200
2. Maffulli N, Longo UG, Gougoulias N, Caine D, Denaro V (2011) Sport injuries: a review of outcomes. Br Med Bull 97:47–80
3. Maffulli N, Longo UG, Spiezia F, Denaro V (2010) Sports injuries in young athletes: long-term outcome and prevention strategies. Phys Sportsmed 38:29–34
4. Malina RM, Meleski BW, Shoup RF (1982) Anthropometric, body composition, and maturity characteristics of selected school-age athletes. Pediatr Clin North Am 29:1305–1323
5. Lippi G, Longo UG, Maffulli N (2010) Genetics and sports. Br Med Bull 93:27–47
6. Maffulli N, Helms P (1988) Controversies about intensive training in young athletes. Arch Dis Child 63:1405–1407
7. Astrand PORK (1986) Textbook of work physiology, 3rd edn. McGraw-Hill, New York

Children, Obesity

▶ Obesity in Children

Children, Principle Components of Motor Fitness

B. HANDS
Institute for Health and Rehabilitation Research, University of Notre Dame, Fremantle, Australia

Synonyms

Motor competence; Motor performance; Skill-related fitness

Definition

▶ Motor fitness is one aspect of the multidimensional construct of physical fitness which is defined as a "set of attributes that people have or achieve that relates to the ability to perform physical activity" ([1], p. 129). The components of motor or skill-related fitness are important for successful performance in all sports and motor skills and include movement control factors of ▶ balance and ▶ coordination, and force production factors of ▶ agility, ▶ power, ▶ speed, and ▶ reaction time. These are distinct from, but interrelated to, the health-related fitness components of cardiovascular fitness, muscle strength, muscle endurance, flexibility, and body composition.

Characteristics

Children's physical fitness and response to exercise is different from adults. Physical fitness has a strong genetic base; therefore, hereditary factors, which affect a person's physiology and rate of maturation along with age, are the major influences in childhood. Measurable changes in fitness will occur in children with normal growth and maturity regardless of external influences, such as opportunity to exercise. Further, there is considerable variation in the timing and tempo of children's growth spurts; therefore, large interindividual physical differences exist between children of the same chronological age. Maturity associated variation can be observed in grouping children by chronological age. Similarly, age differences will be evident in grouping children by stage of development of secondary sex characteristics (e.g., the Tanner stages). For example, two children both aged 11 years will significantly differ in height and weight as well as many motor fitness variables. It is therefore inappropriate to compare fitness components between children of the same chronological age or to predict fitness measures at a later age based on an earlier measure. The complexity resulting from different physiologic patterns and rates of change is further compounded to a lesser degree among children than adults by environmental influences such as physical activity levels or exercise training.

The components of motor fitness variables are strongly interrelated. For example, a child who is agile may also have good coordination, power, speed, and reaction time. In general, those with higher motor fitness will be able to learn faster and perform better in a wider range of skills. The flow on effects of high motor fitness are extensive, and include greater confidence and self-efficacy, and an increased likelihood of being physically active. In contrast, individuals with low motor fitness are more likely to avoid, or withdraw from, participation in many activities.

Motor fitness components or attributes can be measured by laboratory or field-based tests, some examples are shown in Table 1. Many of these tests are routinely included in existing physical education programs, fitness batteries, or motor proficiency tests [2]. To achieve accurate, valid, and reliable test results, children need to be given clear and appropriate information, have an opportunity to practice the test, and be instructed with specific cues, as lack of experience can adversely affect results. Motor fitness test results assist us to identify strengths and weaknesses in children's skill performances; however,

Children, Principle Components of Motor Fitness. Table 1 Common field tests of motor fitness components

Fitness component	Field tests	Important for effective performance in …
Agility	4 × 10 m shuttle run Zigzag run Illinois agility run *T*-test	Rugby, netball, martial arts, tennis
Balance	Stork stand test Line or beam walk	Gymnastics, ballet, diving
Coordination	Alternate hand wall toss test Most of the agility tests	Tennis, baseball, hockey, soccer, juggling
Power	Vertical jump Standing long jump test Seated ball throw	High jump, long jump, shot put, discus, javelin, cycling, rowing, water polo
Reaction time	Ruler drop test	Sprint starts
Speed	30 m sprint 8 s run Swimming 50 m sprint	Sprints, swimming, cycling, basketball

results need to be interpreted in the context of the child's age, physical maturity, and movement experience. In general, the prime focus for children and adolescents needs to be on developing efficient movement techniques, particularly in the preadolescent stages, when movement patterns are being established.

The specific motor fitness components are:

Movement Control Factors
Balance and coordination are particularly important in young children when they are developing mastery of fundamental movements such as running, hopping, and skipping.

Balance
Balance is the ability to maintain equilibrium when stationary or moving and is important in most motor skills. Balance is achieved through the coordinated input from the sensory functions (eyes, ears, and the proprioceptive organs in our joints). There are two types of balance which are quite distinct from each other: static balance and dynamic balance.

Static balance is the ability to maintain equilibrium or retain the center of mass above the base of support in a stationary position, such as standing on one leg or maintaining a handstand. This ability is vital in activities such as gymnastics, ballet, diving, and sports such as wrestling in which the athlete tries to destabilize their opponent. Dynamic balance is the ability to maintain balance while on a moving surface or in motion, such as

hopping, walking along a line, running, or performing a gymnastics routine.

Balance performance can be quite task specific and generally improves with age (preschool to adolescence) and physical maturity. Body structure and factors such as foot length or width are considerations. In growing children, body proportions may change very quickly, which moves the center of gravity and therefore affects balance.

When young, children rely heavily on visual information to maintain balance. By the age of 7–10 years (earlier in females than males), the child is able to integrate information from the proprioceptive system (vestibular apparatus, muscle spindles, Golgi tendon organs, joint receptors) with visual information to inform their balance.

Coordination
Coordination involves the movement of body segments in specific time and space-based patterns in a controlled and accurate manner. It also refers to the integration of sensory information to inform hand-eye and foot-eye movements and is important in a wide variety of games and sports. A highly coordinated person is able to effectively combine a range of different skills into a fluid routine.

Coordination in children is affected by changes in body proportions during growth spurts, for example the ratio between leg and trunk length. These changes alter the biomechanics of simple movements that may have been previously performed in a coordinated manner but now appear clumsy and uncoordinated. The center of gravity of young children is also relatively higher than adults which may affect their ability to move and stop quickly.

Force Production Factors

Agility, power, speed, and reaction time become more important after children have become proficient in fundamental movement skills.

Agility

Agility is the ability to change the direction and position of the body in an efficient and effective manner while moving. It is a combination of coordination, power, balance, and speed [3] and is important in games and sports that require the participant to change direction rapidly in a controlled manner, particularly in an open and changing environment.

Power

Power is the rate at which one can generate maximum muscular force in the shortest time and requires both muscle speed and force. An effective combination of speed and power enables the athlete to produce explosive movements such as jumping, discus throwing, putting a shot, tumbling, or vaulting.

Speed

Speed is the ability to move the body or part of the body quickly in a short period of time. For example, a sprint in running or swimming, a penalty kick in soccer, a baseball pitch, stealing a base in softball. In children, running speed increases with age peaking around 14–15 years for girls and 17 years for boys [4].

Reaction Time

Reaction time is the time that elapses between a person being stimulated to move (receiving a stimulus) and initiating a movement in response. For example, this could be the time between the gun firing to start a sprint race and the body starting to move off the starting block. The stimulus could be received from any sensory system, such as, vision (the ball or position of opponents), hearing (start gun, calls from teammates) or proprioception (body position). Reaction time is important in many play and sporting situations such as avoiding an obstacle in one's path, catching a thrown or hit ball, choosing to shoot rather than pass a basketball, a tennis volley, table tennis, or most martial arts.

Simple reaction time is considered biologically fixed, although choice reaction time can be improved with practice and training. Generally, children react more slowly to stimuli than young adults, but improve with age and experience.

Clinical Relevance

- Motor fitness is an important consideration when assessing or developing overall athletic performance in children and adolescents and is largely based on the maturity of their physiological system. The preferred method to compare children with each other or to norms is to use growth or developmental stage rather than chronological age.
- Outcomes of motor fitness measures are dependent on age and physical maturity.
- Regular participation in physical activity is important to develop motor fitness. Movement programs should provide opportunities to improve all aspects of physical fitness in children and adolescents.
- Motor fitness variables are interrelated and the development of one attribute may have a flow on effect to another. For example, improving muscle power and strength may improve agility and speed.

References

1. Casperson CJ, Powell KE, Christenson GM (1985) Physical activity, exercise and physical fitness: definitions and distinctions for health-related research. Public Health Rep 100:126–131
2. Castro-Pinero J, Artero EG, Espana-Romero V, Ortega FB, Sjostrum M, Suni J et al (2010) Criterion-related validity of field-based fitness tests in youth: a systematic review. Br J Sports Med 44:934–943. doi:10.1136/bjsm.2009.058321
3. Ortega FB, Ruiz JR, Castillo MJ, Sjostrom M (2008) Physical fitness in childhood and adolescence: a powerful marker of health. Int J Obes 32:1–11
4. Payne VG, Isaacs LD (2011) Human motor development: a lifespan approach, 8th edn. McGraw Hill, New York

Cholesterol

Is a complex multicyclic organic molecule whose rigid ring structure provides a structural rigidity to phospholipid membranes by insinuating itself between the PLs. It is also the structural building block for steroid molecules and bile salts.

Cross-References

▶ Lipoproteins

Chondroprotection

Interventions designed to prevent articular cartilage damage, protect the cartilage and slow its deterioration, or repair degenerative cartilage conditions.

Chronic Heart Failure

Stabilized heart function to meet essential systemic demand.

Cross-References

▶ Heart Failure, Training

Chronic Mental Illness

▶ Psychiatric/Psychological Disorders

Chronic Mountain Sickness

Mountain sickness is caused by the lack of O_2. The partial pressure of O_2 (pO_2) declines at an altitude proportional with the barometric pressure as a whole. Thus, the pO_2 of dry air is 100 mmHg at 4,750 m compared to 160 mmHg at sea level. While "Acute Mountain Sickness" (AMS; symptoms: nausea, dizziness, insomnia, headache, dyspnea, tachycardia, pulmonary and cerebral edema) occurs immediately at high altitude, "Chronic Mountain Sickness" (CMS; also known as "Monge's Disease" after its first description by Carlos Monge in 1925) can develop after years of altitude residence, both in natives or in sojourners. Most cases of CMS are seen at over 3,000 m. The pathogenesis of CMS is not fully understood. However, preexisting pulmonary insufficiency, cardiovascular disorder or other diseases that are worsened by inspiratory hypoxia are obviously involved, because only a certain percentage of people living at high altitude suffer from CMS. Severe CMS is characterized by dyspnea, erythrocytosis (high hematocrit), pulmonary hypertension, right heart hypertrophy, and, eventually, congestive heart failure. The arterial O_2 saturation is lowered. The erythrocytosis results from increased erythropoietin production, since this hormone is synthesized in dependence of the O_2 supply of the tissue. The erythrocytosis is associated with an increased blood viscosity, an uneven blood flow through the lungs, and an increased heart burden. In addition, the hypoxia due to the low inspiratory pO_2 causes pulmonary arteriolar constriction, which is the main reason for pulmonary hypertension. In the long term, there is a malorganization of the segments of the pulmonary artery. The afflicted persons suffer from breathlessness, cyanosis, palpitations, headache, dizziness, tinnitus, sleep disturbance, fatigue, and anorexia. Clinical laboratory findings are blood hemoglobin values >200 g/L, hematocrit >0.65, and arterial O_2 saturation <85%. The symptoms will diminish upon descent from altitude and the hematocrit return to normal within about 1 month. Patients who reascent to high altitudes will develop CMS again. Although bloodletting is sometimes proposed as an acute therapeutic option, good clinical practice should aim at restoring the primary alterations of pulmonary, cardiovascular, and renal functions.

Cross-References

▶ Acute Mountain Sickness

Chronic Obstructive Pulmonary Disease

A. R. Koczulla[1], K. Kenn[2], R. Bals[1], C. Franz Vogelmeier[1]
[1]Dept. Pulmonology, University Giessen and Marburg, Marburg, Germany
[2]Klinikum Berchtesgadener Land, GmbH & Co. KG, Prien am Chiemsee, Germany

Synonyms

Endurance training; Exercise training; Muscle training; Rehabilitation therapy in COPD; Strength training

Definition

Exercise training is a part of rehabilitation therapy and the best available therapy for improving muscle function in ▶ COPD. Exercise training contains of endurance and strength training. Strength training is the use of resistance to muscular contraction. Endurance training is the act of deliberation to increase stamina and endurance. A special form of endurance training is interval training which has equal training effects as compared with conventional high-intensity endurance training. Interval training is defined as intensive training, followed by periods of rest.

The exercise training program should be adapted to the patient's limitations and should be, therefore, individually tailored.

Characteristics

Chronic obstructive pulmonary disease is a preventable and treatable disease with some significant extrapulmonary effects (Table 2) that may contribute to the severity in individual patients. Its pulmonary component is characterized by airflow limitation that is not fully

Chronic Obstructive Pulmonary Disease. Table 1 Severity grading of COPD

I: mild	II: moderate	III: severe	IV: very severe
• $FEV_1/VC < 70\%$	• $FEV_1/VC < 70\%$	• $FEV_1/VC < 70\%$	• $FEV_1/VC < 70\%$
• $FEV_1 \geq 80\%$ pred	• $50\% \geq FEV_1 < 80\%$ pred	• 30% pred $\geq FEV_1 < 50\%$	• $FEV_1 < 30\%$ pred or $FEV_1 < 50\%$ plus chronic respiratory failure
Avoiding of risk factors; influenca vaccination, short acting ß-agonists on demand			
Long acting ß-agonists/anticholinergic drugs, rehabilitation			
Accessory inhalative steroids			
Oxygene supplemention therapy at chronic respiratory failure			
Surgical therapy if necessary			

FEV_1 forced expiratory volume in one second, *FVC* forced vital capacity, respiratory failure: arterial pressure of oxygene (PaO_2) less than 8.0 kPa (60 mmHg) with or without arterial partial pressure of CO_2 greater than 6.7 kPa (50 mmHg) while breathing air at sea level

Chronic Obstructive Pulmonary Disease. Table 2 Systemic COPD affection

• Skeletal muscles   • Central nervous system
– Muscle weakness   – Depression
– Muscle atrophy   • Skeletal involvement
• Human body   involvement
– Weight loss   – Osteoporosis
– Cachexia   • Endocrinological involvement
• Heart and circulation   – Dysregulation of hormones
– Coronary heart failure

reversible. The airflow limitation is usually progressive and associated with an abnormal inflammatory response of the lung to noxious particles or gases.

The COPD severity grading and the recommendations regarding therapy are listed in Table 1.

COPD is a lung disease that is characterized by inflammation of the small airways and destruction of the alveolar region resulting in airflow limitation and hyperinflation that are usually progressive. In addition, extrapulmonary effects may occur like cachexia, cardiovascular disorders, muscle atrophy, osteoporosis, depression, and hormone dysregulation (Table 2) [1, 2].

COPD currently ranks as the fourth leading cause of death in the United States and the fifth leading course of death in the world. The death rate for COPD has increased in the recent years despite decreases in the death rates for three other leading causes of death in the United States (heart diseases, malignant neoplasms, and cerebrovascular diseases).

The most important factor in the pathogenesis of COPD is believed to be inflammation of the small airways

caused by the inhalation of inhaled particles and gases. As has been shown in histopathologic studies evaluating small airways of patients with different severities of COPD [3], inflammation is to be found in early stages of the disease and worsens with increasing severity. It is thought that the inflammation causes pathologic changes in the lung tissue by two major mechanisms: production of reactive oxygen metabolites and disturbance of the physiologic protease–antiprotease balance. As a consequence of the inflammation, mediators and cytokines may spill over from the lung tissue into the circulation and thereby affect other organs including peripheral and respiratory muscles. The pathogenetic basis of muscle dysfunction and loss of muscle mass associated with COPD are not well understood. Studies with biopsies from the quadriceps muscle show a significant loss of type I fibers and a relative increase of type II fibers. Microscopically, these muscles show increased apoptosis and oxidative stress as well as inflammatory changes. Further, it could be shown that fiber cross-sectional areas and the capillary contacts to the fiber cross-sectional area are decreased in the course of COPD disease. Muscle metabolic capacity is significantly impaired in COPD patients, and exercise training leads to rapid decline in intracellular pH of the muscle of COPD patients which leads to increasing weakness.

Pulmonary comprehensive rehabilitation is an established mode of treatment for patients with COPD. Rehabilitation programs comprise of education, physical training, psychological support, dietary measures, smoking cessation, and physiotherapy. Rehabilitation is the intervention with the largest effect observed so far regarding health status and exercise capacity in COPD patients [2, 4]. An important part of rehabilitation is physical training.

The combination of endurance training and strength therapy is probably the best strategy to improve peripheral muscle dysfunction and endurance in COPD.

Strength therapy improves muscle mass and strength and induces usually less ▶ dyspnea than endurance training making this training form easier to tolerate.

Endurance training is most commonly performed as cycling or walking. Optimally, patients should exercise for a long time with high intensity. As this is difficult to achieve in most patients with higher degrees of COPD because of limiting dyspnea and fatigue on exertion, interval training can be performed as an alternative, i.e., patients are asked to exercise shorter, but do several sessions that are separated by periods of rest.

Measurements/Diagnostics

Before starting the training therapy, the following diagnostic measurements are recommended: history, physical examination, lung function test, blood gas analysis (capillarized blood), exercise stress test measured by electrocardiogram (ECG), and a 6-min walk test or shuttle walk test.

As many COPD patients are limited by dyspnea and muscle weakness, the exercise training program should be adapted to the patient's limitations and should, therefore, be individually tailored to achieve training goals like control of symptoms, increasing endurance capacity in order to perform activities of daily living (adl) (including work), improving quality of life, and overcoming social isolation.

Strength and endurance training and as special endurance training modality interval training are very important training features. Endurance training is more effective with high intensity compared with moderate or low intensity. Interval endurance training is better tolerated by patients with severe COPD and has equal training effects as compared with conventional high-intensity endurance training. The optimal duration of exercise training has not been sufficiently investigated so far. Studies show that programs with longer training sessions seem to be more effective. Exercising three times per week for a minimum of 4 weeks for at least 30 min per session was effective, but continued training beyond the 4-week period seems to be worthwhile [4].

The training should be of high intensity. This is defined as the intensity that leads to increased blood lactate levels in healthy controls. Patients with respiratory insufficiency often have elevated lactate levels at rest. Therefore, the use of a dyspnea score like the Borg scale may be useful (Table 3). A reasonable target dyspnea intensity is four to six on the Borg scale. A combination of endurance and strength training is recommended.

Chronic Obstructive Pulmonary Disease. Table 3 Borg dyspnea scale

0	Nothing at all
0.5	Very very slight (just noticeable)
1	Very slight
2	Slight
3	Moderate
4	Somewhat severe
5	Severe
6	
7	Very severe
8	
9	Very very severe (almost maximal)
10	Maximal

Upper and lower extremities should be utilized. Treadmill and stationary cycle ergometer are standard devices for endurance training. For upper limb endurance training, arm ergometers may be used. A target heart rate (HR) of 60–80% of the maximum HR is recommended for the arm ergometer or arm cycling without weights. The oxygen saturation should be above 80%. Three to five units per week should be performed. For the lower limb walking, nordic walking, running, treadmill, and bicycle ergometer are recommended exercises. The HR target value should be also 60–80% of the maximal HR and the oxygen saturation above 80%. Three to five units per week with a minimal duration of 30 min. Intensity should be increased stepwise by 5% every five units. Patients with mild to moderate COPD are recommended to exercise beyond the anaerobic threshold, meaning above >80% of the maximum HR.

Free weights, elastic bands, exercise machines, or special isometric exercises without devices are possible for strength training. For the upper limbs elevation against gravity with or without weights are possible training exercises. Using the exercise machine Mm, biceps/triceps training with two to three series and 12–20 repetitions or cycles of 60 s is recommended. The start weights should be weights with 30–50% of the repetition maximum. A stepwise increase after every fifth training unit with ca. 5%.

For the lower limb, M. quadriceps not machine-guided exercises improve coordination and stability better than exercise machine-guided training.

Leg curls using the exercise machine should contain two to three series with 12–20 repetitions. The weight should be stepwise increased. Five percent every five units is a recommended weight increase.

Patients who require oxygen supplementation at rest should perform their training with oxygen insufflation but may need higher flow rates than at rest. It could be shown that supplemental oxygen leads to an improved exercise tolerance. If patients become only hypoxemic during exercise, they should also receive supplemental oxygen therapy to keep SO_2 above 80 mmHg. Even nonhypoxemic COPD patients may benefit from supplemental oxygen therapy.

Noninvasive positive pressure ventilation (NPPV) reduces breathlessness and increases exercise tolerance during exercises. Reasons for the increase in exercise tolerance may be the reduction of the respiratory muscle load. Carefully selected patients may benefit from NPPV therapy during exercise training. Exercise therapy of these patients should be observed by a physician [5]. Training therapy response of COPD patients can be performed with diagnostic tools like history, physical examination, questionnaires like the St. George's Respiratory Questionnaire (SGRQ), 6-min walk test, shuttle walk test, exercise stress tests, and spiroergometry.

In a 7-year follow-up, it could be shown that COPD patients undergoing pulmonary rehabilitation programs did not show significant worsening in exercise tolerance, dyspnea, and HRQL. This could be explained by increases in fat-free mass, the fiber cross-sectional areas, and the capillary contacts. Endurance training therapy increases furthermore the oxidative enzyme capacity and decreases the lactic acidosis and the intracellular pH.

Evidence is growing that rehabilitation therapy including training therapy has a large impact on the COPD disease course and also reduces health care costs.

References

1. Fabbri LM, Luppi F, Beghe B, Rabe KF (2008) Complex chronic comorbidities of COPD. Eur Respir J 31(1):204–212
2. Vogelmeier C, Buhl R, Criee CP, Gillissen A, Kardos P, Kohler D, Magnussen H, Morr H, Nowak D, Pfeiffer-Kascha D, Petro W, Rabe K, Schultz K, Sitter H, Teschler H, Welte T, Wettengel R, Worth H (2007) Guidelines for the diagnosis and therapy of COPD issued by Deutsche Atemwegsliga and Deutsche Gesellschaft fur Pneumologie und Beatmungsmedizin. Pneumologie 61(5):e1–e40
3. Hogg JC, Chu F, Utokaparch S, Woods R, Elliott WM, Buzatu L, Cherniack RM, Rogers RM, Sciurba FC, Coxson HO, Pare PD (2004) The nature of small-airway obstruction in chronic obstructive pulmonary disease. N Engl J Med 350(26):2645–2653
4. Nici L, Donner C, Wouters E, ZuWallack R, Ambrosino N, Bourbeau J, Carone M, Celli B, Engelen M, Fahy B, Garvey C, Goldstein R, Gosselink R, Lareau S, MacIntyre N, Maltais F, Morgan M, O'Donnell D, Prefault C, Reardon J, Rochester C, Schols A, Singh S, Troosters T (2006) American Thoracic Society/European Respiratory Society statement on pulmonary rehabilitation. Am J Respir Crit Care Med 173(12):1390–1413
5. Ambrosino N, Strambi S (2004) New strategies to improve exercise tolerance in chronic obstructive pulmonary disease. Eur Respir J 24(2):313–322

Chronotropic Incompetence

Deficit of increase of heart rate (sinus heart rhythm) in response to various physiologic stimuli like for instance physical exercise.

Chronotropic Response

Increase of heart rate (sinus heart rhythm) in response to various stimuli like for instance exercise.

Cinderella Hypothesis

Motor units with low activation threshold will be activated from early to late without sufficient rest periods and this may result in metabolic overload and subsequent pain perception.

Circadian Rhythms

Refer to the systematic fluctuations in physiological functions that recur over a 24-h period. These changes are normally in harmony with the alternations between sleep and wakefulness but are disrupted during sleep loss, operating on nocturnal shift work schedules or traveling across multiple meridians. The malaise that results from desynchronization while "body clock" time is out of harmony with local time in the new environment is known as jet lag. Normally, it takes about one day per time zone crossed for the normal rhythm to be restored but the time taken is usually shorter after a flight to the west than following an eastward flight. The site of the body clock is a cluster of paired groups of cells in the hypothalamus known as the suprachiasmatic nuclei. These cells have receptors for the hormone melatonin which is secreted by the pineal gland and is suppressed by light. The hormone is responsive to darkness when its actions prepare the body for sleep. The retinohypothalamic tract and the intergeniculate leaflet provide neural pathways for transmission of photic and non-photic signals from the retina to these time-keeping cells which are in turn connected by multisynaptic pathways to the pineal gland. A number of time-keeping genes have been identified from microbiological studies, some of these evident in peripheral tissues. The endogenous rhythm is a result of the interaction of clock genes and clock proteins. The natural period of the endogenous rhythm in isolated or free-running conditions is about 25 h (hence circa diem). In addition to light and melatonin, exogenous factors that set the period to an exact agreement with the light–dark cycle are environmental temperature, physical activity, the timing of meals, and social factors. Heat loss is promoted by the vasodilatory effects of melatonin, and the rhythm in core body temperature that results conforms to a classical cosine function. Due to its large endogenous component, the body temperature curve is used as a marker of circadian rhythms. Many measures of human performance correspond to the curve of body temperature.

Citric Acid Cycle

Citric acid cycle (also known as Krebs cycle or tricarboxylic acid cycle) is a cyclic (i.e., ends at the compound it started from) metabolic pathway that converts the acetyl group to carbon dioxide and hydrogen atoms, taking place in the mitochondria. The primary function of the citric acid cycle is to generate electrons for the electron transport chain, where energy (i.e., ATP) is produced when electrons along with hydrogen atoms are transferred to oxygen. Although oxygen does not directly participate in the reactions of the citric acid cycle, this compound is required for the regeneration of the electron carriers NADH and $FADH_2$ and thus the operation of the pathway. Citrate synthase and succinate dehydrogenase are two enzymes of this pathway catalyzing reactions 1 (conversion of oxaloacetate to citrate) and 7 (conversion of succinate to fumarate), respectively, which have been widely used as read outs for aerobic metabolism adaptations to exercise.

Cross-References
▶ Aerobic Metabolism

Classic Model

A type of periodized training model where the intensity starts off light and the volume low and progresses over time to high intensity and low volume workouts.

Claudication Onset Time

The walking time at which patients first experience leg pain during a treadmill test.

Climacteric

▶ Menopause

Clinical Population

▶ AIDS, Exercise

Clonogenic Survival Assay

The clonogenic cell survival assay determines the ability of a cell to proliferate indefinitely, thereby retaining its reproductive ability to form a large colony or a clone. In this test cells are grown in vitro in soft agar, which reduce cell movement and allow individual cells to develop into cell clones that are identified as single colonies.

Closed Head Injury

▶ Concussion

Clotting

▶ Hemostasis

Coagulation

▶ Hemostasis

Cognition

Charles H. Hillman[1], Kirk I. Erickson[2]
[1]Department of Kinesiology and Community Health, University of Illinois, Urbana, IL, USA
[2]Department of Psychology, University of Pittsburgh, Pittsburgh, PA, USA

Synonyms

Exercise and mental health; Exercise and neurocognitive function

Definition

Cognition means the set of mental processes that contribute to perception, memory, intellect, and action. Cognitive function can be assessed using a variety of techniques including paper-pencil-based tests, neuropsychological testing, and computerized testing methods. Cognitive functions are largely divided into different domains that capture both the type of process as well as the brain areas and circuits that control those functions. Working memory, visual attention, and long-term memory are all examples of different cognitive domains that are dependent on separate neural systems.

Characteristics

Several reviews [3] and meta-analyses [4, 5] have detailed the relationship of exercise to transient and chronic changes in cognition across the human lifespan, including both cognitively intact and impaired individuals. Although there is still much to learn about this relationship, and a consensus has not been reached, the majority of findings suggest that exercise has a small but positive relation with aspects of cognition underlying perception and action. Despite a recognized link between mind and body since at least the ancient Greek civilization, a programmatic study of the exercise–cognition relationship did not emerge until the 1970s [3]. Since that time, the field has grown exponentially due to advances in theory and available measurement techniques as well as a rich literature on nonhuman animal models.

Initially, researchers focused on the relation of exercise to cognitive aging, as a means of understanding lifestyle factors that might improve cognitive health and function, or protect against age-related loss, during the later stages of the lifespan. Empirical evidence for the relation of exercise to cognitive aging has demonstrated benefits across the spectrum of cognitive functions ranging from simplistic motor processes (e.g., finger tapping) to complex cognition (e.g., executive control), leading researchers to suggest that exercise has a generally beneficial relationship to cognition. More recently, researchers have suggested that although exercise appears generally beneficial to cognition, its effects are selectively and disproportionately larger for tasks or task components that require greater amounts of executive control [3]. Such a suggestion has helped shape the understanding of the relation of exercise to cognition as well as the health of underlying neural structures.

Since the initial studies on cognitive aging, researchers have begun to examine the exercise–cognition relationship during earlier periods of the lifespan. Such studies have examined both middle-aged and younger adult populations and demonstrated a similarly beneficial relation of exercise to cognition. The examination of this relationship during the developmental period of the lifespan has been especially interesting in recent years because of the observed benefits to both cognition and scholastic achievement [3, 4]. Specifically, similar benefits of exercise to general and selective aspects of cognition that have been observed in adult populations have been extended to preadolescent childhood, suggesting that exercise is beneficial to cognition and brain health during maturation. Interestingly, the positive relation of exercise has been extended to scholastic achievement, such that more physically active and/or higher aerobically fit children demonstrate better scholastic performance across a variety of standardized and non-standardized tests relative to their less active and fit peers. Again, a consensus on this relationship has not been reached, as other reports have indicated a lack of a relationship between exercise and scholastic performance. Regardless, no reports have indicated that physical activity is detrimental to scholastic performance, suggesting that, at the very least, time spent engaged in exercise does not detract from academic achievement and may lead to improved health of both body and brain.

The advancement of new medical technology, especially magnetic resonance imaging (MRI), provided researchers with the tools to examine the human brain in vivo. These technological advances in human brain imaging, generally referred to as *neuroimaging*, has transformed our view of how the brain gives rise to complex cognitive function and the extent to which various factors influence brain development and affliction. Exercise research has begun to use neuroimaging techniques to determine the extent to which physical activity improves brain function.

This avenue of brain and exercise research began by investigating the effect of exercise and fitness on the aged

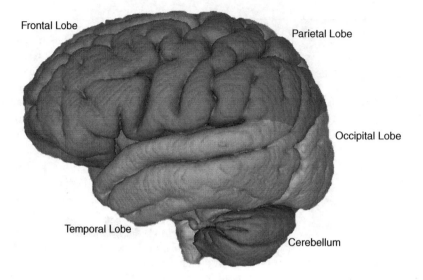

Frontal Lobe

Parietal Lobe

Occipital Lobe

Temporal Lobe

Cerebellum

Cognition. Fig. 1 Lobes of the brain

brain and has since then progressed to earlier periods of the lifespan. During late adulthood, the brain deteriorates in a regionally specific manner, with frontal and temporal regions (see Fig. 1) showing disproportionately faster and greater amounts of decay than other regions. Since the frontal and temporal regions support executive control, the cognitive domain most affected by exercise, it was reasoned that exercise might attenuate age-related deterioration of these regions. Consistent with these predictions, several studies using MRI calculated the amount of brain matter in older adults and found that exercise and higher fitness levels decrease the amount of age-related brain atrophy. That is, older adults with higher fitness levels had more brain tissue in the frontal and temporal lobes than lesser fit adults [1], and greater brain volume leads to better cognitive function [2]. It also appears that only 6 months of moderate intensity exercise is sufficient for increasing the amount of brain tissue in older adults, suggesting that brain tissue remains malleable even well into late adulthood, and that significant increases in brain size can occur relatively quickly with only moderate changes in lifestyle.

The finding that exercise increases the size and amount of brain tissue has been most convincingly demonstrated in healthy older adults; however, evidence is now emerging that exercise also affects the size and shape of brain tissue in other populations. For example, physical activity reduces the risk of developing Alzheimer's disease [3], suggesting that exercise might protect against the heightened loss of brain tissue associated with the disease. Consistent with this, neuroimaging research has demonstrated that aerobically fit adults in the early stages of

Alzheimer's disease have greater amounts of brain tissue than their lesser fit counterparts [3]. Since brain decay is a hallmark for the progression of Alzheimer's disease, these results suggest that exercise might help to prevent or delay the loss of brain tissue, thereby reducing the rate at which the symptoms of Alzheimer's disease progress. Although more research is needed to confirm these results, they are consonant with results in healthy humans and with results in rodent models of Alzheimer's disease that indicate that exercise attenuates the buildup of brain plaques, a putative cause of Alzheimer's disease [3].

Besides being capable of measuring the size and shape of brain matter, neuroimaging methods are also capable of testing how exercise increases brain function and cognitive performance. One technique, called functional MRI, examines brain function by measuring the rapid changes in blood flow to certain brain regions as a result of increased neural activity during the performance of a cognitive task (e.g., memory task). Using this technique in older adults, several studies have found that aerobic exercise increases brain activity during tasks that require attentional focus or memory functions. Increased activity is observed in the prefrontal cortex, which is accompanied by a decrease in brain activity in a region involved with error processing, called the anterior cingulate cortex [3]. Thus, exercise improves cognition by improving brain function in regions that support controlled task performance – the prefrontal cortex, while at the same time reducing brain activity in regions that are no longer necessary for task performance. Although much more research is needed before we fully understand the mechanisms by which exercise improves brain function, neuroimaging research suggests that exercise enhances cognition by influencing the size, shape, and function of particular brain regions.

Similar improvements in brain function have been found in preadolescent children. As described above, there is growing evidence that exercise improves cognitive performance in children, especially on measures of executive control, which is thought to lead to superior academic achievement. In several recent studies, superior cognitive performance in higher fit children was accompanied by elevated brain function, as assessed by event-related potentials (ERPs). ERPs measure the electrical activity emitted from the brain when neurons become active. By using electrodes that are affixed to the scalp surface, neuroelectric signals can be measured during the performance of a cognitive task. Differences in brain activity between high-fit and low-fit children emerge in ERPs during tasks, which require executive control (and presumably the frontal cortex [3]). Similarly, short bouts of aerobic activity improve attentional focus in preadolescent children, and this is related to ERPs measures of brain function.

In sum, there is convincing evidence that exercise and fitness improve cognitive and brain function across the lifespan, but do so in a domain and region specific manner. Executive functions that are supported largely by the prefrontal cortex are the most sensitive to the effect of exercise. Neuroimaging results confirm this finding and suggest that exercise improves cognition by affecting the size, shape, and function of neural circuits involved with successful performance on tasks that measure executive control.

Clinical Relevance

The knowledge that exercise is beneficial to brain health and cognition is relevant for a number of reasons. Specifically, exercise may serve as a non-pharmaceutical option for improving cognition leading to improvements in quality of life, which is especially important during advanced aging. Further, improving brain health and cognition during childhood may serve to build one's cognitive reserve, leading to cognitively healthier adults and less cognitive degradation throughout the aging process. The beneficial relation of exercise to cognitive development may also enhance learning via the derived benefits to brain structure and function. A second argument for the clinical relevance of exercise to brain health may be derived from our ancestry. Specifically, since our ancestors were required to be considerably more active than we are today, having to expend energy to survive, our genome likely developed to support a high level of physical activity on a daily basis. However, contemporary society does not place the same requirements on its members, as recent technological advancements have minimized the need for physical activity that was once necessities in our lives. Thus, decreases in physical activity, along with increases in caloric consumption, have led to an epidemic of poor physical health. It is only recently that researchers have authenticated a link between these unfortunate changes in lifestyle and poorer brain health as well. Accordingly, knowledge of the benefits of exercise to brain health may provide an impetus for increasing participation, leading to benefits in cognitive performance.

References

1. Erickson KI, Kramer AF (2009) Exercise effects on cognitive and neural plasticity in older adults. Brit J Sports Med 43(1):22–24
2. Erickson KI, Prakash RS, Voss MW, Chaddock L, Hu L, Morris KS, White SM, Wojcicki TR, McAuley E, Kramer AF (2009) Aerobic fitness is associated with hippocampal volume in elderly humans. Hippocampus 19:1030–1039
3. Hillman CH, Erickson KI, Kramer AF (2008) Be smart, exercise your heart: exercise effects on brain and cognition. Nat Rev Neurosci 9:58–65
4. Sibley BA, Etnier JL (2003) The relationship between physical activity and cognition in children: a meta-analysis. Pediatr Exerc Sci 15:243–256
5. Smith PJ, Blumenthal JA, Hoffman BM, Cooper H, Strauman TA, Welsh-Bohmer K et al (2010) Aerobic exercise and neurocognitive performance: a meta-analytic review of randomized controlled trials. Psychosom Med 72:239–252

Cognitive Aging

The process of mental decline occurring in late adulthood. This is usually distinguishable from Alzheimer's disease and dementia and is considered to be a normal part of aging, although the extent to which cognitive decline is normal remains a matter of debate. Not all cognitive functions decline with age. The most common cognitive constructs that decline with age include measures of processing speed, episodic and working memory, and executive functions.

Cognitive Reserve

The resilience of adult brain to damage and neurodegeneration by means of new neural resources gained with the experience of the individual. These resources confer capabilities to cope with new and highly complex situations. The component of neural plasticity consisting of neuronal replacement is called neurogenic reserve.

Cold

Hannu Rintamäki
Finnish Institute of Occupational Health, Oulu, Finland
Department of Physiology, Institute of Biomedicine,
University of Oulu, Oulu, Finland

Synonyms
Acclimation; Acclimatization; Adaptation; Habituation

Definition
The terms used here follow the classification presented the Glossary of terms for thermal physiology [1]. The term *adaptation* refers to the changes that reduce the physiological and/or emotional strain produced by stressful components of the total environment. This change may occur within the lifetime of an organism (phenotypic) or be the result of genetic selection in a species or subspecies (genotypic).

The term ▶ acclimation refers to phenotypic adaptive physiological or behavioral changes occurring within an organism, which reduces the strain or enhances endurance of strain caused by experimentally induced stressful changes in particular climatic factors such as ambient temperature in a controlled environment. The term ▶ acclimatization describes the adaptive changes that occur within an organism in response to changes in the natural climate (e.g., seasonal or geographical). The term *habituation* describes the reduction of responses to or perception of a repeated stimulation.

Mechanisms
The thermoneutral ambient temperature for an unclothed resting human is ca. 27°C in the air and ca. 33°C in water. The high thermoneutral temperature points out the tropical origin of human species. With the help of clothing, buildings, heating, and muscular work producing heat, the optimal temperature can be much lower than 27°C. For example, mortality statistics shows that the safest ambient temperature is in Northern Europe (Finland) ca. 14°C, while in Southern Europe (Greece) it is ca. 25°C. In occupational exposures, the limit of ▶ cold work is usually regarded as 10–12°C, at which ambient temperature the tasks requiring fine motor functions start to be hindered. From the other environmental parameters than temperature, especially wind markedly increases the ▶ heat loss in cold environment. Taken together, the body heat balance depends on ambient temperature, ▶ thermal insulation of the clothing, and the magnitude of ▶ metabolic heat production.

For proper physiological functions, core temperature of humans can vary only 4.5°C, between hypothermia (35.0°C) and hyperthermia (39.5°C). Skin temperatures can vary in a much larger range, ca. between 12°C and 40°C without total performance loss.

Stimulation of cold- or heat-sensitive sensors in the skin or deeper tissues sends the message to the thermoregulatory center in the anterior hypothalamus, which further regulates heat production and heat loss. The stimulation of the sensors causes also thermal sensations, which are the driving force for the thermoregulatory behavior (Fig. 1).

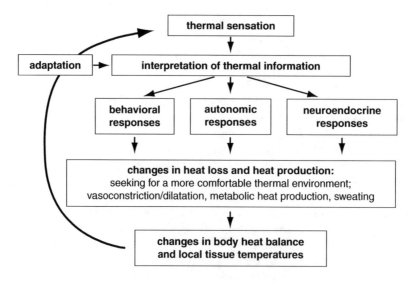

Cold. Fig. 1 Schematic presentation of human thermoregulatory responses

Cold-induced sympathetic stimulation causes vaso-constriction in skin, arms, and legs. Diminished skin and extremity blood flow increases the thermal insulation of superficial tissues more than 300% which could be compared to thermal insulation of 0.9 clo ($0.13°C·m^{-2}·W^{-1}$). With thermoregulatory vasoconstriction/vasodilatation, the body heat balance can be maintained within a range of ca. 4°C.

Cold-induced vasoconstriction increases blood pressure and blood viscosity and decreases plasma volume consequently increasing cardiac work. Cold exposure simulating typical winter activities in subarctic–arctic regions (−15°C, slight wind, good winter clothing) increases within few minutes systolic and diastolic blood pressure by 20–30 mmHg in young subjects and by ca. 60 mmHg in elderly subjects. Face cooling is enough to cause these responses. Acute cold exposure decreases circulating plasma volume while long and repeated cold exposures may increase plasma volume.

In very cold conditions (skin temperature below 2–10°C) the sympathetic stimulation opens the anastomoses connecting arterioles and venules, which increases skin temperatures markedly but temporarily. This cold-induced vasodilatation (CIVD, also called Lewis' reaction or hunting reflex) is most common in fingers and to some extent in face.

At least 80% from the used chemical energy is transformed to heat. Basal metabolic rate is ca. 58 W/m^2 which corresponds to ca. 110 W/individual. Muscular work can increase metabolic rate maximally to 1000–1300 W, but at a continuous work rate the level of 500 W is more probable. Muscular shivering can increase metabolic rate maximally to ca. 300–500 W. In intensive shivering, the energy sources are carbohydrates while in continuous low intensity shivering the energy sources are lipids.

When ambient temperature decreases by 1°C, the 24-h energy expenditure increases 100–130 kJ due to increased amount of clothing, cold-induced heat production, and other factors like snow, ice, and darkness.

There are individual differences in thermal responses. Cold tolerance is increased by large body size (small surface area – body mass ratio), abundant subcutaneous fat, good physical fitness (good ability for heat production, good circulation), male gender (predominantly due to larger body size), young age (via muscle mass and circulation), cold adaptation, and good health. Also personality affects thermal responses: Increased level of neuroticism dampens or slows the autonomic thermoregulatory responses whereas increased extroversion has an opposite effect.

Adaptation to Cold

Behavioral adaptation is most important for the survival of human species in cold climate. It includes, e.g., well-heated houses, good thermal insulation of clothing, warm vehicles, and short exposures to cold.

Human physiological adaptation to cold may comprise either enhanced or dampened responses. Dampened responses (habituation) are much more common. Adaptation to cold can develop in whole body level (general cold adaptation) or locally especially in hands.

Whole Body Adaptation to Cold

Decrease in discomfort and delayed and weakened shivering during cold exposure are usually the first signs of cold adaptation. It takes for about 2 weeks to develop a clear cold adaptation although maximal development of adaptation may last much longer.

The classification of cold adaptations takes into account the changes in core temperature (T_c), mean skin temperature (T_{sk}), and level of metabolism (M). Based on these thermoregulatory responses, four basic types of cold adaptation have been observed: metabolic, insulative, hypothermic, and insulative–hypothermic adaptation. The forms of these classical cold adaptations have been observed from the natives in their natural environments and in Caucasians in laboratory conditions [2].

Metabolic cold adaptation: During cold exposure, metabolic rate is 27–60% higher than in non-adapted ones and it can be higher also at thermal neutrality. T_{sk} is 0.5–1.0°C higher than in non-adapted ones. There is no change in T_c. This feature is found in Alacaluf Indians in Tierra del Fuego, Eskimos, Arctic Indians, and Caucasians living in circumpolar regions and under laboratory conditions. The reason for increased metabolic heat production can be in increased amounts of uncoupling proteins (UCPs), which favor heat production instead of ATP production in mitochondrias. Thyroid hormones stimulate the expression of UCPs. Recent positron-emission tomography (PET) studies have done the role of ▶ brown adipose tissue in adaptive heat production of adult humans very obvious [3].

Insulative cold adaptation: During cold exposure, T_c and metabolic levels are unchanged and T_{sk} is lowered. Found in Aborigines of the north coast of Australia and in people adapted to cold naturally or in laboratory conditions and after repeated immersions in cold water.

Hypothermic cold adaptation: T_c and body heat content are decreased during cold exposure. T_{sk} responses are as in non-adapted subjects. Found in Bushmen of the Kalahari Desert, Quechua Indians living at high altitude in the Andes and Caucasians living for a long time in subarctic areas or after acclimation.

Insulative–hypothermic cold adaptation: Combination of insulative and hypothermic cold adaptations: T_c and T_{sk} are lowered but metabolic rate unchanged during cold exposure. Found in Aborigines of central Australia, nomadic Lapps, people repeatedly immersed in cold water (Ama divers in Japan and Korea) and Caucasians during acclimatization and acclimation studies by water immersions.

Savourey et al. [4] developed a quantitative classification of cold adaptations. The classification is based on T_c, T_{sk}, and M measured during a standard cold air test (2 h at 1°C, wind speed 0.8 m/s, at rest lying on the back, nude) (Table 1).

The factors for developing different types of general cold adaptation are not yet fully understood. It looks like that both environmental conditions, type of exposure (length and severity of exposure, number and frequency of exposures), diet, anthropometry (physical fitness and body fat content), and physical activity can predominate, which kind of general cold adaptation is developed. Launau and Savourey [2] postulate that:

- Metabolic cold adaptation is developed during severe cold stress associated with a possibility of a high energy intake.
- Insulative cold adaptation is developed during light cold stress with low energy intake.
- Hypothermic cold adaptation is developed during a moderate cold stress with very low energy intake.

- Insulative–hypothermic cold adaptation is developed when there is moderate cold stress at night, with very low energy intake, and heat stress during the day.

General cold adaptation is usually developed by whole body cold exposure. However, if the cold exposure of body extremities (e.g., legs) is intensive, it can lead to general cold adaptation, too [2].

Cold winter at high latitudes is not a sufficient to stimulate development of cold adaptation of urban dwellers, as the normal outdoor cold exposures are not long and severe enough. Outdoor work or hobby is required to develop cold adaptation.

Local Cold Adaptation

Local cold adaptation is usually observed in hands and sometimes in feet. Local cold adaptation is a typical dampened response (habituation) to cold: The initially strong vasoconstriction in hands exposed to cold becomes less intensive during adaptation. Also the CIVD response starts earlier in cold adapted hands. Local cold adaptation of hands is sometimes called as "fisherman's hands."

Hormonal and Neuroendocrine Responses to Cold

Acute cold exposure increases plasma noradrenaline concentration as a consequence of sympathetic activation. In some studies also plasma cortisol level has increased. During long-term cold exposure, like winter, aldosterone and thyroid hormone levels tend to increase, although the results are inconsistent. Long-term residence in polar or circumpolar regions in winter in cold and darkness may cause "polar T_3 syndrome" with decreased plasma levels of total and free T_3. This is explained to be a consequence of increased T_3 metabolism. Polar T_3 syndrome is associated with decreased mental and physical performance and can be counteracted by thyroxine supplementation [5].

Exercise Response/Consequences

Adaptation to cold decreases the cooling-induced discomfort and therefore improves performance in cold. Local cold adaptation which dampens the vasoconstriction of hands and facilitate CIVD improve manual performance by keeping the hands warmer, with the costs of increased heat loss. Also metabolic cold adaptation helps to maintain good thermal balance and hence performance. Insulative and hypothermic adaptations, on the other hand, help to save energy. However, the physiological cold adaptations alone are not enough for maintaining homeothermia in cold environments but also behavioral adaptation is needed.

Cold. Table 1 Quantitative classification of cold adaptations [4] (Modified from [2])

Studied change	Observed change	Type of cold adaptation
Difference between T_c observed at the end of standard cold air test and T_c at thermoneutrality	>0 or =	Normothermic
	<0	Hypothermic
T_{sk} after adaptation/T_{sk} before adaptation (measured at the end of the standard cold air test)	<1	Insulative
	=1	Iso-insulative
	>1	Hypo-insulative
M after adaptation/M before adaptation (mean value measured during the standard cold air test)	>1	Metabolic
	=1	Iso-metabolic
	<1	Hypo-metabolic

References

1. Schumacker PT, Rowland J, Saltz S et al (2001) Glossary of terms for thermal physiology. Third Edition revised by the commission for thermal physiology of the international union of physiological sciences (IUPS Thermal Commission). Jpn J Physiol 51:245–280

2. Launay J-C, Savourey G (2009) Cold adaptations. Ind Health 47:221–227

3. Virtanen KA, Lidell ME, Orava J, Heglind M, Westergren R, Niemi T, Taittonen M, Laine J, Savisto NJ, Enerbäck S, Nuutila P (2009) Functional brown adipose tissue in healthy adults. N Engl J Med 360(15):1518–1525

4. Savourey G, Vallerand AL, Bittel JH (1992) General and local cold adaptation after a skin journey in a severe arctic environment. Eur J Appl Physiol Occup Physiol 64:99–105

5. Pääkkönen T (2010) Melatonin and thyroid hormones in the cold and in darkness. Association with mood and cognition. PhD thesis. Acta Univ Oul D 1045. http://herkules.oulu.fi/isbn9789514261213/. Accessed 16 Feb 2010

Cold Work

Ambient temperature, where cold-induced thermoregulatory responses appear. During light physical work, the upper limit of cold work is ca. at 10–12°C.

Collagen

▶ Extracellular Matrix

Comet Assay

Electrophoresis technique for the detection of single-strand and double-strand breaks at the single cell level. It involves the encapsulation of cells in low-melting-point agarose suspension, lysis of the cells in neutral or alkaline conditions, and electrophoresis of the suspended lysed cells.

Compensated Hypertrophy

Adaptive growth of the heart.

Cross-References
▶ Cardiac Hypertrophy, Pathological
▶ Cardiac Hypertrophy, Physiological

Complementary and Alternative Medicine in Inflammatory Bowel Diseases

▶ Inflammatory Bowel Disease, Exercise

Complete Transportation of the Great Arteries

Atrioventricular concordance and ventriculoarterial discordance – i.e., the right atrium connects to the morphological right ventricle which gives rise to the aorta and the left atrium connects to the morphological left ventricle which gives rise to the pulmonary artery. The pulmonary and systemic circulations are connected in parallel rather than the normal in series connection. This situation is incompatible with life unless mixing of the two circuits occurs at birth.

Cross-References
▶ Congenital Heart Disease

Complex Systems

Technically defined as systems composed of two or more interacting parts. Examples include stockmarkets, societies, colonies of ants, schools of fish, flocks of birds, the human body, and sports teams. Complexity refers to the ongoing potential for interactions between components of a complex system which can lead to rich and creative coordinated patterns of behavior emerging. Complex systems can harness inherent processes of self-organization in which system components can adjust their behaviors with respect to each other without regulatory involvement by an executive agent. The rich outcomes of these system interactions can be captured by the well-known phrase 'the whole is greater than the sum of the parts'.

Complex Training

▶ Postactivation Potentiation

Compliance

The change in behavior in comparison to the prescribed regimen, sometimes suggesting making the changes due to pressures from the external prescriber.

Cross-References

▶ Promotion of and Adherence to Physical Activity

Composition of the Human Body

▶ Body Composition

Concentric Activity

During concentric activity, muscular work is performed against gravity, for example by the lifting of weights; in essence, the muscle shortens as it contracts.

Concussion

PAUL VAN DONKELAAR[1], LOUIS R. OSTERNIG[2], LI-SHAN CHOU[2]
[1]School of Health and Exercise Science, University of British Columbia – Okanagan Campus, Kelowna, BC, Canada
[2]Department of Human Physiology, University of Oregon, Eugene, OR, USA

Synonyms

Closed head injury; Mild traumatic brain injury

Definition

Concussion is defined as a complex pathophysiological process affecting the brain, induced by traumatic biomechanical forces. Concussion can be caused by a direct impact to the head or be transmitted to the head via a blow to another part of the body. Typical causes of concussion include falls, contact sporting activities, and car accidents. Following the injury event there is a rapid onset of one or more graded neurological impairments that may or may not involve loss of consciousness and that usually resolve spontaneously over the course of a few days to weeks. These impairments can manifest themselves in a variety of ways including, but not limited to, headache, nausea, balance impairments, difficulty concentrating, heightened sensitivity to sensory stimuli, sleep disturbances, vertigo, confusion, and memory loss. The underlying cause of these impairments is due to neuropathological changes that are physiological rather than anatomical in nature. This is confirmed by the fact that standard clinical structural neuroimaging studies are typically unremarkable following a concussion.

Mechanisms

Concussion occurs when a force is directly or indirectly imparted to the head. The force is transmitted through the brain causing shearing, twisting, and stretching of the neural, glial, vascular, and structural tissues. This has an impact on the physiological functioning of these tissues which, in turn, leads to the functional impairments that are typically observed. In particular, concussion is thought to result in a ▶ neurometabolic cascade of events including abrupt neuronal depolarization, release of excitatory neurotransmitters, ionic shifts, changes in glucose metabolism, altered cerebral blood flow, and impaired axonal function (see Fig. 1 adapted from [1]). At a systems level, this is thought to alter autonomic function and ▶ cerebral autoregulation resulting in an energy crisis in which the metabolic demand induced by the altered neuronal activation is outstripped by the ability of the compromised circulatory system to supply sufficient fuel.

Because of the manner by which the forces induced by the injury event are transmitted through the brain, unlike other neurological injuries such as stroke or Parkinson's disease, the functional disruption induced by a concussion is not localized to a specific area, but rather is widespread and relatively similar across different regions of the brain. Thus, a person suffering a concussion will quite often display a variety of behavioral deficits that are typically associated with one or more different regions in the brain. Moreover, there does not appear to be any evidence of functional deficits associated with the area of the head to which the force was imparted – i.e., visual deficits following a blow to the back of the head, speech deficits with a blow to the left side of the head, etc. However, there are no comprehensive studies that have assessed this in a large enough number of patients to draw any robust inferences. Be that as it may, recent evidence using a variety of modeling and imaging techniques suggests that structures and pathways in the midbrain may be especially susceptible to the twisting and shearing forces induced by the injury event. More specifically, because of the anatomical arrangement of the structures in this part of the brain

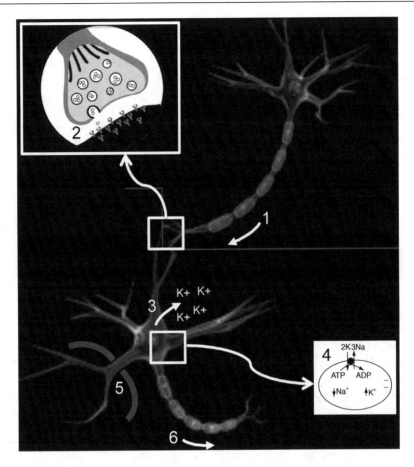

Concussion. Fig. 1 Neurometabolic cascade of events associated with concussion: (*1*) abrupt neuronal depolarization; (*2*) excessive release of glutamate at the synapse; (*3*) disproportionate efflux of potassium; (*4*) hyperglycolysis to fuel increased activity of active membrane ionic pumps; (*5*) altered blood flow due to disrupted cerebral autoregulation; and (*6*) impaired axonal function caused by physical disruption to structural elements

and the biomechanical constraints induced by this arrangement, it is thought that the white matter tracts coursing through the midbrain in particular are more likely to be disrupted than structures and pathways elsewhere in the brain. Because these midbrain tracts carry signals that contribute to widespread brain functions, it is not surprising that a concussion event leads to a wide variety of behavioral disruptions.

It is also apparent that the magnitude of the functional deficits is influenced by the severity of the injury and the complexity of the task. As a general rule, the more severe the initial injury, the more likely it is that the deficits will be more substantial and longer lasting. This relation is weakly but significantly influenced by the impact force occurring during the injury event: the greater the acceleration/deceleration of the head, the more likely it is that a concussion will subsequently be diagnosed – although there appears to be no absolute threshold at which

a concussion is guaranteed to take place. Given these caveats, modeling studies have demonstrated that the best predictor of the likelihood and severity of concussion is the maximum shear stress occurring in the brainstem induced by the shock wave resulting from the force imparted on the head during the injury event [2].

It has also been suggested that concussion history can influence the magnitude and duration of post-injury symptoms. In particular, there are abundant clinical anecdotal examples of repeated concussions resulting in greater and more enduring functional deficits. A corollary of this characteristic is that a smaller impact force is required to induce the injury and subsequent dysfunction with each successive concussion an individual sustains. However, the experimental support for these clinical observations is variable, with some studies demonstrating evidence for such cumulative effects and others unable to do so. A recent meta-analysis on the subject demonstrated that overall there appears to be little influence of concussion history on neuropsychological function several months post-injury except for specific measures related to delayed memory and ▶ executive function [3]. However, it has also been demonstrated that there is a significant functional effect of exposure to blows to the head based on the length of participation in a contact sport. This suggests that cumulative effects are present with long-term exposure to concussive events.

Although concussion history appears to be inconsistently related to the severity and duration of post-injury symptoms, it is clear that it is an excellent predictor of future concussive injuries. In particular, a person who has sustained a single concussion is three times more likely to sustain a second concussion and eight times more likely to sustain a third concussion within a 3 month period after the primary injury event than an individual who has never sustained a concussion [4]. Thus, previous concussions will make an individual more susceptible to subsequent concussions that nevertheless do not result in more severe or longer lasting symptoms at least during the first few months post-injury. However, with repeated exposures over the longer term, such concussive events will eventually result in a cumulative reduction in neuropsychological function.

Part of the challenge in diagnosing and managing a concussion is related to the ability to accurately monitor the nature of the resulting deficits in a sensitive manner. In this regard, there is clear evidence that increasing task complexity exacerbates the effects of a concussion. Thus, whereas simple tasks rarely reveal differences between concussed and non-concussed individuals, more difficult tasks or tasks performed under challenging or complex conditions result in clear performance deficits following a concussive injury. This is most apparent for tasks that engage executive function or cognitive resources. Thus, for example, the simple motor task of pressing a button as quickly as possible in response to a visual stimulus typically does not lead to a reaction time deficit following concussion. However, the same response generated under an executive function constraint (e.g., press the button only when a specific visual stimulus appears in a particular part of the visual display) will quite often cause a significant increase in reaction time in individuals who have recently suffered a blow to the head. Because of these subtleties, a concussion can sometimes be misdiagnosed or mismanaged if a test or tests are used that lack the appropriate level of sensitivity. It is vital for clinicians to keep this in mind when advising athletes, coaches, and parents about the effects of a concussion.

Given the difficulty in diagnosing and managing concussion and the potential for long-term consequences from this injury, the question arises as to what can be done to prevent a concussion from occurring in the context of contact sports settings? Assuming that athletes will continue to participate in high numbers in contact sports such as American football and ice hockey it seems that complete prevention will never be possible. Instead, efforts should be made to reduce the incidence with which concussion occurs and improve the likelihood of complete recovery in the event of an injury. There are a number of areas within the contact sports context in which these goals can be achieved: (1) rule changes that reduce the incidence of violent collisions and promote safer player-to-player contact along with stiffer player and team penalties for infractions of such rules; (2) coaching standards for the appropriate techniques by which to make contact; (3) government legislation which mandates stricter criteria for removing players with suspected concussions and ▶ return-to-play decisions; (4) greater concussion education outreach for players, coaches, parents, and health care providers; (5) improved equipment safety standards and maintenance designed to reduce the concussive effects of impacts when they do occur; and (6) greater awareness of the limitations of current protective equipment (i.e., helmets and mouthguards reduce the incidence of skull, jaw, and dental fractures, but do not protect a player from concussion). By spending time and resources on these specific sets of issues, amateur and professional sports organizations, local and national governments, and allied health care providers will improve the environment surrounding concussion in a contact sports setting.

Exercise Response/Consequences

A common observation in athletes who have suffered a concussion is the exacerbation of symptoms induced by physical exertion. This response is so common that it is often used as an assessment tool by clinicians a part of the return-to-play decision: when the symptoms do not reappear following a bout of exercise, the athlete will be cleared to play as long as they display normalized responses on other clinical assessments (see Diagnostics section).

The mechanism underlying this exercise-induced response is not well understood. It has been suggested that the exacerbation of symptoms results from the disruption to autonomic function and cerebral autoregulation. In particular, the demand for resources induced by the exercise may constrain cortical function because of the dysfunction to the physiological processes helping to maintain homeostasis. This results in a cortical energy imbalance and has functional consequences with respect to a return of symptoms. Thus, when a bout of exercise no longer results in an exacerbation of symptoms, one can deduce that the underlying cortical physiology has recovered to an extent that homeostasis can be maintained successfully. This implies that the structures supporting these physiological processes are no longer overly susceptible to the forces typically present in a contact sports setting and, assuming other clinical assessments have returned to baseline levels, the athlete may be cleared to practice and play.

Diagnostics

As mentioned above, the ability to accurately and sensitively detect that a blow to the head has resulted in behavioral deficits is the key to diagnosing and managing a concussion. Because every athlete is different, it is vital that baseline testing of function be performed ideally prior to the start of every season. By doing so, it becomes possible to compare the athlete to themselves prior to the injury, rather than to a teammate who may have a substantially different level of function. Because such baseline testing will typically include neuropsychological assessments of attention, memory, and executive function, it is important that it occur in a quiet controlled space free from distractions. Once an injury is suspected, the athlete should be tested again in the same environment as soon as possible after the event. If the scores are substantially reduced and the athlete is complaining of symptoms consistent with a concussion then it is very likely that the injury has occurred, even if no loss of consciousness took place. Subsequent testing should be performed at regular intervals over the course of the recovery period to track the return of function.

Sometimes an athlete will continue to complain of symptoms long after a typical recovery period (a few days/weeks) has passed. This has been termed post-concussion syndrome and can be challenging for those providing care and frustrating for the athlete themselves. In such cases, the diagnosis can be difficult because, other than the symptom complaints, the athlete may have no other deficits as revealed by typical clinical assessments. Thus, under such circumstances one may suspect that the individual is malingering. In such cases, a number of more sensitive physiological and microanatomical imaging modalities appear to provide evidence of disruptions/damage that can confirm that the brain is not functioning normally. In particular, transcranial Doppler ultrasound provides a means to quantitate cerebral blood flow and near infrared spectroscopy can assess correlates of cortical metabolism. By using these two physiological techniques, it becomes possible to indirectly make inferences of the energy balance in the brain. Recent research has demonstrated that a mild to moderate brain injury can

substantially alter cerebral blood flow and metabolism as assessed with these tools [5]. In addition to examining cortical physiology, it is also possible to assess microstructural integrity using ▶ diffusion tensor imaging. This variant of magnetic resonance imaging allows one to visualize the extent of disruption to white matter tracts throughout the brain. Using this approach, researchers have demonstrated that mild to moderate brain injury is associated with reduced integrity in a number of white matter tracts and that the extent of this disruption is correlated with deficits in behaviors which rely on the information carried by these pathways [6]. Thus, these state-of-the-art tools provide a more sensitive means by which to confirm that the brain is not functioning properly even if more traditional clinical assessments are unable to do so. By this means, an athlete with post-concussion syndrome, even though they may continue to suffer from long-term symptoms, may nevertheless obtain a confirmed diagnosis. This can then be used to make decisions regarding whether to end a sports career and how best to make accommodations for activities of daily living outside of a sports setting.

In conclusion, research on concussion and the associated public knowledge has increased substantially in the last decade. This has led to marked improvements in the diagnosis and management of concussions and information transfer to athletes, parents, coaches, and health care providers. Despite this increase in knowledge, or perhaps because of it, the dangers inherent in contact sports settings at all levels have been highlighted in both scientific and mainstream media. It is clear, based on this increased knowledge and the associated public awareness, that fundamental changes need to be made in these sports if the incidence of concussions is to be reduced in the future.

References

1. Barkhoudarian G, Hovda DA, Giza CC (2011) The molecular pathophysiology of concussive brain injury. Clin Sports Med 30:33–48
2. Zhang L, Yang KH, King AI (2004) A proposed injury threshold for mild traumatic brain injury. J Biomech Eng 126:226–236
3. Belanger HG, Spiegel E, Vanderploeg RD (2010) Neuropsychological performance following a history of multiple self-reported concussions: a meta-analysis. J Int Neuropsychol Soc 16:262–267
4. Guskiewicz KM, McCrea M, Marshall SW, Cantu RC, Randolph C, Barr W, Onate JA, Kelly JP (2003) Cumulative effects associated with recurrent concussion in collegiate football players: the NCAA concussion study. J Am Med Assoc 290:2549–2555
5. Len TK, Neary JP (2011) Cerebrovascular pathophysiology following mild traumatic brain injury. Clin Physiol Funct Imaging 31:85–93
6. Little DM, Kraus MF, Joseph J, Geary EK, Susmaras T, Zhou XJ, Pliskin N, Gorelick PB (2010) Thalamic integrity underlies executive dysfunction in traumatic brain injury. Neurology 74:558–564

Congenital Cardiovascular Malformations

▶ Congenital Heart Disease

Congenital Coagulopathy

▶ Hemophilia

Congenital Heart Defect

▶ Congenital Heart Disease

Congenital Heart Disease

GEORGE GIANNAKOULAS, SOPHIA-ANASTASIA MOURATOGLOU, HARALAMBOS KARVOUNIS
Cardiology Department, AHEPA University Hospital, Thessaloniki, Greece

Synonyms

Congenital cardiovascular malformations; Congenital heart defect; Cyanotic heart disease; Heart abnormality

Definition

The term congenital heart disease (CHD) represents a number of symptoms and clinical conditions occurring in the presence of a great range of developmental abnormalities that can involve both the heart and/or the great vessels. Congenital heart defects consist one of the most common inborn defects and are one of the main causes of infant death in developed world.

Mechanisms of Exercise Intolerance in CHD

Advances in pediatric cardiology and cardiac surgery have improved the survival of patients with CHD and resulted in an increased number of adults with CHD that live and enjoy a normal qualitative life. However, many CHD patients often experience exercise intolerance regardless of the complexity of their cardiac lesions. Although CHD patients, even those with complex diagnoses, usually underestimate their exercise tolerance, physical limitation is relatively common, affecting more than a third of patients in the Euro Heart Survey, a large European adult CHD registry. It is prominent even in patients with simple lesions, such as atrial septal defects, and becomes more severe in those with ▶ Eisenmenger physiology, univentricular hearts or complex cardiac anatomy. Reduced exercise capacity may occur through a variety of obstructive or/and restrictive cardiac and extracardiac pathogenetic mechanisms.

Limited cardiac output is the main cardiac cause of impaired exercise capacity in patients with CHD. Cardiac output is defined by the product of stroke volume and heart rate and is subjected to their changes. A reduction in stroke volume caused by impaired ventricular function or an inefficiency in adequate heart rate increment (chronotropic incompetence) results in a direct reduction in cardiac output. Ventricular dysfunction is the outcome of long-standing pressure or volume overload conditions resulting from a great variety of abnormalities, such as obstructive or regurgitant lesions, shunts and systemic and/or pulmonary hypertension or through the effects of endothelial and neurohormonal activation, permanent pacing and heart rate-lowering medication. Ventricular dysfunction is therefore commonly seen in CHD as sequela after surgical repair such as atrial switch in complete transposition of the great arteries (TGA) or in patients with a ▶ Fontan circulation. Repeated ventriculotomies and repeated cardiopulmonary bypass operations (especially in previous era) may also contribute to the development of impaired ventricular function. Severe right ventricular volume overload as occurring in patients with large atrial septal defects and to those with severe pulmonary valve regurgitation may eventually result in right ventricular systolic dysfunction, whereas ▶ aortic coarctation, severe aortic valvular/subvalvular stenosis and/or aortic regurgitation, or severe left atrioventricular valve regurgitation as the one resulting after surgical repair of atrioventricular septal defects are the main pathogenetic mechanisms causing left ventricular overload and left ventricular systolic dysfunction. A dilated right heart and a reduced right ventricular output may also impede left ventricular function by impeding its proper filling and causing diastolic dysfunction (ventricular–ventricular interaction). Anomalous coronary circulation often resulting in infarction, ischemia, or sudden cardiac death is a common lesion in patients with CHD and may contribute to the development of ventricular dysfunction. Finally, patients suffering from CHD often experience arrhythmias that lead to worsening of ventricular function. Intrinsic abnormalities of the conduction system and surgical scars that may affect it, can lead to sometimes fatal arrhythmias that impede normal cardiac function and reduce cardiac output, or to a cardiac inability to proper increment of heart rate. Chronotropic incompetence may also result from impaired sympathetic cardiac autonomous nervous activity often seen in patients with single ventricle morphology, aortic coarctation, Eisenmenger syndrome and with ▶ Mustard atrial repair operation in terms of TGA correction, or can be iatrogenic from rate-lowering medication (b-blockers, calcium antagonists, and antiarrhythmic drugs), as well as from permanent pacing.

Limited ventilatory reserve as expressed by reduced forced vital capacity is a common extracardiac cause of reduced exercise capacity in adult patients with CHD. Patients suffering from CHD may experience abnormal pulmonary function owned to pulmonary parenchymal and vascular abnormalities. Atelectasis is not a rare complication of thoracic surgery and results in impaired lung function. CHD is often accompanied by skeletal abnormalities and diaphragmatic hernia and paralysis, conditions obstructing the normal pulmonary deployment and ventilation. Moreover, the development of pulmonary arterial hypertension is an indicator of bad prognosis and is related to impaired exercise capacity due to augmented elevated pulmonary vascular resistance obscuring the normal lung circulation and blood oxygenation. Blood oxygenation and oxygen delivery to the tissues are frequently impaired in patients with CHD. Anemia and secondary erythrocytosis are frequent conditions in CHD patients, both resulting in exercise intolerance using different pathophysiologic mechanisms. Anemia may be the result of medical treatment and especially of anticoagulation therapy, of iron deficiency, of chronic renal disease, of hemolysis provoked by prosthetic valves or may be anemia of chronic disease.

Exercise Intervention

The preventive and therapeutical role of exercise and its beneficial effects in human physical and mental health are well established. However, CHD patients and especially children and teenagers are often subjected to parental restrictions and prohibitions regarding their physical exercise. Overprotection is common in young CHD patients and can lead to lack of competence to their own physical strength and abilities. In most circumstances exercise limitations are unjustified, as current symptoms only account for approximately 30% of all barriers to exercise. Patients suffering from CHD usually underestimate their own capabilities and are unaware of their own possibilities, fact that combined with the overprotection they usually experience from their environment, leads to a restricted physical activity performance.

The 36th Bethesda Conference provided recommendations for determining eligibility for competition in athletes with cardiovascular abnormalities and defined the degree of permitted activity in patients with CHD. In fact, only a minority of CHD lesions are an absolute indication of exercise restriction (Table 1) [1]. Of note, isometric exercise is most difficult to control and less suitable than isotonic exercise in patients with CHD.

Exercise prescription in CHD has been proved to be safe and effective in small studies of various CHD populations (Table 2). The majority of these studies showed that exercise training in adult and pediatric CHD patients resulted in mild to moderate improvement in exercise capacity, as assessed objectively by ▶ cardiopulmonary exercise testing and/or subjectively by questionnaires. However, all these observations are limited by the small sample size and the short duration of training programs [2].

Concerning patients with CHD in clinical practice, exercise training must be classified in accordance to the degree of cardiovascular involvement needed, as expressed by the heart rate, cardiac output, arterial blood pressure, systemic and pulmonary vascular resistances, sympathetic activation, and emotional participation. Exercise intensity and duration of training are also factors that must be taken into account when designing the appropriate exercise program. There is, therefore, a great amount of information needed before choosing the proper training program. The patients' age, concomitant diseases, leisure and working habits, preferences and abilities, the specific CHD diagnosis, the type, the time and the results of the previous surgeries, the biventricular function, possible hemodynamic sequelae and the presence and inducibility of arrhythmias, as well as the patients' cardiovascular and respiratory adaptation capacity in exercise are all parameters that must necessarily be reported before deciding about the optimal exercise program. A clinical and instrumental evaluation is therefore required and in that direction a 12-lead ECG, echocardiography, magnetic resonance imaging, spirometry, 24-h electrocardiographic monitoring, exercise testing, and cardiopulmonary exercise testing can be valuable tools [3].

Cardiopulmonary exercise testing is a useful non-invasive tool which can provide unique information about global cardiovascular performance and patients' objective exercise capacity and is the gold standard method for monitoring and evaluating metabolic workload. A training intensity of 40–50% of the percentage of the ▶ peak oxygen consumption (peak VO2), gradually increased to 70–80%, can be used to determine the most suitable training program for patients with CHD.

Congenital Heart Disease. Table 1 Recommended sport participation in patients with CHD

Lesion	Recommendation
ASD	
With mild PH	Low dynamic and static sports
With pulmonary vascular disease	Low dynamic and static sports, no competitive sports
With tachyarrhythmia or moderate to severe MR	Recommendation after clinical evaluation
VSD	
With mild to moderate PH	Low dynamic and static sports
With severe PH	No sports allowed
With tachyarrhythmia or AV-block	Recommendation after clinical evaluation
PDA	
With mild to moderate PH	Low dynamic and static sports
With severe PH	No sports allowed
AVSD	
Moderate coexisting left atrioventricular valve regurgitation	Low to moderate dynamic and static sports
Pulmonary stenosis	
Moderate/Severe	Low to moderate dynamic and static sports
Pulmonary valve regurgitation	Low to moderate dynamic and static sports
Aortic valve stenosis	
Moderate	Low to moderate dynamic and static sports
Moderate with tachyarrhythmias	Low dynamic and static sports
Severe	No competitive sports
Aortic regurgitation	
Moderate to severe	Low dynamic and static sports
Aortic coarctation	
With high systolic blood pressure	Low dynamic and static sports
Repaired with conduit, interposed graft or on anticoagulation therapy	No sports allowed
Tetralogy of Fallot	
Successfully repaired	Low to moderate dynamic and static sports
Residual disease	Low dynamic and static sports
Repaired with conduit, interposed graft or on anticoagulation therapy	No sports allowed
TGA	
Intra-atrial repair	Low to moderate dynamic and static sports. No competitive sports
Arterial switch operation with ventricular dysfunction	Low to moderate dynamic and low static sports
Repaired with conduit, interposed graft or on anticoagulation therapy	No sports allowed
Congenitally corrected	Low to moderate dynamic and low static sports
Ebstein anomaly	
With tricuspid regurgitation or after surgical repair	Low dynamic and static sports. No competitive sports
Severe disease	No sports allowed
Univentricular hearts/Fontan circulation	Low to moderate dynamic and low static sports. No competitive sports

Congenital Heart Disease. Table 1 (continued)

Lesion	Recommendation
Eisenmenger syndrome	Low dynamic sports. No competitive sports
Congenital coronary artery anomalies	
Unrepaired	No sports allowed

ASD atrial septal defect, *VSD* ventricular septal defect, *PDA* persistent ductus arteriosus, *AVSD* atrioventricular septal defect, *MR* mitral valve regurgitation, *PH* pulmonary hypertension, *TGA* transposition of the great arteries

Congenital Heart Disease. Table 2 Studies of exercise prescription in CHD

Author	Year	Study population	n	Duration	Results
Dua et al. [6]	2009	Various adult CHD	50	10 weeks	Increase in median exercise time, improvement of quality of life
Fredriksen et al. [7]	2000	Children and adolescents with various CHD	55	2 weeks	Increase in peak VO_2
Therrien et al. [8]	2003	TOF	9	3 months	Increase in peak VO_2
Bradley et al. [9]	1985	TOF/TGA	9	12 weeks	Increase in peak VO_2
Moalla et al. [10]	2006	Various pediatric CHD	10	12 weeks	Improved submaximal CPET parameters
Singh et al. [11]	2007	Severe pediatric CHD	14	12 weeks	Improved peak VO_2, heart rate recovery
Rhodes et al. [12]	2005	Severe pediatric CHD	16	12 weeks	Increase in peak VO_2 and peak oxygen pulse
Holloway et al. [13]	2011	Various adult CHD	7	4–6 months	Increase in treadmill time and speed
Minamisawa et al. [14]	2001	Fontan	11	2–3 months	Increase in peak VO_2
Opocher et al. [15]	2005	Pediatric Fontan	10	8 months	Increase in peak VO_2, oxygen pulse, decrease in heart rate curve during submaximal exercise
Brassard et al. [16]	2006	Fontan	5	8 weeks	Positive influence on the neuromuscular function

TOF tetralogy of Fallot, *TGA* transposition of the great arteries, *CPET* cardiopulmonary exercise testing, *peak VO2* peak oxygen consumption

Given that cardiopulmonary exercise testing is usually unavailable in routine training practice, heart rate can be used as an indirect method of metabolic work evaluation and a training intensity of 60–80% of peak heart rate can be used to design a specialized training program [4, 5]. ▶ Accelerometers can be used to access objective information about the frequency, intensity, and duration of physical activity. A two to three times weekly performed training program is usually suggested for CHD patients.

Unfortunately, an adequate discussion of the importance of fitness and a patient-tailored exercise program prescription is rare even in specialized tertiary centers caring for patient with CHD. Advice is more often prohibitive, resulting in an inability to improve patients' health and increase their quality of life by helping to remove or modify many of the perceived barriers to exercise.

Consequences

Although the beneficial effects of exercise are well recognized, there are only few data on its feasibility, safety, and efficacy in patients with CHD. Given that patients with CHD form a heterogeneous group with various anatomic diagnoses and clinical pictures, the type and the intensity of the exercise must be tailored individually, especially when hemodynamic residua, poor functional condition, and increased arrhythmic risk are present. The patients' first steps into physical exercise must always be performed under surveillance. A parent, a teacher, a trainer or a friend must accompany the patient and make him/her feel safe and confident for his/her exercise capacity and physical possibilities. The main goal should be the increase in their effort tolerance, which is fundamental for improving their social integration and permitting employment and sexual relations, especially in young CHD patients. There is a need for future clinical studies, which should shed light on this direction, focusing on the efficacy of various exercise training protocols on the heterogeneous CHD population.

References

1. Graham TP Jr, Driscoll DJ, Gersony WM, Newburger JW, Rocchini A, Towbin JA (2005) Task force 2: congenital heart disease. J Am Coll Cardiol 45:1326–1333
2. Giannakoulas G, Dimopoulos K (2010) Exercise training in congenital heart disease: should we follow the heart failure paradigm? Int J Cardiol 138:109–111
3. Hirth A, Reybrouck T, Bjarnason-Wehrens B, Lawrenz W, Hoffmann A (2006) Recommendations for participation in competitive and leisure sports in patients with congenital heart disease: a consensus document. Eur J Cardiovasc Prev Rehabil 13:293–299
4. Takken T, Harkel AD (2010) Exercise testing and prescription in patients with congenital heart disease. Int J Pediatr. doi:10.1155/2010/791980
5. Piepoli MF, Conraads V, Corra U et al (2011) Exercise training in heart failure: from theory to practice. A consensus document of the heart failure association and the European association for cardiovascular prevention and rehabilitation. Eur J Heart Fail 13:347–357
6. Dua JS, Cooper AR, Fox KR, Graham Stuart A (2009) Exercise training in adults with congenital heart disease: feasibility and benefits. Int J Cardiol 138:196–205
7. Fredriksen PM, Kahrs N, Blaasvaer S et al (2000) Effect of physical training in children and adolescents with congenital heart disease. Cardiol Young 10:107–114
8. Therrien J, Fredriksen P, Walker M, Granton J, Reid GJ, Webb G (2003) A pilot study of exercise training in adult patients with repaired tetralogy of Fallot. Can J Cardiol 19:685–689
9. Bradley LM, Galioto FM Jr, Vaccaro P, Hansen DA, Vaccaro J (1985) Effect of intense aerobic training on exercise performance in children after surgical repair of tetralogy of fallot or complete transposition of the great arteries. Am J Cardiol 56:816–818
10. Moalla W, Maingourd Y, Gauthier R, Cahalin LP, Tabka Z, Ahmaidi S (2006) Effect of exercise training on respiratory muscle oxygenation in children with congenital heart disease. Eur J Cardiovasc Prev Rehabil 13:604–611
11. Singh TP, Curran TJ, Rhodes J (2007) Cardiac rehabilitation improves heart rate recovery following peak exercise in children with repaired congenital heart disease. Pediatr Cardiol 28:276–279
12. Rhodes J, Curran TJ, Camil L et al (2005) Impact of cardiac rehabilitation on the exercise function of children with serious congenital heart disease. Pediatrics 116:1339–1345
13. Holloway TM, Chesssex C, Grace SL, Oechslin E, Spriet LL, Kovacs AH (2011) A call for adult congenital heart disease patient participation in cardiac rehabilitation. Int J Cardiol 150:345–346
14. Minamisawa S, Nakazawa M, Momma K, Imai Y, Satomi G (2001) Effect of aerobic training on exercise performance in patients after the Fontan operation. Am J Cardiol 88:695–698
15. Opocher F, Varnier M, Sanders SP et al (2005) Effects of aerobic exercise training in children after the Fontan operation. Am J Cardiol 95:150–152
16. Brassard P, Poirier P, Martin J et al (2006) Impact of exercise training on muscle function and ergoreflex in Fontan patients: a pilot study. Int J Cardiol 107:85–89

Congestive Heart Failure

Acute failure of the heart to meet systemic demand.

Cross-References
▶ Heart Failure, Training

Connectin
▶ Giant Muscle Proteins: Titin/Nebulin

Connective Tissue
▶ Extracellular Matrix

Constitutive (or Cognate) Protein

A protein that is normally present in the cell, often found at a constant level. In general, these proteins are not highly inducible with stress. Some of the heat shock proteins (such as HSPA8–Hsc70) are considered constitutive.

Constraint Induced Movement Therapy (CIMT)

A therapeutic modality used in stroke rehabilitation, in which repetitive task practice with the paretic limb is coupled with restraint of the non-paretic (ipsilesional) limb.

Continuous Submaximal Training
▶ Endurance Training

Contracture

Abnormal shortening of muscle tissue, rendering the muscle, and associated joint(s), highly resistant to stretching. A contracture can lead to permanent disability. It can be caused by fibrosis of the tissues supporting the muscle or the joint or by disorders of the muscle fibers themselves. Clinically, contracture at a joint or joints is typically observed as flexion and fixation.

Cool Down

Cool down is a period that follows any athletic performance with the aim of facilitating the transition from an exertional state to a resting or near-resting state.

Cooperativity

▶ Coordination, Training

Coordination

The process by which parts of a complex neurobiological system are brought into proper relations with each other during functional goal-directed behavior. A second aspect of neurobiological coordination concerns the process by which the body or parts of the body are organized with respect to environmental objects, events, and surfaces. The study of coordination processes is providing a platform for ongoing research collaborations between motor control theorists and biomechanists in the sports sciences.

Coordination, Training

KEITH DAVIDS[1], DUARTE ARAÚJO[2], CHRIS BUTTON[3]
[1]School of Human Movement Studies, Queensland University of Technology,
Queensland, Australia
[2]Technical University of Lisbon,
Cruz Quebrada, Portugal
[3]School of Physical Education, University of Otago,
Dunedin, New Zealand

Synonyms

Cooperativity; Coordinative structures; Interactions; Learning; Motor system re-organization

Definition

In human movement systems, ▶ coordination refers to the process by which components or degrees of freedom are assembled and brought into functional relationship with each other during goal-directed behavior [1]. There are two other important dimensions to coordination which need to be understood in ▶ neurobiology. First, a functional coordination pattern assembled by an individual to complete a performance goal needs to be organized with respect to important sources of information from the environmental such as objects, other individuals, surfaces, and events. Additionally, groups of performers functioning in a team game need to coordinate their actions with respect to each other as well as key task constraints such as rules, performance area dimensions, and equipment. This process involves coordination between agents in a social neurobiological system [2].

Coordination training refers to "the process of mastering redundant degrees of freedom of the moving organ, in other words its conversion to a controllable system. More briefly, coordination is the organization of the control of the motor apparatus."(p. 127) [3]. Through training and practice motor system degrees of freedom can be reorganized into functionally relevant movement patterns, called coordinative structures. Coordinative structures have been defined as "...an assemblage of many microcomponents...assembled temporarily and flexibly, so that a single microcomponent may participate in many different coordinative structures on different occasions."(p. 344) [4].

Description

Complex neurobiological systems, such as individual athletes or sports teams, are composed of many elements that cohere together and interact with each other during goal-directed behavior. For example, in the human motor apparatus, system elements are the many different, but integrated, subsystems of the human body including the neural subsystem, perceptual subsystem, and skeletomuscular subsystem. In social neurobiological systems like sports teams, system components are the individual athletes who coordinate their actions together in attacking or defensive patterns of play. Such systems exhibit many fundamental attributes including: many independent degrees of freedom or component parts which are free to vary; many different system levels (e.g., neural, hormonal, biomechanical in the human body); nonlinearity of behavioral output; capacity for stable and unstable patterned relationships between system components to emerge through processes of self-organization (i.e., these systems can spontaneously shift between many coordinated states); and the ability of subsystem components to constrain the behavior of other subsystems [5, 6]. In response to Bernstein's degrees of freedom problem, how do complex neurobiological systems organize, maintain, and disaggregate the large-scale (or macroscopic) patterned connections which occur between their components? In fact, a coalition of constraints govern emergence of coordination in neurobiology and neurobiological systems exploit surrounding constraints so that functional patterns of behavior emerge in specific performance contexts. In particular, stable patterns of system organization emerge through intrinsic self-organization processes and a neurobiological system's "openness" to energy flows allows them to use surrounding energy sources to constrain their behavior [6, 7].

Athletes in sports exemplify self-organizing, ► complex systems, using specific information sources to coordinate their actions with respect to important environmental objects, surfaces, and events [1]. These ideas imply that learners need to acquire specific information-movement couplings which they can use to satisfy task constraints in various sports and physical activities. Learners establish information-movement couplings by becoming *attuned* to relevant properties of the environment that produce unique patterns of information flows in different sport contexts. There are two processes involved when learners enhance their attunement to information for action [8]. First, learners educate attention by becoming better at detecting key information variables that specify movements from the myriad of variables that do not. During coordination training, learners become attuned to the minimal information needed to regulate movement from the enormous amount available in the environment. Second, learners calibrate actions by tuning existing coordination patterns to critical information sources and, through practice, establish and sustain functional information-movement couplings to regulate coordinated activity with the environment.

The key idea that information and action constrain each other provides a basis for learning design when training coordination in sport. The mutual interdependence of action and information from the environment suggests that an athlete's perceptual and action systems should not be encouraged to function separately during training and practice tasks by coaches and physical educators (see below [9]). Additionally, since motor system degrees of freedom can be configured in many different ways to achieve a specific movement goal, it is clear that coordination training should give learners opportunities to harness motor system variability and adapt their movement patterns. Individual athletes may benefit from an increased amount of variability in movements or tasks, to enhance stability of performance during coordination training. This idea is counterintuitive to traditional

notions of variability as completely random noise or error in movement systems [10]. Instead, increased movement variability (and subsequent changes to informational constraints of performance) may allow a performer to explore the perceptuo-motor workspace of performance in order to assemble functional movement patterns which satisfy specific task constraints.

During coordination training and performance, the individual elements of the body form recognizable patterns over space and time known as coordinative structures. Coordinative structures are functional synergies that emerge between parts of the body used to achieve specific movement goals such as locomotion, reaching and grasping, and hitting. Coordinative structures were proposed as a solution to Bernstein's degrees of freedom problem [1]. Any change in one component is automatically adjusted for in other system components without jeopardizing the achievement of the task goal. Flexibility in adapting to localized conditions is enhanced by the capacity of microcomponents of a coordinative structure to vary in relation to each so that an action goal can be achieved. The implication is that learning design for coordination training needs to ensure specific, coherent, and realistic environments with relevant information sources available to allow learners to adapt their movements to dynamic performance contexts.

During training, coordinative structures form a kind of "task-specific device" suited for specific performance circumstances. Neurobiological systems "soft-assemble" the coordination solutions to movement problems [11, 12]. Rather than controlling each degree of freedom separately during goal-directed movement, the CNS exploits inherent self-organization processes to form coordinative structures. Due to the regulatory role of information, coordination in a movement system is only completely understood in the midst of the "stream of action" [13]. It was argued that attempting to understand movement coordination separately from its environmental context of forces would result in the amplification of the degrees of freedom problem by this reductionist research strategy. According to Newell [14], coordination is defined as the function that constrains potentially free motor system variables into a behavioral unit, whereas the process of control refers to assigning specific values to the variables in the function. These ideas suggest that the inclusion of movement pattern variability is a useful strategy for training of coordination and control processes in sport. Movement system variability is an important part of learning design in sport and rehabilitation. These ideas imply how during training in sport, an athlete's motor system degrees of freedom (i.e., muscles, joints, limb segments) can be configured into functional coordination solutions to achieve specific goals such as diving off a springboard or kicking a football. The abundance of mechanical degrees of freedom available in the degenerate human movement system can be configured in different ways by athletes to perform a diverse range of tasks. In appropriately designed training environments, athletes can learn how to utilize different system degrees of freedom to stabilize a functional coordination pattern. The suggestion is that movement pattern variability in athletes may be functional in allowing performers to coordinate available motor system degrees of freedom in different ways to satisfy constraints on performance.

This perspective provides a different view on variability than is held traditionally. The traditional negative conception of motor system variability has been based on task outcome measures from behavioral studies (e.g., time spent in balance, variation in reaction time measures), resulting in the interpretation of performance error or noise [15]. The study of complex nonlinear dynamical systems has revealed that variability observed in biological systems needs to be carefully understood since it is often functional [1, 10]. Healthy and adaptive biological systems depend on variability of behavior to ensure optimal functioning and an appropriate level of organizational complexity. Increased variability can provide highly functional exploratory behavior, which reveals useful sources of information to regulate movements [16]. The implication is that coordination training should not be aimed at reproduction of a putative common optimal movement pattern by all learners, but that each individual performer can exploit variability within the movement system in different ways to adapt to changing task constraints over time.

Complex Social Neurobiological Systems

Sports teams have also been considered as complex neurobiological social systems which function in a similar coordinated way as other collectives in nature such as flocks of birds and colonies of ants. In spite of the enormous variability and complexity of team ball game situations, theoretical and experimental evidence points to the existence of patterned interpersonal interactions [2]. In complex biological systems, it has been observed that individual organisms use relatively simple local behavioral rules to create structures and patterns at a collective level that are more complex than the behavior of individual agents. For example, previous work on schools of fish has revealed that individual agents of complex systems have a tendency to spontaneously organize themselves into rich coordinated patterns by modifying their movements on the basis of local social interactions [7, 17].

In team sports, behaviors emerge during performance from individual-environment goal-directed interactions (e.g., from 1-vs-1 subphases to 11-vs-11 in football) and have been established through studying attacker-defender symmetries and symmetry breaking decisions and actions in small-sided subphases of team sports [2, 8]. Self-organization in social neurobiological collectives implies that spatiotemporal patterns between system agents are not externally planned or organized by a coordinating agent according to a pre-existing template, but rather are emergent from the nonlinear interactions of the agents in the system.

In physical terms, these processes are expressed in the emergence of organized structures in phase-space describing the interpersonal interactions in subphases like an attacker-defender dyad. Interpersonal coordination can be studied in the emergence and regulation of coordinated states through inherently perceptual processes, based on the dynamics between individuals in a dyad or group. Team games can be described as a series of sub-goals, each constraining the interpersonal coordination of different players to different extents [2, 8]. In team games, the interaction of an attacker with the ball and a defender in a one-on-one subphase can result in a relatively stable interactive dynamic structure, since the defender may counteract any movement made by an attacker.

Application

How the Training Environment Influences Learning

Variable training conditions can enhance learning because an athlete is required to adapt coordinative structures to changes in constraints. This dynamic process is more representative of many game and competition situations than attempting to reproduce one movement solution under a narrow range of static constraints. For example, Chow et al. [18] showed that early in learning to pass a soccer ball, players can discover and refine appropriate coordination patterns through practice where distance and height constraints of the pass were modified. No direct coaching or instructions were required to elicit learning. Instead the players simply explored different functional solutions that allowed them to satisfy the task goal. Using an individualized movement clustering technique, it was observed that learners switched between different preferred movement patterns both between and within training sessions. Variability in coordination enabled the performers to drive their foot through the ball when kicking for distance or alternatively to create back spin on the ball when lifting it over a barrier. Variable training environments serve to develop the crucial information-movement couplings that athletes require to coordinate their actions.

In contrast to traditional strength or endurance training for athletes, coordination training in sports requires practice conditions that mimic the informational and physical constraints that an athlete might experience in competitive performance. For example, it has been observed that, in triplejump training, athletes that practice components of the coordination pattern separately (as static drills) rather than as a whole (dynamic drills) exhibit less functional coordination patterns [9]. Relative motion plots collected during the hop-step transition showed that, in particular, the upper and lower segments of the free (swing) leg were not coupled as effectively when athletes did not complete a number of strides prior to the crucial transition phase. Clearly, both knowledge and respect of the influential constraints affecting performance of a multi-articular action in sport provides practitioners with a powerful framework to guide exploratory practice of athletes.

These ideas are also relevant for developing coordination between team players. Allowing learners opportunities to work out solutions themselves during game play exploits the idea that team player movements are emergent and self-organized under constraints. The appropriateness of decision and actions are determined by the skill set of individuals, teammates, and opponents, as well as the actions of teammates, opponents, and the state of the game. For example, to enhance coordination between attackers in team games to create scoring opportunities, an important exercise would be to practice small-sided, attacking subphases of the games. Simplified task constraints could provide opportunities for subunits of the team (i.e., attackers) to practice and improve scoring skills involved in creating opportunities for scoring. At the same time, tactical issues can be addressed (i.e., deciding when to initiate an attacking phase) in modified games that are representative of the actual sport. In football for example, one such modified game would be to play five attackers versus three defenders with all players restricted to the middle third of the practice pitch until an offensive passing option presents itself on either flank to open the game up into the attacking third of the pitch [18].

References

1. Turvey MT (1990) Coordination. Am Psychol 45:938–953
2. Schmidt RC, O'Brien B, Sysko R (1999) Self-organization of between-persons cooperative tasks and possible applications to sport. Int J Sp Psychol 30:558–579
3. Bernstein NA (1967) The coordination and regulation of movements. Pergamon, Oxford
4. Kay B (1988) The dimensionality of movement trajectories and the degrees of freedom problem: a tutorial. Hum Mov Sci 7:343–364
5. Kugler PN, Turvey MT (1988) Self-organization, flow fields and information. Hum Mov Sci 7:97–129
6. Kelso JAS (1995) Dynamic patterns: the self-organization of brain and behavior. MIT Press, Cambridge, MA
7. Kauffman SA (1993) The origins of order: self-organization and selection in evolution. Oxford University Press, New York
8. Araújo D, Davids K, Hristovski R (2006) The ecological dynamics of decision making in sport. Psychol Sport Exerc 7(6):653–676
9. Wilson C et al (2009) Movement coordination patterns in triple jump training drills. J Sports Sci 27(3):277–282
10. Latash ML, Scholz JP, Schöner G (2002) Motor control strategies revealed in the structure of motor variability. Exerc Sport Sci Rev 30:26–31
11. Kugler PN, Turvey MT (1987) Information, natural law, and the self-assembly of rhythmic movement. Lawrence Erlbaum, Hillsdale
12. Fitch H, Tuller B, Turvey MT (1982) The Bernstein perspective: III. Tuning of coordinative structures with special reference to perception. In: Kelso JAS (ed) Human motor behavior: an introduction. Lawrence Erlbaum, Hillsdale, pp 271–281
13. Kugler PN, Turvey MT (1988) Self-organization, flow fields and information. Hum Mov Sci 7:97–129
14. Newell KM (1985) Coordination, control and skill. In: Goodman D, Wilberg RB, Franks IM (eds) Differing perspectives in motor learning, memory and control. North-Holland, Amsterdam, pp 295–317
15. Davids K, Glazier P, Araujo D, Bartlett R (2003) Movement systems as dynamical systems: the functional role of variability and its implications for sports medicine. Sports Med 33(4):245–260
16. Davids K, Araújo D, Button C, Renshaw I (2007) Degenerate brains, indeterminate behavior and representative tasks: Implications for experimental design in sport psychology research. In: Tenenbaum G, Eklund R (eds) Handbook of sport psychology, 3rd edn. Wiley, New York
17. Sumpter DJT (2006) The principles of collective animal behaviour. Philos Trans Roy Soc B: Biol Sci 361:5–22
18. Chow JY, Davids K, Button C, Koh M (2008) Coordination changes in a discrete multi-articular action as a function of practice. Acta Psychol 127(1):163–176

Coordinative Structures

▶ Coordination, Training

COPD

Chronic obstructive lung disease, preventable and treatable disease with some significant extrapulmonary effects.

Cross-References

▶ Chronic Obstructive Pulmonary Disease

Core Body Temperature

The temperature of all tissues located at a sufficient depth within the body not to be affected by circulatory adjustments or a temperature gradient through surface tissue. Common indices measured include rectal, esophageal, tympanic, oral and gastro-intestinal.

Core-to-Skin Temperature Gradient

The temperature difference between the body core and the skin. This gradient largely determines non-evaporative heat loss, and can be modified by cutaneous vasomotor tone.

Coronary Artery Disease

▶ Coronary Heart Disease

Coronary Heart Disease

CLAUDIA WALTHER
Department of Cardiology, Kerckhoff Clinic, Bad Nauheim, Germany

Synonyms

Atherosclerosis; Coronary artery disease; Heart attack; Physical exercise training

Definition

Coronary artery disease (CAD) is one of the leading causes of morbidity and mortality in most industrialized countries. During the past years, it has gained increasing importance in developing nations as well. Established cardiovascular risk factors for the development of CAD are arterial hypertension, dyslipidemia, diabetes mellitus, insulin resistance, smoking, age, gender, family history, obesity, mental stress, and physical inactivity. CAD is caused by atherosclerosis, which leads to asymmetric thickening of the inner linings of the coronary arteries.

Such coronary artery lesions are named atheroma and consist of cells, connective-tissue elements, lipids, and debris. Atheromas may lead to a narrowing or blockage of the arteries that provide oxygen to the heart muscle.

Over the last decade, exercise training has emerged as a valid therapeutic measure for primary and secondary prevention of CAD. It enhances physical work capacity, improves clinical symptoms, increases myocardial perfusion, and, most importantly, it reduces morbidity and mortality. Several mechanisms have been proposed to account for the positive effects that are mediated by exercise training: (1) Improvement of ▶ endothelial function, (2) reduction of ▶ oxidative stress, (3) reduction of the inflammatory process, and (4) development of new vessels – and ▶ vascular remodeling.

Pathogenetic Mechanisms

There are different mechanisms on how regular physical exercise leads to positive effects upon the cardiovascular and especially how it leads to its protective effects against atherosclerosis. As such physical exercise positively affects different pathogenetic mechanisms that are all involved in the development of atherosclerosis. These are being described in the following paragraphs.

Exercise and Endothelial Function

The key transmitter in the arterial wall which is responsible for vasodilation is nitric oxide (NO), which is a very small and unstable molecule. NO is produced inside intact endothelial cells by the specific enzyme NO synthase (eNOS) through oxidation of L-Arginine. Nitric oxide reaches the vascular smooth muscle by diffusion and induces a cyclic guanosine monophosphate (cGMP) decrease in the intracellular Ca_2+ concentrations by cGMP-dependent second messengers, which leads to smooth muscle relaxation and, hence, vasodilatation (Fig. 1).

Endothelial NO generation and bioavailability is influenced by mechanical, humoral, and metabolic factors. The regulation of NO synthesis occurs at different levels: (1) eNOS gene polymorphisms are related to eNOS expression and activity and may potentially increase the coronary event rate. (2) eNOS mRNA expression depends on the estrogen status and is influenced by shear stress. (3) eNOS mRNA stability is enhanced by vascular endothelial growth factor (VEGF), and final enzyme activity is regulated by the phosphorylation status of serine/threonine residues.

Exercise training is an instrument to exert mechanical forces at the arterial wall through an increase of shear stress. Shear stress along the endothelium has the potential

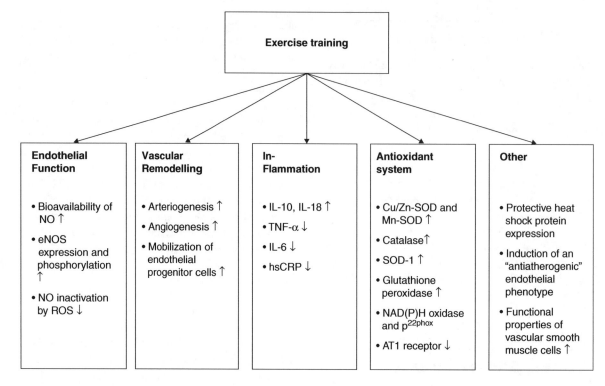

Coronary Heart Disease. Fig. 1 Effects of exercise on endothelial function, vascular remodeling, inflammatory markers, the antioxidant system, and other pathways. *NO* nitric oxide, *eNOS* endothelial nitric oxide synthase, *ROS* reactive oxygen species, *IL* interleukin, *TNF-α* tumor necrosis factor alpha, *hsCRP* high sensitive C-reactive protein, *SOD* superoxide dismutase, *NAD(P)H* nicotinamide adenine dinucleotide phosphate, *AT* angiotensin

to increase eNOS mRNA expression and phosphorylation via AKT (protein kinase B).

NO bioavailability is not only a function of NO production but also of potential NO inactivation by reactive oxygen species (ROS). Several enzymes are responsible for the production of ROS. In case of CAD, especially Nicotinamide adenine dinucleotide phosphatase (NADPH) oxidase, xanthine oxidase, cytochrome P 450, and enzymes of the respiratory chain are the major sources of ROS, which contribute to rapid NO inactivation, thereby causing endothelial dysfunction (Table 1). In the context of NO inactivation, superoxide dismutase (SOD) is a radical scavenger who dismutates ROS, which would otherwise inactivate NO. Exercise training has been shown to increase SOD expression and activity in the vascular bed.

The growing knowledge about the complex regulation of NO synthesis and degradation in cardiovascular diseases and its response to exercise has led to a new understanding of the protective effects of long-term habitual physical activity against atherosclerotic heart disease and vascular aging [1].

Exercise and Antioxidant System

Exercise training is known to protect against atherosclerotic disease, but on the other hand, exercise induces oxidative stress. This is a result of the inefficiency of the mitochondrial respiratory chain and the increase in shear stress on the arterial wall. There is strong evidence that one of the adaptations resulting from exercise is an upregulation of the antioxidant defense mechanisms. Several antioxidant enzymes are upregulated through an increase of laminar shear stress (Table 1).

Exercise and Inflammation

Coronary artery disease is known to be an inflammatory disease, and it is associated with an increase in a lot of inflammatory markers. Some studies suggest that exercise promotes cardioprotection through anti-inflammatory effects. Several authors could demonstrate an inverse relationship between inflammatory markers (hsCRP, IL-6, TNF-α, fibrinogen, and others) and physical fitness and levels of physical activity, especially in patients with cardiovascular disease. The intensity, duration, and type of

Coronary Heart Disease. Table 1 Enzymes producing ROS and radical scavenger enzymes.

Enzymes producing radical oxygen species (ROS)	Radical scavenging enzymes
NAD(P)H oxidase	Superoxide dismutase
Xanthine oxidase	ecSOD
Cytochrome P450	Cu/ZnSOD
Myeloperoxidase	MnSOD
Heme oxygenase	Glutathione peroxidase
Glucose oxidase	Catalase
Cyclooxygenase	Thioredoxin (TRX)
Lipooxygenase	Thioredoxin reductase
Enzymes of the respiratory chain	

In case of CAD, especially NADPH oxidase, xanthine oxidase, cytochrome P450, and enzymes of the respiratory chain were identified as major sources of ROS, which contribute to rapid NO inactivation, thereby causing endothelial dysfunction. However, normally, cells are protected from ROS-mediated damage by radical scavenger enzymes (reported at the *right side*), which are known to decompose ROS

exercise necessary to have an impact on inflammatory markers, however, still is under discussion [2].

Exercise and Vascular Remodeling

Exercise is a powerful stimulus for vascular remodeling and has been shown to increase both the number (angiogenesis) and the diameter (arteriogenesis) of arterial blood vessels in skeletal muscle and the myocardium. These changes of the architecture of the vascular tree are likely associated with functional changes and improved organ blood flow [3].

Angiogenesis

Changes of vascular morphology induced by exercise training in healthy subjects are critically dependent on the initial vessel size. An increased number of vessels in response to exercise training, i.e., angiogenesis, appears to occur on the level of capillaries and very small arterioles (<40 μm in diameter), but not in larger arteries. Vascular remodeling is complex and involves a complex coordination of vascular growth factors, receptors, and modeling factors.

Arteriogenesis

Exercise training has the potential to increase the diameter of large arterioles, small arteries, and conductance arteries, which is an important vascular adaption. Animal studies and clinical observations provide evidence

for a significant correlation between regular physical exercise and increased coronary artery lumen diameter. Arteriogenesis is dependent on activation of endothelial cells and endothelial adherence of monocytes, T-lymphocytes, and bone marrow–derived cells and is mainly dominated by their invasion and production of growth factors in the vascular wall.

Endothelial Progenitor Cells

Endothelial function not only depends on the functional integrity of endothelial and vascular smooth muscle cells, but also on the amount and function of bone marrow–derived stem cells. A subpopulation of these cells, the endothelial progenitor cells, has been shown to improve endothelial function and promote vascular regeneration after damage. Furthermore, these cells have a great capacity for neovascularization. In patients with CAD, the number and function of endothelial progenitor cells is reduced. Exercise training has the potential to mobilize endothelial progenitor cells and to improve their function in patients with CAD, but also in healthy subjects. The impact of EPCs on angiogenesis in ischemic myocardium is still under discussion.

Exercise Intervention

Physical activity helps to ameliorate the potential negative effects of several known atherosclerotic risk factors. Physical activity may be, however, less effective than optimized medical therapy, at least for known risk factors. Nevertheless, an additive effect of medical therapy plus regular physical activity can be postulated. Direct effects of physical activity include weight reduction (in combination with diet), reduction of triglyceride concentrations, and decrease of low-density lipoprotein cholesterol (LDL-C) concentrations. Furthermore, exercise training has the potential to lead to an increase in high-density lipoprotein cholesterol (HDL-C) concentration. Another direct metabolic effect of physical activity is the reduction of insulin resistance and glucose intolerance, which goes along with a risk reduction for the development of metabolic syndrome and diabetes mellitus, respectively [4].

It has been shown in several meta-analyses that exercise-based rehabilitation programs were able to reduce cardiac mortality by 31% in patients with status post myocardial infarction [4]. Despite these beneficial effects of physical exercise upon the prognosis of individual patients, technical advances in percutaneous coronary intervention (PCI) have rendered intracoronary stent implantation the therapy of choice in patients with CAD. However, the risk-benefit-ratio in stable patients with CAD is unclear. Studies comparing an interventional approach including PCI/stent implantation versus a conservative medical therapy strategy show a benefit for PCI concerning relief of symptoms, but no significant difference could so far be detected with respect to reduction of cardiovascular events. In a study comparing exercise training – on top of medical treatment – with PCI/stent implantation, it was demonstrated that exercise training was at least as effective as an interventional approach with PCI and stent implantation with respect to relief of clinical symptoms. In addition, regular exercise training resulted in a better event free survival after 1 year and led to an increased exercise capacity in the exercising patients. An additional approach to an interventional therapeutic strategy may be the implementation of exercise after coronary revascularization, which could reduce the incidence of cardiac events and hospital readmissions compared to patients assigned to usual care.

Although the benefits of regular exercise outweigh its potential risks in patients with stable angina pectoris, it is also recognized that habitually sedentary patients with CHD who engage in strenuous physical activity are at increased risk of myocardial infarction and sudden cardiac death. For this reason, patients with angina who are not routinely active should initially engage in low-intensity activities before engaging in more vigorous physical activity. In addition, patients with CHD who are initiating an exercise program should avoid physical exertion in very cold or hot, humid conditions that might increase the risk of an acute coronary event. Studies performed in supervised exercise programs suggest the risk of major cardiovascular events during exercise training to be between 1/50,000 and 1/120,000 patient-hours of exercise in patients with CHD.

Therapeutical Consequence

Physical inactivity remains a major risk factor for the development of CAD. Therefore, it is of utmost importance that health-care providers support the implementation and maintenance of exercise programs for their patients across the whole lifespan.

Patients with stable angina pectoris should undergo a medical evaluation, including an exercise stress test, for exercise prescription before embarking on an exercise program. General recommendations include low-intensity aerobic training (<40% of maximum aerobic capacity; 50–70% of maximum heart rate) three times per week at the outset. Exercise intensity may progressively be increased as tolerated. Should ischemia or symptoms like angina occur during exercise testing, the target heart rate should generally be fixed at 10 beats/min lower

than the observed ischemic threshold. Each exercise session should consist of three components: (1) a 10 min warm-up period consisting of stretching and low-level calisthenics, (2) a 20–30 min period of aerobic exercise, and (3) a 10 min cool-down period also involving low-level calisthenics and walking. Aerobic exercise (for example, fast walking, jogging, swimming) should be the mainstay of exercise training in patients with CHD. Supervised exercise training programs are also beneficial, especially during the initiation period. They ensure that patients are exercising safely and permit all participants to assess their progress [5].

In conclusion, exercise training is beneficial in patients with chronic stable angina and is associated with an improvement in exercise tolerance, a reduction in angina symptoms, and improved long-term survival. Regular exercise is associated with numerous cardioprotective mechanisms, including effects on endothelial function, inflammation, and improved risk factor control. Patients with angina pectoris should be encouraged to engage in regular physical activity as part of a comprehensive lifestyle intervention for the secondary prevention of CHD.

References

1. Kojda G, Hambrecht R (2005) Molecular mechanisms of vascular adaptations to exercise. Physical activity as an effective antioxidant therapy? Review. Cardiovasc Res 67:187–197
2. Kasapis C, Thompson PD (2005) The effects of physical activity on serum C-reactive protein and inflammatory markers: a systematic review. J Am Coll Cardiol 45:1563–1569
3. Leung F, Yung L, Laher I, Yao X, Chen Z, Huang Y (2008) Exercise, vascular wall and cardiovascular disease. Un update (Part 1). Sports Med 38(12):1009–1024
4. Thompson P, Buchner D, Pina I, Balady G, Williams M, Marcus B, Berra K, Blair S, Costa F, Franklin B, Fletcher G, Gordon N, Pate R, Rodriguez B, Yancey A, Wenger N (2003) Exercise and physical activity in the prevention and treatment of atherosclerotic cardiovascular disease. AHA scientific statement. Circulation 107:3109–3116
5. Fletcher GF, Balady GJ, Amsterdam EA, Chaitman B, Eckel R, Fleg J, Froelicher VF, Leon AS, Piña IL, Rodney R, Simons-Morton DA, Williams MA, Bazzarre T (2001) Exercise standards for testing and training: a statement for healthcare professionals from the American Heart Association. Circulation 104(14):1694–1740

Correlates and Determinants of Physical Activity

Many authors used these words to reflect the factors that affect, or are thought to affect, participation in exercise and physical activity. In other words, they refer to reproducible associations that are potentially causal. Perhaps because it is now recognized that many of the factors discussed are not, or may not be, true determinants (data may show associations but information cannot necessarily be gleaned as to causality), the term "correlates" has now become the standard term to use for this in the literature (see Bauman for a more detailed review). The term "predictor" has also been used in a variety of studies as a synonym of determinant or correlate, that is, not necessarily to mean a causal predictor but a variable statistically associated with a given outcome.

Despite the choice of word, Bauman et al. [1] argued that there are few examples of absolute factors that "cause" the outcome in 100% of cases, and none in the behavioral realm. In behavioral research, there is also the possibility of multiple causal factors (which might "cause" physical activity) and also reciprocal determinism, where the causal relationships are bidirectional – this makes discussion of traditional "causal" pathways more complex. Etiologic variables in behavioral sciences are probabilistic factors that substantially increase the likelihood of the outcomes subsequently occurring, but do not "guarantee" them.**

References

1. Bauman AE, Sallis JF, Dzewaltowski DA, Owen N (2002) Toward a better understanding of the influences on physical activity: the role of determinants, correlates, causal variables, mediators, moderators, and confounders. Am J Prev Med 23(2):5–14

Cortical Plasticity

The ability of the cerebral cortex to adapt to injury and/or environmental stimuli.

Cross-References

▶ Neural Plasticity

Cortical Silent Period

The cortical silent period is a period of reduced or abolished electromyographic activity recorded from a target muscle following transcranial magnetic brain stimulation. The duration of the cortical silent period is used as a measure of cortical inhibition that is thought to be mediated by local GABAergic circuits.

Costal

▶ Diaphragm

CPET (or CXT)

Cardiopulmonary exercise test. A method, which mostly involves analysis of respiratory gas exchange (spiroergometry).

C-Reactive Protein (CRP)

Is one of the plasma proteins known as acute-phase proteins: proteins whose plasma concentrations increase (or decrease) by 25% or more during inflammatory disorders.

Creatine

Louise Deldicque[1], Marc Francaux[2]
[1]Department of Biomedical Kinesiology, Research Centre for Exercise and Health, K.U.Leuven, Leuven, Belgium
[2]Research group in muscle and exercise physiology, Institute of Neuroscience, Université catholique de Louvain, Louvain-la-Neuve, Belgium

Synonyms

(α-Methylguanido)acetic acid; 2-(carbamimidoyl-methyl-amino)acetic acid; Methyl glycocyamine; Methylguanidoacetic acid; N-(aminoiminomethyl)-N-methyl-glycine; N-amidinosarcosine; N-guanyl-N-methylglycine; N-methyl-N-guanylglycine

Definition

Creatine is a nonessential dietary element found in high abundance in meat and fish. Because of its molecular structure, creatine is a member of the ▶ guanidino acid family. It is not an amino acid! Normal daily intake of creatine from an omnivorous diet approximates 1 g [1]. However, creatine is also synthesized within the body, primarily in the liver, from two amino acids by a two-step reaction at a rate of about 1 g per day. In the first step catalyzed by arginine:glycine amidinotransferase, guanidinoacetate is formed from arginine and glycine. In the second step, a methyl group of S-adenosylmethionine is transferred to guanidinoacetate and creatine is formed.

Approximately 120 g of creatine is found in a 70-kg male, 95% in skeletal muscle. Total creatine exists as both free creatine and phosphorylcreatine. The highest levels of creatine and phosphorylcreatine are found in skeletal muscle, heart, spermatozoa, and photoreceptors cells of the retina. Intermediate levels are found in brain, brown adipose tissue, intestine, endothelial cells, and macrophages, and low levels are found in lung, spleen, kidney, liver, white adipose tissue, blood cells, and serum.

Creatine is an important source of chemical energy for muscle contraction because it can undergo phosphorylation with the formation of phosphorylcreatine, and reversible, with donation of the phosphate group to ADP to form ATP. This reaction is catalyzed by the enzyme ▶ creatine kinase and is a rapid source of high-energy phosphate for high-intensity, short-duration physical activity. The initial idea for creatine supplementation in athletes was improving the energy storage under the form of intramuscular phosphorylcreatine.

Creatine kinase activity is higher in skeletal muscle than in others tissues. Evidence exists that the role of the creatine/phosphorylcreatine shuttle system also plays an essential role in energy homeostasis in the heart, brain, and retina to ensure proper development and function.

Mechanism of Action

Since the paper of Roger Harris and collaborators in 1992 who reported for the first time beneficial effects of creatine supplementation, creatine has become one of the most popular dietary supplements in the world. Synthetic supplements exist as creatine monohydrate or various creatine salts, such as creatine citrate or creatine pyruvate, the latter being more soluble than creatine monohydrate.

Muscle creatine content averages 110–120 mmol/kg dry mass and can be increased up to 130–160 mmol/kg dry mass after creatine supplementation, which represents an increase of about 15–30%. Two strategies of supplementation exist. In most conditions, 20 g of creatine is ingested every day for 5 days; thereafter, 3–5 g is consumed daily to maintain muscle uptake. A second strategy omits the loading phase. In this case, the rise in muscle creatine content is slower, but reaches the same level after about 15 days.

To date, several hundred studies have been conducted to evaluate the efficacy of creatine supplementation for improving exercise performance. Nearly 70% of these studies have reported a significant improvement in exercise capacity. The gain in performance can reach up to 10% or 15% depending on the variable of interest, on the exercise mode, and on the exercise intensity. Typically, creatine supplementation seems to be effective in high-intensity, short-duration exercise wherein phosphorylcreatine availability is a limiting factor and not in other situations like in endurance events.

Most, if not all, commercial and anecdotal claims of the beneficial effects of creatine supplementation are focused on the increase in muscle strength and muscle protein mass. Several scientific publications have also emphasized the increase in strength and the higher muscle protein content associated with the increase in body mass or fat-free mass. The pertinent question for researchers and practitioners is whether there is sufficient experimental evidence to support these allegations and what are the mechanisms behind.

After a few weeks of creatine supplementation, the average increase in body mass reported in the literature amounts to 1–2 kg, or 1–2.3% of total body mass, although about 30% of published articles do not report any change. In well-controlled laboratory conditions, creatine supplementation has been shown to improve muscle strength by about 5–20%.

Several hypotheses have been proposed to explain these effects on lean body mass and muscle strength. Creatine per se could induce muscle hypertrophy due to water retention since cellular water content may influence protein metabolism. Creatine has been shown to increase total body water including intracellular water. However, the relative volume of the body water compartments remains unchanged after creatine supplementation. Therefore the gain in body mass cannot be attributed to water retention alone but to an increase in dry matter accompanied by a normal water volume.

Evidence accumulated over the past 15 years suggests that the primary mechanism by which creatine exerts its ▶ anabolic effect in healthy subjects who are weight training is by allowing them to work at a higher proportion of their maximal voluntary contraction force and thus increase the training stimulus. However, this mechanism may not explain all the observations like the higher force production observed in patients suffering from myopathy (see below).

The increase in lean body mass after creatine supplementation could be the result of a larger protein synthesis or a decrease in protein breakdown or both together. However, it has been reported that creatine had no effect on skeletal muscle protein synthesis and breakdown, whether at rest or after resistance exercise suggesting that short-term creatine loading does not have a significant effect on measures of skeletal muscle protein balance.

Other experiments conducted on a longer period of time reported that creatine supplementation resulted in larger increases in type I, IIA, IIAB muscle fiber cross-sectional area compared with placebo after 12 weeks of heavy resistance training and after 2 weeks of leg immobilization followed by 10 weeks of rehabilitation. Creatine supplementation also leads to greater increases in type I and II MHC (myosin heavy chain) mRNA abundance and protein content after 12 weeks of resistance training, suggesting that an increase in MHC synthesis may account in part for the greater increase in muscle size with creatine supplementation. Creatine supplementation has also been shown to amplify the increase in ▶ satellite cell number and myonuclei concentration in human skeletal muscle fibers during 4–16 weeks of resistance training.

In vitro experiments were conducted with the goal of understanding the molecular mechanisms by which creatine stimulates muscle growth. The results indicated that Akt/PKB and p38 MAPK and their downstream targets play essential roles in the enhancement of ▶ myotubes differentiation by creatine [2]. But, the question remains as to how creatine activates the Akt/PKB and the p38 MAPK pathways.

There is a close functional coupling between the ▶ sarcoplasmic calcium ATPase and the creatine kinase system. This functional coupling may explain the faster skeletal muscle relaxation time observed after creatine loading in humans, and the impairment in skeletal muscle excitation/contraction in a mouse model lacking cytosolic and mitochondrial creatine kinase. The increase in calcium uptake may explain the reduction in cytosolic calcium accumulation and enhanced survival of muscular dystrophic myotubes incubated with creatine.

Clinical Use

Creatine supplementation has become one of the most popular ergogenic aids among athletes for enhancing acute performance or training adaptations. In a clinical perspective, the potential exists for creatine to be a therapeutic replacement strategy in neurological and/or muscular diseases as the concentration of phosphorylcreatine in resting skeletal muscle is lower in patients with muscular dystrophy/congenital myopathies, inflammatory myopathies, Huntington's disease, Friedrich's ataxia, and mitochondrial cytopathies, and with normal aging. Brain phosphorylcreatine concentration is lower in patients with mitochondrial cytopathy, cerebral ischemia, and bipolar affective disorders. Creatine supplementation of those patients may result in a partial restoration of intracellular creatine concentration, an increase in type II muscle fiber diameter, improved exercise capacity, increased muscle strength, reduced headache frequency, normalization

of electrocardiogram abnormalities, etc., depending on the type and the severity of the disorder.

Diagnostics

Whereas the determination of the ▶ isoenzymes of creatine kinase or phosphorylcreatine kinase in plasma has been extensively studied and used in the diagnosis of acute myocardial infarction, this paragraph will be focused on the use of creatine itself and its precursors in creatine deficiency syndromes [3] and in neuromuscular diseases [4]. Creatine deficiency syndromes represent a group of inborn errors of creatine synthesis (arginine:glycine amidinotransferase deficiency and guanidinoacetate methyltransferase deficiency) and transport (creatine transporter deficiency). All three defects can be diagnosed by in vivo nuclear magnetic resonance spectroscopy of the brain, which shows a severe reduction or absence of creatine. Laboratory investigations for the diagnosis start with the analysis of guanidinoacetate, creatine, and creatinine in plasma and urine. Measurement of guanidinoacetate, creatine concentrations, and calculation of creatine/creatinine and guanidinoacetate/creatinine ratios in urine makes possible the identification of arginine:glycine amidinotransferase (low creatine with low guanidinoacetate excretion) and guanidinoacetate methyltransferase deficiencies (low creatine with high guanidinoacetate excretion), as well as creatine transporter defects (high creatine/creatinine and guanidinoacetate/creatinine ratios in urine). Moreover, enzyme assays for arginine:glycine amidinotransferase or guanidinoacetate methyltransferase, or a creatine uptake assay for the transporter defect can be performed. DNA mutation analysis of the genes involved can prove the defects at the molecular level. To diagnose patients with creatine transporter deficiency, mutation analysis may be the only choice.

People with neuromuscular disorders such as mitochondrial cytopathies, Huntington's disease, inflammatory myopathies, and Duchenne dystrophy can have lower skeletal muscle total creatine and phosphocreatine concentrations than control subjects. This may be due to lower creatine transporter content or an impairment of energy charge, a measure of the relative amounts of adenosine tri-, di-, and monophosphate in the cell, in these patients. Creatine, phosphocreatine, and adenosine tri-, di-, and monophosphate can be determined in muscle biopsies by biochemical analyses or by nuclear magnetic resonance spectroscopy.

It is of note that guanidinoacetate methyltransferase and arginine:glycine amidinotransferase deficiencies and some neuromuscular disorders are treatable by, or at least benefit from, oral creatine supplementation, but patients with creatine transporter deficiency do not respond to this type of treatment.

References

1. Wyss M, Kaddurah-Daouk R (2000) Creatine and creatinine metabolism. Physiol Rev 80:1107–1213
2. Deldicque L, Theisen D, Bertrand L, Hespel P, Hue L, Francaux M (2007) Creatine enhances differentiation of myogenic C2C12 cells by activating both p38 and Akt/PKB pathways. Am J Physiol Cell Physiol 293:C1263–C1271
3. Nasrallah F, Feki M, Kaabachi N (2010) Creatine and creatine deficiency syndromes: biochemical and clinical aspects. Pediatr Neurol 42:163–171
4. Tarnopolsky MA, Beal MF (2001) Potential for creatine and other therapies targeting cellular energy dysfunction in neurological disorders. Ann Neurol 49:561–574

Creatine Kinase

An enzyme expressed in various cell types that reversibly catalyses the conversion of creatine and adenosine triphosphate to phosphorylcreatine and adenosine diphosphate.

Creatine Phosphate (CP; Phosphocreatine, PC)

A high energy molecule that very rapidly is utilized as payment to re-synthesize ATP.

Critical Power (CP)

The power asymptote of the hyperbolic power–time relationship observed for time-to-fatigue during high-intensity exercise. Critical power represents the highest power output at which it is possible to achieve stable submaximal metabolic (e.g., $\dot{V}O_2$ and blood [lactate]) responses during constant-power exercise.

Crohn's Disease

▶ Inflammatory Bowel Disease, Exercise

Crossbridges

The structures formed when myosin heads bind to actin filaments. This usually happens as a result of activation of the muscle. The crossbridges are responsible for generating the tension on activation.

Crosstalk

Crosstalk refers to the EMG signal detected over a muscle that is generated by a nearby muscle and conducted through the intervening volume of tissue to the recording electrodes. Although crosstalk is an important source of error in interpreting EMG signals, there is currently no accepted approach to prevent crosstalk from contaminating an EMG signal.

Cutaneous Microdialysis

The technique used to assess vascular control mechanisms in the small blood vessels of the skin. These same control mechanisms are found in other tissues and vascular beds, so the skin can be used as a surrogate of microvascular function. This technique involves placing microdialysis fibers (which are small tubes) under the skin using a needle so that drugs (e.g., agonists and antagonists) can be infused into the intradermal space. To determine microvascular function, changes in blood flow to the small vessels of the skin are measured during these infusions.

Cutaneous Vasodilation

The thermo-effector response of the cutaneous vasculature to increase blood flow during hyperthermia. Cutaneous vasodilation increases heat loss by transferring heat from the metabolically active tissues to the periphery via convection. This is largely driven by the core-to-skin temperature gradient. The degree of cutaneous vasodilation reflects the extent of convective heat loss required for thermoregulation.

Cross-References
▶ Thermoregulation

CVA

▶ Stroke

Cyanotic Heart Disease

▶ Congenital Heart Disease

Cycling

GERTJAN ETTEMA, STIG LEIRDAL
Department of Human Movement Science, Faculty of
Social Sciences and Technology Management, Norwegian
University of Science and Technology, Trondheim,
Norway

Synonyms
Bicycling; Biking; Riding a bike

Definition
The narrow definition of cycling is given in one of the
synonyms above, i.e., riding a bike. However, one of the
main characteristics of cycling is that the energy required
for propulsion comes from the human body, not from
artificial devices. Nowadays, there exist various versions of
bicycles that allow for a combination of human and artificially driven propulsion. In the current chapter, the
purely human-powered vehicles are considered. Cycling
is not necessarily restricted to riding a ▶ bicycle, i.e., a two-
wheeled vehicle. Although cycling is usually regarded as
propulsion with the lower extremities, the upper extremities
can be used as well (hand-driven cycling). The UCI (Union
Cycliste Internationale) restricts its activity to cycling on true
bicycles (two wheels) that are driven by the lower extremities
moving in a circular pattern [1].

Description
The first ideas or inventions of a bicycle or bicycle-like
machine may date back to around 1,500. The invention of
the bicycle with a chain-driven rear wheel dates back to
1880–1890 and is referred to as the safety bike. The main
development from safety bicycle to the modern bicycle,
with regard to the driving mechanism, has been the introduction of a gearing system (derailleur), which was
introduced between 1900 and 1910. In modern times,
bicycling has many versions and functions, on or about,
sports (road racing, BMX, mountain biking), recreational
cycling, commuting. Moreover, it is regularly used as
a model for physical activity in performance and health
testing and research.

Cycling cannot be considered a natural form of locomotion for a number of reasons. First of all, it is a non-
weight-bearing activity and thereby likely reduces the
energy cost of locomotion compared to, e.g., gait. Furthermore, in cycling, it is possible to generate propulsive
▶ power almost continuously due to the circular propulsive motion with continuous contact between extremities
and driving system. This is not possible in most other
locomotion forms, such as running, swimming, skating,
cross-country skiing, and rowing, where there is intermittent propulsion, separated by aerial or gliding periods. It
may be that this aspect enhances the ▶ efficiency in cycling
compared to other locomotion forms, as the evenness of
the power distribution over the crank cycle relates closely
to efficiency. Another related characteristic is the lack of an
eccentric muscle action (counter-movement) in the movement cycle, in clear contrast to running.

The energy consumption in cycling has a linear
relation with the produced external power [2], which is
similar to that observed for isolated muscle and referred
to as the Fenn effect. This is likely because cycling
consists of purely concentric muscle contraction. Furthermore, the number of ▶ degrees of freedom in the movement is low and thereby the variation in coordinative
pattern that leads to a cycling movement is limited. This
does not allow for much energy spending in ineffective
muscle action.

Efficiencies, i.e., energy cost per work produced, are
extremely high and may reach 25% [2, 3], which is relatively close to that of isolated concentric muscle contraction and thus indicating very effective transmission of
muscle power to propulsive power.

Because of the gear systems that are available in cycling,
the velocity of the driving movement can be freely chosen,
independent of the locomotion speed. In running this is not
possible; the extension movement of the lower extremity
must exceed the average running velocity as one must accelerate during the push-off. On the other hand, unique for
cycling, movement frequency (cadence) and the velocity of
the propulsive movement are directly coupled.

While cycling, most people adopt a pedal frequency
that is seems to be close to, but still somewhat higher than,
the cadence that leads to the highest efficiency, as opposed
to running where the preferred and most efficient frequencies are similar. Apparently, when cycling, other factors

than energy consumption affect the choice of cadence, e.g., local muscle load and neuromuscular fatigue [3, 4]. Preferred cadence is not a static term, but depends heavily on various factors: external power, body orientation (level vs uphill cycling), and type of regulation of power (e.g., free cycling vs computer controlled ▶ ergometer).

The propulsive power (P) equals the product work per pedal revolution (W_c) and pedal frequency (f_p) and can be presented in different, but equivalent, ways:

$$P = W_c \times f_p = \overline{F}_{\perp p} \times 2\pi r \times f_p = \overline{F}_{\perp p} \times r \times \omega_p$$
$$= \overline{F}_{\perp p} \times v_p = \overline{F}_p \times \cos(\alpha) \times v_p,$$

with $\overline{F}_{\perp p}$ the average pedal force perpendicular on the crank over an entire pedal cycle, r the crank length, ω_p pedal angular velocity (in rad/s), v_p pedal velocity (in m/s), $\overline{F}_p$ the average total pedal force, and α the angle between pedal force and crank. These various options for calculating power in cycling allows for a large variety of variables to choose from that can be measured on a bicycle, both in the laboratory on cycle ergometers or using advanced home trainer systems. This makes this mode of locomotion extremely suitable for research and testing in exercise, physical activity, and health.

Application

Cycling is frequently used in testing of physical performance capacity, both aerobic and anaerobic. This is done by the use of different protocols where external power and thereby metabolic rate are accurately regulated and controlled. Figure 1 shows data for different groups of people with clear different physical capacities. The simple linear relationship allows for easy determination, not only of capacity (i.e., maximally obtainable external power and metabolic rate), but also of any deviation from the relationship for the healthy young adult. In the case of the groups presented in Fig. 1, it is clear that well-trained cyclists have a higher maximal capacity than untrained and ▶ fibromyalgia patients. Patients with ▶ chronic obstructive pulmonary disease (COPD) compare very well with the healthy untrained. Furthermore it is apparent that the fibromyalgia patients deviate to some extent from the general relationship in that they utilize excessive amounts of additional energy when increasing power.

Cycling, including hand-driven cycling, is used regularly in rehabilitative aerobic exercise training for reasons described above: it is a non-weight-bearing form of exercise, it can be performed in a variety of postures, including supine or recumbent position, and it consists purely of concentric work without high-impact phases. Furthermore, extremely low workloads can be applied, which is difficult in, e.g., walking and running. Therefore, cycling is also extremely fitting exercise for weight loss therapy. Ergometer cycling is one of the best exercise modalities for functional electrical stimulation (FES) in

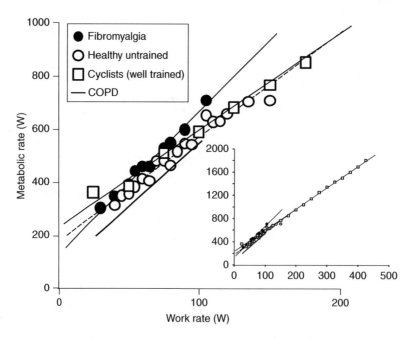

Cycling. Fig. 1 Energy expenditure (metabolic rate) versus work rate in ergometer cycling. □ well-trained cyclists (unpublished, from same experiments as in [5]; ● fibromyalgia patients (unpublished) ○ (untrained, unpublished). Solid fat line COPD [6]

patients with spinal cord injury because it does not require balance control and is a relative easy movement to initiate via FES (by the low number of degrees of freedom).

With regard to training, cycling is mostly used for ▶ endurance training. The effects of cycling training comply with effects of endurance training in general. It is often debated that cycling leads to a lower load of the cardiovascular system than in various other exercise modalities (e.g., running and cross-country skiing) and thereby leads to less training effects. However, there is very little evidence for this notion in the research literature [4]. Still, the maximal ▶ aerobic capacity ($\dot{V}O_{2\,max}$) tends to be higher in (treadmill) running than (ergometer) cycling. Another matter of discussion is if training can improve the efficiency in cycling. Because of the high-efficiency values in general, for reasons stated above, there seems to be little opportunity for improvement. Still, some effects have been documented. Also groups with different training states may show small differences (see Fig. 1). The mechanisms for these training effects are unclear, but muscle fiber-type transformation, changes in the respiratory chain reactions in the mitochondria and improvements of cycling technique, including cadence, are likely candidates. The change in use, rather than transformation, of fiber types may also play a role.

Considering cycling in sports, the most popular discipline is road cycling, consisting of road races (typically 100–250 km taking 3–7 h) and time trials (usually between 10 and 50 km, taking 15–60 min). Stage races consist of several races (varying from 3 days to 3 weeks, usually 1 race per day). The work rate during road races are often low to moderate (100–300 W) but can be very high during critical parts of the race (400–2,000 W) depending on terrain and tactics. Because of the long duration of a race, energy consumption is extremely high, often between 5,000 and 10,000 Kcal/race day [7]. Time trials are typically performed as an individual all-out race. In time trials, work rate can be as high as 450–500 W on average over 1 h [7]. Heart rate is between 88% and 100% of maximal for 95% of the race.

The long duration of competitions forces athletes to perform extreme doses of training, up to 35,000 km per year [7], mostly (about 90% of training time) at low intensity (60–80% maximal heart rate). This includes about 100 races per year for professional cyclists [7]. This extreme dose of exercise is not seen in any other endurance sport. The capability to endure such amount of exercise is likely related to the pure concentric movement nature of cycling. Professional cyclists gain a high aerobic capacity with $\dot{V}O_{2\,max}$ between 75 and 90 ml kg^{-1} min^{-1}.

Cycling technique as a performance factor has come into focus in the last decades. The force effectiveness ratio has gained most interest as a variable describing the quality of technique. The force effectiveness is the ratio between the effective force (perpendicular on the crank arm) and the total force applied to the pedal. This ratio has been shown to be between 40% and 60% depending on work rate and cadence. However, so far, there are no clear indications that this variable is related to performance.

References

1. Union Cycliste Internationale. UCI cycling regulations, version on 02 Jan 2011. http://www.uci.ch/Modules/BUILTIN/getObject.asp?MenuId=MTkzNg&ObjTypeCode=FILE&type=FILE&id=34033&LangId=1 (18 Apr 2011)
2. Ettema G, Lorås HW (2009) Efficiency in cycling: a review. Eur J Appl Physiol 106:1–14
3. Faria EW, Parker DL, Faria IE (2005) The science of cycling. Factors affecting performance – part 2. Sports Med 35:313–337
4. Millet GP, Vleck VE, Bentley DJ (2009) Physiological differences between cycling and running. Lessons from triathletes. Sports Med 39(3):179–206
5. Leirdal S, Ettema G (2009) Freely chosen pedal rate during free cycling on a roller and ergometer cycling. Eur J Appl Physiol 106:799–805
6. Perrault H et al (2007) Cycling efficiency is not compromised for moderate exercise in moderately severe COPD. Med Sci Sports Exerc 39:918–925
7. Jeukendrup AE, Craig NP, Hawley JA (2000) The bioenergetics of world class cycling. J Sci Med Sport 3:414–433

Cyclosporine A

Main immunosuppressive drug in use in heart transplantation in the 1984–2003 era from the class of calcineurin antagonists.

Cystic Fibrosis

BLAKESLEE E. NOYES
School of Medicine, St. Louis University at SSM Cardinal Glennon Children's Medical Center, St. Louis, MO, USA

Synonyms

Cystic fibrosis of the pancreas; Mucoviscidosis

Definition

Cystic fibrosis (CF) is an autosomal recessive disorder recognized as the most common lethal genetic disease in the Caucasian population, with an estimated 30,000 patients in the USA and 27,000 in Europe. CF is most common among Caucasians of northern European descent, with a disease prevalence of ~1 in 3,000 births, and the frequency of being a carrier of a defective CF gene is estimated as 1 in 29. CF affects exocrine glands throughout the body leading to the production of abnormal mucus. Most importantly, the abnormalities in mucus character lead to obstruction of pancreatic ducts, bronchi, and bronchioles. The primary clinical features include protein and fat malabsorption, poor growth, and recurrent respiratory tract infections. CF is caused by mutations in the gene encoding the cystic fibrosis transmembrane conductance regulator (▶ CFTR) protein located on the long arm of chromosome 7. Over 2,500 distinct CFTR mutations have been identified, but deletion of phenylalanine at position 508 (▶ ΔF508) of the CFTR protein is by far the most common.

Pathogenetic Mechanisms

The CFTR protein is expressed primarily on the apical membrane of epithelial cells, where it functions as a regulated chloride ion (Cl^-) channel. However, CFTR has other important regulatory roles in ion movement, notably influencing Na^+ transport and water movement across many epithelial cells (see below). The abnormalities of ion and water movement across epithelial cell surfaces lead to many of the clinical manifestations of CF including symptoms related, primarily, to the respiratory tract, the gastrointestinal tract, and the sweat glands. The CFTR protein is expressed on epithelial cells of many organs, as well as exocrine glands and blood cells, but its most important pathophysiologic consequences involve the respiratory epithelia, the cells lining the ducts of the pancreas, and serous sweat glands.

The mechanism by which CFTR dysfunction leads to the clinical manifestations of CF is based upon the ▶ low-volume hypothesis, one most generally accepted within the CF research community. It postulates that impaired CFTR function causes excessive reabsorption of Na^+ and water. Within the respiratory mucosa, this CFTR defect dehydrates the periciliary layer (PCL) that lies beneath the secreted mucus, thereby slowing or preventing coordinated ciliary movements (Fig. 1).

This defect inhibits normal ciliary movement and cough clearance of mucus allowing hypoxic niches to develop that promote infection with bacteria, notably *Pseudomonas aeruginosa*. Due to this relative dehydration, the mucus of CF patients is thickened and tenaciously sticky, and therefore poorly cleared.

Exercise Intervention

The role of exercise and physical training in cystic fibrosis has been examined closely over the last three decades. Evidence exists that a program of physical fitness in patients with CF may preserve or lessen the rate of decline in lung function, improve survival, and enhance quality-of-life measures. There is considerable debate as to its role as a substitute for chest physiotherapy (CPT) techniques in CF (see below) though systematic reviews have not demonstrated superiority over more traditional forms of airway clearance. However, the addition of an exercise program to CPT significantly improves lung function compared with CPT alone. The mechanism by which exercise might improve airway clearance is not well understood. One

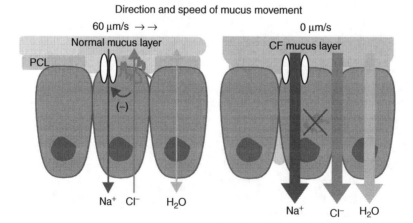

Cystic Fibrosis. Fig. 1 The low-volume hypothesis in CF with a reduced periciliary aqueous layer (PCL) due to excessive salt and water reabsorption because of abnormal CFTR function. Subsequent effects on normal mucociliary transport are shown with a normal epithelium at *left* and CF on *right*

hypothesis suggests that increases in ventilatory demand accompanied by attendant increases in tidal volume and respiratory flow improve clearance of mucus from more peripheral airways. Regardless, most CF practitioners recommend a combined program of physical training along with a daily regimen of CPT to enhance clearance of the thick, tenacious mucus characteristic of CF.

Consequences

The result of the pathogenetic mechanisms described above lead to recurrent respiratory symptoms such as cough, wheeze, and respiratory distress; episodes of bronchitis or pneumonia combined with complications linked to exocrine ▶ pancreatic insufficiency including steatorrhea; failure to thrive; an excessive or "voracious" appetite; malnutrition; and fat-soluble vitamin deficiencies. Up to 15% of patients with CF will present as newborns with ▶ meconium ileus that causes symptoms of small bowel obstruction, including vomiting, abdominal distension, and an absence of bowel movements. However, it bears emphasizing that 5–10% of CF patients have pancreatic sufficiency that permits normal absorption and growth.

The diagnosis of CF can be made in the presence of specific phenotypic features combined with evidence of CFTR dysfunction. The most useful and widely available measure of CFTR dysfunction is the ▶ sweat chloride test. Values for Cl^- over 60 mM are considered diagnostic of CF; values between 40 and 59 mM are graded as intermediate and values <40 mM are considered normal. For infants up to 6 months of age, sweat chloride values <30 mM are normal, and values between 30 and 59 mM are considered intermediate.

Obtaining blood for CF gene mutation analysis is an acceptable alternative to establish a diagnosis of CF, provided that two disease-causing CFTR mutations are identified. However, given the 2,500+ mutations described to date, it is impractical and prohibitively expensive to carry out expanded CF mutation analyses on routine blood samples. Thus, commercial laboratories that screen for a discrete number of the most common mutations may report a falsely negative test. Nevertheless, the sweat test remains the gold standard for diagnosing classic CF.

With the near universal adoption of newborn screening for CF (all 50 states in the USA, the UK, and most European countries), the hope is to identify patients in a presymptomatic stage before the onset of significant malnutrition or pulmonary disease, and to direct early and aggressive interventions at the respiratory and gastrointestinal manifestations of CF.

The respiratory consequences of CF are characterized by excessive airway inflammation developing at a variable period in the first years of life that includes an increase in airway neutrophils and release of pro-inflammatory cytokines such as IL-8. In conjunction with this process, children with CF often become infected with a variety of pathogens, most notably *Haemophilus influenza* and *S. aureus*. Eventually, the majority of CF patients become infected with *Pseudomonas aeruginosa*. Chronic airway infection ensues with mucus plugging, vicious cycles of inflammation and infection, and airway injury with the eventual development of ▶ bronchiectasis. These events worsen lung function, lead to chronic hypoxemia and hypercarbia and, eventually, in the large majority of patients, death from respiratory failure. The goals for treatment of the respiratory manifestations of CF are to prevent or delay progression of the pulmonary lesion through relief of airway obstruction, control of infection, and control of the consequences of infection and inflammation. This entails a multifactorial approach of aggressive airway clearance (chest physical therapy and exercise programs), altering the character of the abnormal mucus (aerosolized therapies such as recombinant human DNase, hypertonic saline), treatment of inflammation (ibuprofen, azithromycin), and treatment of infection (oral, parenteral, and aerosolized antibiotics). In those patients with end-stage respiratory failure, lung transplantation is a potential option.

The GI disease features of CF include evidence of exocrine pancreatic insufficiency in 85–90% of CF patients. Symptoms associated with CF pancreatic dysfunction include large, oily, foul-smelling stools; abdominal distension, discomfort, and flatulence; and increased food and fluid intake. Collectively these symptoms of CF disease in the GI tract lead to poor growth, malnutrition, failure to thrive, and deficiencies of the fat-soluble vitamins A, D, E, and K. Regular replacement therapy with pancreatic enzymes and provision of supplemental vitamins are essential components of proper nutritional management in CF. In some patients, hepatic dysfunction arising from bile duct obstruction secondary to serous gland secretion defects can occur. This may take the form of mild, nonspecific hepatic enzyme abnormalities or in rarer circumstances, biliary cirrhosis with attendant risks of developing portal hypertension, splenomegaly, esophageal varices, and thrombocytopenia. For many years, it has been recognized that better growth is closely linked with improved respiratory outcomes, underscoring the importance of optimizing nutritional management.

Other consequences of CF include the development of CF-related diabetes mellitus arising from auto-digestion of the pancreas and eventual replacement of pancreatic tissue with fat. About 10% of patients develop this complication in the second decade of life with rates as high as 30% in young adults. Oral hypoglycemic agents are generally not helpful in patients with CFRD, such that insulin injections are required. Reproductive system defects in CF include obstructive azoospermia, absence of the vas deferens, and infertility in the large majority of males with CF. While females with CF are reported to have abnormal cervical mucus, they are generally fertile and can successfully deliver a normal infant if they receive appropriate perinatal nutrition and have adequate lung function at parturition.

Survival in cystic fibrosis continues to improve as new basic science knowledge about CFTR and its inheritance, combined with improved understanding of the basic pathophysiology of CF and advances in translational and clinical research have led to increases in median survival among CF patients. Indeed, the latest data available from the US CF Foundation Registry show median survival now extending well into the fourth decade. While this survival reflects a highly significant improvement from just 20 years ago, it still lags far behind survival statistics for the general US population.

References

1. Rowe SM, Miller S, Sorscher EJ (2005) Mechanisms of disease: cystic fibrosis. N Eng J Med 352:1992–2001
2. Orenstein DM, Higgins LW (2005) Update on the role of exercise in cystic fibrosis. Curr Opin Pulm Med 11:519–523
3. O'Sullivan BP, Freedman SD (2009) Cystic fibrosis. Lancet 373:1891–1904
4. Mogayzel PJ, Flume PA (2010) Update in cystic fibrosis, 2009. Am J Respir Crit Care Med 181:539–544

Cystic Fibrosis of the Pancreas

▶ Cystic Fibrosis

Cystic Fibrosis–Related Diabetes Mellitus

Up to 15% of adolescents and 30% of young adults may develop CF-related DM, an entity characterized by insulin deficiency and resistance. Although the exocrine pancreas is primarily involved in CF, in CFRDM, autodigestion of the pancreas with fatty replacement results in islet cell dysfunction. Treatment is with insulin injections as oral hypoglycemic agents are not effective.

Cytochrome C Oxidase (or Complex IV)

It is the last enzyme in the respiratory electron transport chain of mitochondria (or bacteria) located in the mitochondrial (or bacterial) membrane.

Cytokines

Katsuhiko Suzuki
Waseda University, Tokorozawa, Saitama, Japan

Synonyms

Bioactive substances in intercellular signal transduction

Definition

The word "cytokine" is derived from Greek roots meaning "to put cells into motion," and is defined as a diverse family of intercellular signaling molecules that exert important effects on inflammatory and immune responses or hematopoiesis [1].

Basic Mechanisms

Cytokines are produced by a variety of cells and usually act in an autocrine or paracrine manner at extremely low concentrations. Localized ▶ inflammation is considered to be a physiological protective response to initial tissue damage. Subsequently, local inflammatory factors mediate the repair of this damaged tissue as long as the inflammatory process is strictly controlled to keep inflammatory mediators and cells sequestered. The loss of this local control or an overly activated response can result in an exaggerated systemic response, which potentially becomes pathogenic, self-destructive and, at times, fatal to the host. The systemic inflammatory response syndrome (SIRS) is a condition that describes the resultant systemic cytokine release (▶ Hypercytokinemia) associated with numerous acute serious diseases such as severe trauma, thermal injury, shock, systemic infections, adult respiratory distress syndrome, and acute myocardial infarction.

Exhaustive exercise can sometimes cause flu-like symptoms such as fever, chills, fatigue, myalgia, headache, and appetite loss, and these symptoms might be associated with hypercytokinemia. Indeed, it has been suggested that increased cytokine release may underlie the overtraining syndrome in athletes as well as a variety of systemic immune/inflammatory conditions such as the common cold and rheumatoid arthritis [1]. Of the multitude of cytokine mediators operating in SIRS, the three most influential cytokines are considered to be tumor necrosis factor (TNF)-α, ► interleukin (IL)-1, and IL-6. For instance, it has been documented in a sepsis model that TNF-α appears to be the first cytokine released systemically, and peaks within 2 h after the onset of sepsis, followed shortly thereafter by peaks in IL-1, and then IL-6 within 4 h after the onset of illness or infection. These proinflammatory cytokines induce pyrogenesis and promote subsequent acute inflammatory responses such as leukocytosis (neutrophilia) by inducing granulocyte colony-stimulating factor (G-CSF) and ► chemokines (abbreviated from chemotactic cytokines) such as IL-8 and monocyte chemotactic protein (MCP)-1. There are also compensatory anti-inflammatory responses to reestablish homeostasis; some anti-inflammatory cytokines including IL-1 receptor antagonist (IL-1ra), IL-4, and IL-10 are secreted into the circulation, which dampen the proinflammatory cytokine cascade.

Exercise Intervention

Cytokine Kinetics in Case of Exercise

TNF-α has been considered as a primary mediator of the SIRS response. In response to exercise, the plasma concentration has been reported to rise slightly several hours after intensive exercise and following long-lasting endurance exercise, but most studies report no changes in TNF-α [1]. Failure to detect changes in TNF-α after exercise may be attributed to the low intensity of exercise, the delayed secretion, or the rapid clearance from the circulation into the urine. Since exercise stimulates the release of soluble TNF receptor, which inactivates systemic TNF-α, the actions of TNF-α, if any, can be blocked at least in the circulation.

As for IL-1β, several studies have reported that the plasma concentration increases after long-duration exercise. As for short-duration maximal exercise, a slight increase in plasma IL-1β has been reported, but this might be due to the effect of exercise-induced hemoconcentration usually characterized by 20–30% plasma volume changes. The inability to detect changes in IL-1β may also be attributed to a delayed secretion that occurs several hours after exercise. Based on the delayed-onset production, however, there is too little rationale to indicate that TNF-α and/or IL-1β initiate exercise-induced cytokine responses and immune changes.

IL-2 is a potent functional modulator of lymphocytes and there are several reports demonstrating a decrease in plasma concentration after exercise. Endurance exercise induces soluble IL-2 receptor following exercise and this may interfere with the bioavailability of IL-2, and indeed the measurement of systemic IL-2 concentrations. Most ex vivo studies, however, have shown that acute exercise impairs the ability of stimulated lymphocytes to produce IL-2, suggesting that the bioactivity of IL-2 is not easily induced following exhaustive exercise. Interferon (IFN) has been suggested to rise in the circulation following endurance exercise using a bioassay sensitive to IFN-α or neopterin, a biomarker of IFN-γ secretion, but few studies have reproduced the findings with direct measurements using immunoassays specific for IFN-α and IFN-γ. With respect to the effects of acute exercise on ex vivo IFN-α and IFN-γ production by peripheral blood mononuclear cells or whole blood, it is noteworthy that most studies reported decreased responses to exercise. Taken collectively, it is unlikely that the production and actions of IFN are greatly promoted by exercise.

IL-12 was originally identified as a stimulatory factor of natural killer (NK) cells and is now classified as a major immunomodulatory cytokine, driving the production of type-1 cytokines (IL-2 and IFN-γ) and activating NK and T cells. Bioactive IL-12 p70 is a heterodimer composed of two subunits: p35 and p40, whereas the IL-12 p40 homodimer in the absence of p35 expression and free p40 monomer does not mediate IL-12 activity, but acts as an IL-12 antagonist. Endurance exercise increases plasma levels of IL-12 p40, which might block the production of IL-2 and IFN-γ [2].

Anti-inflammatory cytokines also appear after endurance exercise. IL-1ra is a natural antagonistic cytokine that competes with IL-1α and IL-1β for receptor binding without inducing signal transduction. Regardless of whether a small quantity of IL-1 is released after exercise in a delayed-onset manner as described above, the overwhelming increase in IL-1ra should block IL-1 bioactivity in advance, at least in the circulation [3].

IL-4 downregulates TNF-α and IL-1β and upregulates IL-1ra production and thus contributes to the dampening of inflammation. It has been reported that plasma IL-4 increased 2 h after maximal exercise [1]. Since IL-4 is a main inducer of anti-inflammatory and type-2 cytokines (IL-1ra, IL-5, IL-6, IL-10, and IL-13), its involvement in regulating the pro-/anti-inflammatory cytokine balance during exercise is possible.

IL-10 causes the ► immunosuppression associated with various forms of trauma by attenuating the synthesis of proinflammatory and immunomodulatory cytokines and enhancing IL-1ra production. Short-duration near maximal exercise and eccentric exercise do not induce elevations in plasma IL-10, whereas IL-10 is released into the circulation under prolonged, severe exercise conditions [1, 3].

It is known that IL-6 inhibits the release of IL-1β and TNF-α and stimulates the secretion of IL-1ra, IL-10, and soluble TNF receptor, and thus contributes to the termination of immune/inflammatory reactions. On the other hand, IL-6 causes mobilization and functional augmentation of ▶ neutrophils [1, 4]. It is established that endurance exercise increases plasma IL-6 in large amounts. IL-6 is reported to appear in the systemic circulation within 1 h of endurance exercise, and to increase depending on exercise intensity and duration. Pedersen and her colleagues demonstrated that IL-6 is locally produced in contracting skeletal muscles independent of muscle damage [5]. If contracting skeletal muscle is the predominant source of systemic IL-6, the traditional cytokine cascade initiated by TNF-α and/or IL-1 may not necessarily be the initiator of other cytokine induction in the case of exercise. On the other hand, the responses of TNF-α and IL-1β to exercise are smaller, delayed, and less consistent, and there is no corresponding induction of immunomodulatory cytokines. These findings suggest that the exercise-induced cytokine response might differ kinetically from the sepsis-induced prototypical cytokine cascade, although the possibility cannot be excluded that TNF-α and IL-1 are produced and work mainly in local tissues such as skeletal muscle without systemic release [1].

G-CSF, granulocyte macrophage (GM)-CSF and macrophage (M)-CSF are the family of hematopoietic growth factors that control the survival, proliferation, and differentiation of hematopoietic progenitor cells and functionally mature neutrophils, ▶ monocytes, and ▶ macrophages. We reported that marathon running increased plasma and urine concentrations of G-CSF [3]. We further demonstrated that plasma G-CSF concentration increased significantly immediately after maximal exercise, remaining elevated up to 2 h after exercise, and that urine G-CSF levels increased 1 h after exercise [1]. These findings indicate that G-CSF is released rapidly depending on the exercise intensity, and that the increased plasma G-CSF eventually appears in the urine. Similarly, plasma GM-CSF and M-CSF rose immediately but temporarily after maximal exercise, and were also present in urine 1 h later [1].

IL-8 is a potent neutrophil chemotactic and activation protein referred to as neutrophil activating peptide 1 (NAP-1). Moderate-intensity endurance exercise causes no change or a borderline significant rise in plasma IL-8 [4], whereas the marathon race causes a marked increase in plasma IL-8 [3]. These findings suggest that IL-8 is

released into the circulation under prolonged, severe exercise conditions. On the other hand, short-time intensive exercise is also reportedly to enhance plasma IL-8 [1]. These findings suggest that not only the duration but also the intensity of exercise might be important for the IL-8 release.

MCP-1, which is also known as monocyte chemotactic and activating factor (MCAF), facilitates infiltration and activation of monocytes and macrophages. We demonstrated that MCP-1 concentration increased significantly in not only plasma but also urine following a marathon race and immediately after short-duration intensive exercise [1].

Clinical Significance of Cytokine Kinetics

It has been suggested that exercise induces a release firstly of a sequence of proinflammatory cytokines and then of immunomodulatory and anti-inflammatory cytokines. However, it appears that strenuous exercise does not induce proinflammatory cytokines (TNF-α and IL-1) at first but in a delayed-onset manner, if at all. Furthermore, actions of IL-1β, IL-2, and TNF-α can be blocked by IL-1ra and soluble receptors for IL-2 and TNF, or their synthesis might be inhibited by IL-4, IL-6, and IL-10. These antagonistic actions may explain the equilibrium of proinflammatory and immunomodulatory cytokines. On the other hand, a shift from type-1 to type-2 cytokines occurs following acute exhaustive exercise, and this might lead to ▶ allergy reaction and atopic disposition. Indeed, exercise-induced asthma, anaphylaxis, and systemic histamine release are demonstrated to be more prevalent in athletes. Although exhaustive exercise such as marathon and triathlon occasionally result in cellular immunosuppression and increased susceptibility to infection, these pathogenic conditions might be explained partly by the balance of type-1/type-2 (Th1/Th2) cytokines or pro-/anti-inflammatory cytokines.

Exercise is known to generate reactive oxygen species, and inflammatory ▶ oxidative stress caused by neutrophils and monocytes has received growing attention as one of the main pathogenic mechanisms of multiple organ failure in SIRS. Colony-stimulating factors and chemokines that can recruit and activate neutrophils and monocytes are secreted systemically following exercise. This may, at least in part, mediate exercise-induced pathogenesis such as inflammatory-associated muscle damage, exertional rhabdomyolysis, and heatstroke-related multiple organ failure including acute renal dysfunction.

The cytokine responses to exercise are closely associated with stress exposure and energy demands of endurance exercise [1, 5]. With these findings in mind, further

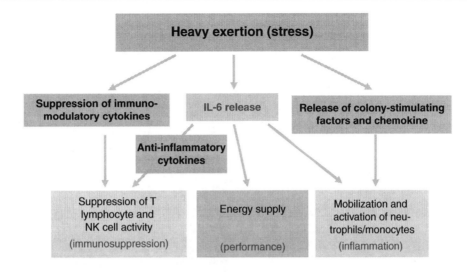

Cytokines. Fig. 1 Biological significance of the exercise-induced systemic cytokine release

studies applying fundamental knowledge to the practical area of sports medicine as well as clinical and preventive medicine are needed (Fig. 1).

Cross-References

▶ Adipose-Tissue-Derived Hormones

References

1. Suzuki K, Nakaji S, Yamada M, Totsuka M, Sato K, Sugawara K (2002) Systemic inflammatory response to exhaustive exercise. Cytokine kinetics. Exerc Immunol Rev 8:6–48
2. Suzuki K, Nakaji S, Kurakake S, Totsuka M, Sato K, Kriyama T, Fujimoto H, Shibusawa K, Machida K, Sugawara K (2003) Exhaustive exercise and type-1/type-2 cytokine balance with special focus on interleukin-12 p40/p70. Exerc Immunol Rev 9:48–57
3. Suzuki K, Yamada M, Kurakake S, Okamura N, Yamaya K, Liu Q, Kudoh S, Kowatari K, Nakaji S, Sugawara K (2000) Circulating cytokines and hormones with immunosuppressive but neutrophil-priming potentials rise after endurance exercise in humans. Eur J Appl Physiol 81:281–287
4. Suzuki K, Totsuka M, Nakaji S, Yamada M, Kudoh S, Liu Q, Sugawara K, Yamaya K, Sato K (1999) Endurance exercise causes interaction among stress hormones, cytokines, neutrophil dynamics, and muscle damage. J Appl Physiol 87:1360–1367
5. Pedersen BK, Febbraio MA (2008) Muscle as an endocrine organ: focus on muscle-derived interleukin-6. Physiol Rev 88:1379–1406

Cytoskeleton

Intracellular meshwork of different types of filaments (microtubuli, actin and intermediate filaments) which is responsible for cellular shape, structure and polarity. It plays important roles in intracellular cell traffic and transport as well as in cell division.

Cytotoxic Therapy

Term used to describe a broad range of therapies (drugs) to kill tumor cells.

D

3,7-Dihydro-1,3,7-Trimethyl-1 H-Purine-2,6-Dione

▶ Caffeine

Daily Energy Expenditure

The energy required throughout a 24 h period that includes resting metabolic rate (RMR), the thermic effect of feeding (the cost of digesting and assimilating nutrients) and physical movement (e.g., exercise and physical activity).

Dalton's Law of Partial Pressures

Described in 1801 by John Dalton, this law states that the total pressure of a compartment is equal to the sum of the partial pressures of the gases present.

D-Dimers

D-dimers are fibrin degradation products released in the process of fibrinolysis. They contain two cross-linked D fragments of the fibrinogen protein. D-dimers are markers of endogenous fibrinolysis and they therefore detected in plasma of patients with thrombosis. While a negative result practically rules out thrombosis (high negative predictive value), a positive result can indicate thrombosis but may also be the outcome of several other clinical conditions. Its main use, therefore, is to exclude thromboembolic disease in patients with low pretest probability.

Cross-References
▶ Hemostasis

Defense of Microorganisms

▶ Immune System

Degeneration

A substantial destruction of the muscle cell, tissue or organ.

Degenerative Joint Disease

▶ Osteoarthritis

Degradative Machinery

▶ Ubiquitin-Proteasome System

Degree of Freedom

One of many elements within a complex system that can exhibit an independent direction of movement through either translation or rotation. How the nervous system is able to regulate and manipulate these elements is often a focus for research in the field of motor control.

Dehydration

The process of reducing the body water content.

Cross-References
▶ Fluid Replacement

Delta F508

It is the most common mutation in cystic fibrosis with ~80% of patients having at least one copy of this mutation and ~50% having two copies. Phenylalanine is deleted at

Frank C. Mooren (ed.), *Encyclopedia of Exercise Medicine in Health and Disease*, DOI 10.1007/978-3-540-29807-6,
© Springer-Verlag Berlin Heidelberg 2012

amino acid 508 of the 1,480 amino acid polypeptide that comprises the CFTR protein. Virtually all patients who are homozygous for delta F508 have evidence of pancreatic insufficiency.

Dendrite

The dendrite is the part of the neuron where electrical and chemical signals are received and integrated.

Dendritic Cells

Mammalian antigen-presenting cells that link the innate and adaptive immune systems. They are found on mucosal membranes and in the blood. There are at least two types: myeloid and plasmacytoid dendritic cells, based on cell characteristics, morphology, substances they secrete, and the innate immune receptors with which they interact. When activated, they migrate to the lymph nodes where they signal lymphocytes to initiate and shape the adaptive immune response to an invading pathogen.

Denervation

The loss of nerve supply to an organ such as skeletal muscle.

Dephosphorylation

Removal of a phosphate group. A dephosphorylation reaction is catalyzed by a phosphatase and reverses the action of a kinase, a protein that catalyzes the transfer of a phosphate group from adenosine 5′-triphosphate (ATP) to its target.

Depression

CHAD D. RETHORST, TRACY L. GREER, MADHUKAR H. TRIVEDI
Department of Psychiatry, University of Texas
Southwestern Medical Center at Dallas, Dallas, TX, USA

Synonyms
Major depressive disorder

Definition
Major Depressive Disorder is characterized by the presence of a Major Depressive Episode. Diagnostic criteria for a Major Depressive Episode includes five or more of the following symptoms, at least one of which being (1) depressed mood or (2) loss of interest or pleasure. Other symptoms (as described in the Diagnostic and Statistical Manual (Fourth Edition –Text Revision) published by the American Psychiatric Association) include: (3) significant weight loss or a decreased or increased appetite, (4) insomnia or hypersomnia, (5) psychomotor agitation or retardation, (6) fatigue or loss of energy, (7) feelings of worthlessness or excessive or inappropriate guilt, (8) diminished ability to think or concentrate, and (9) recurrent thoughts of death or suicidal ideation or suicide attempt.

Pathogenetic Mechanisms
The pathogenesis of depression is not well understood, but it is generally recognized that MDD is characterized by disruptions in several monaminergic neuromodulatory systems, including sertonergic, noradrenergic, and dopaminergic pathways. It has been postulated that disrupted plasticity within these and other neuronal pathways contributes to the development of depression, and that effective treatments for depression work by inducing plasticity in the affected neuronal systems. Recent evidence suggests that decreased expression of growth factors, such as brain derived growth factor and vascular endothelial growth factor, may be causal in the pathogenesis of depression, and that increases in their expression are critical to achieving antidepressant efficacy [1].

Exercise Intervention/Therapeutical Consequences
Analysis of epidemiological data identified the relationship between physical activity and depressive disorders. Higher levels of physical activity have been associated with a lower incidence of future development of MDD. Analysis of the Alameda County Study Data found that individuals who reported low levels of physical activity were at greater risk for developing MDD at 9 years later. A second follow-up, 18 years after baseline assessment, allowed for the examination of the relationship between changes in physical activity and MDD onset. Participants who reported decreased physical activity from baseline to follow-up were at greater risk for MDD at a second follow-up, while participants who increased activity were not at a higher risk for MDD at the 18-year follow-up compared to those who were physically active at baseline and remained physically active [2].

Building on these findings, a number of randomized controlled trials have examined the antidepressant effects of exercise. The results of these studies have been summarized in a number of meta-analyses. These meta-analyses report significant effect sizes for the reduction of depressive symptoms following an exercise intervention, ranging from 0.83 to 1.39 [3]. Analysis of moderating variables through meta-analysis provides further details on the antidepressant effects of exercise. Most trials examining the effects of exercise on depressive symptoms have used aerobic exercise activities (i.e., walking, running, cycling, etc.). Other trials examined the efficacy of resistance training in reducing depressive symptoms. Meta-analytic results have revealed no difference in effect size between the two modalities [3].

Exercise intervention trials in participants with MDD have varied in frequency of exercise sessions (i.e., the number of sessions per week). However, there is no significant difference in effect sizes across trials with different session frequency. Related to exercise frequency is exercise session duration. Typically, exercise has been prescribed in terms of session duration, in which participants exercise for a set amount during each session. The duration of exercise sessions in trials for MDD has ranged from 30 to 90 min. However, the largest effect size is observed in sessions lasting 45–59 min are most effective. Exercise prescriptions have also been defined by a caloric expenditure dose. Dunn et al. [4] found a significant larger reduction in depressive symptoms associated with a high dose of exercise, 16 kilocalories per kilogram of bodyweight (KKW) compared to a lower dose of exercise, 7.5 KKW.

A final variable related to an exercise session is exercise intensity. Exercise intensity for aerobic exercise is typically quantified as a percentage of an individual's maximum heart rate (HRmax). However, some trials have not monitored exercise intensity or have allowed participants to "self-select" exercise intensity. Among those trials that monitored exercise intensity, the prescribed exercise intensity ranged from 50% to 85% of HRmax and no difference in effect size across trials based on exercise intensity.

Acute bouts of aerobic exercise result in transient reductions in depressive symptoms immediately following the session. However, intervention durations of several weeks or months are needed to produce sustained reductions in depressive symptoms. Reductions in depressive symptoms have been observed in trials lasting as little as 4 weeks, though most trials have treatment periods of several months. Larger effect sizes have been observed in trials of 10 weeks or longer compared to those trials with intervention durations of 4–9 weeks.

The studies described above compare exercise to an inactive control group. Other studies have compared exercise to established treatments for antidepressant medications. For example, an RCT conducted by Blumenthal et al [5]. randomized participants to one of three conditions: aerobic exercise, an SSRI (sertaline), or a combination of exercise and medication. The SSRI group showed a more rapid response compared to the exercise and combination groups. However, there were no significant differences in depressive symptoms between the three groups following 16 weeks of treatments. Six months after treatment the exercise group demonstrated lower rates of MDD and participation in exercise was associated with a reduced risk of MDD, while continued use of SSRI did not affect presence of MDD. Results of other studies have been summarized in meta-analysis revealing no difference in effect size in studies comparing exercise to SSRIs [3]. Additionally, exercise is efficacious as augmentation to SSRI treatment [6].

Consequences

MDD annually affects approximately 10% of the population in the United States with a lifetime prevalence of 10% in men and 15% in women. The economic burden associated with depressive disorders is estimated at $83 billion annually [7]. A portion of the burden associated with MDD is due to the limited accessibility and efficacy of current treatments. This indicates the need for more cost-effective, accessible, and alternative treatments for depressive disorders, such as exercise.

Cross-References

▶ Psychiatric/Psychological Disorders

References

1. Nestler E, Gould E, Manji H et al (2002) Preclinical models: status of basic research in depression. Biol Psychiatry 52(6):503
2. Camacho TC, Roberts RE, Lazarus NB, Kaplan GA, Cohen RD (1991) Physical Activity and Depression Evidence from the Alameda County Study. Am J Epidemiol 134:220
3. Rethorst CD, Wipfli BM, Landers DM (2009) The antidepressive effects of exercise: a meta-analysis of randomized trials. Sports Med 39(6):491–511
4. Dunn AL, Trivedi MH, Kampert JB, Clark CG, Chambliss HO (2005) Exercise treatment for depression: efficacy and dose response. Am J Prev Med 28(1):1–8
5. Ja B, Ma B, Ka M et al (1999) Effects of exercise training on older patients with major depression. Arch Intern Med 159:2349–2356
6. Trivedi MH, Greer TL, Church TS et al (2011) Exercise as an augmentation treatment for nonremitted major depressive disorder: a randomized, parallel dose comparison. J Clin Psychiatry 72(5):677
7. Greenberg PE, Kessler RC, Birnbaum HG et al (2003) The economic burden of depression in the United States: how did it change between 1990 and 2000? J Clin Psychiatry 64:1465–1475

Develop

▶ Promotion of and Adherence to Physical Activity

D-Glutamine

▶ Glutamine

Diabetes

▶ Diabetes Mellitus, Prevention

Diabetes Mellitus, Juvenile

M. C. RIDDELL
School of Kinesiology and Health Science, Physical
Activity and Chronic Disease Unit, Faculty of Health,
Muscle Health Research Centre, York University,
York, Canada

Synonyms

Insulin-dependent diabetes mellitus; Type 1 diabetes
mellitus

Definition

Diabetes mellitus is a classification of metabolic diseases
characterized by high blood glucose levels (i.e., hyperglycemia) resulting from an inability of the pancreas to produce enough insulin for the metabolic demands of the
body, or from the body's inability to use the insulin that
it does produce effectively. The most common form of
pediatric (i.e., under the age of 14 years) diabetes is Type 1
diabetes mellitus (T1DM), formally called juvenile diabetes or insulin-dependent diabetes mellitus. T1DM is the
most severe type of diabetes, requiring insulin injections
on a lifelong basis.

T1DM has a global prevalence of 0.02%, with ~70,000
new cases diagnosed each year. The highest prevalence of
T1DM occurs in Scandinavian counties (40 per 100,000
children age <14 years in Finland), Canada, the UK, and
Australia, while the lowest rates occur in Asia and Central
and South America (<4/100,000). T1DM incidence rates
are increasing globally (3% annual increase) with rates
rising dramatically in certain populations such as
post-Gulf War Kuwait (rates have jumped from <4 to
>20/100,000 in a 10 year period).

Pathogenetic Mechanisms

The majority of T1DM cases (~80–90%) result from
autoimmune-mediated beta cell destruction (Type 1a),
while the remaining 10–20% of cases are antibody negative and are termed idiopathic (Type 1b). Inflammation of
the pancreatic islets (insulitis) involves CD4+ and CD8+
lymphocytes, B-lymphocytes, and macrophages. The
recent change in the incidence of T1DM (global rates
growing by >3% per year, with Kuwait jumping from
<4/100,000 to >20/100,000 from pre- to post-Gulf
War), without a major change in population genetics,
suggests that environmental triggers exist for what was
once thought to be primarily a genetically determined
condition. The rate of beta cell destruction is variable
between individuals, lasting from weeks or months to
several years. Recent evidence suggests that even after
50 years of living with the diagnosis, residual beta cell
function may remain in some patients. Regardless of the
etiology, or the severity of beta cell destruction, daily
insulin injections are required, or patients may opt for
a constant subcutaneous insulin infusion device (i.e.,
insulin pump). In instances where beta cell destruction is
rapid and near complete, occurring predominantly in
children and adolescents, the first manifestation of
T1DM may be ketoacidosis, a potentially life-threatening
condition. Vomiting, dehydration, deep gasping breathing, confusion, and occasionally coma are typical symptoms of diabetic ketoacidosis (DKA). Symptoms of
hyperglycemia may include polyuria, polydipsia, lethargy,
weight loss, polyphagia and blurred vision.

Diabetic complications, broadly classified as microvascular or macrovascular, are common in those with long-
standing disease, particularly if they have been under poor
glycemic control [1]. Microvascular complications include
neuropathy (nerve damage), nephropathy (kidney disease),
and vision disorders (e.g., retinopathy, glaucoma, cataract,
and corneal disease). Macrovascular complications include
heart disease, stroke, and peripheral vascular disease (which
can lead to ulcers, gangrene, and amputation). Other complications may include infections, hypoglycemia (low blood
glucose), and hyperglycemia with DKA, impotence, autonomic neuropathy, and pregnancy problems. Although
several mechanisms likely underlie the development of
micro- and macrovascular disease in diabetes, hyperglycemia, dyslipidemia, oxidative stress, and endothelial dysfunction may play a synergistic role.

It is well established that the level of overall glycemic control, as measured by glycated hemoglobin (HbA1c), can partially predict the risk of micro- and macrovacular disease development. Based on data from the Diabetes Control and Complications Trial (DCCT) and the follow-up Epidemiology of Diabetes Interventions and Complications (EDIC) studies, the recommended diabetes management strategy is intensive insulin therapy with the goal of achieving HbA1c levels as close as possible to the normal value (normal being 5–6%). This level of glycemic control is challenging and is largely achieved through insulin pump therapy or multiple daily injections (MDI) with considerable blood glucose monitoring. It is important to note, however, that with intensive treatment, the risk of severe hypoglycemia is increased by two to threefold.

Exercise Intervention/Therapeutical Consequences

Clinicians, exercise physiologists and patients have long wondered if increased physical activity (exercise) can improve T1DM metabolic control and reduce the risk of diabetes-related complications. Surprisingly, there is still insufficient data to answer these very straightforward clinical questions. However, some clues exist to support the notion that, compared to being sedentary, engaging in regular physical activity may enhance glycemic control and overall physical and mental health status.

Physical fitness, as measured by maximal aerobic capacity (VO$_2$max), is indeed associated with HbA1c in several cross-sectional studies of youth with T1DM, such that lower VO$_2$max (i.e., poor fitness) predicts higher HbA1c levels. Interestingly, evidence also exists to support the argument that physical inactivity is associated with poor glycemic control, as evidenced by metrics such as TV viewing time and computer screen time [3]. However, the effects of regular physical training on improving glycemic control in pediatric patients, based on intervention studies, are equivocal with some studies reporting improvements in HbA1c, while others show little or no effect (for a review see Robertson et al. [2]). In adults with the disease, little evidence exists to support the idea that regular exercise improves HbA1c. However, there is good evidence for increased insulin sensitivity and a reduction in total daily insulin dose when exercise is performed regularly [4, 5]. Numerous studies support other health benefits of exercise, including improvements in blood pressure, lipid profile, psychological well-being, cardiovascular fitness, muscle capacity, and weight management.

Based on epidemiological data, regular exercise is associated with lower morbidity rates in individuals with T1DM and may even promote longevity [6]. Although exercise provides many benefits for those with T1DM, adverse events such as hypoglycemia, hyperglycemia, and possibly ketoacidosis occur frequently because the complex physiology that normally occurs during exercise in healthy nondiabetic individuals cannot be easily mimicked in the patient with T1DM (see below). Increased knowledge, awareness, and careful precautions should be taken to ensure sufficient glycemic control in the active youth with T1DM.

Normal Endocrine Responses to Exercise

Glucose homeostasis during prolonged moderate intensity exercise (40–60% VO$_2$max) is primarily regulated by a reduction in insulin secretion and an increase in glucagon release that augments hepatic glucose production. The increased glucagon-to-insulin ratio raises the rate of glucose appearance (Ra) to match the increased rate of peripheral glucose disposal (Rd) into working muscle (Fig. 1). Increased hepatic glucose production occurs through enhanced glycogenolysis and gluconeogenesis, with a greater reliance on the later pathway as the duration of exercise increases. Hypoglycemia occurs, even in nondiabetic individuals, when hepatic glucose production fails to match the elevated glucose uptake by the exercising muscle, which is particularly pronounced during prolonged exercise (usually > than 3 h of activity in the nondiabetic if no food is consumed). If hepatic glycogen stores are depleted during prolonged exercise, gluconeogenesis alone is unable to provide adequate glucose to supply the working muscles.

In healthy individuals, several counterregulatory mechanisms exist to help limit hypoglycemia both at rest when fasting occurs and during prolonged exercise when glucose disposal increases. A slight decrease in glycemia from normal (normal being ~90 mg/dL or 5 mmol/L) lowers insulin secretion and activates the release of various counterregulatory hormones including glucagon, norepinephrine, epinephrine, growth hormone (GH), and cortisol. All of these hormones act to increase hepatic glucose production and lower peripheral glucose disposal. As such, several safeguards need to be breached before hypoglycemia occurs in nondiabetic individuals.

Exercise-Induced Hypoglycemia in Patients with T1DM

For patients with T1DM, the inability to reduce exogenous insulin levels during exercise is a key factor that contributes to an increased risk of exercise-induced hypoglycemia (Fig. 1). A second factor that leads to hyperinsulinemia and hypoglycemia with exercise in patients with T1DM is the accelerated absorption of insulin from subcutaneous tissues, once it has been injected or infused, into the systemic circulation. Relative hyperinsulinemia limits the

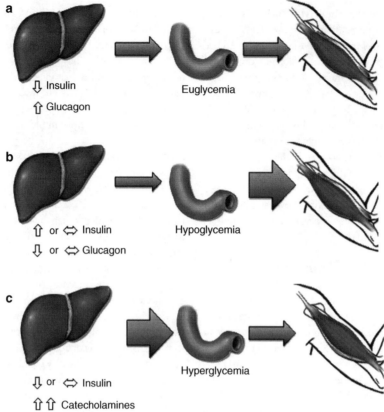

a

⇩ Insulin
⇧ Glucagon

Euglycemia

b

⇧ or ⇔ Insulin
⇩ or ⇔ Glucagon

Hypoglycemia

c

⇩ or ⇔ Insulin
⇧ ⇧ Catecholamines

Hyperglycemia

Diabetes Mellitus, Juvenile. Fig. 1 Blood glucose responses to exercise in nondiabetic or ideally controlled patient with T1DM (**a**), over-insulinized patient (**b**), and under-insulinized patient or patient performing high-intensity exercise under competition stress (**c**). The thickness of the arrows represents glucose flux. In panel a, hepatic glucose production is balanced with muscle glucose uptake and normal blood glucose levels are maintained. In panel b, high insulin concentration reduces hepatic glucose production and increases muscle glucose uptake, resulting in hypoglycemia. In panel c, low insulin concentration or elevated counterregulatory hormones increase hepatic glucose production and decrease muscle glucose uptake, resulting in hyperglycemia

effect of glucagon on hepatic glucose production and promotes insulin-induced peripheral glucose uptake, further decreasing blood glucose levels during exercise. A third factor that may contribute to an increased risk for exercise-associated hypoglycemia in patients with T1DM is the loss in glucagon response to developing hypoglycemia, which typically occurs about 2–4 years after disease onset. Although it has been established that the glucagon response to exercise may be intact in people with T1DM if they are not hypoglycemic, there may be deficiencies in the glucagon response during exercise if the patients were previously exposed to hypoglycemia or if they are, in fact, exercising while hypoglycemic. Some evidence also suggests that there may also be impaired adrenergic responses to exercise in patients with T1DM under hypoglycemic conditions.

Unfortunately, the increased risk of exercise-associated hypoglycemia is not limited to when the exercise is performed. In a multicenter study, children with T1DM ages 11–17 years were twice as likely to have nocturnal hypoglycemia during a night after an exercise day compared to a night after a sedentary day [7]. The main mechanism behind increased insulin sensitivity after exercise appears related to the enhanced recruitment of GLUT-4 transporters, which also increases muscle glucose uptake during exercise. Thus, late-onset hypoglycemia is particularly common and has been reported to occur up to 36 h after exercise in active children with T1DM. The effects of increased insulin sensitivity and the need to replenish glycogen stores likely contribute to the risk of late-onset hypoglycemia. A recent investigation in children with T1DM indicates that increased insulin sensitivity occurs post-exercise and again 7–11 h later [8], which may further elevate their risk for post-exercise hypoglycemia. This implies that blood glucose monitoring after exercise is critical, since late-onset hypoglycemia is such a common risk for those with T1DM.

Insulin Adjustments to Prevent Hypoglycemia

With all insulin therapies, there is the strong possibility that hypoglycemia will occur during exercise, particularly if basal and/or bolus adjustments have not been made in anticipation of the activity. Basal insulin therapy delivers a low dose of insulin, typically over a 12–24 h period, to regulate hepatic glucose production and bolus insulin is administered to control elevations in blood glucose after meals or during periods of hyperglycemia. One potential way to reduce exercise-associated hypoglycemia in those patients who are on insulin pumps is to suspend the basal insulin altogether during the exercise. Because of rapid-acting insulin kinetics, however, it is advisable to do this 60–90 min before the start of prolonged exercise and then to reconnect early in recovery and resume insulin delivery [2]. For MDI patients, it may be better to lower bolus insulin rather than attempt to lower basal insulin in anticipation of exercise, since basal insulin is typically administered via injection early in the mornings and any reduction in basal insulin dosage will influence glycemia over the next 12–24 h. Based on one study conducted in adults with T1DM, it appears that bolus insulin reductions for exercise should range between 25% and 75%, depending on the intensity and/or duration of the activity (Table 1) [2].

In addition to daytime hypoglycemia caused by exercise, post-exercise late-onset hypoglycemia during sleep is also very common. This is particularly problematic as patients may not perceive hypoglycemia during sleep and the hypoglycemic duration may last for several hours. In these situations, a reduction in bedtime basal insulin by ~20% (from bedtime to ~4 AM if on a pump) is recommended [9].

ExCarbs

In certain situations, adjustments to insulin dosages prior to the onset of exercise may be impossible or impractical. For example, if the exercise is unplanned and of a spontaneous nature, with unknown duration, then insulin administration in the meal before the activity may have already been administered. In these situations, patients need to consume "extra" carbohydrates without an insulin bolus to compensate for the increased glucose disposal caused by the activity. An alternative strategy for prevention of hypoglycemia in these cases is to completely disregard any potential contribution of the liver in maintaining blood glucose homeostasis and simply have the patient consume a quantity of oral carbohydrate to match the estimated amount of glucose disposal into working muscle (Fig. 1). ExCarbs, original coined by John Walsh, can be estimated in three ways, according to Perkins and Riddell [10]:

1. The general recommendation for ExCarb consumption is 15–30 g of carbohydrate every 30–60 min of exercise. Although activities vary widely in terms of fuel requirements, this range likely represents a safe starting point for most patients who wish to begin moderate-intensity exercise regimens.
2. A more semiquantitative estimation, based on body mass and average whole body glucose oxidation rates during exercise, is 1 g glucose/kg body weight/h.
3. A more quantitative approach using tables of carbohydrate utilization rates for various physical activities for patients who differ in body mass.

For this last strategy, standardized tables have been devised to help individuals estimate ExCarbs for many different activities with varying intensities according to body weight (Table 2). This activity-specific approach to estimating ExCarbs, although not tested in a clinical trial setting, is a popular resource among active patients with T1DM.

The Alternative ExCarb Approach

As pointed out by Perkins and Riddell [10], the estimated ExCarb amount can be translated from grams of carbohydrate to units of insulin by way of the carbohydrate-to-insulin ratio. For example, an activity that requires 48 g of ExCarbs represents a known amount of insulin, based on the patient's insulin-to-carbohydrate ratio. This number can be calculated by dividing the 48 g of carbohydrates by

Diabetes Mellitus, Juvenile. Table 1 Bolus insulin dose reduction for the meal prior to prolonged aerobic exercise

Intensity of exercise	Duration of exercise and recommended percent insulin reduction	
	30 min	60 min
Low (~25% VO$_2$max)	25%	50%
Moderate (~50% VO$_2$max)	50%	75%
Heavy (~75% VO$_2$max)	75%	–

Diabetes Mellitus, Juvenile. Table 2 Carbohydrate intake recommendations according to body mass and activity performed

	Body mass, lbs (kg)		
	44 (20)	88 (40)	132 (60)
Basketball	23	45	68
Cross-country skiing	10	21	32
Cycling			
10 km/h	7	11	18
15 km/h	10	18	27
Figure skating	18	36	54
Ice hockey	23	45	68
Running			
8 km/h	17	30	41
12 km/h	–	41	55
Snow shoeing	15	30	45
Soccer	17	32	48
Swimming			
30 m/min breast stroke	14	27	52
Tennis	11	19	28
Walking			
4 km/h	9	12	15
6 km/h	12	15	19

Values shown are the estimated number of grams of carbohydrate to consume for 30 min of exercise if the activity is performed during times of peak insulin action and if no adjustments were made. Estimates are based on energy expenditures and on recommendations found in [3]

the patient's carbohydrate-to-insulin ratio (e.g., 12.5 g of carbohydrate is disposed of per unit of insulin). This is the same calculation that a patient would perform in order to determine the food bolus insulin dose of a 48-g carbohydrate meal. However, to accommodate the exercise the patient would administer 3.8 fewer units of insulin in this example (48/12.5 = 3.8 less units of insulin to be administered prior to exercise). This decrease in insulin can be achieved in three ways: a decrease in the food bolus insulin dose for a meal preceding exercise, a decrease in basal insulin just before and during exercise, or a combination of both approaches. This approach is useful if additional calories of ExCarbs are undesired.

Exercise-Induced Hyperglycemia and Ketoacidosis

Although exercise is typically associated with an increased risk for hypoglycemia, certain types of exercise may promote hyperglycemia. Specifically, high-intensity exercise

(i.e., above the lactate threshold) tends to increase blood glucose levels because insulin levels do not rise in the portal circulation of the patient with diabetes to compensate for the normal increase in circulating catecholamine levels [11]. It is well established that exercise-induced increases in catecholamines promote glucose production, free fatty acid release, and increase ketone production while impairing glucose uptake (Fig. 1). If hyperglycemia occurs post-exercise, this phenomenon is usually transient, lasting for 1–2 h in recovery. No current guidelines are available on the amount of insulin to administer in the presence of hyperglycemia after high-intensity exercise for patients with T1DM, although some limited experimental data suggests that a doubling in insulin levels relative to when the vigorous exercise was performed may be needed to counter this transient hyperglycemia.

Young athletes and parents should be aware of the potential for a rise in blood glucose before competition. Even if blood glucose levels are normal in the hours before exercise, anticipatory stress increases counterregulatory hormones and hyperglycemia can occur. Typically, this "stress-related" increase in glycemia at the onset of exercise does not need to be corrected for since the increased glucose utilization rate during the activity, as long as it is aerobic in nature, will often lower blood glucose levels. However, frequent self-monitoring of blood glucose is needed to make sure that any pre-exercise hyperglycemia is not worsened during the exercise, to which continuous glucose monitoring (CGM) may be an asset [12].

In situations of prolonged and severe hypoinsulinemia (missed insulin injections, blocked insulin pump line or site, illness, etc.), patients may have elevations in circulating and urinary ketone bodies. In these situations, vigorous exercise may cause further increases in hyperglycemia and ketoacidosis, particularly if elevated blood ketones are present at the time of exercise. In these situations, hepatic glucose production continues to rise, while glucose utilization remains impaired and glycemic control deteriorates even further [13]. For these reasons, it is strongly recommended to delay exercise if blood glucose is higher than 250 mg/dL (13.9 mmol/L) and if blood or urinary ketones are also elevated. For patients on insulin pump devices with hyperglycemia and elevated ketone levels, infusion sets should be changed and individuals may need to temporarily switch to needles with rapid acting insulin injected until glucose is restored. Hyperglycemia and ketoacidosis may cause dehydration and decrease blood pH, resulting in impaired performance and severe illness. Rapid ketone production can precipitate ketoacidotic abdominal pain and vomiting. In these situations, patients are advised to go to emergency for intravenous insulin and rehydration protocols. With respect to performance, limited evidence suggests that cognitive function and sport performance may be maximized when circulating glucose levels are in the near normal range [14].

Intermittent Exercise and Its Effects on Glycemia

As discussed in the above sections, continuous steady state aerobic exercise typically causes hypoglycemia, while high-intensity anaerobic work can cause hyperglycemia. Good evidence exists to support the notion that the combination of these two discrete forms of exercise can have a moderating effect on glycemia [15]. Even a 10 s all-out sprint either before or after prolonged aerobic exercise can help attenuate hypoglycemia in people with T1DM. If intermittent high-intensity exercise increases, or decreases, post-exercise late-onset hypoglycemia is currently unclear, however.

Summary

Regular physical activity should be considered an important component of the clinical management of T1DM. Glucose management during sport is challenging; however, as several hormonal and neuroendocrine signals exist in the control of glucose homeostasis. Both insulin adjustments and increases in carbohydrate intake may be needed to help promote better glycemia during competition in patients with T1DM.

References

1. Diabetes Control and Complications Trial/Epidemiology of Diabetes Interventions and Complications (DCCT/EDIC) Research Group, Nathan DM, Zinman B, Cleary PA, Backlund JY, Genuth S, Miller R, Orchard TJ (2009) Modern-day clinical course of type 1 diabetes mellitus after 30 years' duration: the diabetes control and complications trial/epidemiology of diabetes interventions and complications and Pittsburgh epidemiology of diabetes complications experience (1983–2005). Arch Intern Med 169(14):1307–1316
2. Robertson K, Adolfsson P, Scheiner G, Hanas R, Riddell MC (2009) Exercise in children and adolescents with diabetes. Pediatr Diabetes 10(Suppl 12):154–168
3. Margeirsdottir HD, Larsen JR, Brunborg C, Sandvik L, Dahl-Jorgensen K, Norwegian Study Group for Childhood Diabetes (2007) Strong association between time watching television and blood glucose control in children and adolescents with type 1 diabetes. Diabetes Care 30(6):1567–1570
4. Austin A, Warty V, Janosky J, Arslanian S (1993) The relationship of physical fitness to lipid and lipoprotein(a) levels in adolescents with IDDM. Diabetes Care 16(2):421–425
5. Wallberg-Henriksson H, Gunnarsson R, Henriksson J, DeFronzo R, Felig P, Ostman J, Wahren J (1982) Increased peripheral insulin sensitivity and muscle mitochondrial enzymes but unchanged blood glucose control in type I diabetics after physical training. Diabetes 31(12):1044–1050
6. Moy CS, Songer TJ, LaPorte RE, Dorman JS, Kriska AM, Orchard TJ, Becker DJ, Drash AL (1993) Insulin-dependent diabetes mellitus, physical activity, and death. Am J Epidemiol 137(1):74–81
7. Tsalikian E, Mauras N, Beck RW, Tamborlane WV, Janz KF, Chase HP, Wysocki T, Weinzimer SA, Buckingham BA, Kollman C, Xing D, Ruedy KJ, Diabetes Research in Children Network Direcnet Study Group (2005) Impact of exercise on overnight glycemic control in children with type 1 diabetes mellitus. J Pediatr 147(4):528–534
8. McMahon SK, Ferreira LD, Ratnam N, Davey RJ, Youngs LM, Davis EA, Fournier PA, Jones TW (2007) Glucose requirements to maintain euglycemia after moderate-intensity afternoon exercise in adolescents with type 1 diabetes are increased in a biphasic manner. J Clin Endocrinol Metab 92(3):963–968
9. Taplin CE, Cobry E, Messer L, McFann K, Chase HP, Fiallo-Scharer R (2010) Preventing post-exercise nocturnal hypoglycemia in children with type 1 diabetes. J Pediatr 157(5):784–8.e1
10. Perkins BA, Riddell MC (2006) Type 1 diabetes and exercise – part II: using the insulin pump to maximum advantage. Can J Diabetes 30:72–80
11. Marliss EB, Vranic M (2002) Intense exercise has unique effects on both insulin release and its roles in glucoregulation: implications for diabetes. Diabetes 51(Suppl 1):S271–S283
12. Riddell MC, Perkins BA (2009) Exercise and glucose metabolism in persons with diabetes mellitus: perspectives on the role for continuous glucose monitoring. J Diabetes Sci Technol 3(4):914–923
13. Berger M, Berchtold P, Cuppers HJ, Drost H, Kley HK, Muller WA, Wiegelmann W, Zimmerman-Telschow H, Gries FA, Kruskemper HL, Zimmermann H (1977) Metabolic and hormonal effects of muscular exercise in juvenile type diabetics. Diabetologia 13(4):355–365
14. Kelly D, Hamilton JK, Riddell MC (2010) Blood glucose levels and performance in a sports camp for adolescents with type 1 diabetes mellitus: a field study. Int J Pediatr 2010:216167. Epub 2010 2 Aug 2010
15. Guelfi KJ, Jones TW, Fournier PA (2007) New insights into managing the risk of hypoglycaemia associated with intermittent high-intensity exercise in individuals with type 1 diabetes mellitus: implications for existing guidelines. Sports Med 37(11):937–946

Diabetes Mellitus, Myopathy

Matthew P. Krause, Thomas J. Hawke
Department of Pathology and Molecular Medicine, McMaster University, Hamilton, ON, Canada

Synonyms

Diabetic myopathy; Insulin-dependent diabetic myopathy; Juvenile-onset diabetic myopathy

Definition

Diabetic myopathy refers to the broad spectrum of pathophysiological alterations to skeletal muscle in response to the diabetic biochemical, hormonal, and cellular environment. This chapter will describe those alterations specific to type 1 diabetes mellitus (T1DM). T1DM causes a host of changes in muscle that can be detected with molecular or biochemical techniques, with microscopy of histochemically prepared tissue samples, or with functional testing (e.g., exercise testing). Typically T1DM is associated with a loss of muscle mass and strength, the former presumably causing the latter [1].

Characteristics

Skeletal Muscle Function in T1DM

Many studies have examined exercise capacity in T1DM, the most common findings being small, but significant losses in maximal aerobic capacity or peak work capacity. The studies that detected significant decreases in aerobic fitness usually found this to correlate to the level of metabolic control as indicated by the level of glycosylated hemoglobin (i.e., worse metabolic control correlating to worse fitness). In older diabetics with a longer disease duration, the severity of ▶ neuropathic symptoms often correlates to the fitness level. In terms of peak contractile strength, it is unequivocally found that there is a loss associated with T1DM which becomes more severe with age and the development of neuropathic symptoms [1]. A generalized summary of diabetic myopathy is illustrated in Fig. 1.

Disease Inception to First Insulin Treatment

Diabetic myopathy may be distinguished into separate stages based on the time course of the disease. T1DM typically presents spontaneously in children or adolescents, which incidentally is a time of accelerated musculoskeletal growth. This period is unique due to the body's requirement for optimal nutritional and hormonal stimulus to support the rate of growth; thus, diabetic myopathy immediately following disease inception is primarily a result of an altered hormonal environment prior to insulin treatment. Studies on young diabetic human skeletal muscle are very limited in number given the ethical limitations in obtaining muscle biopsies from this population, but it has been convincingly demonstrated that loss of skeletal muscle fiber area (a surrogate measure for loss of muscle mass and contractile protein) occurs in a matter of days following disease inception [2]. Unfortunately, it is not unusual for weeks or months to pass before a diabetic is diagnosed and treated, so it is likely that a significant impairment in muscle growth can happen during this time. It is hypothesized that alterations to the hormonal and glycemic environment during this "undiagnosed period" in the young diabetic are the primary mediators of impaired muscle growth. In contrast to the pediatric situation discussed above, neuropathic complications are likely the primary contributor to the loss of muscle mass (atrophy) in the adult diabetic [1].

Effectiveness of Insulin Treatment

Like many diabetic complications (e.g., neuropathy, retinopathy, nephropathy), the severity of diabetic myopathy varies due to the variability in each diabetic's insulin treatment regime. The effectiveness of insulin treatment can greatly vary depending on the patient's consideration to blood glucose values, diet, and exercise schedule. It is important to note however that even the most attentive type 1 diabetics have difficulty maintaining ideal blood glucose levels throughout the day, often experiencing periods of ▶ hyperglycemia during their day (3; see Fig. 2). These periods of hyperglycemia (and hypoinsulinemia) have summated effects on the relevant organs. In particular, uncontrolled ▶ glycation of proteins is known to have negative effects on protein function. For example, in a hyperglycemic environment the contractile protein myosin has been demonstrated to acquire advanced glycation end products (AGE) resulting in a loss of contractile capacity. This contributes to the loss of contractile capacity observed in long-term diabetic skeletal muscle.

Hormonal Environment

It is generally agreed that insulin is an important anabolic hormone because it promotes skeletal muscle protein accumulation through repression of protein catabolism and stimulation of protein synthesis. The loss of insulin with T1DM therefore can have profound effects on skeletal muscle protein balance. Although insulin treatment does not replace a healthy, functioning beta-cell mass in terms of glycemic control, it does provide some anabolic signaling to skeletal muscle. However, the altered hormonal environment in T1DM is not limited to insulin; many hormones that play crucial roles in maintaining skeletal muscle protein balance and metabolism are dysregulated and remain so even during insulin treatment. To name only a few, cortisol (or corticosterone in rodents), interleukin-6 (IL-6), plasminogen activator inhibitor-1 (PAI-1), and insulin-like growth factor-1 (IGF-1) have all been demonstrated to play key roles in muscle growth or atrophy and have been identified as dysregulated with T1DM. Specifically, cortisol, IL-6, and PAI-1 are elevated, and all contribute to muscle protein catabolism and poor muscle growth. Conversely, IGF-1 levels are drastically reduced. IGF-1, similar to insulin, has an anabolic effect on skeletal muscle by promoting accumulation of muscle protein. In experiments using diabetic animals, IGF-1 is also found to be reduced. However, when IGF-1 is restored through supplementation or exercise, myopathic loss of muscle protein is prevented,

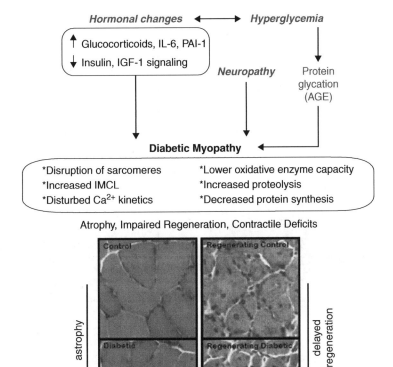

Diabetes Mellitus, Myopathy. Fig. 1 Proposed mechanisms underlying diabetic myopathy. Changes in blood glucose and circulating hormone levels are believed to be the major contributors to the myopathic condition. These alterations in hormonal and glycemic status lead to other pathophysiological changes (e.g., protein glycation) which negatively influence muscle health, ultimately leading to detrimental alterations in muscle phenotype, regenerative capacity, and contractile characteristics. While there are numerous cellular and molecular maladaptations occurring within the muscle, these are manifested as muscle atrophy and impaired regenerative capacity as illustrated by the hematoxylin and eosin (H&E) stained muscle sections displayed. Representative H&E images demonstrate control (nondiabetic) and diabetic skeletal muscle at 8 weeks of diabetes (left column), and 10 days following a cardiotoxin-induced injury (right column) in C57BL/6 and Ins2Akita (+/−) mice (Adapted from Krause and Hawke, unpublished findings). Note reductions in muscle fiber size as indices of muscle atrophy and attenuated regeneration [1]

indicating that IGF-1 may be an appropriate therapeutic target to minimize diabetic myopathy [1].

Diabetic Neuropathy

In long-term T1DM there is an increase in the incidence of neuropathic symptoms. Studies that observe nerve function using clinical tests find that loss of nerve function correlates to the loss of muscle mass and contractile function in older diabetics [4]. On the other hand, neuropathic symptoms have not been readily demonstrated in younger or well-treated diabetics, and loss of muscle mass and function is not as great as in older or poorly treated diabetics.

Fiber Type-Specific Muscle Loss

A host of other physiological changes to skeletal muscle occur with T1DM. The loss of muscle mass has been discussed, but it should be noted that it generally occurs in a muscle fiber type-specific fashion. Type I, or oxidative, muscle fibers appear to be resistant to diabetes-induced atrophy, while fast-twitch, or glycolytic, muscle fibers suffer the greatest loss of fiber size. The mechanism behind this fiber type selectivity is unknown. Studies have demonstrated that muscle groups composed primarily of oxidative fibers do not lose their contractile strength in experimental animal diabetes, while muscle groups

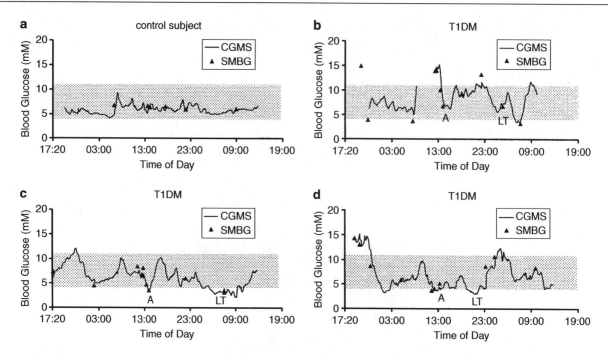

Diabetes Mellitus, Myopathy. Fig. 2 Sample glycemic monitoring using continuous glucose monitoring (*straight line*) and intermittent self-monitoring of blood glucose (*triangles*) over a 48-h period: (**a**) control subject and (**b–d**) three subjects with T1DM. A standardized meal was consumed at 10 a.m. At 1 p.m. all subjects began an exercise session consisting of a 60-min spin class (i.e., cycling with various degrees of resistance and cadence) intended to maintain intensity above 60% of the subjects' predetermined maximal heart rate. "A" indicates acute and "LT" indicates long-term effects of the exercise session on blood glucose. The shaded area represents the optimal glycemic range (between 4 and 11 mmol/L) (this figure has been taken from [3]). Approval needs to be obtained for use of this figure)

composed of glycolytic fibers do exhibit weakness accompanying the atrophy of those muscle fibers. Interestingly, human exercise experiments demonstrate no loss of muscular endurance (a function of oxidative capacity of muscle), but do observe significant losses of strength [4].

Accumulation of Intramyocellular Lipids

Intramyocellular lipid (IMCL) droplets normally are a healthy form of lipid storage in the body, but in diseases such as obesity and type 2 diabetes mellitus (T2DM), these droplets may accumulate excessively and trigger pathological consequences such as insulin resistance. In T1DM it is found that IMCL droplets accumulate as well. It is hypothesized that IMCL accumulate because the skeletal muscle is storing up an alternative energy supply in response to the inevitable hypoglycemic periods. Lipid species such as ceramide and diacylglycerol are found at high levels in IMCL in obesity and T2DM and may be the link between insulin resistance (a hallmark of obesity and T2DM) and IMCL. Interestingly, in T1DM patients with poor metabolic control, there tends to be higher IMCL

accumulation, as well as a tendency toward insulin resistance. It is worth noting that, paradoxically, endurance exercise training also causes accumulation of IMCL but without insulin resistance, indicating that IMCL droplets are not directly pathological to skeletal muscle [1].

Muscle Regeneration

Skeletal muscle has an amazing capacity for regeneration following injury, but this capacity is lost in the diabetic environment. Acute injury causes a loss of muscle mass and fiber size in the diabetic, effectively accelerating the atrophy described above. Fascinatingly, in a diabetic animal experiment where skeletal muscle was surgically removed and transplanted from healthy to diabetic animals and vice versa, regeneration of the healthy muscle in the diabetic environment was impaired, but the diabetic muscle in the healthy environment was not [5]. This study cleverly defines the diabetic hormonal/hyperglycemic environment as the primary pathological influence on skeletal muscle regeneration.

Clinical Relevance

Routine physical activity, whether through sports or a structured training program, is critical for people with T1DM to attenuate or reduce the severity of diabetic complications. Maintaining a healthy, functioning skeletal muscle mass is not only important for one's locomotor abilities but also for the control of glycemic levels and ultimately long-term health in T1DM. Increasing muscle mass and thereby insulin sensitivity through physical exercise improves metabolic control which in turn will impede the progression of diabetic complications, including myopathy itself. However, there are important considerations for the diabetic entering into a new physical activity regime: on one hand are the health benefits bestowed by physical activity including psychosocial benefits, and on the other hand is the possibility of hypoglycemic episodes. The ISPAD Clinical Practice Consensus Guidelines not only outlines the acute and chronic effects of exercise on diabetics but how to effectively implement exercise and sport while safely managing glycemic levels [6].

References

1. Krause MP, Riddell MC, Hawke TJ (2011) Effects of type 1 diabetes mellitus on skeletal muscle: clinical observations and physiological mechanisms. Pediatr Diabetes 12(4 Pt 1):345–364
2. Jakobsen J, Reske-Nielsen E (1986) Diffuse muscle fiber atrophy in newly diagnosed diabetes. Clin Neuropathol 5:73–77
3. Iscoe KE, Campbell JE, Jamnik V, Perkins BA, Riddell MC (2006) Efficacy of continuous real-time blood glucose monitoring during and after prolonged high-intensity cycling exercise: spinning with a continuous glucose monitoring system. Diabetes Technol Ther 8:627–635
4. Andersen H (1998) Muscular endurance in long-term IDDM patients. Diabetes Care 21:604–609
5. Gulati AK, Swamy MS (1991) Regeneration of skeletal muscle in streptozotocin-induced diabetic rats. Anat Rec 229:298–304
6. Robertson K, Adolfsson P, Scheiner G, Hanas R, Riddell MC (2009) Exercise in children and adolescents with diabetes. Pediatr Diabetes 10(Suppl 12):154–168

Diabetes Mellitus, Prevention

GANG HU
Chronic Disease Epidemiology Laboratory, Population Science, Pennington Biomedical Research Center, Baton Rouge, LA, USA

Synonyms

Diabetes; Disorder of carbohydrate metabolism; Type 2 diabetes

Definition

According to the World Health Organization diabetes definition, the term diabetes describes a metabolic disorder of multiple etiology characterized by chronic hyperglycemia with disturbances of carbohydrate, fat, and protein metabolism resulting from defects in insulin secretion, insulin action, or both [1]. There are three main types of diabetes: type 1 diabetes, type 2 diabetes, and gestational diabetes mellitus [1]. Type 1 diabetes, previously encompassed by the term insulin-dependent diabetes mellitus (IDDM) or juvenile-onset diabetes, indicates the processes of beta–cell destruction that may ultimately lead to diabetes mellitus in which "insulin is required for survival" to prevent the development of ketoacidosis, coma, and death [1]. The peak incidence of this form of type 1 diabetes occurs in childhood and adolescence, but the onset may occur at any age [1]. Type 2 diabetes, previously encompassed by non-insulin-dependent diabetes mellitus (NIDDM) or adult-onset diabetes, is the most common form of diabetes and is characterized by disorders of insulin action and insulin secretion, either of which may be the predominant feature [1]. Gestational diabetes is carbohydrate intolerance resulting in hyperglycemia of variable severity with onset or first recognition during pregnancy [1].

Diabetes is one of the fastest growing public health problems worldwide. It has been estimated that the number of individuals with diabetes among adults 20 or more years of age will double from the current 171 million in 2000 to 366 million in 2030 [2]. Type 2 diabetes is by far the most common form, affecting 90–95% of the diabetes population [1,2].

The current World Health Organization criterion for diagnosing diabetes [1] is: one or more classic symptoms plus a fasting plasma $\geq$126 mg/dl (7.0 mmol/l) or a 2-h plasma glucose $\geq$200 mg/dl (11.1 mmol/l) in the oral glucose tolerance test; at least one raised plasma glucose concentration on a fasting plasma $\geq$126 mg/dl (7.0 mmol/l) or a 2-h plasma glucose $\geq$200 mg/dl (11.1 mmol/l) in the oral glucose tolerance test in the absence of symptoms; or treatment with a hypoglycemic drug (oral antidiabetic agents or insulin). In the 2010 American Diabetes Association Diagnosis and Classification of Diabetes Mellitus report, the American Diabetes Association recommended the use of the glycated hemoglobin (HbA1C) test to diagnose diabetes, with a threshold of $\geq$6.5% [3].

Pathogenesis

Diabetes may present with characteristic symptoms such as thirst, polyuria, blurring of vision, and weight loss.

In its most severe forms, ketoacidosis or a non-ketotic hyperosmolar state may develop and lead to stupor, coma, and, in absence of effective treatment, death [1]. Often diabetic symptoms are not severe, or may be absent, and consequently hyperglycemia sufficient to cause pathological and functional changes may be present for a long time before the diagnosis is made [1]. The long-term effects of diabetes include progressive development of the specific complications of retinopathy with potential blindness, nephropathy that may lead to renal failure, and/or neuropathy with risk of foot ulcers, amputation, Charcot joints, and features of autonomic dysfunction, including sexual dysfunction [1]. People with diabetes are at increased risk of cardiovascular, peripheral vascular, and cerebrovascular diseases [1]. Cardiovascular disease accounts for more than 70% of total mortality among patients with type 2 diabetes [1].

The cause of diabetes depends on the type. Type 1 diabetes is partly inherited and then triggered by certain infections [1]. Type 2 diabetes is due primarily to lifestyle factors and genetics [4]. A sedentary lifestyle and obesity are two important lifestyle risk factors for type 2 diabetes [4]. Results from prospective cohort studies and clinical trials have shown that moderate or high levels of physical activity or physical fitness and changes in lifestyle (dietary modification, increase in physical activity, and weight loss) can prevent type 2 diabetes [4]. The levels of physical activity vary considerably among different populations, but regarding the risk of type 2 diabetes, the most important indicator is the proportion of sedentary people. We summarize the current evidence regarding the role of physical activity and physical fitness in the primary prevention of type 2 diabetes.

Training/Exercise Response

Physical Activity and Type 2 Diabetes: Data from Prospective Epidemiological Studies

Results from a lot of prospective epidemiologic studies, conducted among different populations and assessing different domains of activity, indicate that regular physical activity during occupation, commuting, leisure time, or daily life reduces the risk of type 2 diabetes by 15–60%, with most studies showing a 30–50% reduction in the risk. The benefit of physical activity is apparent in both men and women, and in younger and older individuals [4]. These studies generally controlled for age, body mass index, and several other important confounding factors [4]. How much physical activity is required for a reduction in the risk of type 2 diabetes? While the data are sparse, it appears that even moderate-intensity physical activity, such as walking, is sufficient to reduce the diabetes risk as the same as vigorous activity. Perhaps brisk walking 30 min/day is sufficient. Additionally, decreasing the amount of time spent on watching television is helpful for reducing the diabetes risk [4].

Physical Fitness and Type 2 Diabetes: Data from Prospective Epidemiological Studies

Data from several prospective epidemiological studies of physical fitness show similar findings to the studies of physical activity, but with somewhat larger magnitudes of the association between physical fitness and the decreased risk (≥50%) of type 2 diabetes. This may be due to fitness measurements being less prone to measurement error and misclassification. Additionally, factors other than physical activity may influence both physical fitness and health through related biological factors [4].

Change in Lifestyle and Type 2 Diabetes: Data from Clinical Trials

Although observational data suggest a causal association between physical activity/physical fitness, and the risk of type 2 diabetes, experimental evidence is required for a definitive test of the hypothesis that higher levels of activity delay the progression to diabetes. In recent years, several clinical trials have assessed whether regular physical activity, with or without dietary intervention, can reduce progression to type 2 diabetes among adults with impaired glucose tolerance [4]. The available data from clinical trials in Sweden, China, Finland, the United States, India, Japan, and UK have indicated that lifestyle intervention, including counseling for physical activity, dietary modification, and body weight loss, can reduce the risk of type 2 diabetes by 40–60% among adults with impaired glucose tolerance [4]. Moreover, the Finnish Diabetes Prevention Study, the China Da Qing Diabetes Prevention Study, and the American Diabetes Prevention Program [5] further found that the originally-achieved lifestyle changes and risk reduction sustained after discontinuation of lifestyle counseling in the extended follow-up [4,5].

Summary

Diabetes is one of the fastest growing public health problems in the world, and it is a major economic, social, and personal burden. Results from prospective cohort studies consistently indicate that regular physical activity during occupation, commuting, leisure time, or daily life reduces the risk of type 2 diabetes by 15–60%; and lifestyle intervention, including counseling for physical activity, dietary modification, and body weight loss, can reduce the risk of type 2 diabetes by 40–60% among adults with impaired glucose tolerance. Based on the evidence from epidemiological and intervention studies, the US Center for Disease Control and Prevention, the American College of Sports Medicine, the American Heart Association, and the World Health Organization have recommended that adults engage in at least 30 min of moderate-intensity physical activity on most, and preferably all days of the week [6]. Regular physical activity should be an important component of a healthy lifestyle for everyone. Public health messages, health-care professionals, and the health-care system should aggressively promote physical activity during occupation, commuting, leisure time, and all aspects of daily life.

References

1. WHO Consultation (1999) Definition, diagnosis and classification of diabetes mellitus and its complications. Part 1: diagnosis and classification of diabetes mellitus. World Health Organisation, Geneva
2. Wild S, Roglic G, Green A, Sicree R, King H (2004) Global prevalence of diabetes: estimates for the year 2000 and projections for 2030. Diabetes Care 27:1047–1053
3. American Diabetes Association (2010) Diagnosis and classification of diabetes mellitus. Diabetes Care 33(Suppl 1):S62–S69
4. Hu G, Lakka TA, Kilpelainen TO, Tuomilehto J (2007) Epidemiological studies of exercise in diabetes prevention. Appl Physiol Nutr Metab 32:583–595
5. Knowler WC, Fowler SE, Hamman RF, Christophi CA, Hoffman HJ, Brenneman AT, Brown-Friday JO, Goldberg R, Venditti E, Nathan DM (2009) 10-year follow-up of diabetes incidence and weight loss in the Diabetes Prevention Program Outcomes Study. Lancet 374:1677–1686
6. Haskell WL, Lee IM, Pate RR, Powell KE, Blair SN, Franklin BA, Macera CA, Heath GW, Thompson PD, Bauman A (2007) Physical activity and public health: updated recommendation for adults from the American College of Sports Medicine and the American Heart Association. Circulation 116:1081–1093

Diabetes Mellitus, Sports Therapy

MARTIN HALLE, KATRIN ESEFELD, MAXIMILIAN KEMPER
Department of Prevention, Rehabilitation and Sports Medicine, Zentrum für Prävention und Sportmedizin im Olympiapark, Klinikum rechts der Isar, Technische Universität München, Munich, Germany

Synonyms

Exercise in type 2 diabetes mellitus; Type 2 diabetes

Definition

Role of exercise as a therapeutic baseline therapy in the prevention and therapy of type 2 diabetes mellitus.

Pathogenetic Mechanisms

Muscular insulin sensitivity is the key regulatory mechanism that is impaired in prediabetes and clinically manifest type 2 diabetes mellitus. When insulin binds to the insulin receptors located on the muscular cell membrane, a cascade of intracellular pathways is activated, finally inducing the translocation of a glucose transporter (GLUT-4) from the endoplasmatic reticulum to the cellular membrane thereby enhancing the transmembranic flux of glucose intracellularly. This mechanism is normally activated by insulin but is also activated by muscular contraction that also induces the translocation of the GLUT-4-receptor. The latter is, however, independent of the insulin receptor. Thereby physical activity of large muscle groups is capable of improving insulin resistance independent of systemic insulin concentrations [1].

Exercise Intervention

Prevention of Type 2 Diabetes

In recent years several clinical trials have demonstrated that lifestyle interventions can significantly prevent the onset of type 2 diabetes in people with prediabetes. The Chinese Da Qing study [2] was the first large study demonstrating the effects of diet and exercise in preventing type 2 diabetes in persons with impaired glucose tolerance. Thereby, 577 individuals (mean age 45 years) were randomized to receive either standard care or one of the three interventions: diet only (55–65% of total daily calories from carbohydrate, increased consumption of vegetables, reduced intake of simple sugars and alcohol), exercise only (increased leisure physical activity by one unit per day, defined as either 30 min of mild, 20 min of moderate, 10 min of strenuous or 5 min of very strenuous exercise), or a combined diet and exercise intervention. After an observation period of 6 years, diet, exercise, and diet-plus-exercise interventions were associated with 31% (p < 0.03), 46% (p < 0.0005), and 42% (p < 0.005) reductions in risk of developing diabetes compared to standard care, respectively.

Furthermore, the American Diabetes Prevention Program (DPP) [3] and the Finnish Diabetes Prevention Study (DPS) [4], two large prospective randomized intervention studies in patients with impaired glucose tolerance have convincingly demonstrated a relative reduction of diabetes incidence of 58% after 3.2 and 2.8 years of intensive lifestyle intervention. In the DPS 522 adults (aged 40–45 years) were randomized to receive either a control (standard care) or a lifestyle intervention including loss of body weight (≥5%), reduced intake of fat (<30%), saturated fatty acids (<10%), and increased consumption of fibers (>15%) as well as regular moderate

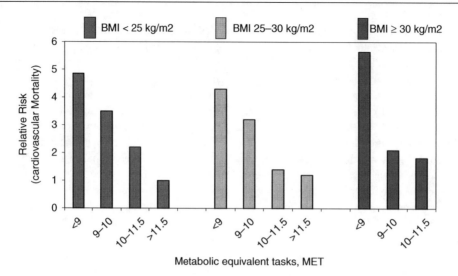

Diabetes Mellitus, Sports Therapy. Fig. 1 Relationship between cardiorespiratory fitness and obesity (Body Mass Index, BMI) in type 2 diabetes on cardiovascular mortality (u = 2,316 Diabetics) [8]

physical activity (>30 min per day endurance and resistance training).

In addition, the DPP compared the effects of a lifestyle intervention and medication intervention receiving metformin in subjects with impaired glucose tolerance. Thereby, at 4 years the lifestyle intervention group showed a weight loss of two times more (−4 kg vs −1.8 kg), and the cumulative incidence of type 2 diabetes was 17% less compared to the metformin group [3].

Therapy of Type 2 Diabetes

Moreover, lifestyle interventions cannot only prevent the deterioration of impaired glucose tolerance to manifest type 2 diabetes as long as the intervention continues, but can even result in sustained lifestyle changes and a reduction in diabetes incidence, which remain beyond the active intervention phase. This has been shown in a follow-up of the DPS. Thereby, participants of the DPS, who were still free of diabetes after a median of 4 years of active intervention period, were further followed up for a median of 3 years. After the total follow-up (median 7 years) the incidence of type 2 diabetes was 4.3 and 7.4 per 100 person-years in the intervention and control group, respectively, indicating 43% reduction in relative risk [5].

Results of the Look Ahead Study [6], a large study on more than 5,000 subjects with type 2 diabetes, showed that regular physical activity (>3 h/week) combined with weight reduction (>7%) led to a significant improvement of cardio-metabolic risk factors, such as waist circumference, hypertension, and levels of blood glucose, cholesterol, and lipids. In addition, both lower fitness and

obesity were associated with lower physical component summary scores in type 2 diabetes. These findings are consistent with previous cross-sectional data showing that improved fitness, rather than reduced fatness, is associated with improved health-related quality of life in those with type 2 diabetes [7] (Fig. 1).

Besides improvements of insulin resistance physical activity improves increased HDL-cholesterol and lipoprotein lipase activity in active skeletal muscle, resulting in an enhanced clearance rate of plasma triglycerides, increased transport of lipids and lipoproteins from the peripheral circulation and tissues to the liver, reduced inflammation, improved endothelial function, and lowered resting heart rate.

Consequences

Exercise has been established as a baseline intervention strategy in the prevention and treatment of type 2 diabetes. Therefore, this approach should be pursued by general practitioners, diabetologists, and others who care for patients with metabolic syndrome or type 2 diabetes. However, medical investigation regarding underlying cardiovascular disease should precede before carefully starting an individually tailored exercise program. This should be accompanied by optimal medical therapy that should be adapted to metabolic changes induced by exercise intervention.

References

1. Wojtaszewski JF, Hansen BF, Gade J, Kiens B, Markuns JF, Goodyear LJ, Richter EA (2000) Insulin signaling and insulin sensitivity after exercise in human skeletal muscle. Diabetes 49:325–331

2. Pan XR, Li GW, Hu YH, Wang JX, Yang WY, An ZX, Hu ZX, Lin J, Xiao JZ, Cao HB, Liu PA, Jiang XG, Jiang YY, Wang JP, Zheng H, Zhang H, Bennett PH, Howard BV (1997) Effects of diet and exercise in preventing NIDDM in people with impaired glucose tolerance. The Da Qing IGT and Diabetes Study. Diabetes Care 20:537–544

3. Knowler WC, Barrett-Connor E, Fowler SE, Hamman RF, Lachin JM, Walker EA, Nathan DM (2002) Reduction in the incidence of type 2 diabetes with lifestyle intervention or metformin. N Engl J Med 346:393–403

4. Tuomilehto J, Lindstrom J, Eriksson JG, Valle TT, Hamalainen H, Ilanne-Parikka P, Keinanen-Kiukaanniemi S, Laakso M, Louheranta A, Rastas M, Salminen V, Uusitupa M (2001) Prevention of type 2 diabetes mellitus by changes in lifestyle among subjects with impaired glucose tolerance. N Engl J Med 344:1343–1350

5. Lindstrom J, Ilanne-Parikka P, Peltonen M, Aunola S, Eriksson JG, Hemio K, Hamalainen H, Harkonen P, Keinanen-Kiukaanniemi S, Laakso M, Louheranta A, Mannelin M, Paturi M, Sundvall J, Valle TT, Uusitupa M, Tuomilehto J (2006) Sustained reduction in the incidence of type 2 diabetes by lifestyle intervention: follow-up of the Finnish diabetes prevention study. Lancet 368:1673–1679

6. Pi-Sunyer X, Blackburn G, Brancati FL, Bray GA, Bright R, Clark JM, Curtis JM, Espeland MA, Foreyt JP, Graves K, Haffner SM, Harrison B, Hill JO, Horton ES, Jakicic J, Jeffery RW, Johnson KC, Kahn S, Kelley DE, Kitabchi AE, Knowler WC, Lewis CE, Maschak-Carey BJ, Montgomery B, Nathan DM, Patricio J, Peters A, Redmon JB, Reeves RS, Ryan DH, Safford M, Van DB, Wadden TA, Wagenknecht L, Wesche-Thobaben J, Wing RR, Yanovski SZ (2007) Reduction in weight and cardiovascular disease risk factors in individuals with type 2 diabetes: one-year results of the look AHEAD trial. Diabetes Care 30:1374–1383

7. Bennett WL, Ouyang P, Wu AW, Barone BB, Stewart KJ (2008) Fatness and fitness: how do they influence health-related quality of life in type 2 diabetes mellitus? Health Qual Life Outcomes 6:110

8. Church TS, LaMonte MJ, Barlow CE, Blair SN (2005) Cardiorespiratory fitness and body mass index as predictors of cardiovascular disease mortality among men with diabetes. Arch Intern Med 165 (18):2114–2120

Diabetic Myopathy

▶ Diabetes Mellitus, Myopathy

Diaphragm

ANDREAS N. KAVAZIS[1], ASHLEY J. SMUDER[2]
[1]Department of Kinesiology, Mississippi State University, Mississippi State, MS, USA
[2]Department of Applied Physiology and Kinesiology, University of Florida, Gainesville, FL, USA

Synonyms
Costal; Inspiratory muscle; Lumbar; Sternal

Definition
The diaphragm and other respiratory skeletal muscles (e.g., external intercostals, pectoralis minor, scalene) are essential for normal ventilation. Importantly, in nearly all mammals, the diaphragm is considered the most important muscle of ▶ inspiration. Thus, maintenance of proper diaphragm function is critical to overall health. Therefore, this review will focus on conditions that lead to diaphragm adaptation. However, we will first provide a short anatomical and biochemical description of the diaphragm.

Anatomically, the diaphragm is a dome-shaped skeletal muscle whose structure provides a means for separating the thoracic and abdominal cavities (Fig. 1). Structurally, the diaphragm can be divided into three parts which include the sternal, costal, and lumbar regions. The coastal region of the diaphragm forms the left and right hemidiaphragms which are the main part of the diaphragm that move during ventilation.

The diaphragm is a skeletal muscle that contracts during inspiration and relaxes during ▶ expiration. According to published reports, the best estimate of the different fiber type distribution in the adult human diaphragm are about 55% slow fibers, 21% ▶ fast oxidative fibers, and 24% ▶ fast glycolytic fibers [1].

Mechanisms
The diaphragm is the primary muscle of inspiration, and therefore decreased diaphragm function could result in inadequate ventilation and ▶ gas exchange. In this regard, a disease (e.g., chronic obstructive pulmonary disease, and sepsis) or other condition (e.g., aging and mechanical ventilation) that leads to diaphragm dysfunction and weakness can result in severe side effects including death.

The diaphragm is chronically active throughout the lifespan. As a result of this activation pattern, the diaphragm has unique functional properties and adaptations that make it a distinctive skeletal muscle. This short essay will address a broad range of issues related to specific adaptations of the diaphragm. Specifically, we will focus on the effects of chronic obstructive pulmonary disease, aging, mechanical ventilation, and exercise on the diaphragm.

Chronic Obstructive Pulmonary Disease and the Diaphragm
Chronic obstructive pulmonary disease is characterized by increased airway resistance which limits the flow of air to and from the lungs. In addition to compromising normal ventilation and gas exchange, chronic obstructive pulmonary disease also results in decreased diaphragm function. This is significant because altered diaphragm function is

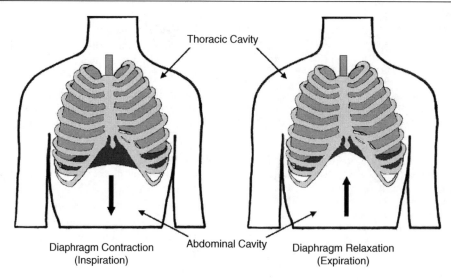

Diaphragm. Fig. 1 The diaphragm is a dome-shaped skeletal muscle which separates the thoracic and abdominal cavities. During inspiration the diaphragm contracts, and during expiration the diaphragm relaxes

directly related to poor clinical status in patients with chronic obstructive pulmonary disease and can result in increased morbidity and mortality. In human chronic obstructive pulmonary disease patients, it has been reported that there are specific adaptations to both the diaphragm muscle quantity and quality. Specifically, patients with chronic obstructive pulmonary disease have a decrease in muscle mass due to a decrease in diaphragm length (i.e., sarcomeric deletion). Furthermore, the diaphragm of chronic obstructive pulmonary disease patients undergoes a fast-to-slow fiber type shift.

In addition to changes in diaphragm muscle mass, there is also a decrease in diaphragm force generating capacity (Fig. 2). Specifically, single diaphragm fibers from patients with chronic obstructive pulmonary disease generated a lower specific force than control subjects. This diaphragmatic remodeling suggests that the diaphragm of patients with chronic obstructive pulmonary disease undergoes alterations to produce a more fatigue resistant phenotype.

Aging and the Diaphragm

It is well known that the mass and force of skeletal muscles are affected by aging. Specifically, in humans, the force produced by limb skeletal muscles decreases with aging and is associated with a loss of muscle mass. This decrease in muscle mass is believed to be due to a reduction in the cross-sectional area of muscle fibers and a reduction in the number of muscle fibers.

Although there is ample information on the effects of aging on limb skeletal muscles, there is only limited information available on the effects of aging on the human diaphragm. Since the diaphragm remains chronically active throughout the lifespan, this suggests that aging might differentially affect respiratory (i.e., diaphragm) and limb muscles.

In this regard, several investigators have reported that the diaphragm maintains its mass throughout life (Fig. 2). Specifically, we have reported that the cross-sectional areas of slow and fast glycolytic diaphragm fibers are not different between young adult (6 months) and senescent (24–26 months) rats. We also noted a small but significant increase in the cross-sectional area of fast oxidative fibers diaphragm fibers [2]. In contrast, investigators have shown aging of limb skeletal muscles causes a shift of fibers toward a slower phenotype. However, the diaphragm does not undergo these fiber type changes with aging [2].

Mechanical Ventilation and the Diaphragm

Mechanical ventilation is used clinically to sustain pulmonary gas exchange in patients that are incapable of maintaining sufficient alveolar ventilation. Although mechanical ventilation is a life-saving measure, prolonged mechanical ventilation is often associated with diaphragm weakness (Fig. 2). In this regard, we and other investigators have shown that the diaphragmatic weakness associated with mechanical ventilation is due to both ▶ atrophy and contractile dysfunction [3].

Importantly, Levine and collaborators have shown that mechanical ventilation leads to atrophy in the human diaphragm [4]. Specifically, this study shows that mechanical ventilation-induced atrophy occurs in both

	Cross-Sectional Area	Contractile Function
COPD	↓	↓
Aging	↔	↓
MV	↓	↓
Exercise	↓	↔

Diaphragm. Fig. 2 The effects of chronic obstructive pulmonary disease (COPD), aging, mechanical ventilation (MV), and exercise on diaphragm cross-sectional area and contractile function

type I and type II human diaphragm fibers. In addition, the data from this study illustrate that only a short period (~18–69 h) of mechanical ventilation in humans leads to a large decline in diaphragm cross-sectional area. Furthermore, several animal studies show that mechanical ventilation also results in a reduction in diaphragmatic maximal tetanic specific force production (i.e., contractile dysfunction).

The changes that occur in the diaphragm following mechanical ventilation are due to both decreased diaphragmatic protein synthesis and increased protein breakdown. However, our data show that mechanical ventilation-induced diaphragmatic proteolysis is a major reason for mechanical ventilation-induced diaphragmatic atrophy and contractile dysfunction. Importantly, we have shown that unloading the diaphragm by mechanical ventilation leads to the activation of several ▶ proteases in the diaphragm (e.g., calpain, caspase-3, ubiquitin proteasome system) [3].

Although the specific molecular signaling pathways that lead to mechanical ventilation-induced diaphragmatic weakness are not fully understood, we and others have shown that increased reactive oxygen species (ROS) production during mechanical ventilation is a critical step in the activation of many pathways involved in diaphragmatic proteolysis. Understanding the specific details of the pathways involved can lead to discoveries to protect patients against MV-induced diaphragm weakness.

Exercise Response/Consequences

Exercise training has been shown to increase the oxidative capacity of the diaphragm. Human studies have shown that respiratory muscle training can result in elevated work capacity by the muscles involved in ventilation. However, it is not clear if this diaphragm muscle training can lead to increased whole body endurance capacity. In addition, the question whether improvement in the oxidative capacity of respiratory muscles is of significant magnitude to cause an improvement in respiratory muscle performance remains unanswered.

Acute exercise increases ROS production and release by skeletal muscle (e.g., diaphragm). The increased diaphragmatic ROS formation can play an important role in the regulation of signaling pathways involved in diaphragm muscle adaptation. In addition, a critical adaptation that occurs in the diaphragm is the exercise-induced upregulation of ▶ antioxidants. Specifically, several studies have shown that endurance exercise training induces increases in diaphragmatic antioxidant enzyme activity. Some of the major and important antioxidant enzymes that are upregulated in the diaphragm following exercise training include copper-zinc and manganese superoxide dismutase, catalase, and glutathione peroxidase. The increased activity of these antioxidant enzymes appears to provide a vital defense against the potentially damaging effects of ROS.

Diagnostics

Measurement of In Vitro Diaphragmatic Contractile Properties

The specific force (i.e., contractile function) of the diaphragm can be measured in vitro. Specifically, a small diaphragm strip is suspended vertically between two lightweight Plexiglas clamps with one end connected to an isometric force transducer within a jacketed tissue bath. The force output is recorded via a computerized data-acquisition system and specific muscle force is calculated [3].

Measurement of In Vivo Diaphragmatic Contractile Properties

A force-frequency curve of the diaphragm is generated by using unilateral phrenic nerve stimulation. The phrenic nerve stimulation can be achieved by either electrical stimulation or cervical magnetic stimulation [5]. Esophageal and gastric pressures are measured, and transdiaphragmatic pressure is obtained by subtraction of esophageal pressure from gastric pressure.

Diaphragm Myofiber Cross-Sectional Area

Sections from frozen diaphragm samples are cut at 10 μm using a cryotome and stained for dystrophin, and slow and fast oxidative myosin heavy chain proteins [3]. Images are then obtained and analyzed to determine fiber cross-sectional area using a computer software program.

References

1. Polla B, D'Antona G, Bottinelli R, Reggiani C (2004) Respiratory muscle fibres: specialisation and plasticity. Thorax 59:808–817
2. Kavazis AN, DeRuisseau KC, McClung JM, Whidden MA, Falk DJ, Smuder AJ, Sugiura T, Powers SK (2007) Diaphragmatic proteasome function is maintained in the ageing Fisher 344 rat. Exp Physiol 92:895–901
3. Powers SK, Hudson MB, Nelson WB, Talbert EE, Min K, Szeto HH, Kavazis AN, Smuder AJ (2011) Mitochondria-targeted antioxidants protect against mechanical-ventilation-induced diaphragm weakness. Crit Care Med 39(7):1749–1759
4. Levine S, Nguyen T, Taylor N, Friscia ME, Budak MT, Rothenberg P, Zhu J, Sachdeva R, Sonnad S, Kaiser LR, Rubinstein NA, Powers SK, Shrager JB (2008) Rapid disuse atrophy of diaphragm fibers in mechanically ventilated humans. N Engl J Med 358:1327–1335
5. Laghi F, Harrison MJ, Tobin MJ (1996) Comparison of magnetic and electrical phrenic nerve stimulation in assessment of diaphragmatic contractility. J Appl Physiol 80:1731–1742

Diarrhea, Exercise Induced

FRANK C. MOOREN
Department of Sports Medicine, Justus-Liebig-University, Giessen, Germany

Synonyms

Exercise associated loose stool; Looseness after exercise; Runner's trots; Runner's diarrhea

Definition

Diarrhea refers to alterations in stool consistency, weight (more than 250 g/day) and frequency (more than 3/day). Additional symptoms may include abdominal cramps, bloating, and any forms of bleedings from occult to macroscopic. Diarrhea is often associated with endurance sports, especially long-distance running, triathlon etc. The prevalence seems to be related to exercise intensity and duration, but also other factors such as age, hydration and training status have to be considered. In some cases severe courses have been reported with symptoms and clinical findings like an ischemic colitis [4].

Mechanisms

Several mechanisms for exercise induced diarrhea have been proposed. However, in most cases detailed experimental evidence is lacking [5].

Intestinal Absorption/Secretion

Diarrheal diseases are characterized by alterations of intestinal absorptive and secretory processes. There is evidence that high intensity exercise affects these processes as detailed described elsewhere in this encyclopedia (term intestinal absorption).

Release of Neuroendocrine Hormones

Some studies report significant increases of neuroendocrine transmitters such as secretin, glucagon, neurotensin, pancreatic polypeptide (PP), motilin, and vasoactive polypeptide (VIP) after endurance exercise. Some of these hormones such as VIP are able to enhance significantly the secretory processes across the intestinal epithelia resulting in a reduced stool consistency. Their release seems to be triggered locally due to either ischemia or mechanical stimulation due to the bowel movement.

Motility

Exercise has been shown to affect intestinal motility. The effect seems to depend on exercise intensity and affects intestinal regions quite different. However, there is evidence that the mean oro-fecal transit time is reduced after intensive and/or long-term exercise resulting in an enhanced stool frequency.

Mechanical Component

The prevalence of gastrointestinal micro-bleedings seems to be higher during running than during other sports like bicycling, rowing, etc. This has led to the suggestion that mechanical alterations may be another causal factor of exercise induced diarrhea. Especially during running vertical movements of the bowel occur which might induce damages of the intestinal epithelia and wall.

Reductions of Intestinal Blood Flow

The most likely pathogenetic mechanisms underlying exercise induced diarrhea are related to exercise associated reductions of intestinal blood flow. Triggered by altered autonomic nerve activity a perfusion shift occurs during exercise which results in an improved perfusion of contractile tissues and skin to support substrate supply and thermoregulation, respectively. In contrast, the perfusion of the GI tract is more and more reduced with values down to about 20% of the resting levels. During exercise in hot environments and dehydration the situation may be even worse. The perfusion shift induces three important pathophysiological factors – hypoxia, oxidative stress, and hyperthermia (Fig. 1; [3]). Local and regional hypoxia results in a depletion of cellular ATP stores leading to reduction of cellular function and metabolism. This includes the loss of

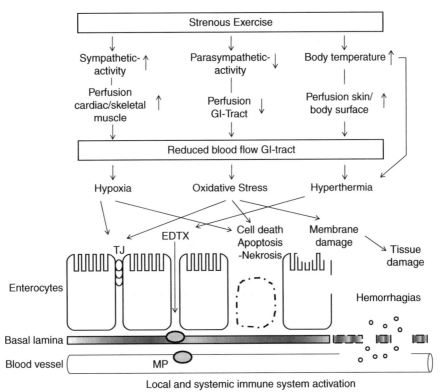

Diarrhea, Exercise Induced. Fig. 1 Schematic diagram summarizing the proposed pathophysiological mechanisms underlying exercise induced alterations of intestinal epithelia structure and function (Modified according [3]). *TJ* tight junctions, *EDTX* endotoxin, *MP* macrophages, *GI* gastro intestinal

intestinal integrity by affecting the sealing function of apical tight junctions (TJ) and results in an enhanced permeability of macro molecules (>150 kDa). TJ are well-known for their function in controlling paracellular traffic of ions and molecules. Moreover, the reduced energetic level impairs any forms of active transport processes and the maintenance of transmembranuous ion gradients. The resulting increase of free intracellular calcium concentration can activate formerly inactive proteases known to induce both necrotic and apoptotic cell death.

Alternatively, the damage of intestinal epithelia can occur via an enhanced oxidative stress. Ischemia and especially the following reperfusion reaction result in a substantial release of reactive oxygen and nitrogen species known to affect directly cellular structures. Finally, it could be shown during both in vitro and in vivo approaches that hyperthermia induces a membrane damage of intestinal epithelial and opens TJ. Together, all three factors are able to induce the various grades of intestinal tissue damage from TJ openings over single cell death toward erosive and hemorrhagic tissue damage of which the latter impresses as a major histologic finding of ischemic colitis. However, it

should be emphasized that already the opening of TJs may have unfavorable consequences. The resulting leakage of endotoxins (lipopolysaccharide (LPS)) into the circulation induces a local and systemic activation of immune cells with the release of inflammatory mediators such as tumor necrosis factor alpha (TNFα) and interleukin-1 (IL-1). With this inflammatory cascade further intestinal tissue damages may result [2]. Furthermore, the systemic immune reaction has been proposed to be involved in the pathogenesis of exercise associated heat stress.

Exercise response/Consequences

Clinical symptoms of exercise associated diarrhea include abdominal cramps, urge to defecate, loos, and bloody stools. Frank hemorrhagic diarrheas are quite rarely reported. The prevalence of micro-bleedings as diagnosed by the biochemical Guajak test varies considerably from 10% to 80%. While after marathon runs values of about 20% have been reported the percentage increased to about 80% after ultramarathon indicating the role of exercise duration and intensity. However, clinical investigations should include also other disorders of the GI tract such as food allergies and intolerances, colon diverticulum, hemangiomas, hemorrhoids, carcinomas, and chronic inflammatory bowel diseases [1]. Therapeutical consequences of gastrointestinal symptoms including exercise induced diarrhea are not presented in this entry as they have been discussed elsewhere in this encyclopedia in more detail.

Diagnostics

For diagnosis of exercise induced diarrhea the close temporal relation of symptoms to the exercise event is often important. Moreover, the relationship between severity of symptoms and exercise intensity/duration may be helpful. As no definitive pathognomonic signs for exercise induced diarrheas exist an exclusion of other reasons might be necessary. Therefore, athletes should be interviewed in depth regarding (1) the use of nonsteroidal antiphlogistics known to induce intestinal epithelial damage, (2) food allergies and intolerances, and (3) stays abroad etc. Further diagnostic tools in order to exclude other GI related may include abdominal ultrasound, hydrogen breath tests, upper and lower GI endoscopy. Laboratory diagnosis should particularly include serology of gastrointestinal viruses and a comprehensive stool analysis in order to detect the presence of pathogenic microorganisms such as yeast, parasites, and bacteria. The measurement of serum levels of thyroxine (T4), triiodothyronine (T3), thyroid-stimulating hormone, gastrin, vasoactive-intestinal polypeptide may be helpful for diagnosis of hormonal induced diarrheas. Eventually radiologic investigations such as double contrast barium enema, abdominal computed tomography and/or endoscopic retrograde cholangiopancreatography may be used in special cases.

References

1. Butcher JD (1993) Runner's diarrhea and other intestinal problems of athletes. Am Fam Physician 48:623–627
2. Jeukendrup AE, Vet-Joop K, Sturk A, Stegen JH, Senden J, Saris WH, Wagenmakers AJ (2000) Relationship between gastro-intestinal complaints and endotoxaemia, cytokine release and the acute-phase reaction during and after a long-distance triathlon in highly trained men. Clin Sci (Lond) 98(1):47–55
3. Lambert GP (2008) Intestinal barrier dysfunction, endotoxemia, and gastrointestinal symptoms: the "canary in the coal mine" during exercise-heat stress? Med Sport Sci 53:61–73
4. Lucas W, Schroy PC 3rd (1998) Reversible ischemic colitis in a high endurance athlete. Am J Gastroenterol 93(11):2231–2234
5. Simren M (2002) Physical activity and the gastrointestinal tract. Eur J Gastroenterol Hepatol 14:1053–1056

Diet

▶ Nutrition

Dietary Reference Intakes (DRIs)

The umbrella term that encompasses the Recommended Dietary Allowances (RDA), Adequate Intakes (AI), Estimated Average Requirement (EAR), and Tolerable Upper Intake Levels (UL). These are the established dietary needs for all required nutrients for healthy individuals in the United States.

Dietary Supplement

▶ Supplementation

Diffusion

Passive movement of molecules down a concentration gradient from one side of a membrane to the other by random thermal motion.

Diffusion Tensor Imaging

A magnetic resonance imaging protocol that allows an assessment of the integrity of white matter tracts in the brain by monitoring the correlated movement of water molecules.

Dihydropyridine Receptors (DHPRs) = L-Type Voltage-Operated Ca^{2+} Channels

▶ Excitation–Contraction Coupling

Direct Calorimetry

Laboratory method that quantifies the amount of heat produced by a subject.

Disability Adjusted Life Years

A summary estimate of population health that measures the difference between a population's health and a normative goal of living in full health.

Disabled Athletes

YAGESH BHAMBHANI
University of Alberta, Edmonton, AB, Canada

Synonyms

Paralympic athletes

Definition

Athletes with disabilities compete internationally in sporting events that are sanctioned by the International ▶ Paralympic Committee (IPC). The following five physical disabilities are represented in these events: ▶ cerebral palsy (CP), ▶ spinal cord injury (SCI), ▶ amputation (AMP), ▶ visual impairment (VI), and "▶ *Les Autres*" (LA, other physical disabilities). At the 2008 Beijing Paralympics, individuals with intellectual disabilities (ID) also competed in these games. The Paralympic Games are hosted by the IPC once every 4 years in the same city and venues as the Olympics. Paralympic athletes compete in 20 individual and team sports at the summer games and five individual and team sports at the winter games (www.paralympic.org). Because athletes with disabilities have impairment in one or more body structures and functions, cardiovascular, neuromuscular, visual, and cognitive performance may be altered, thereby influencing sport performance. In order to ensure that these athletes compete on an equitable basis, the IPC established a functional classification code in 2003. This classification system, which is refined continually, is designed to ensure that success in competition is determined by the athlete's individual physiological and psychological fitness parameters, as is the case for able-bodied sport.

Pathogenic Mechanisms

Cerebral Palsy (CP)

Physical disabilities can be congenital or acquired. CP is a nonprogressive congenital disorder which results in damage to the brain thereby affecting posture and movement. CP can be classified as pyramidal, extrapyramidal, or mixed. In pyramidal CP, the motor cortex which propagates the signal for voluntary movement via the pyramidal tract is damaged. This results in muscle spasticity, the severity of which depends on the location and magnitude of the injury. In extrapyramidal CP, neurological pathways that are external to the pyramidal tract are damaged which result in difficulties in posture and movement. These individuals usually experience frequent, involuntary contractions of the upper and lower extremities. However, contractures and limitations to range of motion are usually not very evident. In mixed CP, damage occurs in both the pyramidal and extrapyramidal tracts. This is the most common type of CP and involves a combination of the conditions described above. Due to the severe brain damage, many of these individuals may have concomitant developmental disabilities. In general, individuals with CP have excess muscle tone which leads to contractures and jerky movements. The lack of reciprocal inhibition can lead to uncoordinated movements and increases the risk for muscle damage.

Spinal Cord Injury (SCI)

SCI can be acquired as a result of motor vehicle accidents, gunshot wounds, assaults, workplace mishaps, and accidents in the sport and recreation environments. These injuries are more prevalent in males compared to females and tend to peak during adolescence or early to middle adulthood. SCI disrupts the motor, sensory, and autonomic nervous system, and therefore has a profound influence on physical and functional capacity. Spina bifida is a congenital disorder which affects the spinal column. The failure of one or more vertebral arches to close before birth results in a protruding spinal cord which can form a sac or tumor. Many of the physical problems associated with this condition resemble those of SCI. Therefore, many of the recommendations for physical activity and fitness programming for these two conditions overlap.

Amputation (AMP)

Congenital deformities of the upper and lower extremities which result in a loss of function occur for a variety of reasons. Upper and lower limb amputations are performed because of trauma, peripheral vascular disease, type II diabetes, tumors, and other medical conditions. Majority of the individuals who undergo amputation tend to be older adults above 55 years. However, many of the individuals who require amputation from trauma and tumors tend to be below 50 years. Anatomically, lower limb amputations can be described as follows: forefoot or midfoot (Syme's amputation), trans-tibial or below knee, trans-femoral or above knee, and hip disarticulation which necessities removal of the femoral hip joint. These amputations can be performed either unilaterally or bilaterally. Obviously the type of amputation will determine the muscle and joints available for exercise, and therefore, influence the individual's capacity for sport participation and physical training.

Visual Impairment (VI)

VI is a sensory disorder that encompasses a wide range of visual acuity. The following terms are commonly used to describe visual impairment: legally blind or "blindness by acuity (clarity)" is the ability to see at 20 ft what the normal eye sees at 200 ft; blind by visual field or "tunnel vision" is having a visual field of less than ten degrees of central vision; total blindness or "no light perception" is the inability to recognize a strong light that is pointed directly to the eye. VI affects individuals of all ages. Excessive oxygenation during incubation has been implicated in childhood blindness. Congenital defects such as cataracts and optic nerve disease are the primary factors for VI in young individuals. Tumors, infectious diseases, and injuries seem to be less likely causes in this age group. In elderly individuals, diabetes, macular degeneration, glaucoma, and cataracts are the leading causes of VI.

Les Autres (LA)

LA refers to the group of physical disabilities that are not included in the previous disabilities. This group includes individuals with traumatic brain injury, post-polio, etc. whose motor function is impaired and are eligible to participate in Paralympic sport.

Physiological Testing of Paralympic Athletes

Theoretical Considerations

In quadriplegic individuals with SCI injury above the first thoracic vertebra (T1 level), sympathetic simulation to the myocardium is disrupted. Consequently, the peak heart rate (HR) that can be attained during exercise is determined by the intrinsic rate of the sinoatrial node which is approximately 115–120 beats/min. In paraplegic individuals with lesion levels below T1, there is no disruption in myocardial stimulation and therefore, these individuals should theoretically be able to attain their age-predicted maximal heart rate (220 – age, years). However, the peak HR that is attained is dependent upon the functional muscle mass available for exercise. In individuals with quadriplegia and paraplegia, stroke volume (SV) during exercise is significantly reduced because of the absence of the active muscle pump (i.e., muscle paralysis) below the lesion level. The reductions in peak HR and SV significantly lower the peak cardiac output (Q) during exercise, thereby lowering the peak oxygen uptake (VO_{2peak}). Typically, there is an inverse relationship between the lesion level and the VO_{2peak} in individuals with SCI [1, 6]. Individuals with CP and AMP have complete innervation of the myocardium and usually are able to attain

their age-predicted maximum HR during incremental exercise. In individuals with CP, the neuromuscular efficiency, defined as the oxygen uptake per unit amount of work, is significantly higher (i.e., reduced efficiency) compared to able-bodied subjects because of the muscle spasticity associated with this condition. Individuals with AMP have a reduced muscle mass available for exercise which could compromise their ability to attain their peak HR, SV, and Q during exercise, thereby reducing their VO_{2peak}. Individuals with VI have no underlying pathology that alters the cardiorespiratory or neuromuscular factors during exercise. However, their neuromuscular efficiency tends to be significantly lower when compared to age-matched controls because of the increased muscle tone associated with exercise that is devoid of visual cues.

Peak Aerobic Power and Ventilatory Threshold

The following principles should be followed when testing the VO_{2peak} of paralympic athletes, regardless of their disability: (1) the testing mode (apparatus) should be specific to their sport. For example, wheelchair athletes (racers, basketball players, tennis players, etc.) should be tested on a wheelchair ergometer (Fig. 1), while CP or AMP runners and cyclists should be tested on a treadmill and cycle ergometer respectively. Nordic skiers with SCI, CP, AP, or VI can be tested using a double poling ergometer in the sitting or standing position (see Fig. 2). Wheelchair ergometers can be independent instruments which are specially modified to quantify the power output, or they can be mounted on a treadmill so that both the velocity and gradient can be controlled during the test protocol; (2) regardless of the testing mode, the incremental test protocol should be designed to recruit as large a muscle mass as possible and elicit the peak physiological responses within 10–12 min. The magnitude of the power output or velocity/slope increments will vary depending upon the nature and degree of severity of the disability. Typically, smaller work rate increments should be utilized for SCI athletes with quadriplegia who have limited upper extremity/trunk function compared to those with paraplegia who have complete use of the upper extremities and are able to recruit a larger muscle mass. An incremental testing protocol is recommended so that the ▶ ventilatory threshold (VT), a measure of submaximal aerobic fitness that is correlated with performance, can be identified. In order to facilitate testing athletes who have a high degree of spasticity, it may be necessary to secure their limbs to the pedal of the wheelchair ergometer for optimal results. The use of medications at the time of testing should be recorded in order to obtain valid and reliable results.

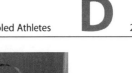

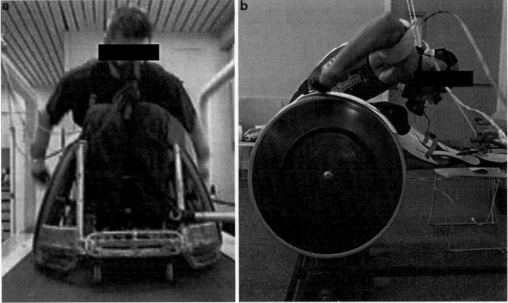

Disabled Athletes. Fig. 1 Paralympic wheelchair athletes being tested on: (**a**) treadmill/roller system; (**b**) frictionless roller system

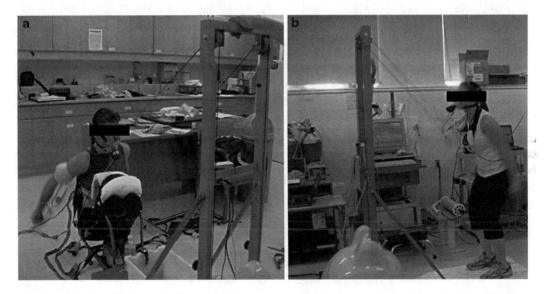

Disabled Athletes. Fig. 2 Paralympic skiers being tested on a double poling ergometer in the: (**a**) sitting position; (**b**) standing position

Representative values for the VO_2 peak and VT are presented in Tables 1 and 2 respectively.

Anaerobic Power and Capacity

The modified 30 s Wingate test that is used for able-bodied subjects is the most popular and reliable test for evaluating these parameters in Paralympic athletes. Arm crank or computerized wheel chair ergometers that are designed to quantify the power output can be used for assessing athletes who lack lower limb function [2]. Athletes with CP and AMP with lower extremity function can be evaluated using cycle ergometry [3, 4]. The peak power attained during the 30 s test is used as an index of the anaerobic power, while the average power generated

Disabled Athletes. Table 1 Typical ranges for the peak aerobic power, peak heart rate, and ventilatory threshold in elite male Paralympic athletes during incremental wheelchair exercise[a]

Disability[b]	Peak VO$_2$ ml/kg/min	Peak HR beats/min	VT ml/kg/min	VT% Peak VO$_2$
Trans-femoral AMP	40–50	180–200	30–40	70–80
CP	30–45	180–200	20–30	60–75
SCI: C5 to C7	15–20	115–122	12–15	80–90
SCI: T1 to T5	25–30	150–170	16–20	65–70
SCI: T6 to T10	30–40	160–180	20–30	65–75
SCI: T11 to L3	40–50	170–190	28–32	70–75
SCI: L4 to S1	40–50	170–190	28–32	70–75
VI[c]	50–65	170–195	35–55	70–80

[a]Values provided are estimated from published wheelchair ergometry studies on male Paralympic athletes. The values for female athletes and athletes will most likely be lower by 10–15%. Athletes with incomplete SCI may demonstrate higher values.
[b]Trans-femoral *AMP* trans-femoral amputation, *CP* Cerebral palsy, *SCI* spinal cord injury, *VI* visual impairment.
[c]Measured during double poling ergometry in three visually impaired male Nordic skiers.

Disabled Athletes. Table 2 Peak oxygen uptake, peak heart rate, and ventilatory threshold in a cross section of Paralympic athletes during incremental arm-cranking exercise[a]

Sport[b]	VO$_{2peak}$ ml/kg/min	HR$_{peak}$ beats/min	VT ml/kg/min	VT% VO$_{2peak}$
Nordic sit skiing (N=5)	51.9±6.9	186.2±11.5	38.3±5.8	73.7±3.2
Wheelchair racing (N=6)	48.1±6.4	187.0±5.7	35.5±6.0	73.5±3.5
Wheelchair basketball (N=13)	36.9±3.7	188.7±10.1	26.0±2.1	70.7±3.5
Wheelchair fencing (N=6)	34.4±5.8	182.0±5.4	23.2±4.0	67.6±1.2
Wheelchair tennis (N=4)	33.1±2.9	176.8±19.7	24.0±2.3	72.6±2.7

[a]Values indicated are Mean±SD reported by Bernardi et al. 2010 [7].
[b]Athletes with the following disabilities participated in these sports: 23 paraplegia, 5 post-poliomyelitis, 3 trasfemoral amputations, and 3 trans-tibial amputations.

during the 30 s protocol is an estimate of the anaerobic capacity. The fatigue index, defined as the decline in power over the 30 s period, is calculated as the ratio between: [(peak power − minimum power)/peak power] × 100. Currently, there is no standardized method for determining the load factor that should be used for the Wingate test in Paralympic athletes because of large differences in functional capacity and the muscle mass that can be recruited during exercise. The appropriate load factor, calculated as a function of body weight, should be estimated during a familiarization session with the athlete. In SCI athletes, the ▶ peak anaerobic power and anaerobic capacity is inversely related to the level of lesion, implying that the lower the injury level the greater the anaerobic fitness and vice versa. The peak anaerobic power of athletes with low level paraplegia (lesion at T8 or lower) can exceed those attained by able-bodied individuals during arm-cranking

exercise [1]. Representative values for various indices of anaerobic power are presented in Table 3.

Body Composition

The hydrostatic weighing method of assessing ▶ body composition, which is based on the two-compartment model (percent body fat and lean body mass), has been validated in able-bodied subjects. However, for practical reasons, this method is not feasible for evaluating body composition in individuals with disabilities. Currently, a variety of noninvasive methods have been validated to evaluate the body composition of athletes with disabilities, including: dual energy X-ray absorptiometry (DEXA) scans, bio-electrical impedance (BIA), and skinfold (SF) methods [5]. DEXA scans provide additional information pertaining to bone mineral density (BMD) and segmental changes in body composition, which is particularly useful

Disabled Athletes. **Table 3** Typical ranges for the anaerobic power and fatigue index in elite male Paralympic athletes during wheelchair ergometry[a]

Disability[b]	Peak power watts	Peak power watts/kg	Average power watts	Average power watts/kg	Fatigue index percent
AMP	120–200	1.7–2.8	100–150	1.4–2.1	Limited research available. Estimated to be within 60–80%.
CP	80–160	1.2–2.3	60–140	0.8–2.0	
SCI: C5 to C7	35–50	0.5–0.7	25–40	0.4–0.6	
SCI: T1 to T5	90–140	1.5–2.0	60–100	0.9–1.4	
SCI: T6 to T10	100–170	1.4–2.4	80–130	1.2–1.9	
SCI: T11 to L3	120–180	1.7–2.5	100–140	1.4–2.0	
SCI: L4 to S1	120–200	1.7–2.8	100–130	1.4–2.1	
VI	No published data available				

[a]Values provided are estimated from published wheelchair ergometry studies on male Paralympic athletes. The values for female athletes and athletes will most likely be lower by 10–15%. Athletes with incomplete SCI may demonstrate higher values.
[b]Trans-femoral *AMP* trans-femoral amputation, *CP* Cerebral palsy, *SCI* spinal cord injury, *VI* visual impairment.

in the SCI population. BIA provides estimates of the absolute and relative values of body fat and lean body mass and can also predict the basal metabolic rate based on these estimates. This method clearly demonstrates that the BMR of athletes with SCI is significantly lower than that of the age-and gender-matched able-bodied counterparts, due to the muscle paralysis in this population. SF methods should be used with caution in athletes with disabilities because of variations in the development of adipose tissue in the active and paralyzed tissue, differences in the mode of ambulation, etc. As well, the validity of the regression equations for predicting the body fat in the different athletic groups has not been well established.

Exercise Intervention/Therapeutical Consequences

Majority of the sport science research on Paralympic athletes has focused on the SCI population with minimal research on the other disabilities. The available evidence suggests that the physiological adaptations are similar to those observed in able-bodied athletes. Cross-sectional evidence on Paralympic athletes indicates that the absolute and relative values for the VO_{2peak} and VT are significantly higher in Paralympians participating in aerobic events compared to those participating in intermittent sports, as indicated in Table 3. Endurance training which meets the minimum criteria for the frequency, intensity, and duration for training [7] induces significant improvements in the central (related to oxygen transport) and peripheral (related to oxygen extraction) factors that determine the VO_{2peak} in SCI athletes. The SV during exercise increases significantly thereby enhancing

Q and overall oxygen transport capacity. Peripheral adaptations include significant improvement in mitochondrial density and oxidative capacity of the trained muscles resulting in a widening of the arteriovenous oxygen difference during exercise. Exercise bradycardia is also observed subsequent to training, implying an improvement in cardiovascular efficiency [1]. In SCI athletes, cardiac dimensions such as left ventricular volume during diastole and left ventricular mass are significantly larger compared to their sedentary counterparts but smaller compared to non-SCI paralympic athletes [8]. Anaerobic power is also significantly higher in paralympic athletes compared to their untrained counterparts [2]. This may be attributed to peripheral adaptations such as enhanced muscle mass and improved synchrony of motor unit recruitment during exercise. DEXA scans have shown that the BMD of the active limbs in SCI athletes is significantly higher than the paralyzed limbs, implying that regular exercise promotes the development of BMD or attenuates the rate of decline in BMD in these athletes [5]. In athletes with SCI, respiratory function is compromised and may be a limiting factor during endurance events [9]. In these athletes, respiratory muscle training seems to be effective in improving localized functional capacity and sport performance [10].

Cross-References

▶ Spinal Cord Injury

References

1. Bhambhani Y (2002) Physiology of wheelchair racing in athletes with spinal cord injury. Sports Med 32:23–51

2. van der Woude LHV, Bakker WH, Elkhuizen JW, Veeger HEJ, Gwinn T (1997) Anaerobic work capacity in elite wheelchair athletes. Am J Phys Med Rehabil 76:355–365
3. Chin T, Sawamura S, Fujita H, Nakajima S, Ojima I, Oyabu H et al (1997) The efficacy of the one-leg cycling test for determining the anaerobic threshold (AT) of lower limb amputees. Prosthet Orthot Int 21:141–146
4. Dwyer GB, McMahon AD (1994) Ventilatory threshold and peak exercise responses in athletes with CP during treadmill and cycle ergometry. Adapt Phys Activ Q 11:329–334
5. Mojtahedi MC, Valentine RJ, Evans EM (2009) Body composition assessment in athletes with spinal cord injury: comparison of field methods with dual-energy X-ray absorptiometry. Spinal Cord 47:698–704
6. van der Woude LH, Bouten C, Veeger HE, Gwinn T (2002) Aerobic work capacity in elite wheelchair athletes: a cross-sectional analysis. Am J Phys Med Rehabil 81:261–271
7. Bernardi M, Guerra E, Di Giacinto B, Di Cesare A, Castellano V, Bhambhani Y (2010) Field evaluation of Paralympic athletes in selected sports: implications for aerobic training. Med Sci Sports Exerc 42:1200–1208
8. Gates PE, Campbell IG, George KP (2002) Absence of training-specific cardiac adaptation in paraplegic athletes. Med Sci Sports Exerc 34:1699–1704
9. Leicht CA, Smith PM, Sharpe G, Perret C, Goosey-Tolfrey VL (2010) The effects of a respiratory warm-up on the physical capacity and ventilatory response in paraplegic individuals. Eur J Appl Physiol 110:1291–1298
10. Mueller G, Perret C, Hopman MT (2008) Effects of respiratory muscle endurance training on wheelchair racing performance in athletes with paraplegia: a pilot study. Clin J Sport Med 18:85–88

Disorder of Carbohydrate Metabolism

▶ Diabetes Mellitus, Prevention

Disorders of Fat Metabolism

▶ Lipid Metabolism Disorders

Disturbance of the Heartbeat

▶ Cardiac Arrhythmias

Dizziness Upon Standing

▶ Orthostatic Intolerance

DNA Damage

DNA is under constant siege from a variety of damaging agents. Damage to DNA and the ability of cells to repair that damage has broad health implications, from aging and heritable diseases to cancer.

Dominant Negative

A form of an enzyme that is inactive and also dampens the enzymatic activity of other forms of the enzyme.

DOMS

Delayed onset muscle soreness.

Cross-References

▶ Eccentric Muscle Damage

Dopamine

The neurotransmitter dopamine belongs to the class of catecholamines. It is involved in regulating functions like movement, mood, and attention. Examples for diseases with changes in dopaminergic neurotransmission are Parkinson's disease (loss of dopaminergic neurons) and Schizophrenia (excess of dopamine in the limbic system and dopamine deficit in frontal areas).

Doping

MARIO THEVIS, WILHELM SCHÄNZER
German Sport University Cologne, Institute of Biochemistry – Center for Preventive Doping Research, Cologne, Germany

Synonyms

Drug abuse in sports; Manipulation of performance

Definition

Doping in sports has been defined by the WADA as the "occurrence of one or more anti-doping rule violations" that have been further detailed in the WADC [1]. Those rules include the presence of a prohibited substance or its metabolites or markers in an athlete's bodily specimen, the use or attempted use of a prohibited substance or method, refusal or failing to provide a doping control sample, violation of requirements regarding out-of-competition testing, and athlete's availability including failure to provide whereabouts information, tampering or attempting to tamper with any part of doping control, possession of as well as trafficking in any prohibited substances and methods, and administration or attempted administration of a prohibited substance or method.

Description

Substances and methods of doping have been applied to artificially enhance physical performance presumably since athletes have started competing in sports. Reports from the ancient Olympic Games described specific diets and techniques to improve strength and stamina of sportsmen, and also numerous contemporary competitions have been accompanied by doping scandals, confessions, and adverse analytical findings in sports drug testing. Hence, doping control is an important aspect allowing for clean and fair sports, and WADA-accredited drug testing laboratories currently measure approximately 200,000 doping control samples per year in competition and out-of-competition [2]. These analyses include the search for numerous classes of drugs prohibited in sports such as anabolic agents (group S1, further categorized into exogenous anabolic-androgenic steroids, endogenous anabolic-androgenic steroids, and other anabolic agents); peptide hormones (group S2) such as EPO, hGH, insulin-like growth factor-1 (IGF-1), insulins, etc., and their respective releasing factors; beta-2-agonists (group S3) such as fenoterol and reproterol; hormone antagonists and modulators (group S4), for example, aromatase inhibitors and selective estrogen receptor modulators (SERMs); diuretics and other masking agents (group S5) including for instance furosemide and plasma volume expanders; stimulants (group S6) such as amphetamine, sibutramine, and strychnine; narcotics (group S7) such as morphine and fentanyl; cannabinoids (group S8) including hashish; glucocorticosteroids (group S9); alcohol (group P1); and beta-blockers (group P2) such as atenolol and metoprolol. In addition, methods enabling the enhancement of oxygen transfer (group M1, including for instance blood doping), chemical and physical manipulation (group M2, e.g., urine substitution), and gene doping (group M3) are prohibited. While the application of compounds and use of methods belonging to the categories S1–S5 and M1–M3 are not allowed at any time, S6–S9 and P1–P2 are prohibited in competition only [3].

In order to enable athletes, who suffer from particular diseases, to participate in competitions, therapeutic use exemptions (TUEs) for selected drugs are to be obtained. For instance, the use of insulin is prohibited only for sportsmen demonstrably not suffering from insulin-dependent *diabetes mellitus* (IDDM) but allowed for those who received TUE approval due to the need to substitute the hormone for treating IDDM. This applies also to other substances such as glucocorticosteroids (group S9), selected beta-2-agonists (group S2), etc. if the necessity and route of administration is in accordance with respective regulations [3].

Application

The compliance of athletes with the anti-doping rules is tested by frequent doping control analyses that are conducted in- as well as out-of-competition. Major tools for the detection and identification of drugs are chromatographic-mass spectrometric systems and immunological methods that enable the screening for approximately 500 drugs and agents relevant for doping control purposes [4]. Target analytes are extracted or concentrated from provided bodily specimens and subjected to analytical procedures, which unambiguously prove the presence or absence of banned compounds.

Gas or LCs are commonly interfaced to various mass spectrometric analyzers such as single- or triple-stage quadrupole, ion trap, orbitrap, time of flight or sector field mass spectrometers. By means of chromatography, target compounds are characterized by means of their retention behavior and separated from the vast majority of other analytes present in doping control samples. After elution from the chromatographic system, substances are introduced into the ion source of mass spectrometers (MS). In case of gas chromatography (GC), ionization is commonly accomplished at reduced pressure by means of electron impact (electron ionization, EI) or protonation/deprotonation/adduct formation by means of chemical ionization (CI). Generated ions are subsequently detected by mass analyzers and recorded as spectra that display the mass-to-charge ratios (m/z) versus relative abundances. At 70 eV, EI represents a high energy ionization technique resulting in a considerable degree of fragmentation of analytes, and the dissociation pattern is highly informative enabling the structural characterization and unambiguous identification of target compounds. A typical example of an EI mass spectrum derived from testosterone is presented in Fig. 1.

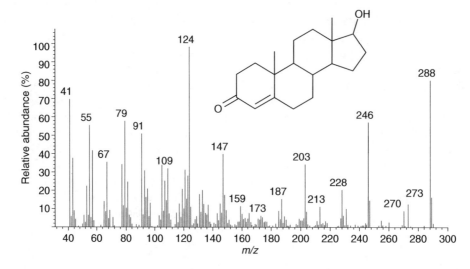

Doping. Fig. 1 EI-mass spectrum of testosterone. The molecular ion is found at *m/z* 288 and informative fragment ions characterizing the analyte are observed for instance at *m/z* 246 and 124

LCs are usually coupled to mass spectrometers at atmospheric pressure using electrospray ionization (ESI), atmospheric pressure chemical or photo ionization (APCI or APPI, respectively) in positive or negative modes. In contrast, ESI, APCI, and APPI are so-called soft ionization techniques that usually yield protonated or deprotonated molecules as well as adduct ions that are subsequently dissociated either by tandem MS (e.g., ion trap or triple-stage quadrupole mass spectrometers) yielding product ion mass spectra that also contain detailed structural information for compound characterization and identification. The advantage of LC-MS(/MS) over GC-MS is the capability to measure heavy- or nonvolatile without the need of derivatization as well as peptides and proteins such as insulin, which has become an invaluable tool for doping control purposes and complements the utility of GC-MS. A product ion mass spectrum of human insulin obtained after collision-induced dissociation of the fivefold charged precursor ion is depicted in Fig. 2.

A special version of GC-MS is gas chromatography/combustion/isotope ratio mass spectrometry (GC/C/IRMS), which allows the distinction of endogenous compounds from chemically derived counterparts. Synthetic testosterone has been frequently misused in sports, and the only currently available option to unambiguously differentiate between the human urinary testosterone or its metabolites and those derived from pharmaceutical preparations is the determination of carbon isotope ratios. Those differ between natural and synthetic steroids in relative compositions of ^{13}C and ^{12}C, which is measured

from carbon dioxide generated by combustion of analytes after GC separation [4].

In addition to mass spectrometric methods, selected immunological assays are employed in doping controls to determine peptide hormones such as EPO, hGH, or human chorionic gonadotrophin (hCG) as well as homologous blood transfusion. The low concentration of intact EPO in urine samples necessitates the use of sensitive methods utilizing monoclonal antibodies to visualize the target protein. In addition, the separation of human urinary EPO from its recombinant counterpart in doping control specimens requires isoelectric focusing (IEF) and/or sodium dodecyl sulfate – polyacrylamide gel electrophoresis (SDS-PAGE). While hCG is also detected in urine samples (males only) using immunoassays, hGH and homologous blood transfusion are revealed only by means of blood sampling. In case of hGH, several isoforms (22, 20, 17, and 5 kDa) circulate in humans while the recombinant analog is composed of the 22 kDa version only. Hence, administration of recombinant hGH results in an impaired ratio of the isoforms, which are determined using two different quantitation assays. Homologous blood transfusion is detected by means of flow cytometry in doping control blood samples utilizing the uniqueness of red blood cell surface antigen patterns. The membranes of erythrocytes bear numerous complex oligosaccharides and rhesus (Rh) polypeptides that compose a virtually unique and identifying set of parameters. The genetically defined combination of at least 45 independent antigens (e.g., C, c, E, e, K, k, Fya, Fyb, Jka, Jkb, etc.) characterizes an individual's erythrocytes and allows the unambiguous

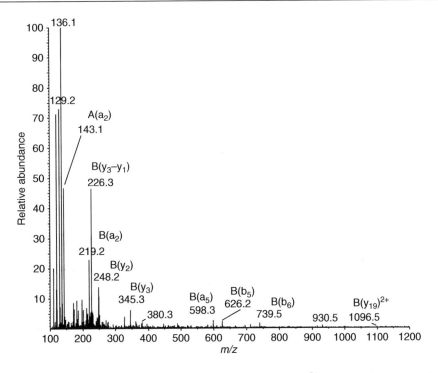

Doping. Fig. 2 ESI-MS/MS spectrum of the fivefold charged precursor ion $[M+5H]^{5+} = 1162.4$ of human insulin. Sequence information is obtained from diagnostic product ions derived from N- and C-termini such as m/z 219 and 226

discrimination of those from a second population, which would be present after homologous blood transfusion [5].

Finally, the attempt of sample manipulation is an issue of doping controls, in particular with regard to urine specimens. Several cases of urine substitution (e.g., by means of catheterization or hidden containers filled with "clean" urine) or confessions of urine adulteration by proteases were reported and demonstrate another dimension of anti-doping rule violations. If urine samples are suspicious for substitution, DNA analysis can be applied for individualization and, thus, verification or falsification of the suspect. The use of proteases to mask the presence of prohibited peptide hormones is detected by abnormal protease activities in urine specimens and subsequent identification of xenobiotic proteases [5].

References

1. World Anti-Doping Agency (2008) The World Anti-Doping Code. 2003. http://www.wada-ama.org/rtecontent/document/code_v3.pdf. (02–14–2008)
2. World Anti-Doping Agency. Laboratory Statistics (2008) http://www.wada-ama.org/rtecontent/document/LABSTATS_2006.pdf (02–15–2008)
3. World Anti-Doping Agency (2008) The 2008 Prohibited List. 2008. http://www.wada-ama.org/rtecontent/document/2008_List_En.pdf (28–11–2007)
4. Thevis M, Schänzer W (2007) Mass spectrometry in sports drug testing: structure characterization and analytical assays. Mass Spectrom Rev 26:79–107
5. Thevis M, Kohler M, Schänzer W (2008) New drugs and methods of doping and manipulation. Drug Discov Today 13:59–66

Double Periodization

Refers to two competitive periods within a year. For example, this may consist of a winter or summer competitive period or an indoor and outdoor competitive phase.

Doxorubicin

A common type of chemotherapy used in the treatment of many cancer types, including breast cancer and lymphoma.

Drafting

To swim, cycle, or run close behind another athlete so as to benefit from the reduction in air pressure created behind the athlete ahead.

Drinking Behaviors During Long Distance Events

▶ Long Distance Running

Drug Abuse in Sports

▶ Doping

Dual Task Balance

Balance during performance of two tasks, one of which involves a challenge to the balance system. The dual/secondary task may be cognitive or motor.

Duchenne Muscular Dystrophy

CHAD D. MARKERT[1], MARTIN K. CHILDERS[2],
ROBERT W. GRANGE[3]
[1]Wake Forest Institute of Regenerative Medicine, Wake Forest University, Winston-Salem, NC, USA
[2]Department of Neurology and Institute for Regenerative Medicine, Wake Forest University, Winston-Salem, NC, USA
[3]Department of Human Nutrition, Foods and Exercise, Virginia Polytechnic Institute and State University, Blacksburg, VA, USA

Synonyms

Neuromuscular disease; X-linked degenerative muscle disease

Definition

Duchenne muscular dystrophy (DMD): A progressive, lethal, X-linked disease of skeletal and cardiac muscle affecting nearly 1 in 3,500 males born each year in the United States. In healthy individuals, muscle damage is repaired by resident muscle progenitor/"stem" cells (satellite cells). However, in DMD, continuous cycles of damage eventually overwhelm the body's capacity for regeneration.

Exercise: A planned, structured, and repetitive physical activity intended to condition the body. A well-rounded training program including aerobic and resistance training, and flexibility exercises, is recommended by the American College of Sports Medicine for healthy adults. The potential for exercise to ameliorate symptoms of degenerative muscle diseases has not been well studied.

Exercise in Duchenne muscular dystrophy: The use of properly prescribed exercise as a palliative treatment to counter the pathophysiologic mechanisms of Duchenne muscular dystrophy.

Pathogenetic Mechanisms

Introduction

Duchenne muscular dystrophy (DMD) results from the absence of the large (427 kD) protein dystrophin and associated proteins in the dystrophin-glycoprotein complex (DGC) at the muscle sarcolemma. The loss of dystrophin is a direct consequence of mutations in the dystrophin gene found on the X-chromosome that yield premature stop codons; these mutations result in expression of non-functional dystrophin protein. The absence of dystrophin leads to the absence of the other DGC proteins. DMD is therefore considered an X-linked degenerative muscle disease that affects boys.

Although the precise pathophysiologic mechanisms are not presently known, five mechanisms have been proposed [1]. The absence of dystrophin is thought to leave muscle cells vulnerable to contractile activity. Nevertheless, patients with this disease would like to use their muscles just as all boys do – for completing routine activities of daily living, for playing, for independence, for physical exercise; indeed, these are some of the reasons we have muscles in the first place. Unfortunately, the scientific literature shows that a consensus does not exist regarding whether exercise improves or worsens DMD. Understanding the five pathophysiological mechanisms might help the DMD research community to design studies to define and refine guidelines for appropriate and inappropriate physical stresses that DMD patients place on their muscles. Herein, we briefly review the five mechanisms, followed by the potential interactions of exercise with each.

The five pathologic mechanisms are: (1) mechanical weakening of the sarcolemma, (2) inappropriate calcium influx, (3) aberrant cell signaling, (4) increased oxidative stress, and (5) recurrent muscle ischemia [1]

Mechanical Weakness of the Sarcolemma

Several lines of evidence, including immunolocalization and physiologic studies of dystrophic muscle in vitro or ex vivo, support the notion that dystrophin stabilizes the membrane (sarcolemma) of muscle cells [1]. Furthermore, in vivo studies of two chronically active muscles that are critical to sustaining life – the diaphragm and heart – show increased sarcolemmal permeability, and thus fragility, in dystrophic mdx mice. So it would be expected that an exercise challenge could exacerbate this effect.

Inappropriate Calcium Influx

Excessive influx of calcium into dystrophic muscle cells may occur either due to the sarcolemmal tearing described above or possibly due to increased permeability of calcium leak channels or stretch-activated channels. In either case, intracellular concentration of Ca^{2+} is increased, with pathologic consequences. Underlying the pathology may be calcium-sensitive proteases or mitochondria-mediated cell death. In the first case, calpains may exaggerate proteolysis of contractile proteins, leading to muscle cell necrosis. In the second, mitochondria, which are sensitive to abnormally high Ca^{2+}, are overloaded, causing muscle cell necrosis.

Aberrant Cell Signaling

Recent evidence indicates that signaling not only within but between cells may be pathologically disrupted as a result of dystrophin deficiency [2]. These data also suggest that the various cells interacting with the muscle progenitor cell niche must be considered. Because a given muscle cell's neighbors are not only other muscle cells but a wide variety of other cell types, study of their effects on signaling cascades offers daunting complexity. The various cells of the muscle progenitor cell niche may be considered based on the tissues in which they reside [2]. For example, microvessels interact with muscle cells, and microvessels are composed of various endothelial cells, perivascular cells, and smooth muscle cells. Similarly, nerves, macrophages, neutrophils, and even extracellular matrix (ECM) interact with differentiated muscle cells and muscle progenitor cells. These interactions are mediated by signaling cascades.

Increased Oxidative Stress

Oxidative stress is the accumulation of destructive reactive oxygen species (ROS), which damage lipids, proteins, and DNA. Whether ROS are produced by muscle cells undergoing crisis, infiltrating inflammatory cells, or both, the outcome is oxidative stress if the ROS are not quenched by the body's antioxidant defenses. The ROS contribute to myofiber injury by damaging lipid-enriched membranes, such as mitochondrial and nuclear membranes, and the sarcolemma itself.

Recurrent Muscle Ischemia

The alpha-adrenergic system mediates constriction of the microvessels that supply striated muscle. During exercise,

a decrease in sympathetic drive in addition to local regulation of vascular tone by metabolites produced by contracting muscles helps to match blood flow to working muscles (i.e., exercise or functional hyperemia). In healthy muscle, one of the local regulators of vascular tone is nitric oxide (NO), the product of neural nitric oxide synthase (nNOS). nNOS is associated with the DGC in healthy muscle. In dystrophic muscle, contracting muscle is supplied by blood vessels that are constricting more than dilating, and muscle ischemia follows. Absence of dystrophin and the DGC is associated with loss of nNOS activity, and so the diminished production of NO is thought to contribute to the muscle ischemia.

Exercise Intervention

Introduction

For each of the five pathologic mechanisms described above, the potential influences of exercise as an intervention are described below. Due to a dearth of guidelines for exercise prescription in DMD, further research studies are warranted. Experimental designs of these studies may benefit from consideration of how the five mechanisms interact with a given exercise regimen and which outcome measures are most informative (Table 1).

Exercise and Sarcolemmal Weakening

Certain forms of increased muscle activity may be beneficial in DMD to improve muscle contractility and energetic efficiency, depending on the intensity of the exercise. This conclusion is supported following a review of several studies in animal models and in human patients. Past animal studies, and more recent work, suggest that voluntary exercise is less damaging to dystrophic muscles than forced exercise. The human studies focused on inspiratory muscle training in DMD patients. Since then, several other studies have shown that the function of respiratory muscles improves with training. Importantly, respiratory muscle training is most effective when initiated in the early stages of DMD, suggesting an age-dependent effect. This set of training studies (e.g., [3]) is particularly relevant because the studies were performed using human patients, not animal models of the disease.

Exercise and Inappropriate Calcium

Systematic studies of exercise effects on expression of calpain, calpastatin, and Ca^{2+} channels in DMD patients or animal models are lacking; however, several lab groups are poised to complete these experiments. Exercise shifts the myosin heavy chain (MHC) signature, with effects on calcium handling, and Western blot experiments are

Duchenne Muscular Dystrophy. Table 1 Potential benefits of appropriate exercise in DMD: representative methods, outcome measures, and specific effects

Pathophysiology	Method to evaluate	Outcome measure	Potential effect of appropriate exercise
Mechanical weakening of the sarcolemma	Evans blue dye injection	Percentage of degenerating fibers	Membrane protection
Inappropriate Ca^{2+} influx	Current clamp, voltage clamp; zymography	Cell/membrane electrical properties; calpain level and activity	Improved Ca^{2+} handling
Aberrant cell signaling	Staining cells for presence of growth factors	Amount of growth factors/cytokines	Activation of compensatory or antagonistic signaling pathways
Increased oxidative stress	Zymography, ferricyanide staining	Glutathione peroxidase, manganese superoxide dismutase expression/activity	Increased mitochondrial antioxidant capacity
Recurrent muscle ischemia	Forearm blood flow, NIR spectroscopy	Muscle oxygenation	Angiogenesis, improved ability to blunt alpha-adrenergic vasoconstriction, increased NOS activity

Methods and outcome measures listed have primarily used animal models, although most are feasible in human studies
Ca^{2+} calcium, *NOS* nitric oxide synthase, *NIR* Near-infrared

routinely completed in exercise biochemistry laboratories. Whether MHC shifts correlate with improved Ca^{2+} handling and with improved functional outcomes in DMD patients is, however, speculative [4].

Exercise and Aberrant Cell Signaling

Exercise may influence the identity of cells in the muscle progenitor cell niche. Exercise can induce shifts in MHC expression and alter the capillary-to-fiber ratio. Excessive accumulation of cells of the immune system, such as neutrophils and macrophages, is seen in histologic sections of DMD muscle; however, it is unclear whether exercise may alter the identity and amount of immune cells in the muscle, or specifically in the muscle progenitor cell niche, and whether this would have a beneficial effect. Recent data correlates the frequency of mesenchymal stromal cells (MSCs) and blood vessel density. Future studies of dystrophic muscle may focus on interactions of exercise, the immune system, MSCs, and functional outcomes. The field of MSCs as therapeutic for DMD is burgeoning, but few studies of exercise effects on MSCs, in health or in disease, have been performed.

Exercise and Increased Oxidative Stress

Exercise appears to elicit an upregulation of mRNA of endogenous antioxidant enzymes. Thus, endogenous antioxidant activity appears sensitive to exercise, while exogenous antioxidants are supplied via diet. Recent evidence

in mdx mice suggests that voluntary exercise and dietary antioxidants independently improve muscle function [5]. Future research should be directed to confirm that antioxidant activity levels remain elevated following a given regimen of physical activity in patients with DMD and that functional benefits follow.

Exercise and Recurrent Muscle Ischemia

Further research is needed to determine whether exercise may ameliorate recurrent muscle ischemia in DMD patients [6]. Exercise may improve tissue oxygenation chronically, but impaired vascular control may mean that exercise has detrimental acute effects – so benefits versus costs must be considered. Dynamic contacts between muscle fibers and capillaries exist, and further studies of the developmental interactions of the muscle progenitor niche with the circulation are warranted [2].

Consequences

If a given intervention, such as exercise, confers a benefit to a patient with DMD, how is the benefit measured? Table 1 summarizes methods and measurements and how they may be applied to each of the five mechanisms of DMD pathophysiology.

Outlook

Future research must present explicit descriptions of physical activity/exercise regimens studied, and investigators in the field should appreciate the differences that exist between animal models of DMD and human patients. The goal is to design experiments that inform, rather than confound, our ability to devise appropriate exercise prescription for DMD patients.

The type of exercise, how frequently it is performed, its intensity, and how much time is spent exercising are all worthy of further study in animal models and DMD patients. Presently, few exercise/physical activity guidelines exist to guide parents and caretakers. However, like the disease itself, physical activity regimens are dynamic, and across the lifespan of a DMD patient, exercise can be adapted as appropriate. For example, breathing exercises may help with the function of respiratory muscles at a young age. Older patients may benefit from stretching exercises, to ameliorate contractures that accompany progression of the disease and transition to a wheelchair. Methodical studies of physical activity will require clear definitions of physical activity, making the term less conceptual and more operational, especially in the face of disease. The defined outcome measures of bench research, whether at the nucleic acid or tissue level, will benefit from corroborative outcome measures of clinical/translational research, focused on function. As methodical studies of exercise in DMD are awaited, parents, healthcare professionals, and patients can use their discretion to tailor exercise.

References

1. Petrof BJ (2002) Molecular pathophysiology of myofiber injury in deficiencies of the dystrophin-glycoprotein complex. Am J Phys Med Rehabil 81(11 Suppl):S162
2. Gopinath SD, Rando TA (2008) Stem cell review series: aging of the skeletal muscle stem cell niche. Aging Cell 7(4):590
3. Topin N et al (2002) Dose-dependent effect of individualized respiratory muscle training in children with Duchenne muscular dystrophy. Neuromuscul Disord 12(6):576
4. Fraysse B et al (2004) The alteration of calcium homeostasis in adult dystrophic mdx muscle fibers is worsened by a chronic exercise in vivo. Neurobiol Dis 17(2):144
5. Call JA et al (2008) Endurance capacity in maturing mdx mice is markedly enhanced by combined voluntary wheel running and green tea extract. J Appl Physiol 105(3):923
6. Lai Y et al (2009) Dystrophins carrying spectrin-like repeats 16 and 17 anchor nNOS to the sarcolemma and enhance exercise performance in a mouse model of muscular dystrophy. J Clin Invest 119(3):624

Dynamic Balance

Maintaining stability or equilibrium during movements such as reaching, turning, and stepping.

Dynorphin

▶ Opioid Peptides, Endogenous

Dyslipidemia

ULF G. BRONAS[1], ARTHUR S. LEON[2], HENRY L. TAYLOR[2]
[1]University of Minnesota, School of Nursing, Minneapolis, MN, USA
[2]Laboratory of Physiological Hygiene and Exercise Science, School of Kinesiology, Minneapolis, MN, USA

Synonyms

Dyslipoproteinemia

Definition

Dyslipidemia is defined as an elevated level of total cholesterol, low-density lipoprotein (LDL) cholesterol, and triglycerides (TG), and reduced levels of high-density lipoprotein (HDL), alone or in combination. It is a major risk factor for coronary heart disease (CHD). Cholesterol and TG are transported through the blood stream as part of lipoproteins. The principal transporter of cholesterol is LDL, which delivers cholesterol to tissue cells via specialized cell receptors; HDL transports cholesterol away from peripheral tissues to the liver for conversion to bile salts and its elimination via the gastrointestinal tract. Triglycerides are primarily transported from the gastrointestinal tract to the blood stream by chylomicrons following a meal and by very low-density lipoprotein (VLDL) formed in the liver in the fasting state.

Characteristics

Dyslipidemia is a highly prevalent major risk factor for coronary heart disease (CHD) in the United States. The supporting evidence is strongest for the role of LDL. LDL infiltration of the linings of coronary and other large – and medium-sized arteries and its subsequent oxidation initiates atherosclerosis, the underlying cause of CHD, as well as of stroke and peripheral arterial disease. Aggressively lowering LDL cholesterol by dietary and pharmacologic interventions, particularly by HMG-coenzyme A reductase inhibitors (so-called statin drugs), has been shown to stop the progression and partially reduce the severity of atherosclerosis, thereby reducing the risk of initial or recurrent CHD clinical events.

Dyslipidemia. Table 1 National Cholesterol Education Panel's classification of total, LDL, and HDL cholesterol and triglyceride concentrations (mg/dl)

Total cholesterol	
<150:	Optimal
<200:	Desirable
200–239:	Borderline high
≥240:	High
LDL cholesterol – primary target of therapy	
<100:	Optimal
100–120:	Near optimal/above optimal
130–159:	Borderline high
160–189:	High
≥190:	Very high
HDL cholesterol	
<50 (for women):	Low
<40 (for men):	Low
≥60:	High
Triglycerides	
<100:	Optimal
<150:	Normal
150–199:	Borderline high
200–499:	High
≥500:	Very high

Values for non-HDL cholesterol are 30 mg/dl higher than the value for LDL-C

To convert mg/dl to international unit mmol/L, divide cholesterol values by 38.7 and triglycerides by 88.54

Conversely, HDL cholesterol levels have been shown in observational epidemiologic studies to be inversely related to risk of CHD. In these studies, each 1 mg/dl decrease in HDL cholesterol was associated with a 2–3% higher risk of CHD. The postulated primary mechanism for its apparent cardioprotective effect is its ability to remove cholesterol deposits from diseased arteries. However, there currently is only limited clinical trial evidence that raising HDL cholesterol levels by either lifestyle and/or pharmacologic interventions reduces risk of CHD.

The evidence that elevated levels of TG (i.e., hypertriglyceridemia) is an independent risk factor for CHD is not as strong as for LDL and HDL cholesterol. This is because TG measurements are subject to greater biological and laboratory variability. Further, hypertriglyceridemia is commonly accompanied by multiple other major risk factors for CHD, particularly the components of the so-called proatherogenic metabolic syndrome. This syndrome consists of a combination of elevated TG with reduced levels of HDL cholesterol, hypertension, elevated blood glucose, obesity, and a sedentary lifestyle.

Table 1 shows the current National Cholesterol Education Panel's classification of fasting blood lipid levels in the fasting state.

Following blood lipid assessment, individuals found to have dyslipidemia should be screened for the presence of cardiovascular disease or diabetes mellitus and for other major risk factors in addition to dyslipidemia, i.e., cigarette smoking, age, family history of CHD events in first-degree relatives, and hypertension. These data can be used to provide a global risk score for probability of future CHD events and to determine the intensity of subsequent risk factor interventions.

Clinical Relevance

Therapeutic lifestyle interventions, concurrent with or preceding pharmacologic management of dyslipidemia, include dietary modification, smoking cessation, weight reduction, and aerobic exercise. A high prevalence of dyslipidemia and the metabolic syndrome is attributed to the Western diet, characterized by an excessive intake of red and processed meat, high-fat milk and dairy products, fried and salty foods, refined grains, and high-calorie sugar-laden desserts and soft drinks. Dietary modification to reduce total, saturated, and trans fats; cholesterol; and excess calories is the cornerstone for lipid management. Weight management, including employing increased physical activity, will have a favorable impact on total and LDL cholesterol as well as all of the components of the metabolic syndrome.

About 30% of all CHD deaths in the United States are attributed to cigarette smoking, and the risk is related to the quantity smoked. Among the multiple mechanisms contributing to this increased risk of CHD is its negative impact on HDL cholesterol. People who discontinue smoking generally have an improvement within as little as 30 days in HDL cholesterol with an average increase of 6–8 mg/dl.

A moderate alcohol intake of one to two drinks or ounces a day is associated in observational studies with a reduced risk of CHD. This is postulated to be in part due to its ability to raise HDL cholesterol levels more than 12%. However, alcohol also raises TG and blood pressure levels, can be addictive, and in excess can contribute to numerous other health problems. Thus, for ethical reasons, nondrinkers should not be encouraged to start using alcohol for prevention of CHD.

Observational studies have consistently reported a strong inverse association between physical activity and physical fitness and risk of CHD. Research has demonstrated multiple plausible protective effects of aerobic PA against CHD at all stages of its development. These

Dyslipidemia. Table 2 Lipid-modifying effects of major types of lipid-regulating drugs

Class	LDL-C	HDL-C	TG
HMG-CoA reductase inhibitors (statins, e.g., atorvastatin)	↓20–63%	↑5–15%	↓10–37%
Bile acid sequestrants (e.g., cholestyramine)	↓15–30%	↑5%	±
Fibric acid derivatives (e.g., gemfibrozil)	↓10–15%	↑5–20%	↓20–50%
Niacin (e.g., sustained release)	↓5–25%	↑15–35%	↓20–50%
Cholesterol absorption inhibitor (ezetimibe)	↓20%	↑5%	±

↑ increase, ↓ decrease, ± variable if any

include beneficial effects on dyslipidemia. The most consistently observed effect of aerobic exercise training on blood lipids is a modest increase in HDL cholesterol of 2–3 mg/dl or about 4–5%. However, there is a great deal of variability in this response, apparently primarily related to genetic factors. Exercise also can reduce TG levels in both the postprandial and fasting state. However, LDL cholesterol levels generally are not significantly reduced by exercise training, unless there is a concomitant weight loss. Most of the studies reporting a favorable effect of exercise on HDL cholesterol consisted of 30–60 min of aerobic forms of exercise, three times per week, with a weekly energy expenditure of 900–2000 kcal. This is equivalent to 15–20 miles per week of brisk walking or jogging.

Generally individuals with moderate or severe dyslipidemia will require drug therapy in addition to lifestyle intervention for its management. Table 2 summarizes the current types of pharmacologic agents and their effects on dyslipidemia components.

Dyslipidemia is a major contributor to risk of CHD. Lifestyle interventions to help manage this condition include diet, weight management, smoking cessation, a moderate alcohol consumption, and regular aerobic exercise. Therapeutic lifestyle intervention should precede drug therapy in milder cases and be included along with drug therapy as adjunctive treatment of this condition. The principal contribution of exercise is a modest raising effect on HDL cholesterol and as a component of a sound weight management program. Attention also needs to be paid to aggressive management of other modifiable risk factors for primary or secondary prevention of CHD.

References

1. Adult Treatment Panel III (2001) Executive summary of the third report of the national cholesterol education program (NCEP). Expert panel on the detection, evaluation, and treatment of high blood cholesterol in adults. JAMA 285:2486–2497
2. Leon AS, Bronas UC (2009) Dyslipedemia and risk of coronary heart disease: Role of lifestyle approaches. Am J Lifestyle Med 3(4):257–273
3. Chiuve SE, McCullough ML, Saclks FM, Rimm EB (2000) Healthy lifestyle factors in the prevention of coronary heart disease among men. Benefits among users and nonusers of lipid-lowering and antihypertensive medications. Circulation 114:160–167
4. Fletcher B, Berra K, Braun L et al (2005) Managing abnormal blood lipids. A collaborative approach. Circulation 112:3184–3209
5. U.S. Department of Agriculture and U.S. Department of Health and Human Services Dietary Guidelines for Americans (2005). www.healtierus.gov/dietary guidelines. Accessed 19 July 2008
6. U.S. Department of Health and Human Services (2009) Your guide to lowering cholesterol with TLC. (Therapeutic Lifestyle Changes). NIH Publication No. 06–5235. Bethesda
7. Varady KA, Jones PJH (2005) Combination diet and exercise interventions for the treatment of dyslipidemia: an effective preliminary strategy to lower cholesterol levels? J Nutr 135:1829–1835
8. Lichenstein AH, Appel LJ, Brands M et al (2006) Diet and lifestyle recommendations revision 2006. A scientific statement from the nutrition committee. Circulation 114:82–96
9. Iestra JA, Kromout D, Van der Schouw YT et al (2005) Effect size of lifestyle and dietary changes on all-cause mortality in coronary artery disease patients. A systematic review. Circulation 112:924–939
10. Danttilo AM, Kris-Etherton PM (1992) Effects of weight reduction on blood lipids and lipoproteins: a meta-analysis. Am J Clin Nutr 56:320328
11. Craig W, Palomaki G, Haddow J (1989) Cigarette smoking and serum lipids and lipoprotein concentrations: analysis of published data. BMJ 298:784–788
12. Durstine SL, Grandjean PW, Cox CA, Thompson PD (2002) Lipids, lipoproteins, and exercise. J Cardiopulm Rehabil 22:389–398
13. Leon AS, Sanchez OA (2001) Response of blood lipids to exercise training alone or combined with dietary intervention. Med Sci Sports Exerc 33(Supple):S502–S515
14. Leon AS, Rice R, Mandel S et al (2001) Blood lipid response to 20 weeks of supervised exercise in a large biracial population: the HERITAGE family study. Metabolism 49:S13–S20
15. Leon AS, Gaskill SE, Rice T et al (2001) Variability in the response of HDL cholesterol to exercise training in the HERITAGE family study. Int J Sports Med 22:1–9

Dyslipoproteinemia

▶ Dyslipidemia
▶ Lipid Metabolism Disorders

Dysmetabolic Syndrome

▶ Metabolic Syndrome

Dysoxia

▶ Hypoxia, Focus Hypoxic Hypoxia

Dyspnea

The word dyspnea comes from the Greek "dys-," difficulty + "pnoia," breathing = difficulty of breathing. Dyspnea may be caused by pulmonary and non-pulmonary reasons. Dyspnea is commonly referred to as shortness of breath. It can be defined as air hunger, or the sensation of having the urge to breathe, that is caused by lack of oxygen in the bloodstream. Dyspnea is the most common symptom of COPD.

Dysregulation of Energy Balance

▶ Obesity: Signals of Energy Balance

Dystrophin

A 427 kDa protein, associated with the DGC, that serves as a critical link between the muscle cytoskeleton and the extracellular matrix. Loss of dystrophin is the cause of Duchenne muscular dystrophy.

Dystrophin-Glycoprotein Complex (DGC)

A set of proteins in muscle cells which spans the sarcolemma, permitting physical linkage between filamentous actin of the intracellular cytoskeleton and merosin of the extracellular matrix. Important components of the DGC include dystrophin, neuronal nitric oxide synthase (nNOS), dystrobrevin, dystroglycan, sarcoglycan-sarcospan, and syntrophin.

Dystrophy

▶ Myopathy

E

E3 Ubiquitin Ligases

Class of enzymes catalyzing the last step in ubiquitination reaction: the transfer of activated ubiquitin to the target protein, forming covalent bond between ubiquitin and lysine of target protein and hydrolyzing ATP.

EAH

▶ Hyponatremia, Exercise Associated

Eccentric Activity

During eccentric activity, the muscle supports a weight as it is lowered; this may be a training weight, or simply the weight of the individual when running downhill. In essence, the muscle is lengthened as it contracts. This places a strain on the contracting muscle that may be seen as delayed muscle soreness and the release of enzymes such as creatine kinase.

Cross-References

▶ Eccentric Muscle Damage

Eccentric Muscle Damage

UWE PROSKE, DAVID L. MORGAN
Department of Physiology, Electrical & Computer Systems Engineering, Monash University, Clayton, VIC, Australia

Synonyms

Plyometric exercise

Definition

Eccentric muscle damage is often associated with DOMS (delayed onset muscle soreness) which is more accurately defined as a symptom of the damage rather than the damage itself. Eccentric exercise is sometimes known as plyometric exercise.

Eccentric muscle damage results from exercise where muscles are used as brakes to slow down a movement. In this process, the muscle is lengthened while generating tension. The forced lengthening leads to damage including areas of disrupted sarcomeres which can be as small as a single sarcomere in a single myofibril as well as larger areas of hyper-contracted myoplasm, known as contraction clots, extending across a single muscle fiber and running along its length for many sarcomeres. Fibers with disrupted sarcomeres, leaking membranes, and no resting membrane potential are removed by macrophages and replaced by new fibers during the subsequent days or weeks. Unaccustomed eccentric exercise is accompanied by other damage indicators, including increased resting tension, shorter rest length, reduced ability to generate force, swelling, and DOMS.

Basic Mechanisms

It is generally agreed that there are two microscopic signs of damage in a muscle immediately after eccentric contractions. These are the presence of disrupted sarcomeres in myofibrils and damage to the excitation–contraction (EC) coupling system. Here, the view is taken that the damage begins with overstretch of sarcomeres since a specific hypothesis exists which is able to account for such a process [3].

It is well known that the descending limb of the sarcomere length–tension curve is a region of potential sarcomere length instability where sarcomere inhomogeneities can develop. During stretch of a contracting muscle fiber, all sarcomeres will be stretched while bearing the same tension, so "weaker" sarcomeres (those with smaller isometric tension capabilities) will stretch more rapidly. If the muscle fiber is on the descending limb of its total length–tension relation (passive plus generated tension, Fig. 1, left panel), these weaker sarcomeres will become progressively longer and weaker, in a vicious circle effect, as they move down the descending limb of the curve. This process continues until such sarcomeres reach the yield point in their

Frank C. Mooren (ed.), *Encyclopedia of Exercise Medicine in Health and Disease*, DOI 10.1007/978-3-540-29807-6,
© Springer-Verlag Berlin Heidelberg 2012

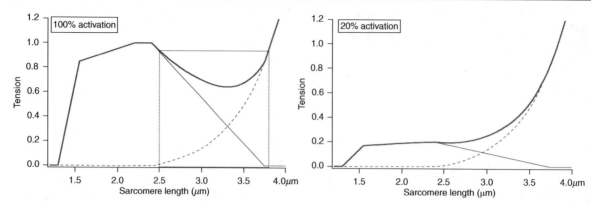

Eccentric Muscle Damage. Fig. 1 Schematic length-tension curves for half-sarcomeres. Total active tension (*thick line*) is the sum of the passive tension (*dashed*) and the tension developed by the cross-bridge array (*thin line*). For 100% activation (*left panel*), this will result in a region where total tension decreases with increasing length, the descending limb. Sarcomeres around 2.5 μm will have the same total isometric tension as sarcomeres at 3.8 μm, beyond filament overlap. If the developed tension is reduced to 20% (*right panel*), there is no descending limb, and hence no instability is predicted. This is likely to happen in experiments using isolated myofibrils. Note that reduced activation also shifts the optimum length for tension generation to the right, contributing further to the loss of a descending limb

force–velocity relation for lengthening. Beyond this point, they will continue to lengthen rapidly, uncontrollably, to the point where tension in passive structures rises (dashed line, Fig. 1) to balance the active tension in adjacent non-lengthened sarcomeres. This usually occurs beyond filament overlap, depending on initial length and the passive length–tension curve. During a lengthening contraction, this process is repeated, iteratively, from the weakest to the next weakest sarcomere and so on. If the muscle is activated submaximally or at low temperature, there may be no inflection in the total length–tension curve, no descending limb and, therefore, no sarcomere instabilities, that is, all sarcomeres become progressively stronger with length (Fig. 1, right-hand panel).

The evidence suggests that overstretched sarcomeres are distributed at random along the middle portion of fibers while sarcomeres in the end regions are typically shorter and stronger. At the end of the stretch, as the muscle relaxes, myofilaments in most overstretched sarcomeres reinterdigitate and are able to resume their normal contractile function. A few fail to do so, perhaps because of incorrect realignment, and they become "disrupted." It is postulated that during repeated eccentric contractions, the number of disrupted sarcomeres grows until a point is reached where the EC coupling machinery becomes damaged. Here, the first sign is the shearing of t-tubules whose torn ends then seal off [5]. That, in turn, leads to inactivation of some sarcomeres, thereby helping to spread the damage. Since sarcomere length instability only occurs on the descending limb of the length–tension

curve, indicators of damage show a strong length dependence, that is, the longer the starting length of the active stretch, the greater the damage.

There are many reports of the structural signs of muscle damage from eccentric contractions. These include sarcomeres out of register, Z-line streaming, regions of overextended sarcomeres or half-sarcomeres, regional disorganization of the myofilaments, and t-tubule damage.

A characteristic structural feature in an area of disruption is an overstretched half-sarcomere facing a half-sarcomere that has shortened to very short lengths. Such a pattern of disruption can be explained as a result of the actions of the two elastic proteins in sarcomeres, titin and desmin [4]. Titin anchors the ends of the thick filaments to the Z-lines; desmin spans the length of the sarcomere from Z-line to Z-line. If the only elastic filament present in the sarcomere was titin, the two half-sarcomeres would operate completely independently of one another, and one half-sarcomere could become overstretched, leaving its partner unaffected. However, the presence of the desmin means that with one half-sarcomere overstretched, this also stretches the desmin, reducing the force on the crossbridge array. Since the force generating capability of the other half-sarcomere remains close to normal, it shortens down to a point where the tension in its titin has fallen to zero and myofilament overlap is somewhere on the ascending limb of its length–tension relation. The structural outcome of all of this is what is observed under the electron microscope, a very short half-sarcomere facing an overstretched half-sarcomere. Ultrastructural features of disruption of the EC coupling machinery include more longitudinal t-tubule segments, changes in disposition of triads, caveolar clusters, and apposition of multiple t-tubule segments with terminal cisternae elements [5].

It has been proposed that the presence of overstretched sarcomeres in muscle fibers increases their series compliance as sarcomeres change from having an active stiffness (many relatively stiff ▶ crossbridges) to only a passive stiffness, represented by the slope of the passive length–tension curve. A consequence of an increase in series compliance is an immediate shift in the muscle's active length–tension relation in the direction of longer muscle lengths [3]. This immediate shift should not be confused with the delayed shift that occurs within a week as part of the adaptation process (see below). Two consequences of the increase in series compliance from damage are a slowing of the rate of rise of active tension and a fall in the twitch: tetanus ratio. Interestingly, the increase in series compliance, expressed as a shift in the muscle's optimum length for contraction, reaches its peak shortly after a series of eccentric contractions and then gradually reverses back to original values over the next 48 h. Our interpretation is that, with time, some of the overstretched sarcomeres contributing to the series compliance are able to gradually re-interdigitate to resume their normal function, while those that are irreversibly damaged may lead myofibrils or even whole fibers to stop functioning altogether, removing their contribution from the overall increase in series compliance.

Immediately after a series of eccentric contractions, there is a rise in ▶ passive tension, as well as a fall in active tension and shift in optimum length. This rise in passive tension is postulated to result from activation of sarcomeres by uncontrolled release of Ca^{2+} in the damage areas, that is, an injury contracture. Subjects who have undergone unaccustomed eccentric exercise become sore next day (DOMS). This is thought to result from high Ca^{2+} levels in damage areas stimulating the release of prostaglandins and tachykinins which trigger an inflammatory response including swelling and soreness. The swelling is from local extravasation, leading to edema. The soreness is the result of sensitization of muscle nociceptors.

Exercise Intervention

One of the most interesting features of damage from eccentric contractions is the rapid training effect. Unaccustomed eccentric exercise at long length causes damage. Repeating the same exercise a week later produces much less damage. Efforts to reveal the source of this acquired protection, using biopsies, have so far been unsuccessful

(for references, see [4]). Any explanation for the damage from eccentric contractions needs to be able to account for the training effect. Explanations based on the elimination of inherent structural defects within sarcomeres, or on increases in muscle strength from training, are not supported by the evidence. In recent years, increases in the optimum length of muscles a week after eccentric exercise have been shown in both animals [2] and humans [1]. If damage is caused by sarcomere length instability when the muscle is stretched to beyond optimum length, then a shift in optimum to longer lengths as a result of training will increase the length at which instability becomes apparent. In other words, it will increase the length to which the muscle must be stretched before damage results. Alternatively, it will decrease the amount of damage at a given length. How could this shift in optimum come about? The most plausible mechanism is an increase in the number of sarcomeres in series in myofibrils. This has previously been shown to be a mechanism that has the required timescale, that is, new sarcomeres can be grown within a few days [2]. The optimum fiber length for peak active tension is a product of the number of sarcomeres and the optimum sarcomere length. Increasing the number of sarcomeres therefore increases the optimum length. This, in turn, means that exercise covering the same length range as before the damage is no longer beyond optimum, so that the sarcomere length distribution remains stable and no damage results.

Some frequently asked questions about the training effect are: Why does the muscle "un-adapt" over time? Why does a period of no eccentric exercise cause the muscle to become vulnerable again? A mechanism based on growing extra sarcomeres provides an obvious explanation. Extra sarcomeres in series add to the mass of the muscle and to the metabolic cost of generating tension but not to the tension generated, which scales with the number of myofibrils in parallel. Shortening velocity at a given load, and hence the available rate of work, does scale with the number of sarcomeres in series, but for postural and slow locomotor tasks, this is not an important consideration. Hence, in the interests of minimizing metabolic cost, it is generally advantageous to reduce the number of sarcomeres in series, unless they are needed to prevent muscle damage from eccentric contractions. So the number of series sarcomeres present in a muscle to protect it against eccentric damage is determined by the length range over which eccentric exercise normally occurs. Hence, the observation that when we walk downstairs one at a time, we don't normally become sore next day, but walking down the same number of stairs two steps at a time leaves us sore next day in our knee extensors.

The sarcomere addition theory also raises the question of whether susceptibility to damage from eccentric contractions can be increased by non-eccentric exercise, namely, high energy consumption concentric exercise. There is at least anecdotal evidence that this is so, namely, cyclists who exercise predominantly concentrically are particularly susceptible to exercise induced damage in knee extensors. Lynn and Morgan [2] have shown the corresponding trend of decreased sarcomere numbers in rats trained to run uphill compared with increased sarcomere numbers in rats trained to run downhill. So eccentric training prevents eccentric damage. Concentric training increases the risk of eccentric damage. Optimum length and series sarcomere counts change in line with the kind of exercise, supporting the explanation given for the damage.

References

1. Brockett C, Morgan DL, Proske U (2001) Human hamstring muscles adapt to damage from eccentric exercise by changing optimum lengths. Med Sci Sports Exerc 33(5):783–790
2. Lynn R, Morgan DL (1994) Decline running produces more sarcomeres in rat vastus intermedius muscle fibers than incline running. J Appl Physiol 77(5):1439–1444
3. Morgan DL (1990) New insights into the behavior of muscle during active lengthening. Biophys J 57:209–221
4. Proske U, Morgan DL (2001) Muscle damage from eccentric exercise: mechanism, mechanical signs, adaptation and clinical applications. J Physiol 537(2):333–345
5. Takekura H, Fujinami N, Nishizawa T, Ogazawara H, Kasuga N (2001) Eccentric exercise-induced morphological changes in the membrane systems involved in excitation-contraction coupling in rat skeletal muscle. J Physiol 533:571–583

Eccentric Strength

Peak force exerted by players while lowering or breaking an overcoming load.

Ecologic Model of Physical Activity

Theoretical model offered by Spence and Lee that describes mechanisms of a complex ecologic system that contribute to physical activity in humans.

Efficiency

The ratio between energy expenditure and work production.

Efficiency of Locomotion

The ratio of mechanical work (per unit distance) to the cost of transport (per unit distance).

Eisenmenger Physiology

Severe pulmonary hypertension in the presence of a reversed central shunt. A congenital heart disease defect causing large left-to-right shunt leads to a progressive, finally irreversible rise in pulmonary vascular resistance. This, in turn, results in reversal of or bidirectional shunt flow with hypoxemia and cyanosis. Pulmonary vascular obstructive disease induced by the high shunt flow is responsible for the progressive rise in pulmonary vascular resistance.

Elastic Strength

Elastic strength or reactive strength is dependent on the stretch-shortening cycle and is the ability to exert maximal force during a high-speed movement.

Electrolyte Disorder

▶ Hyponatremia, Exercise Associated

Electrolytes

TAMARA HEW-BUTLER
Exercise Science School of Health Science, Oakland University, Rochester, MI, USA

Synonyms
Free ions; Mineral salts

Definition
An electrolyte is any substance that will dissolve into free ions and thereby conduct electricity within body fluids, tissues, and cells. Most electrolytes exist as an ionic solution, whereas a ▶ solute is dissolved in a ▶ solvent. Water is

the principle solvent of the human body and constitutes ~60% of a normal individual's total body weight. When solutes dissolve within body water, each solute generally disassociates into positively charged (▶ *cations*) and negatively charged (▶ *anions*) ions. Electrolytes serve mainly to conduct electrical impulses and affect acidity within bodily tissues. Although ions dissociate and migrate freely within a solution, electroneutrality (overall balance between positively and negatively charged particles) generally exists in both the extracellular and intracellular body water compartments under physiological conditions.

Mechanism of Action

Electrolytes play important physiological roles in Exercise Medicine with regard to health, performance, and disease. Cellular processes, metabolism, and fluid homeostasis all require a tightly regulated and specific quantity of positively and negatively charged electrolytes in plasma to continue functioning properly. ▶ *Hormones* singularly or in combination sustain plasma electrolyte concentrations within a normal range by regulating intake (ingestion and absorption in the gastrointestinal tract), distribution (between bodily tissues and compartments), and output (mainly through the kidney) at rest through conditions of extreme physical stress. If the dietary intake of electrolytes is sufficient to accommodate need, health and performance are likely maximized. However, if intake (acute or chronic) and/or output (gastrointestinal, urinary or sweat) is either insufficient or exuberant, pathophysiology or disease will most likely occur.

Five abundant macrominerals – all serving dual physiological roles as electrolytes of particular importance in the field of Sports Medicine – will be highlighted in this section. These highlighted mineral ions include four cations: calcium (Ca^{++}), magnesium (Mg^{++}), potassium (K^+), and sodium (Na^+) plus one common anion of salt: chloride (Cl^-). Collectively, the active and passive movements of these electrolytes play critical roles in: (1) bone metabolism (Ca^{++} and Mg^{++}), (2) muscle contraction (Ca^{++}, K^+, Na^+, Cl^-), (3) nerve conduction (Ca^{++}, Mg^{++}, K^+, and Na^+), and (4) fluid homeostasis (K^+, Na^+, Cl^-). The physiological importance of these highlighted electrolytes within each specific tissue and fluid compartment are briefly touched upon below:

1. *Bone metabolism*: Approximately 99% of calcium [1] and 50% of total body magnesium [2] are stored within and contribute to the inorganic structural integrity of bone. When blood levels of ionized calcium fall below normal, the parathyroid gland is stimulated which facilitates secretion of parathyroid hormone (PTH) into the bloodstream. Parathyroid hormone then stimulates the release of calcium from bone (via mobilization of calcium ions into the extracellular fluid) which re-elevates blood calcium levels back into the normal physiological range. Like calcium, low magnesium levels also stimulate PTH secretion while high magnesium concentrations may suppress PTH secretion. Thus, blood magnesium concentrations affect bone metabolism and blood calcium concentrations by independently modifying the release of parathyroid hormone. Conversely, the thyroid hormone, calcitonin, opposes the actions of PTH and protects against skeletal calcium loss.

2. *Muscle contraction*: In order for a muscle to contract, an ▶ *action potential* must be generated down the muscle membrane, which activates calcium release and triggers myofilament sliding. Local passive influx of Na^+, efflux of K^+, and diffusion of Cl^- are necessary to generate voltage signals which result in muscle contraction. Active transport (requiring ATP) of Na^+ and K^+ across the muscle cell membrane by sodium-potassium ATP-ase pumps is then required to restore the functional resting membrane potential required for subsequent depolarization(s). Local interstitial and intracellular disturbances of Na^+, K^+, and Cl^- (presumably by lactic acid production) are believed to have implications in the generation of muscle fatigue [3].

3. *Nerve conduction*: The transmission of electrical signals throughout the nervous system largely occurs through the selective activation of voltage-gated ion channels which traverse the neuronal cell membrane. Generally speaking, voltage-gated sodium channels generate action potentials lasting less than 1 ms, while calcium-gated channels generate action potentials lasting longer than 100 ms. When specific ion channels – largely selective for Na^+, K^+, or Ca^{++} – are activated, ions flow across the nerve cell membrane down their concentration gradient which alter membrane voltage. This voltage change may lead to an action potential which propagates the transduction of nerve signals. The divalent cation, magnesium, alternatively contributes to nerve conduction by participating in a number of enzymatic reactions which influence the stability of nerve tissue.

4. *Fluid homeostasis*: Plasma concentrations of both sodium ($[Na^+]$) and potassium ($[K^+]$) play critical roles in fluid homeostasis. The sodium cation represents the body's main *extra*cellular solute which cannot passively cross the cell membrane. Similarly, the potassium cation represents the body's main

*intra*cellular solute and can only cross the cell membrane through an active transport process (sodium-potassium ATP-ase pump). Thus, sodium largely exists in the fluids outside the cells, while potassium is largely located within cells. Conversely, body water can flow freely across cell membranes and thereby flows down an ▶ *osmotic gradient* from areas of low solute concentration into areas of high solute concentration. Thus, changes in [Na$^+$] and/or [K$^+$] (and to a lesser degree [Cl-] which is the main anion associated with Na$^+$) profoundly affect fluid homeostasis by altering: the amount of fluid located in various tissue compartments, fluid volume, and secondarily cellular size. The hormones arginine vasopressin (AVP) and aldosterone serve to primarily regulate water and sodium balance, respectively, when fluid balance perturbations occur.

Clinical Use

Electrolytes are essential for maintaining health, ensuring peak performance, and preventing disease. Therefore, it is prudent for exercise specialists to be able to identify: (1) the primary function for each macromineral electrolyte, (2) natural dietary sources for each electrolyte, (3) signs and symptoms of each particular electrolyte deficiency, and (4) signs and symptoms of each particular electrolyte excess. These four clinically relevant sub-points are briefly highlighted below and should be considered when performing comprehensive health and nutritional screenings of athletes.

Calcium (Ca^{++}) is the most abundant mineral in the body.

Function: Primarily (99%) builds and maintains the structural integrity of bone and teeth. Secondarily (1% total body stores) supports muscle contraction, nerve impulse transduction, normal heart rhythm, blood clotting, enzyme function, and hormone secretion.

Dietary Sources: Dairy products, sardines and salmon (with bones), tofu, green vegetables are good natural dietary sources of calcium.

Deficiency: Moderate hypocalcemia generally presents with neurological symptoms such as confusion, memory loss, delirium, depression, and hallucinations which are reversible with restoration of normal blood calcium levels. Critically low blood calcium levels may elicit tingling sensations, muscle spasms and stiffness, seizures, and abnormal heart rhythms.

Excess: Moderate hypercalcemia generally causes gastrointestinal symptoms such as nausea/vomiting, constipation and abdominal discomfort, and loss of appetite but increased thirst. Severe hypercalcemia is life threatening and can cause delirium, hallucinations, coma, arrhythmias, and muscle weakness.

Magnesium (Mg^{++}) is the fourth most abundant mineral in the body. Magnesium deficiency can impair physical performance. However, when body magnesium states are normal, supplemental intake has not been shown to enhance physical fitness or performance.

Function: Most (50%) total body magnesium is stored in bone, while the other 49% is stored in a variety of tissues, participating in more than 300 diverse enzymatic reactions. Less than 1% of total body magnesium actually circulates within the bloodstream but important in a variety of physiological functions relating to energy metabolism, immune, cardiovascular, and nerve system functioning.

Dietary Sources: Green leafy vegetables, beans, peas, and unprocessed grains are good natural dietary sources of magnesium.

Deficiency: Moderate hypomagnesemia can cause vague symptoms such as nausea, vomiting, sleepiness, fatigue, personality changes, muscle spasms, weakness, and loss of appetite. Critically low levels of magnesium may cause seizure activity, particularly in children.

Excess: Moderate hypermagnesemia may cause low blood pressure and difficulty breathing along with generalized weakness. Severe hypermagnesemia may trigger cardiac arrest.

Potassium (K$^+$) is the principle cation found within cells.

Function: Potassium levels are 30 times higher inside than outside of cells. Active transport of potassium across the cell membrane (via sodium-potassium ATP-ase pumps) utilizes 20–40% of resting energy expenditure; underscoring the importance of maintaining constancy of the intracellular to extracellular ratio of potassium. Maintenance of the cell resting membrane potential is necessary for nerve transmission, muscle contraction, and normal heart rhythms. The potassium cation also participates in carbohydrate metabolism (cofactor in the enzyme pyruvate kinase) as well as fluid homeostasis (osmotic equilibrium).

Dietary Sources: Fruits (bananas, oranges, prunes, raisins) and vegetables (potatoes and tomatoes) provide the best natural dietary sources of potassium.

Deficiency: Moderate hypokalemia generally presents with fatigue, muscle weakness, and cramps. Hypokalemia-induced intestinal paralysis may also cause symptoms of bloating, constipation, and abdominal discomfort.

Severe hypokalemia may result in muscle paralysis and fatal cardiac arrhythmias.

Excess: Moderate hyperkalemia generally presents with symptoms such as tingling in the hands and feet plus muscle weakness leading to paralysis. Severe hyperkalemia may also trigger fatal cardiac arrhythmias.

Sodium (Na$^+$) is the principle cation found outside cells (extracellular).

Function: Sodium levels are ten times higher outside the cell than inside the cell and largely contribute to the maintenance of plasma volume and fluid homeostasis. More locally, sodium is a critical electrolyte which contributes to proper nerve and muscle functioning.

Dietary Sources: Table salt, meat, and processed foods constitute the largest source of dietary sodium intake.

Deficiency: Moderate hyponatremia (either from excessive salt loss and/or water retention) may cause neurological symptoms such as confusion and sluggishness and/or muscle cramps. Severe hyponatremia generally produces altered mental status changes and can lead to seizures, coma, pulmonary edema, and death. Athletes who drink more water than their body can excrete during exercise have died from brain swelling (encephalopathy) as a direct result of exercise-associated hyponatremia.

Excess: Moderate hypernatremia stimulates increased sensations of thirst and may be associated with nausea and vomiting. Severe hypernatremia may also produce symptoms of confusion and muscle twitching as well as result in seizures, coma, and death. There have been no known reported deaths directly attributed to exercise-associated *hyper*natremia.

Chloride (Cl$^-$) is the principle anion of sodium, with the combined solute (NaCl) commonly referred to as table salt.

Function: Chloride contributes to acid–base balance, fluid homeostasis, and nerve and muscle functioning.

Primary Dietary Sources: Table salt, meat, and processed foods generally contain an equal amount of chloride to every sodium ion.

Deficiency: Hypochloremia rarely causes symptoms nor likely occurs without additional electrolyte imbalances. Breathing difficulties (hypoventilation) and/or muscle twitching may be signs of hypochloremia, but low blood chloride levels are generally associated with and clinically overshadowed by more life-threatening symptoms associated with low blood sodium levels.

Excess: Hyperchloremia rarely produces symptoms, but may be associated with labored breathing, weakness, and intense thirst in association with other electrolyte abnormalities.

Diagnostics

An electrolyte imbalance can usually be diagnosed by routine blood tests evaluating plasma electrolyte concentrations. The normal ranges for plasma calcium, magnesium, potassium, sodium, and chloride concentrations are detailed in Table 1. In otherwise healthy individuals (i.e., no liver, kidney, gastrointestinal, cardiovascular, or respiratory problems), the primary source of electrolyte loss in exercising athletes occurs via sweating. Sweat electrolyte losses vary widely among individuals and can be dynamically affected by exercise intensity, climate, diet, fitness, and degree of acclimatization. The identified ranges of sweat electrolyte excretion in normal individuals are detailed in the table below [4]. In most cases, if dietary intake and total body stores of electrolytes is sufficient to match losses, supplemental intake is not necessary to prevent disease or enhance performance. The recommended dietary intakes formulated by the National Institutes of Health [1, 2] the Food and Nutrition Board at the Institute of Medicine of the National Academies [5] should be sufficient to accommodate daily losses for healthy individuals participating in recreational physical activity. However, if sweat electrolyte losses are exuberant (high training load, extreme climates, etc.) increased daily macromineral intake may be necessary.

Electrolytes. Table 1 Normal plasma and sweat concentrations as well as recommended daily adequate intake for the five macrominerals

Macromineral/ electrolyte	Normal range in [plasma] (mEq/L)	Typical range in [sweat] (mEq/L)	Recommended daily adequate intake (AI) (mg)	Tolerable upper intake limit (UL) (mg)
[Ca^{++}]	4.3–5.3	0.3–2	1,000 *(25 mEq)*	2,500 *(63 mEq)*
[Mg^{++}]	1.5–2.0	0.2–1.5	Males: 400 *(17 mEq)* Females: 310 *(13 mEq)*	*None established* 350 *gUL supplements*
[K$^+$]	3.5–5.0	3–15	4,700 *(120 mEq)*	*None established*
[Na$^+$]	135–145	10–70	1,500 *(65 mEq)*	2,300 *(100 mEq)*
[Cl$^-$]	98–106	5–60	2,300 *(65 mEq)*	3,500 *(100 mEq)*

References

1. National Institutes of Health Office of Dietary Supplements (2010) Dietary supplement fact sheet: calcium: health professional fact sheet. http://ods.od.nih.gov/factsheets/Calcium_pf.asp. Accessed 5 Aug 2010
2. National Institutes of Health Office of Dietary Supplements (2010) Dietary supplement fact sheet: magnesium. http://ods.od.nih.gov/factsheets/Magnesium_pf.asp. Accessed 9 Aug 2010
3. McKenna MJ, Bangsbo J, Renaud JM (2008) Muscle K^+, Na^+, and Cl^- disturbances and Na^+-K^+ pump inactivation: implications for fatigue. J Appl Physiol 104:288–295
4. Sawka MN, Burke LM, Eichner ER, Maughan RJ, Montain SJ, Stachenfeld NS (2007) American College of Sports Medicine Position Stand: exercise and fluid replacement. Med Sci Sports Exerc 39:377–390
5. National Academy of Sciences, Institute of Medicine, Food and Nutrition Board (2004) Dietary reference intakes for water, potassium, sodium, chloride, and sulfate. National Academies Press, Washington, DC

Electromyography

KEVIN G. KEENAN[1], ROGER M. ENOKA[2]
[1]Neuromechanics Lab, Department of Human Movement Sciences, College of Health Sciences University of Wisconsin-Milwaukee, Milwaukee, WI, USA
[2]Department of Integrative Physiology, University of Colorado, Boulder, CO, USA

Synonyms

Myoelectric signal

Definition

Electromyography is the technique used to record the electrical signals generated by muscle (myo) fibers in response to activation by the nervous system [1]. The electrical signals measured with electromyography correspond to the ▶ field potentials associated with the currents that underlie muscle fiber ▶ action potentials. The recording obtained with this technique is known as an electromyogram (EMG).

Description

A typical EMG obtained during a muscle contraction comprises the summed field potentials due to the activation of many muscle fibers. The number of muscle fibers activated during a muscle contraction depends on the intensity of the contraction and is related to the number of motor neurons that are recruited for the task. A motor neuron and the few hundred muscle fibers it innervates is known as a ▶ motor unit and the nervous system controls muscle force by varying the amount of motor unit activity.

Because there is usually a high fidelity between the generation of an action potential by a motor neuron and its subsequent appearance as muscle fiber action potentials, electromyographic recordings provide information about the activation of muscle by the nervous system. As the amplitude of the signal increases with the number of muscle fibers involved in an action, the EMG signal provides a global measure of muscle activation.

Depending on the geometry and location of the recording electrodes, an EMG can range from a recording of the muscle fiber potentials belonging to a single motor unit to those produced by many motor units. Two common approaches involve recording EMGs with electrodes either on the surface of the skin or inserted into a muscle. The first approach involves attaching a pair of electrodes to the skin, connecting the electrodes to a differential amplifier, and recording the field potentials as the action potentials propagate along many muscle fibers. The subsequent recording, which is known as a surface EMG, comprises waveforms with varying numbers of positive and negative phases that result from the field potentials approaching, passing under, and then traveling away from the electrodes. Because the EMG comprises the sum of these waveforms, the field potential associated with each action potential is distorted by the summation of the overlapping positive and negative phases and the composite signal is referred to as an interference EMG. The second approach involves inserting either fine wires or a needle electrode into a muscle and recording motor unit activity. The selectivity of the intramuscular EMG can be varied greatly by changing the size, location, and geometry of the electrode, and can detect activity from single motor units up to the interference pattern produced by activity in many motor units. In addition to these two common approaches, the advent of multichannel EMG approaches has made it possible to record many single motor unit action potentials concurrently with intramuscular electrodes and to detect single motor unit activity from the surface of the skin.

Several measurements can be used to characterize the interference EMG and thereby infer characteristics of the activation signal sent from the spinal cord [2]. In general, the measurements include quantifying the amplitude and estimating the spectral properties of the interference EMG. Both assessments begin by band-pass filtering the recording in the range of 10–500 Hz to attenuate the contributions from sources other than the muscle of interest. Although filtering can reduce the contributions by movement artifacts and signals generated by radio frequency sources, it does not alter contributions from neighboring muscles, which are referred to as crosstalk. To estimate EMG amplitude, the filtered signal is commonly rectified to obtain the absolute values and averages are calculated over specified intervals (Fig. 1). EMG amplitude is reported in volts or as a percentage of the value obtained during a reference contraction. The standards advocated by the International Society of Electrophysiology and Kinesiology for reporting EMG data can be found at www.isek-online.org/standards_emg.asp.

Many investigators determine the spectral content of the electromyogram. Due to the significant influence of the shape of the recorded field potentials on the distribution of power in the density spectrum, changes in the shapes of the potentials, such as those that can occur during fatiguing contractions, cause the distribution to shift. Aside from the influence of such global effects on the activated muscle fibers, however, a spectral analysis provides limited information about the motor units that are activated during a contraction. The factors that also influence the frequency spectrum include: (1) distortion of the field potentials by the summation of overlapping positive and negative phases; (2) the distribution of the rates at which the motor neurons discharge action potentials; (3) the amount of correlation in the discharge times of the activated motor units to the frequency spectrum; (4) the anatomical properties of the muscle fibers

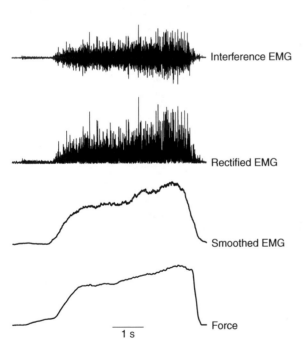

Electromyography. Fig. 1 The interference electromyogram (EMG) from first dorsal interosseus was full-wave rectified and averaged (50 ms smoothing window), and the average EMG signal closely relates to the force produced during an isometric contraction during index finger abduction

(e.g., length, angle of inclination to the surface, and location of the neuromuscular junctions); (5) the distance between the activated muscle fibers and recording electrodes; and (6) rectification. Due to the multiple factors that can influence the frequency spectrum, a spectral analysis of the electromyogram does not provide information about such properties as average discharge rate, changes in the discharge rate of low-threshold motor units, the upper limit of motor unit recruitment, the types of motor units recruited during a contraction, the fiber-type proportions of a muscle, the amount of ▶ motor unit synchronization, fluctuations in muscle force, or the decrease in muscle force during fatiguing contractions [3].

Applications

An EMG signal can provide useful information about the timing and amount of muscle activation and, when normalized, an estimate of the force exerted by the muscle. These features are useful for applications that range from the control of prosthetic devices to the assessment of strategies used by the nervous system to perform various tasks.

Neurorehabilitation

The EMG signal is used as a control signal to drive many types of neurorehabilitation devices, including prosthetic, orthotic, computer-assisted, robotic, exoskeletal, and wheelchair devices. The purpose of this approach is to preserve, improve, or replace neuromotor function. The control signal can be based on information related to the timing, amplitude, or frequency content of the EMG signal. The EMG-derived signal is used to control a mechanical motor to influence neuromotor function, or in combination with electrical stimulation to influence muscle function directly. Although single-channel techniques, such as EMG amplitude and on/off times, can be successful in single muscle systems, the development of realistic neurorehabilitation devices demands the use of multichannel EMG approaches with advanced signal-processing techniques (e.g., pattern-recognition algorithms) to provide realistic control of multidimensional systems.

Biofeedback

There are a number of tools available to provide feedback to individuals about physiological function, including parameters estimated from the surface EMG. Application of the EMG as a biofeedback tool is common in the fields of clinical psychology, physical medicine and rehabilitation, and sport performance. The typical reason for this application is to increase awareness of muscle activity, often with the goal of improving an imbalance due to inappropriate levels of muscle activation. The sources of this imbalance in muscle activity (reviewed in [1]) can include weakness, postural deficit, improper reflex function, chronic pain, and stress. The general approach in many biofeedback applications is to first identify an inappropriate amount of activity in a muscle and then to design a training intervention that will restore normal levels of muscle activation.

Ergonomics

Ergonomics involves the optimization of workplace conditions and job demands to the capabilities of the workers. One important consideration in the design of work environments is the physical load that individuals encounter on a daily basis. Because of the association between EMG amplitude and load, albeit with some limitations, surface EMG can identify and estimate the loads experienced by specific parts of the musculoskeletal system. This is important because internal loads and forces are difficult to measure directly (in contrast to external forces) and can only be estimated by biomechanical analyzes. For example, EMG is routinely used to estimate the amount of muscle involvement in different tasks and to assess the potential etiology of workplace problems, including musculoskeletal disorders, stress and increased muscle tension, pain, and muscle fatigue. This approach is being extended with long-term (>4 h) recordings of EMGs in work environments to assess potential workload problems. As an

example of this approach, Fig. 2 depicts the first hour of a 10-h EMG recording (μEMG; OT Bioelettronica, Torino, IT) from tibialis anterior and biceps brachii, in addition to accelerometry recordings from the hip (GT3x+, Actigraph, Pensacola, FL). The subject performed a battery of simulated activities of daily living (ADLs) in the lab and then went about their normal workday (free-living) while the signals were recorded.

Clinical EMG

Intramuscular and surface EMG signals are used as diagnostic tools for neuromuscular disorders. Needle and fine-wire electrodes, for example, can be inserted into the muscle being investigated to quantify different parameters of the EMG signals. Because of the increased selectivity of this type of EMG recording, details about muscle fiber and motor unit properties can be inferred [4]. The parameters most commonly used in diagnostic EMG, in addition to nerve conduction velocity estimates, include motor unit action potential amplitude and duration, turns, zero-crossings, and the number of phases. Each of these parameters can provide useful information to the skilled clinician in the diagnosis of myopathies and neuropathies. In addition to these invasive approaches, surface EMG is routinely used for the assessment of movement disorders, including tremor, myoclonus, dystonia, dyskinesia, and gait abnormalities.

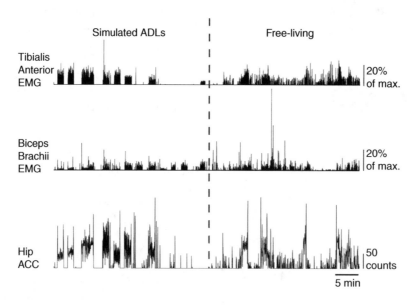

Electromyography. Fig. 2 Surface electromyograms (EMGs) from tibialis anterior and biceps brachii were detected for 10 h (only 1 h shown for clarity) from a subject performing a set of 12 simulated activities of daily living (ADLs) in the lab and a free-living period of typical activities. For comparison, an acceleration signal (ACC) was also detected with a hip worn 3-axis accelerometer and data were converted to the metric of "counts" as routinely done in physical activity assessment to represent the intensity of the activity being performed

The EMG signal is routinely used to estimate neuromuscular activity by associating the parameters estimated from the EMG with the activity of the muscle fibers contributing to the signal. This approach is valid for many applications, though useful information can only be obtained by considering all the different factors that can influence the EMG signal. More advanced methods are currently being developed that involve multichannel EMG and advanced signal-processing techniques to improve the extraction of physiologically relevant information from the EMG signal.

References

1. Merletti R, Parker P (2002) Electromyography: physiology, engineering, and non-invasive applications. Wiley, Hoboken
2. Farina D, Holobar A, Merletti R, Enoka RM (2010) Decoding the neural drive to muscles from the surface electromyogram. Clinical Neurophysiology 121:1616–1623
3. Heckman CJ, Enoka RM (2011) The motor unit. In: Wagner P, Edgerton VR, Baldwin KM (eds) Handbook of physiology: exercise in health and disease. American Physiological Society (in press)
4. Stålberg E (2003) Clinical neurophysiology of disorders of muscle and neuromuscular junction, including fatigue. Elsevier B.V, Amsterdam

Electron Transport Chain

Electron transport chain (also known as respiratory chain) is the biochemical process where electrons are transferred from NADH and $FADH_2$ to oxygen yielding NAD^+, FAD, and water, thus generating large amounts of cellular energy (ATP). This process takes place in the inner mitochondrial membrane and is coupled to oxidative phosphorylation, where ATP is synthesized from ADP and P_i.

Electrophysiologic Study (EPS)

An invasive test in which one or more catheter(s) are passed through the veins (or arteries) from the groin and/or neck into the heart, in order to define the etiology of the arrhythmia, thus enabling how to best treat it.

Cross-References

▶ Implantable Cardioverter Defibrillator

Eleven-a-Side 0–9 Soccer

▶ Soccer

Elite Swimmer

Swimmer that participates in main international competitions (e.g., continental championship, world championships, Olympic Games) on regular basis while young adult.

Elongation

Elongation is measure of deformation and is defined as the displacement of a given reference point:

$$\Delta L = L' - L, \ Unit : [m]$$

Where ΔL the elongation, L is the initial length and L' is the length after stretching.

Encourage

▶ Promotion of and Adherence to Physical Activity

Endocrines

▶ Steroid Hormones

Endothelial Dysfunction

Sebastian Sixt[1], Josef Niebauer[2]
[1]Herz-Zentrum Bad Krozingen, Deparment of Angiology, Bad Krozingen, Germany
[2]University Institute of Sports Medicine, Prevention and Rehabilitation; Institute of Sports Medicine of the State of Salzburg; Sports Medicine of the Olympic Center Salzburg-Rif, Paracelsus Medical University, Salzburg, Austria

Synonyms

Altered modulation of vasomotor tone

Definition

The endothelium is a complex endocrine and paracrine organ that controls secretion of various inflammatory markers aside from vasoregulation, smooth muscle cell proliferation, platelet aggregation, monocyte and leuko-cyte adhesion, and thrombosis all of which are cardinal features in the pathogenesis and progression of atherosclerosis. The health of the vasculature critically depends on normal functioning of the endothelium. Endothelial dysfunction is defined as an imbalance in which the effects of vasoconstrictors outweigh the effects of vasodilators. Endothelial vasodilator dysfunction has been observed in patients with traditional coronary risk factors including hypercholesterolemia, low levels of high-density lipoprotein (HDL) cholesterol, smoking, hypertension, diabetes, and hyperhomocystemia, and further associated with environmental factors including ingestion of a high-fat meal and physical inactivity even in the absence of evidence for atherosclerotic lesions. All over, this suggests that the endothelium is both a target and a mediator of atherosclerosis. Moreover endothelial dysfunction is an independent predictor of atherosclerotic disease progression and coronary event rates.

Mechanisms

The endothelium synthesizes a host of vasoactive substances that induce vascular smooth cell relaxation, the most potent is described to be nitric oxide (NO) [1]. In fact impaired endothelium-dependent vasorelaxation has been primarily attributed to the reduced bioavailability of NO. There is accumulating evidence that the consequences are an increase of acute phase proteins such as fibrinogen and high sensitivity C-reactive protein, which possesses an important prognostic impact. NO not only exerts its well-known vasodilatory and vasoprotective effects but also has anti-inflammatory and anti-thrombotic properties. NO production by endothelial NO synthase (eNOS) is increased in response to shear stress and potent vasodilatory hormones such as acetyl-choline and bradykinin. As mentioned, a reduced vasodilatation response to exogenous acetylcholine (or methacholine) and to reactive hyperemia have been demonstrated in the presence of cardiovascular risk factors. The impairment of endothelium-derived NO action has been explained by means of reduction in eNOS stability by increased reactive oxygen species, elevated vascular superoxid production, and also by impairment of endothelium NADPH oxidase activity. ▶ Hyperglycemia per se can also adversely affect endothelial function, including leukocyte adhesion, intercellular permeability, growth, and the production of vasoactive substances. It was proposed, that insulin resistance and the accompanying defects associated with the ▶ metabolic syndrome are dependent on a defect in the phosphatidylinositol 3-kinase (PI3-K) pathway and thus directly alter

endothelial vasoreactivity by oxygen-derived free radicals. Furthermore, the peroxisome proliferator-activated receptor-γ (PPAR-γ), which is a member of the nuclear receptor superfamily and is activated by ligands regulating gene expression, plays a pivotal role in the pathogenesis of atherosclerosis [2]. PPAR-γ is expressed on the majority of vasculature cells, including endothelial cells. Recently, PPARs were considered the nuclear transcriptional regulators of atherosclerosis.

In the following, approaches to improve endothelial function will be addressed.

Consequences

Physical exercise is an underused and effective treatment strategy in patients with atherosclerosis [1]. It has been shown to improve endothelium-dependent vasodilation in a variety of populations with different cardiovascular risk factors. More recent evidence suggests that ▶ exercise training not only improves vascular function in the exercising musculature but also induces generalized improvement in endothelial function, most likely as a result of shear stress-mediated changes [3]. Furthermore, there is evidence that exercise not only induces improved endothelial function but furthermore attenuates progression and in some patients induces regression of coronary artery disease in normoglycemic patients [4].

As a therapeutic strategy, exercise has been shown to improve endothelial function, most likely due to a direct effect on endothelial NO activity and production. In earlier exercise training studies some investigators proposed that the improvement in endothelial function was secondary to amelioration of the cardiometabolic risk factor profile. There is accumulating evidence that the repeated exposure of the vasculature to increased shear stress, and not so much an attenuation of the cardiometabolic risk factor profile, is the primary physiological stimulus for an increase in NO-synthase upregulation and NO production. These changes may already occur after short periods of exercise training. In agreement, we saw after 4 weeks and after 6 months of supervised, intensive ambulatory ergometer training a significant increase of the flow-mediated dilatation (FMD) of the brachial artery [5]. Effects of physical exercise versus rosiglitazone on endothelial function in coronary artery disease patients with prediabetes [8]. This is also in line with other investigators who found in patients with stable CAD an improved FMD of the brachial artery in a randomized crossover study of 8 weeks of combined aerobic and resistance exercise training. As expected, this improved endothelial vasoreactivity in a conduit artery of a trained and also untrained limb was related to a constitutive upregulation of the NO-synthase expression and secretion. Furthermore, the increase in blood flow led to flow-mediated shear stress on the vessel wall, which further liberates NO from the endothelium. Consistently, an improvement of the endothelial function occurs even in the absence of changes in cardiometabolic profile, which further lends support to the hypothesis of an independent effect of exercise training on the vessel wall [1]. Long- but not short-term multifactorial intervention with focus on exercise training improves coronary endothelial dysfunction in diabetes mellitus type 2 and coronary artery disease [7]. Exercise training, however, does not change the endothelium-independent glycerol-trinitrat (GTN) induced dilatation neither in healthy subjects as reported elsewhere nor in patients with heart failure, diabetes mellitus, and hypertension.

Current guidelines on the management of the individual components of the metabolic syndrome emphasize that lifestyle modification (▶ multifactorial intervention) is a first-line therapy (see also Fig. 1). Additional consumption of a Mediterranean-style diet leads to a modest reduction in body mass and beneficial effects on endothelial dysfunction and vascular inflammatory markers. This intriguing evidence is also supported by the ability of antioxidant vitamins or food antioxidants to improve the transient endothelial dysfunction seen in healthy individuals after consumption of a single high-fat meal.

Adjunctive medical therapy plays also an important role. Thiazolidinediones, for example, bind to the above-mentioned peroxisome proliferator-activated receptor-y (PPAR-y), with high affinity to enhance insulin-mediated glucose transport into adipose tissue and skeletal muscle to control hyperglycemia. Already short-term treatment with Thiazolidinediones has anti-atherogenic propensities.

To address the question whether thiazolidinedione might exert direct effects on the endothelium, some investigators were able to demonstrate in healthy subjects that rosiglitazone significantly increased FMD already on the first day of treatment and it had an even more pronounced effect on day 21 independent of its effects on glucose metabolism and lipid profile. Conclusive with in vitro data thiazolidinedione may directly modulate the endothelium via NO release. In patients with metabolic syndrome the results, however, are conflicting. There are data that thiazolidinedione enhances FMD after 8–16 weeks of treatment, whereas other authors did not find any improvement even after 20 weeks of treatment despite an obvious effect on metabolic parameters. The last data were collected in patients with metabolic syndrome and thus in patients with profound alterations in the metabolic profile. It is also in these patients with an unfavorable metabolic profile and coronary disease in whom values of FMD are lowest. This may explain why baseline

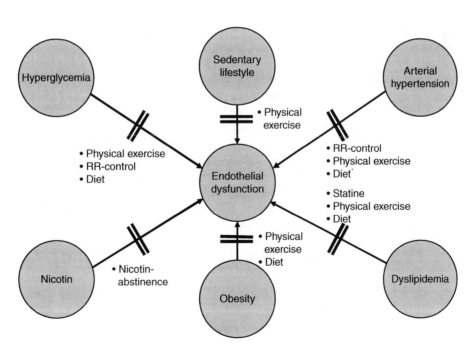

Endothelial Dysfunction. Fig. 1 Multifactorial intervention and endothelial dysfunction. RR = blood pressure

endothelium-dependent FMD of the brachial artery in prediabetic patients with only mild alterations in metabolic parameters and an optimal medical therapy for ▶ dyslipidemia and ▶ arterial hypertension (including statins and ACE-inhibitors) is very similar to that otherwise seen in healthy subjects. Indeed, it has previously been shown that a combination therapy that includes statins and ACE-inhibitors does lead to an improved effect on endothelial function and inflammatory markers.

Further PPAR-γ activators are known to have anti-inflammatory properties and lead to a reduced thrombogenicity. Some investigators found in healthy subjects a rapid and significant reduction of the vascular biomarker hs-CRP within 1 day of an intake of 8 mg rosiglitazone, accompanied by an increase in FMD. Similarly in patients with metabolic syndrome markers of inflammation were reduced and endothelial function was ameliorated. Furthermore, an improvement of the serum CRP was observed after short-term treatment with rosiglitzone, which correlated with a reduction in insulin resistance, despite a significant elevation of the levels of triglyceride and low-density lipoptrotein.

Overall the prognostic value of the endothelial function was demonstrated in the largest population-based study in older adults with or without cardiovascular disease (CVD) (Cardiovascular Health Study) [6]. The authors concluded that brachial FMD is a predictor of future clinical cardiovascular events, even after adjustment for other conventional CVD risk factors; however, brachial FMD added very little to the prognostic accuracy of current traditional cardiovascular risk scores.

Diagnostics

Brachial flow-mediated dilation (FMD) is a validated, noninvasive physiological measure widely used to quantify endothelial function. The measurements need to be taken in subjects in supine position after a pneumatic cuff is positioned immediately distal to the olecranon process to provide forearm ischemia. After 10 min of rest by means of B-mode and Doppler ultrasound baseline diameter and arterial flow velocity are measured in the brachial artery proximal to the antecubital fossa before the blood pressure cuff is inflated on the forearm for 5 min to 50 mmHg above systolic blood pressure. Velocity of blood flow is recorded then for 15 s immediately after cuff release and diameter measurements were made continuously during the 2 min after cuff release.

References

1. Niebauer J, Cooke JP (1996) Cardiovascular effects of exercise: role of endothelial shear stress. J Am Coll Cardiol 28(7):1652–1660
2. Plutzky J (2003) Medicine. PPARs as therapeutic targets: reverse cardiology? Science 302(5644):406–407
3. Green D, Cheetham C, Mavaddat L, Watts K, Best M, Taylor R, O'Driscoll G (2002) Effect of lower limb exercise on forearm vascular function: contribution of nitric oxide. Am J Physiol Heart Circ Physiol 283(3):H899–907
4. Niebauer J, Hambrecht R, Velich T, Hauer K, Marburger C, Kalberer B, Weiss C, von Hodenberg E, Schlierf G, Schuler G, Zimmermann R, Kubler W (1997) Attenuated progression of coronary artery disease after 6 years of multifactorial risk intervention: role of physical exercise. Circulation 96(8):2534–2541
5. Sixt S, Rastan A, Desch S, Sonnabend M, Schmidt A, Schuler G, Niebauer J (2008) Exercise training but not rosiglitazone improves endothelial function in prediabetic patients with coronary disease. Eur J Cardiovasc Prev Rehabil 15(4):473–478
6. Yeboah J, Crouse JR, Hsu FC, Burke GL, Herrington DM (2007) Brachial flow-mediated dilation predicts incident cardiovascular events in older adults: the Cardiovascular Health Study. Circulation 115(18):2390–2397
7. Sixt S, Beer S, Blüher M, Korff N, Peschel T, Sonnabend M, Teupser D, Thiery J, Adams V, Schuler G, Niebauer J (2010) Eur Heart J 31(1):112–119, Epub 2009 Sep 30
8. Desch S, Sonnabend M, Niebauer J, Sixt S, Sareban M, Eitel I, de Waha S, Thiele H, Blüher M, Schuler G (2010) Diabetes Obes Metab 12(9):825–828

Endothelial Function

The endothelium is a unique structure building up the inner layer of the vasculature, thus forming an interface between circulating blood and the various organ systems. In contrast to previous concepts the endothelium is not just a passive interior lining of the blood vessels but a vital dynamic tissue involved in many other active functions, such as secretion and modification of vasoactive substances or participation in the process of contraction and relaxation of vascular smooth muscle.

Endothelial Progenitor Cells

Endothelial progenitor cells are bone marrow–derived (or vascular wall–derived) *cells* that can circulate in the blood and have the ability to differentiate into *endothelial cells*.

Endothelium

Vascular endothelium is the continuous monolayer of specialized cells on the inner surface of blood vessels. These cells are linked to each other by a variety of adhesive structures and control the permeability of the vessel wall and hence exchange between intravascular and interstitial compartments. The endothelial surface has been known to have anticoagulant, anti-inflammatory, and antithrombotic properties. In addition the endothelium plays an active role in vascular homeostasis through its role in controlling vascular tonus via the production of nitric oxide; a powerful vasodilator.

Endurance

JOHN A. HAWLEY[1], MARTIN J. GIBALA[2]
[1]Exercise Metabolism Group, School of Medical Sciences, Health Innovations Research Institute, RMIT University, Bundoora, VIC, Australia
[2]Department of Kinesiology, McMaster University, Hamilton, ON, Canada

Definition

Endurance is the ability of an individual to perform repeated skeletal muscle contractions at a prescribed submaximal power output or speed. The capacity of an organ system to adapt to repeated bouts of physical activity so that their exercise capacity is improved is termed physical training [1]. In this regard, previously healthy, but sedentary individuals can, after only a few weeks of endurance training, exercise comfortably for prolonged periods at intensities that, prior to training, they could sustain for only a few minutes. For many years, it was believed that this increased capacity for endurance was solely the result of training-induced cardiovascular adaptations such as an increase in cardiac output and stroke volume accompanied by an enhanced delivery of oxygen to the working muscles. However, it is now well accepted that the substantial increase in endurance in the trained state is, in large part, due to metabolic consequences of biochemical adaptations in the skeletal muscles rather than to improved delivery of oxygen [2]. This chapter will provide an overview of the adaptation of skeletal muscle to endurance training with reference to both healthy athletic and diseased populations.

The Goals of Endurance Training

The goals of endurance training differ depending on the population being discussed. For the competitive endurance athlete, the goal of endurance training is to increase the ability to sustain the highest average speed of movement or power output for a given distance or time [3]. This, in turn, depends on the rate and efficiency at which chemical energy can be converted into mechanical energy for skeletal muscle contraction. In the case of individuals with pathology or disease states (such as cardiovascular disease, obesity, or type 2 diabetes), the goal of endurance exercise training is to improve health outcomes by attenuating the decline in physiological capacity (such as skeletal muscle insulin resistance) and restoring physiological function. It is now well accepted that regular endurance exercise offers an effective therapeutic intervention to improve insulin action in skeletal muscle in insulin-resistant individuals [4], while epidemiological data have established that physical inactivity increases the incidence of at least 17 unhealthy conditions, almost all of which are chronic diseases or considered risk factors for chronic diseases [5]. Irrespective of the outcome goals and the population, training for enhancement of endurance should aim to induce multiple physiological and metabolic adaptations that enable an individual to (1) increase the rate of energy production from aerobic pathway, (2) maintain tighter metabolic control (i.e., match ATP production with ATP hydrolysis), (3) minimize cellular disturbances, (4) increase economy of motion, and (5) improve the resistance of the working muscles to fatigue during exercise [3].

Components of an Endurance Training Program

The key components of any endurance training program are the volume (duration), intensity, and frequency of exercise sessions. The sum of these inputs can be termed the training stimulus or training impulse that either enhance (fitness) or decrease (fatigue) endurance capacity. Training responses are directly related to the volume of exercise undertaken [6], although there is obviously a maximum duration beyond which additional stimulus does not induce further increases in functional capacity (i.e., increases in mitochondrial and capillary density or enzyme activity). This implies that the control mechanism(s) signaling adaptive responses are eventually titrated by exercise duration [7]. For endurance athletes, the plateau in adaptive response phenomenon is important because many athletes undertake prodigious volumes of training in the belief of a direct relationship between the amount of work performed and subsequent performance enhancement [8]. Of note is that in the case of sedentary, overweight individuals, Houmard et al. [9] showed that an exercise prescription that incorporated approximately 170 min of exercise/week improved insulin sensitivity more substantially than a program utilizing approximately 115 min of exercise/week, regardless of exercise intensity and volume. Accordingly, these workers recommended that total exercise duration should be considered when designing training programs with the intent of improving insulin action.

Independent of exercise volume/duration, it is important to note that in order for major adaptations to occur, the training stimulus must be progressively increased until it exceeds the capacity for endurance exercise in the untrained state. If an endurance training program is well within the capacity of the untrained organism, it will not provide a major adaptive stimulus [2]. In this regard, rats undertaking more intense work bouts for a shorter time induced similar increases in enzyme activity (i.e., cytochrome c) to those observed after more prolonged submaximal exercise training [10]. The paradigm that high-intensity interval training is a time-efficient strategy to increase endurance and skeletal muscle oxidative capacity is discussed subsequently [11].

Mechanisms

Over 40 years ago, Holloszy [12] reported that endurance exercise training induced substantial increases in the mitochondrial content of rats. After 3 months of progressive training during which running speed and duration were gradually increased, submaximal exercise time to exhaustion improved over 600% (from ~30 to ~190 min). In subsequent studies, it was demonstrated that skeletal muscle undergoes many adaptive changes which increase its capacity to oxidize fatty acids and ketones. Underlying these increases in respiratory capacity are marked increases in the levels of many enzymes responsible for the activation, transport, and β-oxidation of long-chain fatty acids as well as the enzymes of the citric acid cycle, components of the respiratory chain involved in the oxidation of NADH and succinate, and mitochondrial coupling factor I (for review [2, 12, 13]). Collectively, the adaptive increase in the capacity to oxidize fatty acids results in a greater reliance on fat oxidation for energy during submaximal work of the same relative intensity in the trained, compared to the untrained state: this adaptation helps to protect against the rapid depletion of endogenous glycogen stores and improves endurance capacity and/or performance.

During the past two decades, considerable progress has been made in our understanding of the cellular and molecular factors regulating fuel metabolism during endurance exercise [14, 15]. Advancements in the fields of exercise biochemistry and cell signaling have elucidated the mechanism(s) by which perturbations in energy status are monitored inside contracting muscle cells, and helped identify target molecules that increase fuel supply to maintain

adenosine triphosphate (ATP) concentration. Exercise produces a multitude of time- and intensity-dependent physiological, biochemical, and molecular changes within skeletal muscle. With the onset of contractile activity, cytosolic and mitochondrial Ca^{2+} concentrations are rapidly increased and, depending on the relative intensity of the exercise, metabolite concentrations change (i.e., increases in adenosine diphosphate concentration and adenosine monophosphate (AMP) concentration, decreases in muscle creatine phosphate and glycogen). These contraction-induced metabolic disturbances activate several key kinases and phosphatases involved in signal transduction. Chief among these are the calcium-dependent signaling pathways that respond to elevated Ca^{2+} concentrations (including Ca^{2+}/calmodulin-dependent kinase, Ca^{2+}-dependent protein kinase, and the Ca^{2+}/calmodulin-dependent phosphatase calcineurin), the 5'-AMP-activated protein kinase (AMPK), several of the mitogen-activated protein kinases, and protein kinase B/Akt [15, 16].

The AMPK has been implicated as a critical signaling protein involved in the regulation of multiple metabolic and growth responses in skeletal muscle in response to endurance exercise. This "fuel-sensing" enzyme is involved in acute exercise-induced events and also plays an obligatory role in adapting skeletal muscles to repeated bouts of exercise during training [3, 16, 17]. The AMPK cascade is turned on by cellular stresses that deplete ATP (and consequently elevate AMP), either by accelerating ATP consumption (e.g., muscle contraction) or by inhibiting ATP production (e.g., hypoxia, ischemia). Once activated, the AMPK cascade switches on catabolic processes both acutely (by phosphorylation of downstream metabolic enzymes such as acetyl coenzyme A carboxylase) and chronically (by effects on gene expression), while concomitantly switching off ATP-consuming processes. Chronic activation of AMPK enhances the protein expression of glucose transporter-4, hexokinase, and several oxidative enzymes, as well as increasing mitochondrial density and muscle glycogen content. Accordingly, many of the chronic endurance training-induced adaptations in skeletal muscle have been proposed to involve AMPK [3, 16, 17]. Results from cross-sectional studies demonstrate that AMPK protein levels are increased in muscle from endurance-trained athletes, while AMPK activation during exercise undertaken at the same relative intensity is blunted in trained compared with untrained individuals [18].

Exercise Response

High-intensity interval training (HIT) refers to repeated sessions of relatively brief, intermittent exercise, often performed with an "all out" effort or at a constant work-load that elicits ≥85% of peak O$_2$ uptake (VO$_2$peak). Depending on the intensity, a single effort may last from a few seconds to up to several minutes, with multiple efforts separated by up to a few minutes of rest or low intensity exercise. While it has long been recognized that "sprint"-type training can increase muscle oxidative capacity [19], recent evidence suggests that many adaptations normally associated with traditional endurance training can be induced faster than previously thought with a surprisingly small volume of HIT. Gibala et al. [20] compared changes in muscle oxidative enzymes and endurance exercise performance after low-volume HIT and high-volume endurance training. The sprint protocol consisted of six sessions of brief, repeated "all out" 30-s cycling efforts, interspersed with a short recovery, over 14 days. The endurance protocol consisted of six sessions of 90–120 min of moderate intensity cycling, with 1–2 days of recovery interspersed between training sessions. As a result, subjects in both groups performed the same number of training sessions on the same days with the same number of recovery days; however, total training time was 2.5 versus 10.5 h, respectively, for the sprint and endurance group, and training volume differed by 90% (~630 versus 6,500 kJ). Muscle biopsy samples obtained from the vastus lateralis before and after training revealed similar increases in muscle oxidative capacity, as reflected by the maximal activity of cytochrome c oxidase (COX) and COX subunits II and IV protein content, as well as similar changes in endurance cycling time trial performance. A subsequent study from the same group [21] showed that 6 weeks of sprint or endurance training produced similar changes in metabolic control during matched-work exercise (e.g., reduced phosphocreatine and glycogen utilization) despite large differences in total exercise volume and training time commitment.

The potency of HIT to elicit rapid changes in muscle oxidative capacity comparable to endurance training is no doubt related to its high level of motor unit recruitment, and the potential to stress type II fibers in particular. As noted, contraction-induced metabolic disturbances in muscle activate several kinases involved signal transduction, which in turn are believed to play a role in promoting specific coactivators involved in mitochondrial biogenesis and metabolism [16]. Given the oxidative phenotype that is rapidly upregulated by HIT [20], it is plausible that metabolic adaptations to this type of exercise could be mediated in part through signaling pathways normally associated with endurance training. Terada et al. [22] showed in rats that a single session of exercise that consisted of either high-intensity swimming (14 × 20 s

intervals while carrying a load equivalent to 14% of body mass, with 10 s of rest between intervals) or low-intensity swimming (2 × 3 h with no load, separated by 45 min of rest) produced similar increases in the protein expression of peroxisome proliferator activated receptor γ coactivator 1α (PGC-1α), the transcriptional coactivator that functions as a regulator of mitochondrial biogenesis. It was recently shown that four 30-s bouts of intense cycling increased phosphorylation of AMPK and p38 MAPK and increased the mRNA expression of PGC-1α [23]. Activation of these specific signaling cascades may therefore explain in part the metabolic remodeling induced by HIT, including mitochondrial biogenesis and an increased capacity for glucose and fatty acid oxidation [24].

Diagnostics

High-intensity interval training is often dismissed outright as unsafe, unpractical, or intolerable for many individuals, but there is growing appreciation of the potential for this type of training to stimulate improvements in health and fitness in a range of populations, including persons with various disease conditions [25, 26]. For example, Tjønna and colleagues [25] recently examined the efficacy of aerobic interval training (AIT) or continuous moderate exercise (CME) to reverse features of the metabolic syndrome. Thirty-two patients with a mean age of 52 years were randomized to equal volumes of either AIT (4 × 10 min at 90% of heart rate maximum, HRM) or CME (continuous exercise at 70% of HRM) or three times a week for 16 weeks, or to a control group. AIT increased maximal aerobic capacity more than CME (35% versus 16%) and was associated with removal of more risk factors that constitute the metabolic syndrome. AIT was also superior to CME in enhancing endothelial function, insulin signaling in fat and skeletal muscle, and the protein content of PGC-1α and maximal rate of sarcoplasmic reticulum Ca2+ uptake in skeletal muscle. These and other findings have important practical implications for exercise training in rehabilitation programs and suggest that high-intensity interval training programs may yield more favorable results than traditional endurance training programs that encompass greater volumes of exercise undertaken at moderate to low intensities.

References

1. Booth FW, Thomason DR (1991) Molecular and cellular adaptation of muscle in response to exercise: perspectives of various models. Physiol Rev 71:541–585
2. Holloszy JO, Coyle EF (1984) Adaptations of skeletal muscle to endurance exercise and their metabolic consequences. J Appl Physiol 56:831–838

3. Hawley JA (2002) Adaptations of skeletal muscle to prolonged, intense endurance training. Clin Exp Pharmacol Physiol 29:218–222

4. Hawley JA (2004) Exercise as a therapeutic intervention for the prevention and treatment of insulin resistance. Diabetes Metab Res Rev 20:383–393

5. Booth FW, Gordon SE, Carlson CJ, Hamilton MT (2000) Waging war on modern chronic diseases: primary prevention through exercise biology. J Appl Physiol 88:774–787

6. Fitts RH, Booth FW, Winder WW, Holloszy JO (1975) Skeletal muscle respiratory capacity, endurance, and glycogen utilization. Am J Physiol 228:1029–1033

7. Booth FW, Watson PA (1985) Control of adaptations in protein levels in response to exercise. Fed Proc 44:2293–2300

8. Hawley JA, Stepto NK (2001) Adaptations to training in endurance cyclists: implications for performance. Sports Med 31:511–520

9. Houmard JA, Tanner CJ, Slentz CA, Duscha BD, McCartney JS, Kraus WE (2004) Effect of the volume and intensity of exercise training on insulin sensitivity. J Appl Physiol 96:101–106

10. Dudley GA, Abraham WM, Terjung RL (1982) Influence of exercise intensity and duration on biochemical adaptations in skeletal muscle. J Appl Physiol 53:844–850

11. Hawley JA (2008) Specificity of training adaptation: time for a rethink? J Physiol 586:1–2

12. Holloszy JO (1967) Biochemical adaptations in muscle. Effects of exercise on mitochondrial oxygen uptake and respiratory enzyme activity in skeletal muscle. J Biol Chem 242:2278–2282

13. Holloszy JO, Rennie MJ, Hickson RC, Conlee RK, Hagberg JM (1977) Physiological consequences of the biochemical adaptations to endurance exercise. Ann N Y Acad Sci 301:440–450

14. Coffey VG, Hawley JA (2006) Training for performance. Insights from molecular biology. Int J Sports Physiol Perform 1:284–292

15. Coffey VG, Hawley JA (2007) The molecular bases of training adaptation. Sports Med 37:737–763

16. Hawley JA, Hargreaves M, Zierath JR (2006) Signalling mechanisms in skeletal muscle: role in substrate selection and muscle adaptation. Essays Biochem 42:1–12

17. Aschenbach WG, Sakamoto K, Goodyear LJ (2004) 5′ adenosine monophosphate-activated protein kinase, metabolism and exercise. Sports Med 34:91–103

18. Nielsen JN, Mustard KJ, Graham DA et al (2003) 5′-AMP-activated protein kinase activity and subunit expression in exercise-trained human skeletal muscle. J Appl Physiol 94:631–641

19. Ross A, Leveritt M (2001) Long-term metabolic and skeletal muscle adaptations to short-sprint training: implications for sprint training and tapering. Sports Med 31:1063–1082

20. Gibala MJ, Little JP, van Essen M, Wilkin GP, Burgomaster KA, Safdar A, Raha S, Tarnopolsky MA (2006) Short-term sprint interval versus traditional endurance training: similar initial adaptations in human skeletal muscle and exercise performance. J Physiol 575:901–911

21. Burgomaster KA, Howarth KR, Phillips SM, Rakobowchuk M, Macdonald MJ, McGee SL, Gibala MJ (2008) Similar metabolic adaptations during exercise after low volume sprint interval and traditional endurance training in humans. J Physiol 586:151–160

22. Terada S, Kawanaka K, Goto M, Shimokawa T, Tabata I (2005) Effects of high-intensity intermittent swimming on PGC-1α protein expression in rat skeletal muscle. Acta Physiol Scand 184:59–65

23. Gibala MJ, McGee SL, Garnham A, Howlett K, Snow R, Hargreaves M (2009) Brief intense interval exercise activates AMPK and p38 MAPK signaling and increases the expression of PGC-1α in human skeletal muscle. J Appl Physiol 106(3):929–934

24. Gibala MJ, McGee SL (2008) Metabolic adaptations to short-term high-intensity interval training: a little pain for a lot of gain? Exerc Sport Sci Rev 36:58–63

25. Tjønna AE, Lee SJ, Rognmo Ø, Stølen TO, Bye A, Haram PM, Loennechen JP, Al-Share QY, Skogvoll E, Slørdahl SA, Kemi OJ, Najjar SM, Wisløff U (2008) Aerobic interval training versus continuous moderate exercise as a treatment for the metabolic syndrome: a pilot study. Circulation 22:346–354

26. Wisløff U, Støylen A, Loennechen JP, Bruvold M, Rognmo Ø, Haram PM, Tjønna AE, Helgerud J, Slørdahl SA, Lee SJ, Videm V, Bye A, Smith GL, Najjar SM, Ellingsen Ø, Skjaerpe T (2007) Superior cardiovascular effect of aerobic interval training versus moderate continuous training in heart failure patients: a randomized study. Circulation 115:3086–3094

Endurance Capacity

A concrete measure of maximal ability for endurance performance, usually determined by a maximal oxygen uptake test.

Endurance Training

KATHRYN H. MYBURGH

Department Physiological Sciences, Fellow of the American College of Sports Medicine, Stellenbosch University, Stellenbosch, South Africa

Synonyms

Aerobic training; Continuous submaximal training; High-intensity submaximal interval training; Oxidative capacity training; Physical Training

Definition

Endurance training consists of multiple bouts of purposeful exercise training with intensity and duration that requires increased demands on aerobic energy provision. The intended result of a program of endurance training may be to enhance endurance capacity, to improve fatigue resistance during exercise, to exercise at the same workload with lesser disturbance in homeostasis or positive modification of disease or risk of developing disease.

Characteristics

Endurance training can take on many forms. The design of an endurance training program will depend on the goals of the individual and will vary (as all training does) in intensity and duration of the workloads during each session, as well as the total duration and the frequency of sessions. As workloads increase, the duration of the bout will decrease until it is necessary to change a continuous session into an interval training session. Even intervals at maximal intensity lasting only 30 s require energy provision by the aerobic system during the work and the rest phases. Such disturbances in homeostasis activate mechanisms for physiological coping and adaptation. Some adaptations may occur within one or very few sessions, but most will require at least 3–12 weeks of consistent training. Since detraining can set in rapidly, long-term health benefits rely on months, sometimes years, of regular participation in endurance training.

Participants in endurance training will usually fit into one of the following three categories:

1. Athletes participating in a wide variety of sports where performance is enhanced by endurance training. These sports are not only those characterized by long duration of continuous exercise at submaximal exercise intensities. Here one can include elite and subelite athletes, as well as individuals participating seriously in competition and training with the intention of improving their performance or maintaining their performance despite increasing age and many daily commitments other than training.
2. Generally healthy individuals undertaking endurance training as a modality for health maintenance or improvement of health status.
3. Patients whose exercise capacity is compromised, but who can improve their functional capacity and health status within the constraints of their disease by undertaking purposeful, usually supervised, training that includes endurance training. In some instances, the endurance training may impact positively on the specific disease status, or progression of the disease.

Design of Endurance Training Programs

1. At present, scientists are still trying to understand how to translate research results into training advice for elite athletes. It is clear that high-intensity training interventions in subelite endurance athletes can improve endurance performance, particularly with intervals lasting 2–5 min at intensities from ~80% to 95% of maximum workload. However, elite athletes spend a substantial portion of their training time in lower intensity zones [1]. More research is required to elucidate clearly the adaptations more responsive to greater volume vs. greater intensity of endurance training, so that evidence-based training prescription can be tailored for sport-specific and event-specific

requirements. Using fiber type adaptation as example, it is well known that endurance training causes a transformation of type IIX to type IIA fibers. However, a proportion of fibers remain as hybrids of these two fast twitch fiber types if training volume is not too high. Increasing running training volume above 70 km/week has been associated with a decrease in the more powerful hybrid fibers in favor of the more oxidative, fully converted type IIA fibers [2]. Therefore, the design of endurance training programs for elite athletes must be tailored relative to the importance of muscle power output vs. the duration of effort.
2. In untrained individuals or individuals starting to increase their volume of endurance training, a training intensity of 50–60% is sufficient to elicit improvements in endurance performance if training frequency is ~5 times per week. The duration of sessions should slowly increase to ~45 min. If the primary goal of endurance training is not related to improving performance, but rather health maintenance, 150 min per week of moderate intensity may be sufficient, although a greater volume would be required if body fat loss was a goal. These general recommendations on endurance training load are also applicable for prevention of chronic disease. Practical advice suggests that moderate-intensity endurance training should elevate heart rate significantly, whereas increasingly elevated breathing frequency is considered a sign of higher intensity that can be sustained for a shorter duration. The volume and intensity of endurance training required to prevent chronic disease may in future be influenced by a better knowledge of the interaction among family history (genetic background), risk profiles (current), and the extent of physiological adaptation required to successfully reduce either morbidity or mortality or both. At present, the recommendation is that the higher the dose of endurance activity, the greater the benefit for prevention of chronic diseases, especially those exacerbated by inactivity [3].
3. Endurance training was first described as a rehabilitation modality following cardiovascular events, due to the well-known resultant improvements in cardiac function and blood lipid profile. On one end of the scale of cardiac function, endurance athletes have greatly adapted myocardium with increased left ventricular mechanical function and compliance. At the other end, it is now accepted that endurance training can safely and effectively be prescribed for patients with chronic heart failure [4]. In patient populations, the design of endurance training

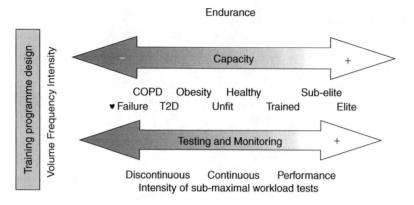

Endurance Training. Fig. 1 Endurance training can be prescribed for individuals anywhere on the continuum of endurance capacity phenotypes. Although testing and monitoring may differ, program design considers the same elements of volume, intensity, and frequency

programs could include only submaximal continuous exercise, whilst others rely on intervals with somewhat higher intensity, or a combination. If interval training is used, both the work intensity and the rest intervals must be planned.

Planning an endurance training program is usually preceded by assessment of current endurance capacity and followed (in many cases) by monitoring of improvements in endurance performance. However, the principles of program design (volume, frequency, and intensity) are consistently considered in all groups (see Fig. 1).

Measurements/Diagnostics

Purposeful, regular endurance training will result in physiological alterations at many levels: genes, proteins, cells, tissue, and organ changes summate to improve whole body performance.

Testing and Monitoring Endurance Capacity

Endurance capacity has typically been measured during incremental exercise to exhaustion with workloads increasing every 30 s up to every 180 s. Both submaximal and maximal parameters are considered as indicators of endurance capacity. But the exercise test and parameters of greatest interest will vary depending on which group is tested.

1. Most elite endurance athletes have already achieved an extremely high maximal rate of oxygen consumption (VO_2max) and their endurance capacity improvements in response to training are better determined by other tests such as: all-out time trials of a distance appropriate for the athlete's competition or training phase; number of intervals at a controlled work-to-rest

ratio that can be completed before exhaustion; duration that fatigue can be resisted at a set relative workload (% of peak, usually of intensity close to or at VO_2max); physiological responses to absolute submaximal workloads (set workload and duration) and finally, the ability to return to the resting state after a set quantity and intensity of work. When the changes expected are small, as would be the case in already well-trained athletes, it is important to note that the validity of changes in these parameters depends on the athlete's familiarity with the test and the day-to-day biological variation that is typical of the specific population and test.

2. There is substantial inter-individual variation in the response of VO_2max to a similar endurance training program. Perhaps more important than absolute improvements is how laboratory testing might be used for training prescription. Exercise tests can be used to determine three or four categories of workload: below the first lactate breakpoint in incremental tests, between this point and the point that steady state exercise can be maintained for long durations; workloads inducing drifts in physiological variables within 10–20 min; and workloads inducing rapid fatigue. Representative heart rates are used for training program design. Changes in these parameters are useful to monitor improvements, but also to adjust the training as the capacity improves.

3. In individuals suffering from chronic disease, endurance capacity may initially be very low, but any improvement will allow for a greater volume and intensity of further endurance training. The importance of this point is that the improvements in health

status are dose-dependent. Improvements in exercise capacity should translate into improvements in ability to perform activities of daily living, which should therefore also be assessed.

Physiological Parameters Improved by Endurance Training

Some of the adaptations to endurance training are measurable during well-designed exercise tests, whilst others are apparent even at rest. Since increased endurance capacity is so closely related to oxygen flux, the most well-known adaptations to endurance training in all populations are related to the various systems involved: decreased submaximal minute ventilation (mainly due to decreased breathing frequency), decreased resting and submaximal heart rate (improved cardiac contractility and positive left ventricular morphology), less reduction of arterial oxygen saturation at maximum aerobic workload and increased arteriovenous oxygen difference across the working muscle bed (efficiency of gas transfer and increased peripheral capillarization), and greater oxidative enzyme activity (increased mitochondrial volume).

For each of the groups discussed above, a few research problems and recent interesting findings will be mentioned.

1. Much research on the effects of endurance training on muscle and metabolic adaptation is done in subelite athletes, and it is unclear if results are directly applicable to elite athletes. Statistical analyses of experimental results may not highlight which changes are significant to elite athletes where very small margins of improvement may clinch victory. This remains a problem when the nature of the experiment requires invasive sample collection or multiple exhaustion-inducing tests that could interfere with training. Nonetheless, experimental evidence should influence the principles on which endurance training programs are based. The tools of molecular biology indicate clearly that the intramuscular signaling proteins respond rapidly to exercise and ultimately influence gene expression and protein production in two phases: early responses and later secondary responses. It is currently clear that the acute responses of the signaling networks differ between untrained and well-trained subjects. Of importance is also how quickly the response to a particular type of training session is no longer apparent, because ultimately, the cumulative response will result in significant changes.

2. In healthy noncompetitive adult exercisers, the main benefit of regular endurance training is related to reduced chronic disease morbidity and mortality. Since several chronic diseases of lifestyle are associated with obesity, there is a tendency to relate benefits of endurance exercise to reductions in body fat. However, independent effects of moderate-intensity endurance training include improvements in: autonomic cardiovascular regulation (improving control of blood pressure and regular heart rate), reduced reactivity of platelets and enhanced breakdown of fibrin (positively modifying the risk of thrombotic events), and an increase in insulin-sensitive glucose transporter isoform in skeletal muscle (improving blood glucose clearance). Maintaining the motivation to train could rely on more concrete observations of improved endurance capacity itself. In healthy individuals, gradual improvements in VO_2max of 10–20% can be expected over the first 12 months of an endurance training program. However, reduction in resting and submaximal heart rates plateaus earlier within 6 and 3 months, respectively [5].

3. In patient populations, some of the well-known specific adaptations to endurance training include lowered blood pressure in patients with hypertension, lower fasting triglycerides, and higher high density lipoprotein cholesterol in patients with dyslipidemia and improved insulin sensitivity in patients with type II diabetes (T2D). Current research results are beginning to elucidate many additional physiological markers that are adapted by endurance training and their beneficial implications, for example, reduced C-reactive protein in patients with impaired glucose tolerance indicating reduced chronic inflammation which is important for reducing atherosclerosis, normalization of plasma adiponectin in patients with T2D indicating an improved endogenous anti-inflammatory profile, and improved work capacity for respiratory effort in patients with chronic obstructive pulmonary disease. In summary, perhaps one of the greatest benefits of improved endurance capacity is greater quality of life, and this is particularly relevant in diseases where quality of life is significantly reduced, such as in fibromyalgia where endurance training reduces some of the symptoms.

Cross-References

▶ Chronic Obstructive Pulmonary Disease

▶ Diabetes Mellitus, Sports Therapy

References

1. Esteve-Lanao J, San Juan AF, Earnest CP, Foster C, Lucia A (2005) How do endurance runners actually train? Relationship with competition performance. Med Sci Sports Exerc 37(3):496–504
2. Kohn TA, Essen-Gustavsson B, Myburgh KH (2007) Exercise pattern influences skeletal muscle hybrid fibers of runners and non-runners. Med Sci Sports Exerc 39(11):1977–1984

3. Haskell WL, Lee IM, Pate RR, Powell KE, Blair SN, Franklin BA, Macera CA, Heath GW, Thompson PD, Bauman A (2007) Physical activity and public health: updated recommendation for adults from the American college of sports medicine and the American heart association. Med Sci Sports Exerc 39(8):1423–1434

4. Meyer T, Kindermann M, Kindermann W (2004) Exercise programmes for patients with chronic heart failure. Sports Med 34(14):939–954

5. Scharhag-Rosenberger F, Meyer T, Walitzek S, Kindermann W (2009) Time course of changes in endurance capacity: a 1-yr training study. Med Sci Sports Exerc 41(5):1130–1137

Energetics

A branch of physiology dedicated to the study of the flow, transformation, and expenditure of different energy sources in a biological system.

Energy

In the nutrition field, the term "energy" refers to "kilocalorie (kcal)," or "Calorie." Energy is required by the body and is obtained from the macronutrients (carbohydrate, fat and protein). Within the body, energy is produced as adenosine triphosphate (ATP).

Energy Balance

The state in which the amount of stored energy (mainly body fat) of an organism is stable due to a matching of energy intake and energy expenditure over some period of time. Energy balance is achieved via the convergence of a multitude of peripheral signals on hypothalamic circuits that modulate both feeding behavior and energy expenditure.

Energy Consumption

▶ Energy Expenditure

Energy Cost of Locomotion

The energy expended to cover one unit of distance (the cost of transport).

Energy Cost of Running

Energy cost of running represents the energy required for running at a given submaximal speed. It is determined by several factors including training, environment, physiology, biomechanics, and anthropometry.

Energy Demands

The costs required to perform biological and physical work, from a cellular to whole-body levels.

Energy Expenditure

C. Capelli, P. Zamparo
Department of Neurological, Neuropsychological, Morphological and Movement Sciences, School of Exercise and Sport Sciences, University of Verona, Verona, Italy

Synonyms
Energy consumption; Metabolic expenditure

Definitions
Body weight remains constant if the amount of energy introduced with the nutrients (carbohydrates, lipids, and proteins) is equally matched by the energy spent. Total energy expenditure (TEE) is the sum of the ▶ resting metabolic rate (RMR), of the diet induced thermogenesis (*DIT*, i.e., the increment in energy consumption following the ingestion of nutrients) and of the ▶ physical activity energy expenditure (PAEE). If *TEE* is evaluated per day, it is defined as ▶ daily energy expenditure (DEE).

▶ Basal metabolic rate (BMR) is an entity different from *RMR*, as it is a clinical definition for metabolism measured under strictly standardized conditions. BMR, expressed in kilocalories per hour per square meter of body surface, is less than RMR and quantifies the minimal amount of energy sufficient to preserve the basic vital functions of the subject. It decreases with age, it is higher in male than in female, and it is also influenced by several factors such as race, climate, eating habits, and living style.

Characteristics
All the metabolic energy produced by a given subject *via* the energetic transformations is converted into heat.

Therefore, it can be determined measuring the heat produced and exchanged with the environment.

▶ Direct calorimetry quantifies the amount of heat produced by the subject. With this method, we measure in a human calorimeter the increase in temperature of the water or assess the state transitions that water and ice undergo consequently. The direct calorimeter of Atwater and Benedict is usually utilized to this aim. The water circulating in a heat exchanger installed inside the thermically insulated calorimeter where the subject is located absorbs the heat produced. The quantity of heat produced is calculated by measuring the increase of the water temperature flowing through the heat exchanger knowing the specific heat of the water. Additional information for a precise calculation of heat production are the specific heat of the objects inside the chamber and the latent heat of vapor production (measured form the amount of water vapor extracted from the expired air).

With the ▶ indirect calorimetry the energy is measured by assessing the volume of O_2 and CO_2 exchanged by our body. This method is based on the thermochemistry of the oxidative processes in vivo. The amount of metabolic energy produced when our body takes up a liter of O_2 (▶ metabolic equivalent of O_2) depends on the oxidized substrate. For instance, when carbohydrates are utilized, it amounts to 5.046 kcal·l^{-1}; when lipids are oxidized it equals to 4.578 kcal·l^{-1}. For proteins, it amounts to 4.48 kcal·l^{-1}. The ratio of the produced CO_2 ($\dot{V}CO_2$) to the consumed O_2 ($\dot{V}O_2$) (i.e., the ▶ respiratory quotient QR) is different for each of the nutrients depending on their chemical structure: for carbohydrates RQ is equal to 1, for lipids 0.7 and for proteins 0.8. Therefore, the value of RQ in vivo, since we usually utilize a mixture of nutrients, may assume any intermediate value between 1 and 0.7. In addition, a RQ of 0.8 may derive from the oxidation only of protein or from the oxidation of lipids and carbohydrates in different proportions. Therefore, the energy equivalent of oxygen depends on RQ. However, before adopting the proper value of the energy equivalent of O_2, also the volumes of O_2 utilized and of CO_2 produced to oxidize proteins must be computed. To this aim, knowing that: (a) 1 g of urinary N_2 corresponds to the oxidation of 6.25 g of protein, (b) the physiological caloric value of protein is 4 kcal/g, (c) the RQ for proteins is 0.8, and (d) the energy equivalent of O_2 for proteins is 4.48 kcal/g; one can calculate: (a) the amount of oxidized proteins, (b) the kcal produced during the oxidative breakdown of proteins, and (c) the $\dot{V}CO_2$ and $\dot{V}O_2$ involved in the process. These two values are subtracted from the measured $\dot{V}CO_2$ and $\dot{V}O_2$ to obtain to the non-proteic RQ that can be finally referred to the correct equivalent energy of O_2 obtained from standard tables or by means of simple numeric manipulations.

In several instances, BMR may also be estimated by using regression equations developed for general or special populations.

To calculate DEE, the day is usually divided in three periods of 8 h each:

1. In the first period the subject is at rest or is sleeping. The energy expenditure is equal to RMR (Resting Metabolic Rate) or slightly lower.
2. In the second period the subject is busy in his/her working and professional activities.
3. In the third period the subject is involved in recreational and domestic physical activities (PAEE).

The energy expenditure related to physical activity (PAEE) may be assessed by using several methods. First, the energy expenditure of several work/recreational activities has been assessed and presented in tables and handbooks. Popular measuring methods include the doubly labeled water, or free-living indirect calorimetry, indirect calorimetry by using portable calorimeters, the use of triaxial or uniaxial accelerometers, the recording of the heart rate, the utilization of validated questionnaires. More recently, instruments that simultaneously record and analyze several physiological signals have been introduced and validated [1]. Each of the proposed methods has pros and cons. In general, however, they should allow the assessment of PAEE over long periods of time in ecological conditions, be safe for the subject and be validated against gold standard methods for measuring EE.

An alternative method that utilizes the technique of differential positioning system (dGPS) for recording movement and speed during locomotion has been proposed. Thanks to portable and cheap devices that implement this tracking technology, the most important factors influencing the economy of popular standardized types of human locomotion (walking, running, cycling), that is, inclination and speed, are measured.

Clinical Relevance

Physical Activity Prescription

Physical inactivity is one of the leading risk factors for global mortality and several international and national agencies (e.g., WHO, ACSM) have proposed guidelines for promoting physical activity to different populations (e.g., males and females, young and elderly) [2]. Any type of physical activity should be tailored to the individual needs and could be prescribed on the basis of the known relationship between the "dose" (intensity and duration of exercise) and the corresponding "response" elicited on the cardio-ventilatory and muscular systems. On these guidelines the intensity of different forms of exercise is defined by categories (e.g., light, moderate, severe, and vigorous) that are characterized by a range of *MET* values (1 *MET* = 3.5 ml·min^{-1}· kg^{-1}) or by a range of absolute or relative (in% of maximum) values of $\dot{V}O_2$ and heart rate.

As an example, an exercise of moderate intensity, in young adult females, is in the range of 5.4–7.5 *METs* [2], corresponding to a $\dot{V}O_2$ of 18.9–26.2 ml·min^{-1}· kg^{-1}; for a subject of 60 kg of body mass, exercising for 30 min, the energy expended would be 34–47 l of oxygen; assuming an energy equivalent of 4.578 kcal·l^{-1} (see above). This corresponds to the consumption of 155–216 kcal.

A certain level of exercise intensity could be accurately prescribed by "utilizing" different forms of "exercise" of which the *EE* is known. Several forms of human locomotion are particularly suited to this aim, as the relationship between speed and metabolic power, and hence cardiopulmonary and metabolic responses, is mediated via the interposition of the so-called ▶ energy cost of locomotion *(C)*. Namely, by knowing *C* and the speed, the corresponding metabolic power ($\dot{E}$) can be calculated (see below). This is of particular importance, since a great fraction of the PAEE during leisure time refers to popular sports and activities like walking, jogging, running, or cycling.

The Energy Cost of Human Locomotion

C of several forms of human locomotion can be calculated as:

$$C = \dot{E}/v \qquad (1)$$

where $\dot{E}$ is the metabolic power (the energy expenditure in the unit of time) and *v* is the speed of progression [3]. If the speed is expressed in m·s^{-1} and $\dot{E}$ in kJ·s^{-1}, *C* results in kJ·m^{-1}: it thus represents the energy expended to cover one unit of distance (the cost of transport) in analogy with the liters of gasoline needed to cover a km for a car: the larger this value, the less economical the car.

C is generally expressed per kilogram of body mass and above resting values (J·m^{-1}·kg^{-1}) because the cost of transport depends, among the others, on the mass of the subject and on his/her RMR (see Definitions).

Values of *C* as a function of *v* are reported in the literature for several forms of locomotion (in land and on water), mainly for cyclic activities such as walking, running, cycling, swimming, rowing, kayaking, skiing, and skating (Fig. 1). In all these forms of locomotion, it is sufficient to measure *v* in order to obtain an accurate estimate of PAEE on the basis of the appropriate *C* versus *v* relationship. This allows prescribe physical activity as

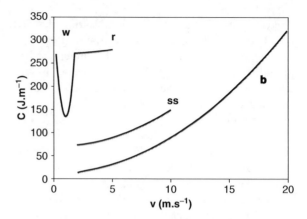

Energy Expenditure. Fig. 1 Net energy cost per unit of distance (*C*, J·m^{-1}) for different forms of human locomotion on land as a function of speed *v* (m·s^{-1}): *w* walking, *r* running, *ss* speed skating (on ice, dropped posture), *b* bicycling (standard racing bike, dropped posture). Data apply to a 70 kg, 175 cm subject at sea level, in calm air and on flat, uniform terrain (Adapted from di Prampero [3])

a scientifically based therapy since the metabolic power elicited by the exercise at stake is known and quantified.

As an example, when walking at the "self selected speed," net energy cost is of about 2 J·m^{-1}·kg^{-1}; in running the energy cost is almost independent of the speed and amounts to about 4 J·m^{-1}·kg^{-1}. Thus, a subject of 70 kg of body mass that covers 1 km by walking at his/her self selected speed (about 1.25 m·s^{-1} in healthy adults) will consume 140 kJ of energy, which correspond to a PAEE of 33.5 kcal (1 kJ = 0.239 kcal); if he covered the same distance by running he would consume 67 kcal.

Besides body mass and RMR, several other factors could affect *C*. This should be taken into account for a proper prescription of PAEE in particular populations of subjects. For sake of simplicity, these factors will be summarized for walking only (the most simple way of human locomotion).

The net energy cost of walking:

- Changes as a function of the speed: *C* is minimum at the self selected speed (see Fig. 1) and increases at slower and faster speeds (at 0.1 and 2 ms^{-1} *C* is of about 4 J·m^{-1}·kg^{-1}).
- Is affected by the slope: *C* is of about 4 and 8 J·m^{-1}·kg^{-1} at 10% and 20% of upward slope and about 1.5 J·m^{-1}·kg^{-1} at 10% downhill.
- Changes as a function of the surface's compliance: *C* is about 10–20% larger than on a blacktop surface on a dirt road or light brush and up to 2–3 times larger than on firm terrain when walking on loose sand or deep snow.

- Increases when the subject has to carry additional masses (such as a knapsack or heavy boots), the more so the more distant to the body center of mass (BCOM) are the added masses.
- Increases with the use of walking aids (such as crutches): in these condition C is up to 2–4 times greater, for any given speed, than in "normal walking."
- Is larger in pathological gait, the more so the more pronounced the spasticity (such as in spastic paresis or cerebral palsy), the loss of flexibility (such in cases of cast immobilization or joint fusion), the level of amputation, and the neural impairment (e.g., in multiple sclerosis and spinal cord injury).

The reader is referred to these reviews for further details on "normal gait" [4] and "pathological gait" [5].

The changes in the energy cost of walking reported above can be understood by knowing that, at any given speed, the mechanical determinants of C are the work per unit distance (W, kJ·m^{-1}) and the efficiency (η):

$$C = W/\eta \qquad (2)$$

It follows that, for any given speed and form of locomotion, C will be lager the lager W and the lower η. For instance, on a incline (upward slope) additional work is required to raise the BCOM so that W (and hence C) is larger than on flat terrain at the same speed; spasticity, on the other hand, is a condition where efficiency is decreased due to the presence of co-contractions and where W is increased, among the others, by the presence of jerky motions and this results in a proportional increase in C.

The relationship between C, W, and η is also useful to understand how locomotory passive tools "work."

As indicated in Fig. 1, compared to walking and running, locomotory tools such as skies, skates, and bicycles allow for a reduction in C; these tools reduce W because they allow for a "gliding phase" thus reducing intra-cyclic variations in v (e.g., reducing the horizontal component of W); in addition, bicycles reduce to a minimum the vertical displacement of BCOM thus reducing the vertical component of W.

The considerations reported above can thus be summarized as follows:

- PAEE can be accurately measured when C of a given form of locomotion is known.
- C depends on the speed and the mode of locomotion.
- C of a given form of locomotion, and at a given speed, depends also on all those factors that can further affect W or η.
- The literature provides all data needed to calculate C in cyclic-type forms of locomotion and in all possible

"conditions" (e.g., sedentary and athletes, males and females; young and elderly; healthy or impaired; flat terrain or incline; firm or compliant surfaces . . .).
- Thus, even if some care is needed to take into account all these variables it is indeed possible to accurately prescribe physical activity to different populations according to their specific needs.

References

1. Brage S, Brage N, Franks PW, Wong MY, Andersen LB, Froberg K, Wareham NJ (2003) Branched equation modelling of simultaneous accelerometry and heart rate monitoring improves estimate of directly measured physical activity energy expenditure. J Appl Physiol 96:343–351
2. American College of Sports Medicine (2009) ACSM guidelines for exercise testing and prescription, VIII editionth edn. Lippincott Williams & Wilkins, Baltimore
3. di Prampero PE (1986) The energy cost of human locomotion on land and in water. Int J Sports Med 7:55–72
4. Saibene F, Minetti AE (2003) Biomechanical and physiological aspects of legged locomotion. Eur J Appl Physiol 88:297–316
5. Waters RL, Mulroy S (1999) The energy expenditure of normal and pathological gait. Gait Posture 9:207–231

Energy Intake

Energy intake, often referred to as food intake, is the integrated consumption of food per unit time. It is often described by the kcals eaten per day, per meal, or per feeding bout Energy Expenditure- Energy expenditure is the amount of energy expended in a given period of time. Energy expenditure includes the energy used to sustain the body (basal metabolic rate) and energy used during physical activity (both exercise and non-exercise activity), as well as energy expended via adaptive thermogenesis.

Cross-References

▶ Athlete's Diet

Energy Metabolism

JIE KANG
Human Performance Laboratory, Department of Health and Exercise Science, The College of New Jersey, Ewing, NJ, USA

Synonyms

Bioenergetics; Energy transformation

Definition

Energy is defined as the ability to produce change and can be measured by the amount of work performed during a given change. In the body, energy is first obtained from energy-containing nutrients in food and, in most circumstances, then being converted as potential energy stored in the body tissues. Via cellular respiration, this potential energy is then converted to the high-energy compound ▶ adenosine triphosphate (ATP) as well as heat. The energy in ATP is used for a variety of biological work, including muscle contraction, synthesizing molecules, and transporting substances.

Basic Mechanisms

ATP: Biologically Usable Energy

ATP is the most important carrier of the energy that is necessary to perform many complex functions. This energy-containing compound stores potential energy extracted from food and can yield such energy to power various biological activities. ATP is the only form of chemical energy that is convertible into other forms of energy used by living cells. As such, ATP is often regarded as energy currency. Fats and carbohydrate are main storage forms of energy in the body. However, energy derived from oxidation of these two fuels does not release suddenly or sufficiently fast enough to meet the energy demand of those activities that are short and explosive. In this context, ATP may be viewed as a temporary reservoir of energy which functions to provide instant energy to the cells whenever it is needed. The body can store a very limited amount of ATP. Most activities are powered by ATP mainly produced through oxidation of carbohydrate and fat. The example that the body relies on its stored ATP is those moments of holding breath during a short sprint or lifting.

Bodily Energy Stores

Energy is stored in the body primarily as fat in the form of ▶ triglycerides, though a much smaller amount is also stored as ▶ glycogen in the muscle and liver. The body must have a steady supply of energy, and some of it comes from ▶ glucose, the simplest form of carbohydrate. As we eat, energy is supplied by the diet. Between meals, the breakdown of stored glycogen and fat help in meeting energy needs. If no food is eaten for more than several hours, the body must shift the way it uses energy to ensure that glucose continues to be available. This is accomplished by increasing the use of stored fat and by mobilizing liver glycogen. The maintenance of blood glucose is of particular importance to the survival and functioning

Energy Metabolism. Table 1 Availability of energy substrates in the human body

Energy substrates		Weight (g)	Energy (kcal)
Carbohydrates	Muscle glycogen	400	1,600
	Liver glycogen	100	400
	Plasma glucose	3	12
	Total	503	2,012
Lipids	Adipose tissue	12,000	108,000
	Intramuscular triglycerides	300	2,700
	Plasma triglycerides	4	36
	Plasma fatty acids	0.4	3.6
	Total	12,304	110,740

Note: These values were estimated based on an average 80-kg man with 15% body fat. 1 g carbohydrate = 4 kcal, 1 g fat = 9 kcal

of the central nervous system. Glycogen stores are limited, and for an 80-kg person, the body contains approximately 500 g or 2,000 kcal of glycogen (Table 1), which in theory could be depleted within several hours of strenuous exercise [3]. As glycogen stores decrease significantly, there will be an increase in protein degradation that produces amino acids. Some amino acids are converted to glucose, while others are directly metabolized for energy. Protein is not stored as an energy fuel in the body. As such, a breakdown of protein for producing glucose and hence energy can result in the loss of muscle and other lean tissues.

Of the three energy-containing nutrients, the fat molecule carries the largest quantities of energy per unit weight. In a well-nourished individual at rest, ▶ catabolism of lipids provides more than 50% of the total energy requirement [5]. Although most cells store small amounts of fat in their cytosol, most of the body's fat is stored in adipose tissue. The potential energy stored in fat molecules for an 80-kg individual can be well over 100,000 kcal (Table 1). Given an energy expenditure of 100 kcal per mile, this amount of energy can fuel an individual to run over 1,100 miles [2]. This contrasts sharply to the limited 2,000 kcal of stored carbohydrate, which could only fuel a 20-mile run. During prolonged energy restriction, substantial amounts of fat are used to provide energy. However, when the supply of glucose is limited such as during starvation or under the diabetic state, fatty acids cannot be completely oxidized, chemical ▶ ketones are produced. Ketones are the by-products produced mainly in the mitochondrial matrix of liver cells when carbohydrates are so scarce that energy must be obtained from breaking down fatty acids. Ketones can be used as an energy source by many tissues. In sustained starvation, even the brain adapts to meet some of its energy needs from utilizing ketones [4].

Exercise Intervention

Bioenergetic Pathways

The amount of ATP the body stores can only sustain maximal exercise for several seconds such as 60-yard sprint, high and long jump, base running, and football play. Consequently, in most sporting events and daily physical activities, ATP is always replenished continuously through a series of chemical reactions involving energy transformation. Three distinctive bioenergetic pathways have been identified to play a role in replenishing ATP and they are: ATP-PCr system, glycolytic system, and oxidative system.

The ATP-PCr system is also known as the phosphagen system because both ATP and PCr contain phosphates. This system serves as the immediate source of energy for regenerating ATP. With some ATP being resynthesized from PCr, this system is able to fuel all-out exercises for approximately 5–10 s such as 100-m sprint. If maximal effort continues beyond 10 s, or more moderate exercise continues for longer periods, ATP replenishment requires energy sources in addition to PCr.

The glycolytic system uses strictly the energy stored in carbohydrate molecules such as glucose or glycogen for replenishing ATP the cell needs. This system is also referred to as ▶ glycolysis, which contains a cascade of chemical reactions, each of which is catalyzed and regulated by a specific enzyme. This system is rather inefficient in terms of how much of the energy stored in a glucose molecule can result in ATP resynthesis. In fact, the amount of ATP produced from anaerobic glycolysis is only 5% of what a glucose molecule is capable of generating. This system, however, has the advantage of replenishing ATP rapidly. With this system, most cells are able to withstand short periods of low oxygen by using anaerobic glycolysis. Consequently, this energy system plays a major role in fueling sporting events in which energy production is near maximal for 30–120 s, such as 200–800 m run.

Most of the energy used daily comes from oxidation of carbohydrate, lipid, and, in rare cases, protein consumed in the diet. Such aerobic production of energy occurs within mitochondria, "the powerhouses of the cell." As mentioned earlier, the glycolytic system captures only a very small portion of the energy stored in a glucose molecule. However, the oxidative system makes possible for the remaining energy to be extracted from the glucose molecule. The oxidative system involves a complex series of chemical reactions that utilize oxygen as part of their respiration

process. Unlike the glycolytic pathway, which only applies to carbohydrate, the oxidative system allows participation of not only carbohydrate, but also lipid and protein. Due to its potential of extracting energy from all three macronutrients, the oxidative pathway produces a majority of energy throughout the day. This energy system is used primarily in sports emphasizing endurance such as distance running ranging from 5 km to the marathon and beyond.

Brooks et al. [1] have attempted to classify athletic activities into one of the three groups: power, speed, and endurance. Such a classification has an advantage of allowing us to identify a predominant energy system for many different athletic activities. According to this classification, intramuscular high-energy phosphate compounds ATP and PCr supply most of energy for power events such as short distance sprinting and weight lifting. For rapid, forceful exercises that last about 1 min or so, muscle depends mainly on glycolytic energy sources. Intense exercise of longer duration (i.e., >2 min) such as middle distance running and swimming requires a greater demand for aerobic energy transferring. Table 2 illustrates energy sources of muscular work for various types of athletic activities.

For most activities energy needed is not provided by simply turning on a single energetic pathway, but rather a mixture of several energy systems operating in a sequential fashion but with considerable overlap. For example, in the transition from rest to moderate intensity exercise, oxygen consumption does not increase instantly to the desirable level. This suggests that energy systems other than oxidative pathway contribute to the overall production of ATP at the beginning of exercise. There is evidence to suggest that at the onset of exercise, the ATP-PCr system is the first bioenergetic pathway being activated, followed by glycolysis, and finally aerobic energy production. However, after a steady state is reached, the body's ATP requirement can be met primarily via aerobic metabolism.

Carbohydrate and Fat Utilization During Exercise

Carbohydrate is often regarded as the most preferable energy source by the body. During intense exercise of sufficient duration, carbohydrates such as muscle glycogen and blood glucose derived from liver ▶ glycogenolysis are the primary energy substrates. Glycogen is a large polymer, comprised of many glucose residues and readily degradable upon the action of enzyme. Glycogen undergoes a process of glycogenolysis that yields free glucose molecules. This glucose can then enter the glycolytic pathway in which energy is transformed. The importance

Energy Metabolism. Table 2 Energy source of muscular work for different types of sporting events

	Power	Speed	Endurance
Event	Shot put	200–800 m run	1,500 m run
	Discus	100–200 swim	10 K
	Weight lifting		400–800 m swim
	High jump		Cross-country
	40 yard dash		Road cycling
	Vertical jump		Marathon
	100 m run		
Duration of event	0–10 s	10 s – 3 min	>3 min
Source of energy	ATP	ATP	Muscle glycogen
	PCr	PCr	Liver glycogen
		Muscle glycogen	lipids
Energy system	Phosphagen	Glycolysis	Oxidative pathway
Rate of process	Very rapid	Rapid	Slower
Oxygen involved	No	No	Yes

of their availability during exercise is demonstrated by the observation that fatigue is often associated with muscle glycogen depletion and/or hypoglycemia. With respect to energy provision, carbohydrates are superior to fat in that (1) they can be used for energy with and without oxygen, (2) they provide energy more rapidly, (3) they must be present in order to use fat, (4) they are the sole source of energy for the central nervous system, and (5) they can generate 6% more energy per unit of oxygen consumed.

Triglycerides represent another major source of energy stored primarily in adipose tissue, although they are also found in muscle tissue. Via ▶ lipolysis, a triglyceride is split to form a glycerol and three fatty acids. These products can then enter metabolic pathways for energy production. Despite the large quantity of lipid available as fuel, the processes of lipid utilization are slow to be activated and proceed at the rates significantly lower than the processes controlling carbohydrate utilization. They also require oxygen, so to maximize fat utilization a low to moderate intensity exercise is recommended. Lipids are important segment of energy substrates used during prolonged exercise or during extreme circumstances such as fasting or starvation when carbohydrate stores decline significantly. To endurance athletes, even small increases in the ability to use lipid as fuel during exercise can help slow muscle glycogen and blood glucose utilization and delay the onset of fatigue. An increase in the ability to use lipid can be realized by improved oxidative capacity of skeletal muscle following endurance training.

Summary

ATP is the most important form of potential energy that is necessary to perform many biological functions. Due to limited storage, ATP needs to be replenished instantly from the use of energy stored in foods such as carbohydrate and fat in order to power most activities. ▶ Biosynthesis of ATP is accomplished via operation of three energy yielding systems: (1) ATP-PCr system, (2) glycolytic system, and (3) oxidative system. The three energy systems differ considerably in terms of rate and capacity of producing ATP. Such differences among the three energy systems provide the ability for the body to be able to derive energy under various circumstances whether generating explosive power, enduring a long distance event, or simply performing a household activity. Energy is stored in the body primarily as fat in the form of triglycerides, though a much smaller amount of carbohydrate is also stored as glycogen in the muscle and liver. Carbohydrate and fat are the two primarily sources of energy used in the event where there is a need to replenish ATP in order to meet the energy demand. While carbohydrate represents a major energy fuel used in most circumstances, fat can be of importance especially under conditions in which carbohydrate stores decrease significantly.

References

1. Brooks GA, Fahey TD, Baldwin KM (2005) Exercise physiology-human bioenergetics and its applications. McGraw Hill, New York
2. Kang J (2008) Bioenergetics primer for exercise science. Human Kinetics, Champaign

3. McArdle WD, Katch FI, Katch VL (2005) Sports and exercise nutrition, 2nd edn. Lippincott Williams and Wilkins, Baltimore
4. Powers SK, Howley ET (2001) Exercise physiology-theory and application to fitness and performance. McGraw Hill, New York
5. Vander AJ, Sherman JH, Luciano DS (2001) Human physiology-the mechanisms of body function, 7th edn. McGraw Hill, New York

Energy Source

Is a system which makes energy; for instance, in living cells where there are many metabolic pathways that produces ATP as an end product.

Energy Substrates

Energy substrates are compounds that can be utilized for the production of energy. Dietary energy substrates contain fats, carbohydrates, and proteins which are digested to smaller molecules that can be used as cellular energy substrates e.g., lipids and fatty acids, glycogen and glucose, and amino acids, respectively. Fatty acids have the highest caloric equivalent with 1 g of fatty acid generating 9 kcal, while 1 g of carbohydrates and amino acids are equivalent 4 kcal each.

Energy Transformation

▶ Energy Metabolism

Energy-Dense Foods

Foods containing a high amount of energy per gram.

Engagement

▶ Promotion of and Adherence to Physical Activity

Enhancement of Performance Capacity in Long Duration Events

▶ Training, Aerobic

Enkephalin

▶ Opioid Peptides, Endogenous

Enteral Nutrition

Enteral nutritional support includes both oral ingestion and tube feeding. The latter constitutes a way to provide food through a tube placed in the nose (nasogastric/nasoenteral), the stomach (percutaneous endoscopic gastrostomy – PEG tube), or the small intestine (nasojejunal).

Environmental Heat Stress

Refers to the heat load induced by the ambient conditions. Considerable effort has been made in occupational contexts in devising appropriate indices of heat load. These have been based either on subjective responses to different combinations of environmental variables or the prediction of physiological responses necessary for heat balance. These have included the rise in body temperature and in predicted sweat rate. The most frequently used tool for indicating environmental heat stress is the wet-bulb and globe thermometer (WBGT Index) which takes radiant heat, relative humidity, and dry-bulb temperature into account. The weighted formula is as follows:

$$WBGT = 0.7 \; WB + 0.2 \; GT + 0.1 \; DB$$

Where T stands for temperature, WB indicates wet bulb for recording humidity, GT represents globe temperature for registering radiant load, and DB means dry ambient temperature.

The clothing worn and the indoor heating and ventilation systems are also relevant. Cloud cover and precipitation are relevant outdoors.

A WBGT value of 28°C is considered dangerous for distance races over 16 km, but sports throughout the world are often contested in more arduous climatic conditions.

Epidermal Growth Factor Receptor (EGFR)

Activating of the EGFR signalling pathway has been linked with important mechanisms of tumor progression such as proliferation, angiogenesis, metastasis and decreased apoptosis. EGFR is frequently expressed at elevated levels in multiple cancers, affecting adversely the treatment outcome and prognosis of patients.

Epigenetics

Epigenetics is a new field that examines how the shape of DNA and the position of markers on DNA modulate gene transcription.

EPOC

Excess postexercise O_2 consumption; refers to the amount of recovery O_2 uptake above the pre-exercise baseline. Although this term more accurately describes recovery O_2 uptake, because of tradition, it remains interchangeable with "O_2 debt."

Eppendorf Microelectrode

Eppendorf Microelectrode allows to measure directly the oxygen tension in tumor tissue.

Equilibrium

▶ Balance

Ergogenic Aids

Ergogenic refers to "performance-enhancing," and thus, "ergogenic aids" refers to any supplement that is purported to enhance performance. These ergogenic aids are not always legal.

Ergogenic Effect

Any external influence or compound that can be determined to enhance athletic performance.

Ergometry

HERBERT LÖLLGEN[1], RUTH LÖLLGEN[2]
[1]Sana-Klinikum Remscheid, Johannes-Gutenberg-University, Mainz, Remscheid, Germany
[2]Soins intensifs pédiatriques, Département médico-chirurgical de pédiatrie- DMCP, Bâtiment hospitalier, Lausanne, Switzerland

Synonyms
Exercise ECG; Exercise testing; Stress testing

Definition
Ergometry is the quantitative measurement and evaluation of physical capacity and cardiopulmonary exercise tolerance ($>$ stress and $>$ strain) of both of healthy and diseased subjects as well as of trained athletes.

Description
Exercise testing is mostly performed with bicycle or treadmill testing, with bicycling in supine or sitting position. Other modalities are arm cycling with rotating cranks in the standing position, 6- (or 12) minutes' walk test (6 MWT or 12 MWT). A recent development is the shuttle-walking test with an audio signal from a cassette tape pacing the subjects walking speed. In sports medicine, field tests are further modes of testing. Step testing (Master two step) or stair climbing are older, historical forms of exercise testing but no longer in use today.

Stress can also be applied by coldness (ice water), drugs (e.g., dobutamine or arbutamine), electrical (atrial) stimulation of the heart by a pacing catheter, and by psychological or mental stress.

Mode of Exercise Testing
Bicycling testing is the modality of choice in Europe whereas treadmill testing is widely used in the US. Bicycling testing is mostly done in the sitting or semisupine-position with steps of 2 min' duration and increments of 25 or 50 W every 2 min, according to the subject's physical fitness: low fitness: increments of 25 W or 50 W every, high fitness 50 W. Exercise should be continued until exhaustion as symptom limited incremental exercise testing (Fig. 1). For treadmill testing, the Bruce protocol is among many protocols the widespread one and consists of five progressive stages of 3 min' duration each with increasing grades until exhaustion.

FUNCTIONAL CLASS	CLINICAL STATUS	O₂ COST ml/kg/min	METS	BICYCLE ERGOMETER	Treadmilll

| | | | | | BRUCE |
| | | | | | 3 MIN STAGES MPH / %AGR |

FUNCTIONAL CLASS	CLINICAL STATUS	O_2 COST ml/kg/min	METS	BICYCLE ERGOMETER	MPH	%AGR
NORMAL AND I	HEALTHY, DEPENDENT ON AGE, ACTIVITY	73.5	21	Watts		
		70	20		5.5	20
		66.5	19			
		63	18			
		59.5	17		5.0	18
		56.0	16			
		52.5	15			
		49.0	14	246 (250)		
		45.5	13		4.2	16
		42.0	12	221 (225)		
		38.5	11	197 (200)		
		35.0	10	172 (175)	3.4	14
	SEDENTARY HEALTHY	31.5	9	148 (150)		
		28.0	8	123 (125)		
		24.5	7	98 (100)	2.5	12
II		21.0	6			
	LIMITED / SYMPTOMATIC	17.5	5	74 (75)	1.7	10
		14.0	4	49 (50)		
III		10.5	3	24 (25)		
		7.0	2			
IV		3.5	1			

Ergometry. Fig. 1 Recommendation of exercise testing protocols. Figure shows functional class, clinical finding, oxygen costs, METs, and protocol for bicycling and treadmill testing (Bruce protocol) (Modified from [1]). Data for bicycle testing in brackets are rounded off or up

Indications for Exercise Testing

There are four fields of indications

- Examinationofphysicalfitness(physicalcapacityorfitness)
- Diagnostic indication, mainly of heart and lung diseases
- Control of interventions by therapy (drugs, rehabilitation or percutaneous coronary interventions (PCI), coronary artery bypass grafting(CABG), or control of rate responsive pacemakers(PM))
- Assessing of prognosis

Physical fitness examination concerns healthy subjects, athletes, or patients for example, before surgery or rehabilitation program or physical training program. Diagnostics mainly address detection of cardiopulmonary disease (coronary artery disease (CAD), chronic obstructive lung disease (COLD), arrhythmias, or hypertension. Prognosis as to course of disease or length of life and other hard endpoints will be estimated for example, after acute MI, in hypertension, in cardiac failure, and after intervention (see above). Evidence based indications (class, grade) in detail are reported in the guidelines of cardiology or sports medicine societies [1, 3, 4, 6].

Contraindications

Acute or severe chronic cardiac or pulmonary diseases are absolute contraindications for exercise testing such as decompensated cardiac failure, unstable angina pectoris or decompensated hypertension. In addition, acute thrombosis or malignant arrhythmias, acute or severe diseases of other organs such as kidney and liver are clearly contraindications for ergometry. Relative indications are less severe status of disease. In any case, indication for examination with exercise testing has to be determined by the supervising physician.

Parameters to Be Measured

The following parameters can be recorded and/or calculated during exercise testing and may help in evaluating health and/or fitness status.

- *Physical capacity or physical fitness*: To be measured as work load in watt (or formerly mkp).
- *MET*: In addition, *metabolic equivalent* (MET) should be calculated. MET is the metabolic equivalent, that is, oxygen consumption at rest (1 MET = 3.5 ml/kg/min) and a manifold of resting value. Both parameters yield physical capacity (Fig. 1).
- *RPE*: Ratings of perceived exertion (Borg, 3, 4, 6) reflect the subjective sensation of exertion and corresponds well to exercise capacity. Similarly, ratings of dyspnea can be obtained.

- *Heart Rate*: Heart rate is a basic parameters to be measured during exercise testing and serves as a monitoring parameter during ergometry. Heart rate also serves as a reference value for calculation of other parameters and as a value per se for assessing cardiac response to stress. Heart rate can be within normal range (60–100 bpm), below or above. "Normal" values show a large interindividual variation, the term reference value should be preferred. Normal values reflect "normal" cardiac rate response.
- *Tachycardia* or exaggerated heart rate during exercise test may indicate
  - Lack of training, hyperkinetic situation
  - Hyperthyreotic status
  - Cor pulmonale
  - Anemia or
  - Cardiac failure
- *Bradycardia* during exercise test can be seen in.
  - Trained subjects, athletes
  - patients with chronotropic incompetence
  - Or during drug treatment (e.g., ß-receptor or calcium channel blockers)

    Maximal heart rate serves as reference estimate either exhaustion or to calculate training recommendation using percentage of maximum heart rate for endurance training.
- *Blood pressure* during exercise testing serves as a kind of monitoring to avoid overshooting of blood pressure. This then might be of danger for the patient, though such a complication is rather rare. Blood pressure beyond reference values indicates a so-called exercise – induced hypertension or a latent hypertension. This then leads to further diagnostic procedure or to therapy. Hypotensive blood pressure reaction is to been seen in heart failure or even in hypertrophic cardiomyopathy. A diagnostic procedure should be initiated in any case.
- *ECG* is the most important parameter to be measured during ergometry. ECG is used for monitoring to see early any possible complication such as arrhythmias or signs of ischemia [2]. Exercise testing with ECG recording in asymptomatic and symptomatic subjects is predominantly performed to detect coronary artery disease. There are typical changes of stress ECG with a ST-segment depression as the mainstay indicating ischemia (Table 1).

    Sensitivity of exercise ECG is about 68% (+/−16%), Specificity about 77% (+/−17%) giving a predicting value of 91% (87–96%). Validity of exercise ECG is much higher in symptomatic subjects

Ergometry. Table 1 Interpretation of ECG responses to exercise indicating ischemia

ST-segment displacement
Ischemia may be present with:
Horizontal or downsloping ST-segment depression of the J-point (> 0.1 mV) and the slope between 0.06 and 0.08 s past J point (>0.1 mV)
Slowly upsloping ST-segment displacement with ST-segment depression >0.2 mV at 0.06–0.08 s past J, slope should be < 1.0 mV/s
J-point displacement: >0.2 mV possibly pathological
ST-elevation (>0.1 mV):
Without preceding myocardial infarction: indicates ischemia at proximal LAD or coronary spasm in LAD
With previous myocardial infarction (Q-wave infarction): may indicate wall motion abnormalities

according to the Bayes rule than in asymptomatic persons. Reasons for false-positive and false-negative responses have to be taken into consideration. In addition, analysis of heart rate will be taken mostly from registered ECG signal. Detection of arrhythmia is another indication of exercise testing. However, ambulatory ECG (Holter monitoring) from 1 to 7 days is by far more reliable than stress testing. On the other hand, occurring arrhythmias during exercise, give some valuable informations, especially when evaluating syncope in athletes. Supraventricular or ventricular tachycardia, intermittent atrial fibrillation or new left bundle branch block are pathological and further examination should be started. These observations also may disqualify athletes from competitive sports. In any case, structural heart disease such as ion channel diseases or cardiomyopathy has to be excluded if severe arrhythmias do occur during exercise.

- *Respiratory gas exchange.* Spiroergometry is one of the oldest methods used in exercise testing, since 1928. However, introducing small sized measurement devices together with computer supported evaluation made this method simple and cost-effective. Spiroergometry is for most parameters independent from subject's cooperation. One important parameter is the maximum oxygen uptake (VO2max), one of the major endpoint besides anaerobic threshold. This value serve as a measure of physical capacity in all subjects. In patients with severe cardiopulmonary diseases, peak VO2 is often used to characterize maximal power or capacity. This latter parameter depends on the cooperation of the subject and has some arbitrary value. The respiratory gas exchange method gives a lot of additional parameters such as dead space ventilation, respiratory equivalent, and more. Together with blood gas analysis, information on respiratory gas exchange in the lung can be calculated in depth.

- *Cardiac pressures and flow (Right heart catheter).* By means of a semi-floating right heart catheter, analysis can be performed of right and left heart measuring pressure, flow, cardiac output, and vascular resistance (total and pulmonary).

  Besides of physiological questions, right heart catheter gives valuable information on pulmonary artery pressure in pulmonary artery hypertension, on left ventricular load and reserve both with regard to diagnosis and prognosis. This method however, is invasive and has to be performed by an experienced physician.

- *Lactate analysis.* Evaluating physical fitness, lactate measurement is widely used to determine the lactate threshold. This is sometimes done a preparticipation examination in highly trained athletes but also in monitoring athletes over time to evaluate training effects and estimation of competition qualities. In addition, lactate measurement is often used in field tests for monitoring training intensity for avoiding overtraining.

- *Cardiac Imaging.* There are many modalities for cardiac imaging during ergometry. Imaging is performed to analyze cardiac function and structure.

  - *Stress echocardiogram* with ergometry or using drugs or pacing to increase heart rate and cardiac output. Stress echocardiogram is worldwide most often used to examine structure and function of the heart in normal subjects, athletes, and patients with cardiac diseases. With good experience, stress echo is the method of choice to examine the heart noninvasively.

  - Analysis is concerned with wall-motion anomalies due to systolic heart failure or ischemia, tissue doppler for analyzing ischemic response to stress, and changes of left and right heart dimensions indication heart failure and vitality of the myocardium. In addition, stress echo gives information on heart valve competence or insufficiency during exercise, thus improves indication für surgery or conservative approach.

  - *Radionuclide imaging* (>PET,>SPECT) will be performed to evaluate for myocardial ischemia due to coronary artery disease. This can be seen with perfusion defects in the scan, for residual necrosis after myocardial infarction, to control effects of coronary interventions and to analyze left ventricular function at rest and exercise (nuclide angiography). In contrast to stress echo and MRI, radionuclide examination exposes the subject to radiation [1, 3, 4, 6].

– *Magnet resonance imaging* (MRT or MRI, cardiac magnetic resonance imaging) is using drugs or pacing for cardiac stimulation. Comparable to stress echo, MRT gives reliable information on myocardial ischemia, myocardial viability, alterations of heart valve function (stenosis or insufficiency). Stress to the heart in most cases is induced via drugs (dobutamine, adenosine, regadenoson) or cardiac pacing. Using gadolinum as contrast agent, MRI may show late enhancement as sign of myocarditis or necrosis.

Guidelines for Exercise Testing
There are specific and many guidelines for exercise testing in different populations and patients group according to class and stage as proposed by the AHA/ACC and partly bei ACSM [1, 2, 4, 7, 8].

Total Quality Management (TQM)
TQM means prevention and detection of faults (so-called poka yoke in Japan). Today, TQM contains (1) quality of structure: ergometer calibration, precision of analysators etc., (2) quality of process: written indications and contraindications, guidelines when to stop ergometry, general guidelines available, documentation of protocol, and results, and (3) quality of results: benchmarking, correct and false- positive/negative, criteria for validity, evidence criteria, predictive value etc.

Clinical Use and Applications

Subjects and Environments
In athletes, exercise testing is performed in almost any of clinical and sports medicine situations. Usually, ergometry is used to evaluate exercise capacity thus giving prognosis of performance capacity in training and competition. Exercise testing in women has some specific differences compared to those parameters used in men. Women have more ECG abnormalities at rest, a lower prevalence of CAD, lower voltage criteria, and more hormonal induced reactions making the interpretation especially of exercise ECG more difficult. There is now a general agreement that stress echo in this situation is very useful to evaluate suspected diseases in women. Exercise testing in children

can be done using special child adapted ergometers. Indications are similar to those in adults whereby CAD is a rather rare indication. Evaluating physical capacity, even during long-term observation, is often done in children. Standardization and reference values have to be applied for the pediatric population [4, 5]. Exercise testing is now also done in older subjects to evaluate physical capacity, to detect diseases and to evaluate prognosis, but also to recommend regular physical activity. Preoperative evaluation is one more indication as surgical procedures are done in octogenarians or even older patients. Exercise testing is widely used for rehabilitation purpose when starting rehabilitation, and to see overall improvement of exercise capacity after reconditioning. This holds mainly true for cardiac and pulmonary rehabilitation, but also for metabolic diseases. For occupational medicine, exercise testing has a strong physiological basis and rational for impairment and disability evaluation. Further, fitness for special occupations such as fireworker, depends on exercise capacity. Exercise testing is also done for monitoring impairment in workers exposed to inhalation or toxic substances (e.g., miners, dust exposed workers). Exercise testing for screening is often done for screening asymptomatic subjects for latent diseases such as CAD or pulmonary diseases. Guidelines for this procedure have been developed in cardiology, where males over 45 and females over 55 years can be tested by exercise. Also, preparticipation examination in leisure time athletes is an indication for active subjects.

Diseases
Indications for exercise testing in congenital and in valvular heart disease are mainly given to examine the severity of the defect during exercise when cardiac functional rest is compensated. Also, indication for surgery (cardiac or noncardiac) is strongly supported by results of exercise testing. Besides, long-term prognosis of congenital heart disease with and without cardiac surgery is an important indication of exercise testing. Heart failure without decompensation at rest is now a clear-cut indication for exercise testing, especially by spiroergometry. Severity, control of effects of interventions (drugs, biventricular pacing (CRT or cardiac resynchronization therapy)) and prognosis are the mainstay of stress testing in heart failure. In any case, exercise testing is always done before heart transplantation is to considered. Exercise testing with regard to Ischemia is described above. Exercise testing to detect or control arrhythmias is complimentary to ambulatory ECG to detect arrhythmias (see above). New methods such as t-wave alternans give by far more reliable information on the potential thread by maligne arrhythmias, especially in

cardiac patients. In subjects with peripheral artery disease (pad), treadmill testing and walking tests are the methods of choice for analyzing the severity of the disease and to examine the effects of therapy, either intervention such as surgery, dilatation and stenting, walking training or drugs. Bicycle testing is of little value in these patients. In lung diseases, exercise testing is a standard and often used approach. Indications are: examination of severity of the disease, e.g., COLD, before pulmonary or non-pulmonary surgery, to analyze the possible risk of anesthesia, for examination of impairment and disability, when there is a compensation claim, and to observe prognosis over long time.

References

1. American College of Sports Medicine (2006) ACSM's guidelines for exercise testing and prescription, 7th edn. Lippincott, Philadelphia
2. Ellestad MH (1996) Stress testing, 4th edn. Davis, Philadelphia
3. Froelicher V, Myers J (2006) Exercise and the heart, 5th edn. Saunders, Philadelphia
4. Gibbons RJ (2002) AHA/ACC gudielines update for exercise testing. J Am Coll Cardiol 40:1531–1540
5. Löllgen H (2005) Cardiopulmonary function diagnostic (in German), 4th edn. Novartis, Nürnberg
6. Löllgen H, Erdmann E, Gitt A (eds) (2009) Ergometry (in German), 3rd edn. Springer, Heidelberg
7. Myers J (2009) Recommendations for clinical exercise laboratories. Circulation 119:3144–3161
8. Weisman IM, Zeballos RJ (eds) (2002) Clinical exercise testing. Karger, Basel

ERK

Extracellular signal-regulated kinases belong to the group of serine/threonine kinases. Eight isoforms (ERK 1–8) are known. Associated signaling pathways are involved in regulating diverse cellular processes such as proliferation, differentiation, growth, inflammation, and apoptosis.

Erythrocytes

Main blood oxygen and carbon dioxide carriers in blood and source of signals for blood flow regulation.

Erythrocytopoiesis

▶ Erythropoiesis

Erythropoiesis

WOLFGANG JELKMANN
Institute of Physiology, University of Luebeck, Luebeck, Germany

Synonyms

Erythrocytopoiesis; Production of erythrocytes

Definition

The term erythropoiesis derives from the Greek stems "*erythros*" (red) and "*poiein*" (making) and describes the process of the production of erythrocytes (red blood cells). Erythrocytes are filled with ▶ hemoglobin for O_2 transport. Erythropoiesis balances the physiological loss of aged erythrocytes (life span 100–120 days). In adults, erythropoiesis usually takes place in the marrow of the flat bones. Erythrocytes are the progeny of myeloid ▶ stem cells, which produce erythrocytic progenitors and precursors (the "erythron") in a series of multiplication, differentiation, and maturation steps. Erythropoiesis involves cell–cell as well as cell–matrix interactions and soluble factors. An essential growth factor is erythropoietin (EPO), a glycoprotein hormone that is mainly of renal origin. EPO binds to specific receptors of erythrocytic progenitors, primarily the "colony-forming units-erythroid" (CFU-E), thereby inhibiting their apoptotic death and promoting their proliferation. Young erythrocytes (reticulocytes) are increasingly released beginning 3–4 days after a rise in circulating EPO. Secondary erythrocytosis develops on high altitude residence, as tissue hypoxia is the main stimulus for EPO synthesis. In contrast, anemia due to insufficient erythropoiesis results from the lack of EPO, ▶ iron, ▶ vitamin B_{12}, or folic acid.

Characteristics

Erythrocytes and Their Ancestors

The red blood cells make up about 42% of the blood volume in females and 47% in males (hematocrit), with mean counts of 4.8, respectively, 5.3 Mio. red cells/µL blood. Human erythrocytes are flexible round disks without nuclei. Their greatest thickness (at the edge) is only 2 µm and their diameter about 7.5 µm (normocytes). The biconcave shape enables them to pass through narrow, curved capillaries, and it facilitates the gas transfer because of the large surface and the small diffusion distances. Erythrocytes are filled with hemoglobin (Hb), the O_2 transport protein. Hb is composed of two α and two β globin chains, each attached to a heme group containing ferrous iron to which O_2 can bind. The mean Hb concentration is normally 140 g/L blood in females and 160 g/L in males, with 1 g Hb binding maximally 1.34 mL O_2 (O_2 transport capacity). Erythrocytes also contain the enzyme carbonic anhydrase that catalyzes the reversible reaction of CO_2 with H_2O yielding H_2CO_3 (carbonic acid), which dissociates to HCO_3^- and H^+, the latter being buffered by Hb.

Erythrocytes circulate in the blood for 100–120 days. Then, they are engulfed by phagocytes in the bone marrow, and under pathological conditions also in the liver and the spleen. The globin and the heme are separated and the iron is salvaged for reuse. To keep the total red cell mass constant, young erythrocytes are continuously generated in the hemopoietic tissues – the yolk sac of the embryo, the liver, and spleen of the fetus, and the red marrow of the flat bones in adults. About 1% of the 25×10^{12} erythrocytes of an adult are renewed every day. This implies an erythropoiesis rate of $2–3 \times 10^6$ red cells per second. The rate of erythropoiesis can increase about tenfold after a loss of blood or when the erythrocyte life span is pathologically shortened. Erythropoiesis requires iron, vitamin B_{12}, and folic acid in addition to basic nutrients (amino acids, lipids, carbohydrates). Iron availability is regulated by the hepatic peptide hormone ▶ hepcidin.

Erythrocytes are the offsprings of a small pool of self-perpetuating myeloid stem cells called "CFU-GEMM" (colony-forming unit generating granulocytic, erythrocytic, megakaryocytic, and monocytic progeny) or CD34$^+$ cells (CD means "cluster of differentiation," with the number indicating specific membrane marker proteins). Their proliferative activity depends on the local environment and the presence of cytokines such as interleukin-3 [1]. In the erythrocytic line (the "erythron"), at the next level of differentiation are the committed erythrocytic progenitors (Fig. 1). First are the "BFU-E" (burst-forming units-erythroid), which can generate several hundred erythroblasts within 10–20 days. The more differentiated "CFU-E" (colony-forming units-erythroid) generate 8–64 erythroblasts within 7–8 days, forming erythroblastic islands with a central macrophage. The process involves adhesive reactions as well as various

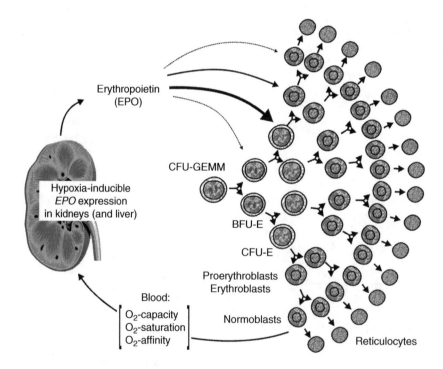

Erythropoiesis. Fig. 1 Simplified scheme of the feedback control of erythropoiesis. Erythrocytes transport O_2 in blood. Lack of O_2 (hypoxia) is a stimulus for the synthesis of erythropoietin (EPO), primarily in the kidneys. EPO is a survival, proliferation, and differentiation factor for the erythrocytic progenitors, particularly the colony-forming units-erythroid (CFU-E). Strictly speaking, the development from a pluripotent myeloid CFU-GEMM to the normoblasts involves about 10^{12} cell divisions. The O_2 capacity of the blood increases with the enhanced release of reticulocytes

cytokines and chemokines. The proerythroblasts, which express ferritin, are the first cells of the erythron that are microscopically identifiable. As development progresses, the nuclei of the descendants become smaller and the cytoplasm more basophilic, due to the presence of ribosomes. The cells in this stage are called basophilic erythroblasts. These possess cell membrane receptors for binding the iron delivering protein, ▶ transferrin. As the descendants begin to synthesize Hb, they are called polychromatic erythroblasts, because their cytoplasm attracts both basic and eosin stains. Hb synthesis involves three major substrates: protein, protoporphyrin, and iron. Orthochromatic erythroblasts (syn. normoblasts) do not divide any more but extrude their nuclei and enter the circulation as reticulocytes. These lose their filaments and organelles (mitochondria, polyribosomes) within 2 days, thus becoming mature erythrocytes. Under normal conditions 0.3–1.8% of the red blood cells are reticulocytes. Acceleration of erythropoiesis increases this percentage and repression decreases it. Erythrocytes have no intracellular structures visible by light microscopy. The mean corpuscular volume (MCV) of a normocytic erythrocyte amounts to 87 fl (compared to 900 fl of the proerythroblast) and the mean corpuscular Hb mass (MCH) of a normochromic erythrocyte to 30 pg.

The Hormone Erythropoietin

The specific stimulus for erythropoiesis is a fall in the tissue O_2 pressure (pO_2). Hypoxic stress (an imbalance between O_2 supply and demand) causes an increase in the synthesis of the hormone erythropoietin (EPO) [2]. The human EPO gene (*EPO*) is located on chromosome 7 (q11–q22). *EPO* expression is controlled by transcription factors. GATA-2 inhibits the *EPO* promoter. ▶ Hypoxia-inducible factors (predominantly HIF-2) activate hypoxia-response elements (HRE) of the *EPO* enhancer [3]. HIF are heterodimeric proteins (α/β). In the presence of O_2, the HIFα subunit is prolyl-hydroxylated and undergoes immediate proteasomal degradation. Under hypoxic conditions, HIFα translocates to the nucleus and heterodimerizes with HIFβ. Hence, *EPO* transcription increases when the O_2-capacity of the blood is reduced (anemia), when the arterial pO_2 is lowered (hypoxemia), or when O_2 unloading is impaired (high Hb-O_2-affinity). The stimulation of EPO production by hypoxia is used in sports to increase the O_2-capacity (living and/or training at altitude, respectively, in rooms with artificially reduced O_2-concentrations at sea level). *EPO* gene produces a translation product of 193 amino acids. Prior to the secretion of EPO, an *N*-terminal leader peptide of 27 amino acids and a *C*-terminal arginine are cleaved.

Circulating EPO is composed of 165 amino acids that form a globular structure of four α-helical bundles. In addition, EPO possesses four glycans (carbohydrate chains), which amount to 40% of EPO's total molecular mass of 30.4 kDa. There are three complex-type *N*-glycans (at Asn^{24}, Asn^{38}, and Asn^{83}), which are permissive for the secretion and stability of EPO, and a small *O*-glycan (at Ser^{126}) that lacks functional importance. The microheterogeneity of endogenous and recombinant EPO results from differences in the composition of the glycans.

EPO amounts are usually expressed in International Units (IU), with 1 IU eliciting *per definition* the same erythropoietic response as 5 µmol cobaltous chloride. The plasma concentration of EPO is 6–32 IU/L (about 10^{11} mol/L) in healthy humans. The levels vary greatly between individuals, but there are no major gender- or age-specific differences. Of note is the diurnal fluctuation of the plasma EPO level, with a nadir in the morning. Plasma EPO increases exponentially, when the Hb concentration falls below $\sim$125 g/L. Although acute physical work has no major influence on circulating EPO levels, reticulocytosis may develop 1–2 days thereafter, because stress hormones (catecholamines, cortisol) stimulate the release of reticulocytes from the bone marrow.

EPO is of hepatic origin in fetuses. After birth the kidneys become the main sites of its production. EPO mRNA is expressed mainly in peritubular interstitial fibroblasts in the renal cortex. In addition, some EPO mRNA is detectable in brain, liver, spleen, lung, and testis. Brain EPO is a separate entity, as it exerts local neuroprotective effects. In the bone marrow, EPO stimulates the proliferation and differentiation of the erythrocytic progenitors, particularly the CFU-E. Mechanistically, EPO prevents them from undergoing apoptosis (programmed cell death) and enables them to generate colonies of erythroblasts. CFU-E express the major erythroid-specific transcription factor, GATA-1. While EPO is strictly required for erythropoiesis, it is supported by other hormones, namely, testosterone, thyroid hormone, somatotropin, and insulin-like growth factor 1. The differences in red cell counts and Hb in women compared to men result from the stimulation of erythropoiesis by androgens [2].

EPO acts through binding to a transmembrane receptor (EPO-R) of its target cells. The mature human EPO-R is a 484 amino acid glycoprotein of about 60 kDa. The EPO-R belongs to the cytokine class I receptors, which are characterized by an extracellular *N*-terminal domain with conserved cysteines and a WSXWS-motif, a single hydrophobic transmembrane segment, and a cytosolic domain that lacks enzymatic activity. Two of the membrane-spanning EPO-R molecules form a homodimer that binds one EPO molecule. As a result, cytoplasmic Janus kinases 2 (JAK2) phosphorylate tyrosine residues of the EPO-R, which provide docking sites for signaling proteins (enzymes and transcription factors). The effect of EPO is terminated by the action of the hemopoietic cell phosphatase (HCP), which catalyzes JAK2 de-phosphorylation. The EPO/EPO-R complex is eventually internalized and degraded.

Clinical Relevance

Pathophysiology of Erythrocytoses

Erythrocytosis (syn. polycythemia) results from persistent overstimulation of erythropoiesis [4]. Red cell counts, Hb value, and Hct are abnormally high. Consequently, the blood viscosity is increased, which raises the cardiac afterload and disturbs the microcirculation. Primary erythrocytosis is a myeloproliferative disorder. Secondary erythrocytosis results from overproduction of EPO, commonly due to tissue hypoxia. In fact, excessive EPO production causes the erythrocytosis in ▶ chronic mountain sickness. Disorders associated with an increased O_2 affinity of the blood may also lead to abnormally high plasma EPO levels and erythrocytosis. Of note, changes in renal blood flow have little influence on the rate of EPO synthesis and rarely cause erythrocytosis. Paraneoplastic EPO formation may occur in patients suffering from renal carcinoma, Wilms' tumor, hepatocellular carcinoma, or cerebellar hemangioblastoma [2].

Pathophysiology of Anemias

Anemia means, literally, bloodlessness. In clinical usage the term refers primarily to a lack of Hb and the diminished ability of the blood to transport O_2. There can be a reduction in the number of erythrocytes and/or in the Hb content of the individual erythrocytes [4]. Of note, Hb levels and Hct are often below normal in athletes (sports anemia) due to an increase in the blood plasma volume (pseudoanemia). The most common reason of true anemia is iron deficiency. This can be produced by a diet with inadequate iron content, diminished iron absorption from the digestive tract, or chronic loss of blood due to, for example, ulcers and heavy menstrual bleeding. In iron deficiency anemia the blood contains small erythrocytes with a subnormal Hb content (hypochromic microcytic anemia). In contrast, megaloblastic anemias are generally caused by a deficiency of vitamin B_{12} (pernicious anemia) and/or folic acid, due to inadequacies in either diet or absorption. When these vitamins are lacking cell division

Erythropoiesis. Table 1 Pathophysiology of erythropoiesis

A. Increase → Erythrocytosis (syn. Polycythemia)
• Polycythemia *vera* (due to myeloid stem/progenitor cell abnormality)
• Secondary polycythemia (due to increased plasma EPO)
B. Decrease → Anemia
• Increased loss of red blood cells
– Acute bleeding
– Hemolysis (toxins; spheroid cells, sickle cells)
• Defect in red blood cell production
– Iron deficiency (due to insufficient intestinal resorption, chronic bleeding, inflammation)
– Vitamin B_{12} deficiency
– Folic acid deficiency
– Primary bone marrow failure (due to cytotoxic drugs, radiotherapy)
– Lack of EPO (due to chronic kidney disease, inflammation)
– Thalassemia

is impaired, and abnormally large erythrocytes with a shortened life span arise (hyperchromic macrocytic anemia). Normochromic normocytic anemia due to insufficient EPO production develops in patients with chronic renal failure (renal anemia), systemic inflammations, or malignancies (anemia of chronic disease). The anemias of patients with chronic renal failure or cancer in combination with chemotherapy can be corrected by replacement therapy with ▶ recombinant human EPO (rhEPO, Epoetin) or analogs thereof [5]. The target Hb in blood is clinically set at 100–120 g/L. rhEPO is identical to endogenous EPO with regard to its amino acid sequence. However, there are distinct differences in the composition of the *N*- and *O*-glycans of rhEPO compared to endogenous EPO. Other reasons for anemia are summarized in Table 1.

References

1. Dessypris EN, Sawyer S (2003) Erythropoiesis. In: Greer JP, Foerster J, Lukens JN, Rodgers GM, Paraskevas F, Glader B (eds) Wintrobe's clinical hematology, vol 11. Lippincott Williams & Wilkins, Baltimore, pp 195–216
2. Jelkmann W (1992) Erythropoietin: structure, control of production, and function. Physiol Rev 72:449–489
3. Smith TG, Robbins PA, Ratcliffe PJ (2008) The human side of hypoxia-inducible factor. Br J Haematol 141:325–334
4. Hodges VM, Rainey S, Lappin TR, Maxwell AP (2007) Pathophysiology of anemia and erythrocytosis. Crit Rev Oncol Hematol 64:139–158
5. Jelkmann W (ed) (2003) Erythropoietin: molecular biology and clinical use. FP Graham, Johnson City

Erythropoiesis-Stimulating Agents

Substances which stimulate the erythropoiesis.

Erythropoietin (EPO)

EPO is a glycopeptide hormone that stimulates erythropoiesis, that is, the production of red blood cells. The misuse of EPO in particular in endurance sports has been reported several times. Major effect is the increase of erythrocyte concentration in the blood and, thus, an enhanced oxygen transport capacity.

E-Selectin

Is a cell adhesion molecule expressed only on endothelial cells activated by cytokines. Like other selectins, it plays an important role in inflammation. It is also known as CD62 antigen-like family member E (CD62E).

Essential Hypertension

▶ Hypertension
▶ Hypertension, Training
▶ Hypertension, Physical Activity

Estrogen

A class of hormone formed from androgen precursors, secreted chiefly by the ovaries, placenta, adipose tissue, and testes, and that stimulate the development of female secondary sex characteristics and promote the growth and maintenance of the female reproductive system. The most biologically active estrogen is 17-β estradiol. Estrogens appear to impact endothelial function.

Euhydration

The state of having a normal body water content.

Eupnea

Normal, unlabored, or relaxed breathing.

Evaporation

Evaporation is the vaporization of a liquid occurring at its surface. Evaporation requires the addition of sufficient kinetic energy (i.e., heat) to break intermolecular forces within a liquid. The rate of evaporation is determined by the difference between the partial vapor pressure of the substance on the evaporative surface and within the surrounding gas. Evaporation is also accelerated by an increased rate of flow of a gas across an evaporative surface. The amount of heat required to vaporize 1 g of water at 30°C is 2,430 J. Similarly, the amount of heat required to vaporize 1 g of eccrine sweat is 2,426 J. This value is not altered by ambient temperature and relative humidity, or by the concentration of solutes present in human sweat.

Evaporative Heat Loss

The rate of heat dissipated by evaporation. Includes sensible and insensible evaporative heat loss from the skin, respiratory tract and all other mucosal membranes. In humans, during hyperthermia cutaneous evaporative heat loss is controlled via thermal sweating.

Event-Related Potentials

Neuroelectric activation that is measured using electroencephalography and time-locked to an event such as a stimulus or response. Individual components of event-related potentials are often associated with specific cognitive processes that occur between the perception of a stimulus and response execution.

Magnetic Resonance Imaging-A noninvasive medical device that provides detailed images of soft biological tissues such as the brain. By using the natural magnetic properties of the body, high resolution images can be generated and can act as diagnostic information or as outcome variables from scientific research. By changing sequence parameters, different types of images can be generated. In relation to brain function, images that focus on white matter, gray matter, or functional characteristics of blood flow or neural activity can be identified.

Excess Postexercise Oxygen Consumption

CHRISTOPHER B. SCOTT
Department of Exercise, Health and Sport Sciences, University of Southern Maine, Gorham, ME, USA

Synonyms

Oxygen debt; Recovery oxygen uptake

Definition

Exercise raises ▶ metabolic rate, typically represented by an elevated oxygen (O_2) uptake that accompanies the increase in ▶ energy demands. When exercise stops elevated O_2 uptake levels fall, eventually attaining previous resting levels. The timing of this decrease is affected by the duration and especially the *intensity* of the previous exercise [1]. The volume of O_2 consumed between the completion of exercise and the return to resting levels has been termed Excess Postexercise Oxygen Consumption or EPOC (Fig. 1) [2].

Description

Product and by-product formation and removal occur at accelerated rates as muscle ▶ metabolism rises, fueling the energy demands of contraction. Because exercise is varied in the type, intensity, and duration of participation, so too are the associated costs. The extent of EPOC is likewise quite variable as working muscles (and the whole body) gradually return to a "normal" resting state. After a single bout of weight lifting for example, EPOC may last minutes; after moderate intensity jogging or bicycling for 60 min or more it may last hours; and following an intense competitive sporting event or physical workout EPOC may last days.

Regarding the history of EPOC, changes in interpretation continue, with terminology serving as a primary example. The original term applied to EPOC was ▶ O_2 debt – some physiology textbooks still use this descriptor. Original interpretations of the O_2 debt were based on a "balance sheet" description of physiological events: "...*the body has to 'go into debt' for oxygen, to obtain its energy on the 'security' of a concentration of lactic acid which it will require future 'oxygen income' to eliminate*"

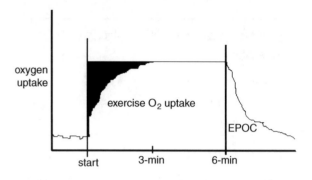

Excess Postexercise Oxygen Consumption. Fig. 1 Oxygen uptake is shown at rest, immediately preceding the start of low to moderately intense aerobic exercise. When exercise abruptly starts, O_2 uptake rises quickly, eventually becoming proportional to energy demands; this is known as the ▶ aerobic exercise energy expenditure. The area in black represents ▶ anaerobic energy expenditure contributions that end when O_2 consumption reaches a steady state (at minute 3). When exercise abruptly stops, EPOC is shown rapidly, then gradually returning to resting levels. The volume of O_2 consumed during aerobic exercise represents the largest energy cost

[3, p. 442]. It was later discovered that an O_2 debt could be incurred without any increase in ▶ blood lactate levels, when exercise was both brief and intense. This finding provided the still prevalent rationale of a fast phase (lasting minutes) and longer-term phase (lasting hours) as parts of the O_2 debt. Comparative investigations likewise revealed dissociation between blood lactate levels and the amount of O_2 consumed in the recovery from physical activity. Lack of an apparent cause-and-effect scenario – lactate removal increases O_2 uptake – prompted a terminology change and the acronym EPOC was coined [2].

An accounting of all physiological costs associated with EPOC has not been successful, yet there are undeniable factors involved that have undergone attempted quantification [1]. Expended fuel reserves during exercise, for example, are replaced during recovery: contracting muscle uses limited stores of high-energy phosphates ▶ adenosine triphosphate (ATP) and ▶ creatine phosphate (CP) at the initiation of exercise (as part of anaerobic metabolism) and these are aerobically resynthesized immediately after the cessation of exercise (the so-called fast phase). Restoration of O_2 within hemoglobin and myoglobin (oxygen carrying proteins) occurs rather immediately postexercise. Costs of elevated ventilation rates (muscles required for breathing) along with cardiac

E

(heart) rate and contractility as part of O_2 delivery also have immediate effects on EPOC volume.

Over a longer period of time other factors are at play (the slow phase) that require increases in aerobic energy exchange: fat stores broken down to fatty acids during exercise are removed from the blood stream in recovery, being oxidized for fuel or reconverted back to triglycerides for storage – the latter being an example of fatty acid-triglyceride ▶ substrate cycling [1]. Because the energy costs of recovery are met by aerobic ATP resynthesis, fat may be a favored fuel. Moreover, small amounts of lactate can be converted back to glucose and glycogen (another example of substrate cycling) though the majority appears also to fuel recovery [2]. The effect of hormones released during exercise as well as any protein synthesis, repair, or turnover resulting from exercise delay EPOC's return to resting O_2 uptake levels.

Application

While it is obvious that the recovery from exercise increases O_2 consumption above resting levels, how much of an increase this represents in terms of ▶ daily energy expenditure remains unclear. The question of how much is important because the majority of daily energy expenditure – 60–75% – is accounted for by *resting* O_2 uptake; exercise and physical activity adds a significant albeit often minimal increase to daily energy expenditure [4]. Whether regular exercise or a prolonged EPOC better explains an increased ▶ resting metabolic rate (RMR) in active individuals is not known. Regardless, an elevated RMR only is found in highly trained individuals [5]. It is further apparent that athletic performance or ability – sedentary versus trained individuals – has a minimal influence on the extent of EPOC [6].

Early EPOC studies almost exclusively followed an aerobic exercise format, that is, exercise preceding EPOC was typically defined in terms of a large muscle mass moving rhythmically and continuously over periods of time in terms of a relative percentage of VO_2 max. To the contrary, intermittent anaerobic-type exercises (e.g., resistance training) involving small and large muscle masses, and defined in terms of a percentage of maximum repetition (RM) number have been shown to promote EPOC to an extent that can exceed that of aerobic exercise [7].

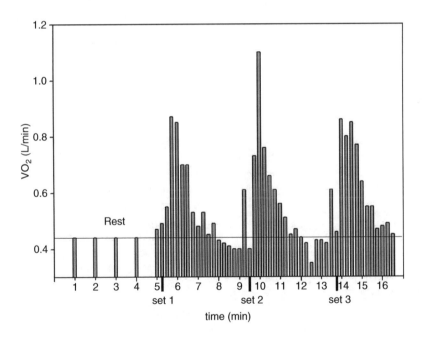

Excess Postexercise Oxygen Consumption. Fig. 2 Oxygen uptake data are at first shown for 1–5 min of rest, each vertical bar represents a 15-s measurement period (I min^{-1}). At minute 5, the start of three sets of bench press exercise begins (the *black line* at *bottom*), with five repetitions comprising each set (70% of a 1-RM). The lifting period for each set is 15 s, recovery between sets is 4 min. Note that exercise O_2 uptake is minimal during resistance training, with EPOC (i.e., rest/recovery periods) representing the largest aerobic energy cost. EPOC rises and peaks in the rest/recovery after each set [12]; with aerobic exercise it plummets immediately toward resting levels. These data are from a single subject

Comparisons, however, between intermittent work and steady-state power (e.g., isometric vs isotonic) as well as exercise intensity descriptions of both (% VO$_2$ max vs% 1-RM) are difficult to standardize between anaerobic and aerobic exercise [8]. As an example, the energy costs of aerobic exercise are dictated by the rate of O$_2$ consumed during the exercise period, always exceeding anaerobic energy expenditure and EPOC (Fig. 1). To the contrary, the lowest amount of O$_2$ is consumed during sets or bouts of anaerobic-type exercise, with the largest energy cost estimates coming from anaerobic energy expenditure and one or more EPOC (i.e., recovery) periods [9, 10] (Fig. 2). Interestingly, exercise scientists often average the O$_2$ uptake of the rest/recovery periods after weight lifting sets with exercise O$_2$ uptake; for aerobic exercise, recovery O$_2$ uptake (i.e., EPOC) is kept separate [6]. Metabolic differences between exercise and recovery have the potential to affect O$_2$ uptake and energy expenditure relationships for both so that this practice may need to be changed [1, 11].

References

1. Borsheim E, Bahr R (2003) Effect of exercise intensity, duration and mode on post-exercise oxygen consumption. Sports Med 33:1037–1060
2. Gaesser GA, Brooks GA (1984) Metabolic bases of excess post-exercise oxygen consumption: a review. Medicine and Science in Sports and Exercise 16:29–43
3. Hill AV, Long CNH, Lupton H (1924) Muscular exercise, lactic acid and the supply and utilization of oxygen – parts I-III. Proceedings of the Royal Society Bulletin 96:438–475
4. Danforth E (1981) Dietary-induced thermogenesis: control of energy expenditure. Life Sci 28:1821–1827
5. Poehlman ET (1989) A review: exercise and its influence on resting energy metabolism in man. Medicine and Science in Sports and Exercise 21:515–525
6. LaForgia J, Withers RT, Gore CJ (2006) Effects of exercise intensity and duration on the excess post-exercise oxygen consumption. Journal of Sport Sciences 24:1247–1264
7. Elliot DL, Goldberg L, Kuehl KS (1992) Effect of resistance training on excess post-exercise oxygen consumption. J Appl Sport Sci Res 6:77–81
8. Meirelles CM, Gomes PSC (2004) Acute effects of resistance exercise on energy expenditure: revisiting the impact of the training variables. Rev Brazilian Med Esporte 10:131–138
9. Scott CB, Croteau A, Ravlo T (2009) Energy expenditure before, during, and after the bench press. J Strength Cond Res 23:611–618
10. Scott CB, Learay MP, Ten Braak AJ (2011) Energy expenditure characteristics of weight lifting: 2 sets to fatigue. Appl Physiol Nutr Metab 36:115–120
11. Scott CB (2011) Quantifying the immediate recovery energy expenditure of resistance training. J Strength Cond Res 25:1159–1163
12. McArdle WD, Foglia GF (1969) Energy cost and cardiorespiratory stress of isometric and weight training exercises. J Sports Med Phys Fitness 9:23–30

Excitation–Contraction Coupling

Ioannis Smyrnias[1], Martin D. Bootman[2], H. Llewelyn Roderick[2,3]
[1]Department of Cardiology, The James Black Centre, King's College London, London, UK
[2]Laboratory of Signalling and Cell Fate, Babraham Institute, Cambridge, UK
[3]Department of Pharmacology, University of Cambridge, Cambridge, UK

Synonyms

Ca^{2+} release channels; Dihydropyridine receptors (DHPRs) = L-type voltage-operated Ca^{2+} channels; Myoplasm = cytoplasm; Protein kinase A (PKA) = cyclic AMP-dependent kinase A

Definition

▶ Excitation–contraction (EC) coupling in striated (skeletal and cardiac) muscle physiology is a term broadly used to define the physiological process of transduction of an electrical stimulus (action potential) to a mechanical response (contraction). The EC-coupling cycle involves the following sequence of events: (1) depolarization of the plasma membrane and its membrane invaginations (the t-tubular system) by an action potential; (2) transduction of the depolarization signal to the ▶ sarcoplasmic reticulum (SR) membrane; (3) activation of Ca^{2+} release from the SR and subsequent global elevation of intracellular [Ca^{2+}]; (4) transient interaction of Ca^{2+} with contractile proteins leading to muscle contraction; and (5) return of [Ca^{2+}] back to levels at resting conditions and muscle relaxation. The macromolecular complex that defines the EC-coupling apparatus mainly consists of the 1,4-dihydropyridine receptors (DHPRs) serving as voltage sensors, the ▶ ryanodine receptor (RyR) Ca^{2+} release channels in the SR membrane, calsequestrin acting as a Ca^{2+} binding/sensing protein, and troponin-C as the Ca^{2+} sensor for induction of contraction (Fig. 1).

Basic Mechanisms

Skeletal Muscle

Mammalian skeletal muscle fibers are mainly characterized by the transient contractions ("twitches") caused by propagated action potentials in response to neural stimulation. The EC-coupling cycle dictates the actions of slow- and fast-twitch fibers, with the former contracting for long periods

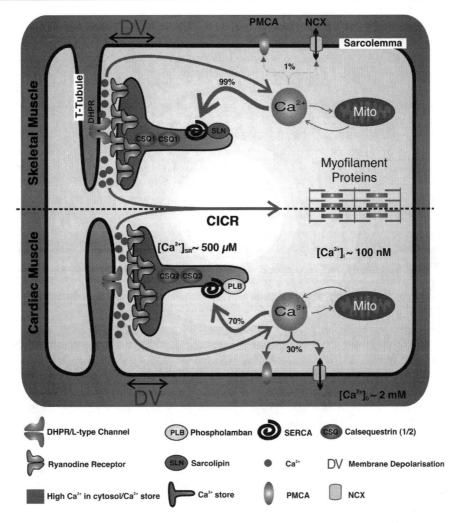

Excitation–Contraction Coupling. Fig. 1 *Schematic of EC-coupling in skeletal and cardiac muscle.* An *idealized* representation of a cell is shown that illustrates the plasma membrane, its t-tubular invaginations, the sarcoplasmic reticulum Ca^{2+} store, and the machinery responsible for Ca^{2+} signal generation and modulation. The Ca^{2+} concentration in the SR ($[Ca^{2+}]_{SR}$), cytosol ($[Ca^{2+}]_i$), and extracellular space ($[Ca^{2+}]_0$) are indicated. In skeletal muscle, the action potential (ΔV) depolarizes the plasma membrane causing a change in conformation of the a_{1S} subunit of DHPR (L-type Ca^{2+} channels) leading to the induction of Ca^{2+} release from the SR via associated type 1 RyRs. Ca^{2+} diffuses from its site of release to the myofilaments inducing contraction. Ca^{2+} is sequestered back into the SR via SERCA1. SERCA1 is modulated by sarcolipin. Ca^{2+} is also taken up by mitochondria. In cardiac muscle, the action potential causes the opening of the a_{1c} subunit of DHPR allowing Ca^{2+} influx into the dyadic cleft. An increase in Ca^{2+} in this region activates its own release from the SR via RyR2. Ca^{2+} diffuses from its site of release to the myofilaments inducing contraction. Ca^{2+} is sequestered back into the SR via SERCA2a. SERCA2a is modulated by phospholamban in a PKA-dependent manner. Ca^{2+} is also extruded across the plasma membrane via NCX and PMCA. The relative contributions of the mechanisms for plasma membrane extrusion and SR Ca^{2+} sequestration to Ca^{2+} clearance are indicated. The mitochondria also participate in Ca^{2+} clearance from the cytosol

of time and with little force, whereas the latter contract quickly and powerfully but fatigue very rapidly.

The excitation process in skeletal muscle begins with release of acetylcholine (ACh) from nerve terminals at the neuromuscular junction. Binding of the neurotransmitter to its receptor causes depolarization of the plasma membrane leading to waves of action potentials that spread out from the motor end plate along the sarcolemma and into the t-tubular system. The t-tubular system in skeletal muscle consists predominantly of complex transverse and longitudinal tubular networks and acts to sustain propagated action potentials. The t-tubular network forms a junctional region with the SR membranes (the "triad"), generating protein complexes that transmit excitation to the SR (Fig. 1). The action potential waves spread to the surface/▶ t-tubules, where they are sensed by four positively charged transmembrane segments in DHPRs, subsequently depolarizing the membrane. A cytoplasmic loop between repeats II and III in the $\alpha1$ subunit of DHPRs transmits the signal to the RyR1 Ca^{2+} release channels at the cisternae of the SR. This communication is considered to occur through a physical coupling between the DHPRs and RyR1s via junctional "feet" formed by RyR1s spanning the gap between the SR and the t-tubule membrane. The physical coupling (also known as mechanical or conformational coupling) between DHPRs and RyR1s causes a conformational change and opening of the SR Ca^{2+} release channels [1]. Unlike cardiac muscle, Ca^{2+} entry from the extracellular space is not a prerequisite for EC-coupling in skeletal muscle. DHPR complexes at the surface/t-tubular membranes are arranged in groups of four ("tetrads") for every homotetrameric RyR1 they face [2]. The complex molecular network that regulates Ca^{2+} release from the SR also includes calsequestrin, a low affinity, high capacity Ca^{2+} storage/binding protein localized in the SR terminal cisternae, which is anchored with triadin and junctin providing a direct link with RyR1s [3]. Additional proteins (e.g., junctophilin-1, JP-45, and FK506-binding protein) have been shown to be required for both for the structural formation of the machinery involved in skeletal muscle EC-coupling and for its fine-tuning.

The rate of Ca^{2+} release from the SR depends on the number of RyR1s occupied with activated DHPR tetrads and the average open probability of RyR1s. Ca^{2+} release from the SR causes a rise in $[Ca^{2+}]$ in the myoplasm from approximately 100 nM for both the slow- and fast-twitch muscle fibers at resting conditions to near 1 mM when stimulated [4]. Elevated levels of Ca^{2+} in the myoplasm allow for its interaction with the contractile protein troponin-C on actin filaments, unmasking the inhibitory effects of tropomyosin and revealing cross-bridge binding sites on the actin filament. ADP-bound myosin binds to the newly uncovered actin binding sites, releasing ADP and allowing for sliding of actin over myosin and shortening of the muscle fiber (contraction). ATP binding on myosin allows myosin heads to release actin and return it to the low affinity site. Hydrolysis of ATP returns myosin to its ADP-bound state [5].

For relaxation to occur, myoplasmic $[Ca^{2+}]$ needs to return to resting levels. This is achieved predominantly by sequestration of Ca^{2+} back into the SR. Notably, the plasma membrane Ca^{2+} ATPases (PMCA) and ▶ Na^+/Ca^{2+} exchangers (NCX) confer only modest importance in cellular Ca^{2+} homeostasis, as over 99% of the activating Ca^{2+} in skeletal muscle fibers originate from the SR. Ca^{2+} transport across the SR membrane is mediated by the action of the SR Ca^{2+} ATPase (SERCA). SERCA activity is governed by its protein regulator sarcolipin (also phospholamban in slow-twitch muscle) and by SR luminal and myoplasmic $[Ca^{2+}]$. Feedback inhibition due to high luminal $[Ca^{2+}]$ is observed only in slow-twitch skeletal muscle fibers, which affects the fatigue capacity of the muscle fiber [6].

Cardiac Muscle

The molecular components that govern the contractile apparatus in cardiac muscle are broadly similar to those in skeletal muscle fibers (Fig. 1). However, the mechanism of EC-coupling between skeletal and cardiac muscle is different. Each contractile cycle in cardiac myocytes is initiated by the generation of action potentials by pacemaker cells in the ▶ sinoatrial (SA) node. Action potentials are rapidly propagated throughout the heart via specialized conduction fibers and from cell to cell via gap junction intercellular channels. Ventricular and atrial myocytes are connected to each other by a series of intercalated discs made up of an array of gap junctions, which conduct the action potential directly between the cytoplasm of adjacent cells.

Depolarization of the plasma membrane in cardiac myocytes leads to activation of the abundantly expressed sarcolemmal Ca^{2+} channels (DHPRs) and subsequent Ca^{2+} influx from the extracellular space. Ca^{2+} entry through DHPRs occurs into a narrow cleft formed by sarcolemmal and t-tubular membranes (the "dyad") [7]. The structural architecture of the dyad in ventricular and, to a lesser extent, atrial myocytes accommodates key Ca^{2+} handling proteins in the EC-coupling process. As a result, DHPRs are in close proximity to RyR2s defining the profile of Ca^{2+} release in cardiac myocytes. Importantly, depolarized DHPRs mediate the initial elevation in $[Ca^{2+}]$, which acts as a trigger to activate Ca^{2+} release via juxtaposed RyR2s on the SR membranes. Activation of RyR2s is followed by their coordinated opening, thereby releasing a tenfold greater amount of Ca^{2+} from the SR than the initiating trigger, significantly amplifying $[Ca^{2+}]$ in the cytoplasm. This process is known as ▶ Ca^{2+}-induced Ca^{2+} Release (CICR) [8]. The Ca^{2+} dependency of the release of Ca^{2+} from the SR ("chemical coupling") and the absence of a physical interaction between DHPRs and RyR2s (no "mechanical coupling") constitute the major differences in the mechanisms of EC-coupling between skeletal and cardiac muscle. Summation of the EC-coupling events at each dyad and their diffusion out of the dyad gives rise to an increase in global intracellular Ca^{2+}. As a result, Ca^{2+} ions engage myofilament proteins, which then stimulate myocyte contraction via the actin–myosin contractile machinery, similarly to that described for skeletal muscle fibers [9].

EC-coupling events are short-lived. Atrial and ventricular myocytes reach peak contraction within a few tens of milliseconds after generation of the action potential at the SA node [10]. In order for cardiac myocytes to relax and the heart to enter diastole to allow for the next heartbeat, $[Ca^{2+}]$ needs to return to baseline levels. Indeed, to allow for the 500 beats per minute of a mouse heart, the cycle needs to be complete in around 100 ms. Unlike skeletal muscle fibers, reduction in $[Ca^{2+}]$ occurs by Ca^{2+} sequestration back into the SR and/or mitochondria, as well as extrusion from cell. The SERCA pump directs Ca^{2+} back into the SR and the plasma membrane NCX and Ca^{2+} ATPases transport Ca^{2+} to the extracellular space utilizing an electrochemical gradient. Ca^{2+} can also be sequestered into the mitochondria via the mitochondrial Ca^{2+} uniporter. Importantly, the relative contribution of SERCA and NCX in Ca^{2+} sequestration and removal varies between species. In rats, the activity of SERCA is higher in ventricle than in human ventricle and Ca^{2+} removal through NCX is lower (i.e., 92% for SERCA and 7% for NCX in rats vs. 70% for SERCA and 28% for NCX in humans) [11].

Exercise Intervention

Skeletal Muscle

Differences in certain steps of the EC-coupling cycle determine the ability of fast- and slow-twitch skeletal muscle fibers to withstand excess activity (e.g., exercise). For instance, repetitive excitation of the muscle fiber may lead to a less negative resting membrane potential and reduced depolarization caused by a decreased $[K^+]$ gradient across the sarcolemma, resulting in decreased fiber excitability. In addition, fewer RyR1s are under the direct control of the voltage-sensing DHPRs in slow- compared to fast-twitch fibers, explaining the slower and smaller Ca^{2+} transients measured in the former [12]. Finally, physiological factors, such as temperature, osmolality, $[H^+]$, and $[Mg^{2+}]$, affect the contractile apparatus and relaxation phase and determine the fatigue capacity of fast- and slow-twitch muscle fibers [13].

Cardiac Muscle

To accommodate the changing needs of the organism from states of rest to activity (i.e., exercise), the output of the heart is modified. This change in output is signaled by the sympathetic and parasympathetic branches of the autonomic nervous system, which act at the level of the pacemaker, conduction fibers, and individual myocytes. Many of the effects of these pathways are mediated through regulation of cellular cyclic AMP levels (cAMP), which act via protein kinase A (PKA) to phosphorylate proteins involved in EC-coupling. As a result of phosphorylation, activity of these proteins is changed [14]. For example, activation of β-adrenergic receptors by the sympathetic pathway leads to an increase in cAMP, which activates PKA, which then phosphorylates many targets including phospholamban (PLB) (the cardiac equivalent of sarcolipin). Phosphorylation of PLB causes its dissociation from SERCA relieving its inhibitory effect and allowing SERCA to sequester Ca^{2+} from the cytosol at a higher rate. Sympathetic stimulation increases heart rate (positive chronotropy), contractility (positive inotropy), and conduction velocity (positive dromotropy). Parasympathetic stimulation acts to bring the heart back to normal after the actions of the sympathetic nervous system by slowing down the heartrate, reducing contractility of the atrial cardiac myocardium, and reducing conduction velocity at the sinoatrial and atrioventricular nodes.

References

1. Meissner G (1994) Ryanodine receptor/Ca2+ release channels and their regulation by endogenous effectors. Annu Rev Physiol 56:485–508
2. Protasi F, Paolini C, Nakai J, Beam KG, Franzini-Armstrong C, Allen PD (2002) Multiple regions of RyR1 mediate functional and structural interactions with alpha(1 S)-dihydropyridine receptors in skeletal muscle. Biophys J 83:3230–3244
3. Guo W, Campbell KP (1995) Association of triadin with the ryanodine receptor and calsequestrin in the lumen of the sarcoplasmic reticulum. J Biol Chem 270:9027–9030
4. Williams DA, Head SI, Bakker AJ, Stephenson DG (1990) Resting calcium concentrations in isolated skeletal muscle fibres of dystrophic mice. J Physiol 428:243–256
5. Gordon AM, Homsher E, Regnier M (2000) Regulation of contraction in striated muscle. Physiol Rev 80:853–924
6. Fryer MW, Stephenson DG (1996) Total and sarcoplasmic reticulum calcium contents of skinned fibres from rat skeletal muscle. J Physiol 493(Pt 2):357–370
7. Bootman MD, Higazi DR, Coombes S, Roderick HL (2006) Calcium signalling during excitation-contraction coupling in mammalian atrial myocytes. J Cell Sci 119:3915–3925
8. Roderick HL, Berridge MJ, Bootman MD (2003) Calcium-induced calcium release. Curr Biol 13:R425
9. Sham JS, Cleemann L, Morad M (1995) Functional coupling of Ca2+ channels and ryanodine receptors in cardiac myocytes. Proc Natl Acad Sci USA 92:121–125
10. Luss I, Boknik P, Jones LR, Kirchhefer U, Knapp J, Linck B, Luss H, Meissner A, Muller FU, Schmitz W et al (1999) Expression of cardiac

E

calcium regulatory proteins in atrium v ventricle in different species. J Mol Cell Cardiol 31:1299–1314

11. Bers DM (2002) Cardiac excitation-contraction coupling. Nature 415:198–205

12. Fryer MW, Neering IR (1989) Actions of caffeine on fast- and slow-twitch muscles of the rat. J Physiol 416:435–454

13. Pate E, Bhimani M, Franks-Skiba K, Cooke R (1995) Reduced effect of pH on skinned rabbit psoas muscle mechanics at high temperatures: implications for fatigue. J Physiol 486(Pt 3):689–694

14. Klabunde RE (2005) Cardiovascular physiology concepts. Lippincott Williams & Wilkins, Philadelphia

Executive Control

A set of cognitive operations underlying the selection, scheduling, coordination, and monitoring of complex, goal-directed processes involved in perception, memory, and action. These processes are dependent on a variety of brain circuits with the most important being the prefrontal and parietal regions. Executive control operations allow for the modulation and control of perceptual and emotional processes allowing for self-regulation of impulsive and sensation-seeking behaviors. Executive control functions mature late in development and decline earlier in late adulthood.

Executive Functions

Executive functions are a group of cognitive functions that are crucial for goal formation, planning, carrying out goal-directed plans, and effective performance. The frontal lobes and their connections to other brain areas are the crucial neural substrates. Executive functions are most vulnerable to brain damage and the effects of aging.

Exercise

Exercise refers to planned, structured, and repetitive movement to improve or maintain one or more components of physical fitness and/or to enhance motor task performance. It covers all forms of conscious and active muscle movements. These movements can be part of different activities like laboring, training, sports activities, lifestyle activities, and warfare. Exercise performance is of two types: rhythmic (aerobic exercise) and isometric (anaerobic exercise). The latter form of exercise is of short duration. In many physical activities, both forms of exercise are involved.

Cross-References

► Speed Training
► Training, Aerobic

Exercise Acidosis

► Acidosis

Exercise and Cancer-Related Side Effects

► Cancer, Therapy

Exercise and Immune Function

► Immune System
► Mucosal Immunity

Exercise and Mental Health

► Cognition

Exercise and Neurocognitive Function

► Cognition

Exercise and Prognosis After Cancer Diagnosis

► Cancer, Therapy

Exercise and Risk of Upper Respiratory Tract Infection

▶ Immune System
▶ Mucosal Immunity

Exercise Associated Loose Stool

▶ Diarrhea, Exercise Induced

Exercise Capacity

Is the peak level of aerobic work one can perform. It is expressed in milliliters of oxygen utilized per kg of body weight per minute (Peak VO_2) or metabolic equivalents (METs; 1-MET = 3.5 ml of O_2/kg/min). This is equivalent to the amount of energy expended per kg of body weight, during 1 min of rest. Any activity above resting requires greater oxygen consumption, and therefore, yields a higher MET level.

Cross-References

▶ Maximal Oxygen Uptake
▶ Pulmonary System, Performance Limitation

Exercise ECG

▶ Ergometry
▶ Exercise Electrocardiogram

Exercise Electrocardiogram

JONATHAN N. MYERS
VA Palo Alto Health Care System, Stanford University, Palo Alto, CA, USA

Synonyms

Cardiopulmonary exercise test; Exercise ECG; Stress testing

Definition

The exercise electrocardiogram (ECG) is a well-established tool that has been used in cardiovascular medicine for much of the last century. While the exercise ECG is primarily designed to assess the presence of coronary artery disease (CAD), it has many applications. The majority of exercise ECGs are performed in adults with symptoms of CAD or those who have a high probability of having CAD. The procedure is usually conducted as part of a symptom-limited exercise test on a treadmill or a cycle ergometer. The test is often considered the "gatekeeper" to more expensive and/or invasive procedures, since it is usually the first diagnostic evaluation when an individual is suspected of having CAD.

Description

The clinical exercise test and accompanying exercise ECG is a widely used, noninvasive procedure that provides diagnostic, prognostic, and functional information for a wide spectrum of patients with cardiovascular, pulmonary, and other disorders. Graded exercise tests are used to assess a patient's ability to tolerate increased physical exertion, while ECG, hemodynamic, and symptomatic responses are monitored in a controlled environment. Graded, progressive exercise can produce abnormalities that are not present at rest, the most important of which are manifestations of myocardial ischemia, including ST segment changes on the ECG, symptoms, and electrical instability. The test is also commonly used to evaluate other system disorders, such as ventilatory gas exchange abnormalities in patients with pulmonary disease or chronic heart failure, symptoms associated with peripheral vascular disease, and even neurologic disorders.

In cardiovascular medicine, the exercise test is commonly used for evaluating the efficacy of medical therapy, for the assessment of interventions, and as a first-choice diagnostic tool in patients with suspected CAD. In its role as a "gatekeeper" to more expensive and invasive procedures [1, 2], the test has become even more important in the current era of health care cost containment. Although originally developed as a diagnostic tool, numerous studies have established the role of the exercise test in the selection of patients for cardiac transplantation, risk stratification after a myocardial infarction (MI), and the assessment of disability [1, 2]. Despite the burgeoning of related diagnostic techniques, guidelines have recommended that the exercise test remain the first-choice modality for diagnosis of CAD [1]. This is because the use of the exercise ECG prior to other, more technological, imaging techniques has been demonstrated to be effective

E

in eliminating costly and unnecessary diagnostic procedures.

The exercise test has numerous indications. The most common reason patients are referred for exercise testing is for the evaluation of chest pain, or more generally, to assess signs and symptoms of coronary disease. Other common clinical objectives include the following:

- Physiologic response of post-MI and post-revascularization patients to exercise
- Functional capacity for the purpose of exercise prescription
- Exercise capacity for the purpose of work classification (disability evaluation) and risk stratification (prognosis)
- The efficacy of medical, surgical, or pharmacologic treatment
- The presence and severity of arrhythmias
- Preoperative physiologic status
- Intermittent claudication

Clinical Applications

In patients with CAD, exercise can cause an imbalance between myocardial oxygen supply and demand (ischemia), which can result in an alteration (decrease or elevation relative to the baseline) in the ST segment of the electrocardiogram. These changes are the foundation of the exercise test clinically. Typical normal and abnormal ST segment responses to exercise are illustrated in Fig. 1. Ever since electrocardiographic changes were first associated with myocardial ischemia in the 1920s, the diagnostic ECG criteria and leads that exhibit abnormalities during exercise have been the source of significant debate. Numerous ECG criteria, including complex mathematical constructs, combined scores, and ST areas during

exercise and recovery, have been proposed to optimally diagnose the presence of CAD. However, guidelines on exercise testing from national and international organizations have continued to suggest the application of a traditional diagnostic criterion: 1.0 mm or greater ▶ ST segment depression that is horizontal or down-sloping 60–80 milliseconds after the J-point (a "positive" response). ST segment depression greater than 1.0 mm that is down-sloping is generally indicative of more severe CAD. The vast majority of ischemic ST changes occur in the lateral precordial leads, although on rare occasion ST abnormalities may be isolated to the inferior leads. When the latter occurs, the ▶ predictive value of the test is lower.

The significance of ▶ ST segment elevation depends on the presence or absence of Q waves. When ST elevation occurs in the presence of a normal resting ECG, it is usually indicative of severe transmural ischemia, it can be arrhythmogenic, and it localizes the ischemia. Conversely, exercise-induced ST segment elevation occurring in leads with Q waves is more common and is related to the presence of dyskinetic areas. This response is relatively common in patients after an MI and is of much less concern.

There are several important nuances concerning the proper measurement of exercise-induced ST segment changes. ST segment depression is measured as a change from the isoelectric line (PR segment) and is considered abnormal if the next 60–80 ms after the J-point is flat or down-sloping. However, in patients who exhibit ST segment depression at rest, exercise-induced ST depression is measured from the baseline (resting) level. In contrast, ST segment elevation is measured from the level at which the ST segment starts, and slope is not considered. Examples of these are illustrated in Fig. 2. The significance of up-sloping or horizontal ST segment depression with T-wave inversion

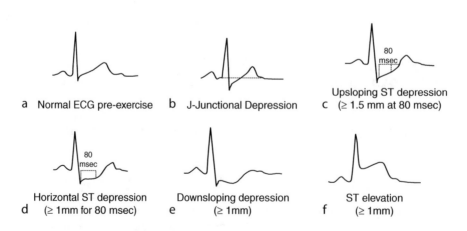

a Normal ECG pre-exercise   b J-Junctional Depression   c Upsloping ST depression (≥ 1.5 mm at 80 msec)

d Horizontal ST depression (≥ 1mm for 80 msec)   e Downsloping depression (≥ 1mm)   f ST elevation (≥ 1mm)

Exercise Electrocardiogram. Fig. 1 Examples of normal and abnormal ST segment responses to exercise

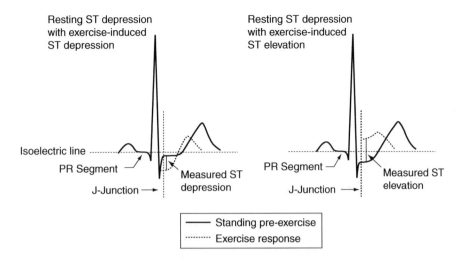

Exercise Electrocardiogram. Fig. 2 Example of exercise-induced ST segment *depression* when the ST segment is depressed at rest (*left*) and an example of ST *elevation* when there is resting ST segment depression (*right*)

has been debated. Infarction, ventricular aneurysm, bundle-branch block, hypokalemia, ventricular hypertrophy, abnormal oxygen-carrying capacity of blood caused by anemia, pulmonary disease, and drugs such as digoxin and quinidine may all influence the ST segment response; these and other conditions may cause exercise-induced ST segment depression that is not caused by CAD.

Diagnostic Characteristics. How accurately the exercise ECG distinguishes those with disease from those without disease depends on the population tested, the definition of disease, and the criteria used for an abnormal test. The most common terms used to describe test accuracy are ▶ sensitivity and ▶ specificity. Sensitivity is the percentage of times a test correctly identifies those with CAD. Specificity is the percentage of times a test correctly identifies those without CAD. Sensitivity and specificity are inversely related and are affected by the choice of discriminant value for abnormal, the definition of disease, and, most importantly, by the prevalence of disease in the population tested. For example, if the population has a greater prevalence or severity of disease (such as coronary disease in multiple vessels), the test will have a higher sensitivity. Alternatively, the test will have a higher specificity (and low sensitivity) when performed in a group of younger, healthier subjects. Studies have shown that the exercise ECG more accurately diagnoses CAD when combined with other pre-test risk information and other exercise test responses (e.g., using multivariate *scores*) [3].

A widely cited meta-analysis of the exercise testing literature indicates that the exercise ECG has, on the average, a sensitivity of approximately 68% and a specificity of approximately 77% [4]. However, these

values range widely in the various studies; the diagnostic performance of the exercise ECG depends highly upon the pre-test probability of disease. For example, sensitivity can be as low as 40% among patients with single-vessel disease, but greater than 90% among those with triple-vessel disease. Conversely, the specificity of the test is usually quite low (i.e., 50–60%) in patients who have more severe CAD but is quite high in populations that are relatively healthy. These values reported in the literature and the inverse relationship between sensitivity and specificity underscore the importance of considering the patient's pre-test characteristics (chest pain and CAD risk factors) before beginning the test. No test result can be interpreted accurately without considering the patient in the context of his or her pre-test characteristics.

Another important term that helps define the diagnostic value of a test is the predictive value. The predictive value of an abnormal test (positive predictive value) is the percentage of people with an abnormal test result who have disease. Conversely, the predictive value of a normal test (negative predictive value) is the percentage of people with a normal test result who do not have disease. The predictive value of a test cannot be determined directly from the sensitivity and specificity but is strongly associated with the prevalence of disease in the population tested. The calculations used to determine sensitivity, specificity, and predictive value are presented in Table 1.

Summary. Although there have been many advances in technologies related to the diagnosis of CAD, the numerous applications and widespread availability of the exercise test continue to make it one of the more important tools in cardiovascular medicine. Advantages of the

Exercise Electrocardiogram. Table 1 Terms used to demonstrate the diagnostic value of a test

Sensitivity	$\frac{TP}{TP+FN} \times 100$
Specificity	$\frac{TP}{TN+FP} \times 100$
Positive predictive value	$\frac{TP}{TP+FP} \times 100$
Negative predictive value	$\frac{TN}{TN+FN} \times 100$

TP true positives, or those with abnormal test results and with disease; *FN* false negatives, or those with normal test results with disease; *FP* false positives, or those with abnormal test results and no disease; *TN* true negatives, or those with normal test results and no disease.

exercise ECG relative to other diagnostic procedures include the fact that it is noninvasive, inexpensive, and that the test is often performed by non-cardiologists in the office setting. Therefore, it continues to have an important place as a first-choice modality in determining the presence of CAD, in which the test is often used to determine which patients require further work-up or referral to a cardiologist or another specialist. Guidelines recommend that the exercise ECG be performed prior to more expensive and invasive diagnostic procedures since this approach has been shown to avoid unnecessary procedures and to be cost-effective. In addition to the diagnostic information from the ECG, the exercise test contains a wealth of other clinically useful information. For example, exercise capacity is a powerful prognostic marker [5], and symptoms, ECG abnormalities, rate-pressure product achieved, and heart rate in recovery from exercise all provide important information for stratifying risk in patients with or at risk for cardiovascular disease. Other applications include the assessment of therapy, exercise prescription, and helping to guide medical/surgical management decisions for the patient.

References

1. Gibbons RJ, Balady GJ, Bricker JT, ACC/AHA et al (2002) Guideline update for exercise testing. A report of the ACC/AHA task force on practice guidelines (Committee on Exercise Testing). J Am Coll Cardiol 40:1531–1540
2. Froelicher VF, Myers J (2006) Exercise and the heart, 5th edn. W.B. Saunders, Philadelphia
3. Ashley E, Myers J, Froelicher V (2002) Exercise testing scores as an example of better decisions through science. Med Sci Sports Exerc 34:1391–1398
4. Gianrossi R, Detrano R, Mulvihill D, Lehmann K, Dubach P, Colombo A, Mcarthur D, Froelicher V (1989) Exercise-indiced ST depression in the diagnosis of coronary artery disease. A meta-analysis. Circulation 80:87–98
5. Kodama S, Saito K, Tanaka S et al (2010) Cardiorespiratory fitness as a quantitative predictor of all-cause mortality and cardiovascular events in healthy men and women: a meta-analysis. JAMA 301:2024–2035

Exercise in Type 2 Diabetes Mellitus

▶ Diabetes Mellitus, Sports Therapy

Exercise Preconditioning

A cardiac phenotype that is resistant to IR injury subsequent to the therapeutic condition of exercise.

Cross-References
▶ Ischemia-Reperfusion Injury, Exercise-Induced Cardioprotection

Exercise Prescription

The *F*requency (how often), *I*ntensity (how hard), *T*ime (how long), and *T*ype (what modality) of physical activity or *FITT*.

Exercise Testing

PETER H. BRUBAKER
Department of Health and Exercise Science, Wake Forest University, Winston-Salem, NC, USA

Synonyms
Graded exercise testing (GXT); Stress testing

Definition
A test used to provide information about how the cardiovascular and pulmonary systems respond to physical stress. It usually involves walking on a treadmill or pedaling a stationary bike at increasing levels of difficulty, while the electrocardiogram, heart rate, and blood pressure are monitored. In some situations, expired pulmonary gas measurements are also obtained. Thus, the "stress" test can be used to: evaluate the presence of ▶ myocardial ischemia, evaluate the effectiveness of medical/pharmacologic therapy, determine the need for further invasive diagnostic testing, determine ▶ functional capacity/physical fitness, and obtain data to generate an individualized "exercise prescription."

Description

Of the many advances in the diagnosis of coronary artery disease (CAD), exercise testing remains an indispensable tool. When performed appropriately, exercise testing yields valuable diagnostic, prognostic, functional, and therapeutic information at a relatively low cost and with minimal risk. Data from several studies indicate that exercise testing is safe, even in high-risk patients, with no more than one death, four myocardial infarctions, and approximately five hospital admissions per 10,000 exercise tests [1]. Prior to an exercise test, a complete medical history and a physical examination to identify contraindications for exercise testing should be standard practice. When any absolute contraindications to exercise are identified, the patient should be referred to a primary physician for further medical management. Patients with relative contraindications may be tested after careful evaluation of the risk-benefit ratio for the exercise test. Major CAD risk factors and signs, and symptoms of cardiopulmonary disease should be used to stratify patient risk and to determine the appropriate level of medical supervision. The patient should be advised prior to the test to refrain from food, alcohol, caffeine, or tobacco within 3 h of testing. Patients should be well rested for the exercise test; therefore, they should also be advised to avoid vigorous activity on the day of testing. Patients should continue any prescribed medical regimens, unless instructed otherwise by a physician. The exercise test administrator should explain the potential risks and discomforts associated with exercise testing to the patient as thoroughly as possible. Specific steps should be taken to ensure patient safety during the test, such as a demonstration of the safe use of the testing modality. Steps should also be taken to reduce patient anxiety, such as answering questions and describing expectations (reporting symptoms, level of exertion expected, test endpoints, etc.). Informed consent should be obtained, as it has important ethical and legal implications and ensures the patient is aware of the purposes and risks associated with test. To ensure patient comfort during the testing procedure, patients should be advised to wear clothing that is comfortable and that provides freedom of movement. Suggestions should be made regarding clothing that allows the technician to place electrocardiogram (ECG) electrodes and the blood pressure cuff appropriately. Proper fitting shoes with rubber soles should also be recommended to ensure good traction, particularly for treadmill testing.

The specific exercise test should be selected on the basis of the purpose of the test, the health and fitness status of the client, and should consider the most appropriate exercise modality and the most appropriate exercise protocol. In many exercise laboratories, these issues are determined by the availability of equipment and by custom; however, each can have a profound effect on the response to the exercise test. The purpose of exercise testing is to increase total body and myocardial oxygen demand at safe increments within a reasonable time period. This requires dynamic exercise that uses major muscle groups, permitting a large increase in cardiac output, oxygen delivery, and gas exchange. The modalities used for diagnostic testing include cycle ergometers, treadmills, arm ergometers, steps, and, in some cases, chemical stressors (aka "pharmacologic" stress testing). The bicycle ergometer and treadmill are the most commonly used exercise testing modalities. A bicycle is generally less expensive, occupies less space, and is less noisy. During cycling, upper body motion is decreased, making blood pressure and ECG recording easier. The workload on simple, mechanically braked bicycle ergometers is not always accurate, however, and is dependent upon pedaling speed, which may vary. This variation in workload can be overcome by using electronically braked bicycle ergometers, which maintain a constant workload over a wide range of pedaling speeds. In either case, bicycle ergometer work is typically expressed in kilogram-meters per minute (kgm/min), or watts. The treadmill is used mainly in North America. It is more expensive than a cycle ergometer, is relatively immobile, and noisier. Researchers comparing treadmill and bicycle ergometry report that maximal oxygen uptake is 10–20% higher (range, 6–25%) and maximal heart rate is 5–20% higher on the treadmill compared with the cycle ergometer [2]. A slightly higher incidence of ST segment changes and angina has been reported during treadmill testing. Exercise-induced myocardial ischemia identified by thallium scintigraphy has been reported to be greater after treadmill testing than after cycle ergometry. Although most of the differences between the two modalities are minor, the treadmill may be preferred when the major goals of the test are to optimally assess the patient's functional limits and to identify ischemia. It is most appropriate to select an exercise protocol based on the patient being tested and the purpose of the exercise test. Figure 1 presents many of the protocols used for either the treadmill or bicycle ergometer [1]. Electrocardiography (ECG) and blood pressure are integral parts of cardiopulmonary assessment during exercise testing. Proper skin preparation techniques and precise electrode placement are critical in obtaining an accurate electrocardiograph. In clinical settings, the 12-lead Mason-Likar placement is generally used because it produces fewer artifacts and

Exercise Testing. Fig. 1 Common exercise protocols and associated metabolic costs of each stage

Functional class / clinical status (left margin):

- FUNCTIONAL CLASS: NORMAL AND I, II, III, IV
- CLINICAL STATUS: HEALTHY, DEPENDENT ON AGE, ACTIVITY — SEDENTARY HEALTHY — LIMITED — SYMPTOMATIC

METS	O_2 COST ml/kg/min	BICYCLE ERGOMETER for 70 KG body weight Kpm/min (WATTS)	BRUCE 3 MIN STAGES MPH / % GR	BRUCE RAMP PER MIN MPH / % GR	USAFSAM MPH / % GR	"SLOW" USAFSAM MPH / % GR	MODIFIED BALKE MPH / % GR	ACIP MPH / % GR	MOD. NAUGHTON (CHF) MPH / % GR
21	73.5		5.5 / 20	5.8 / 20					
20	70			5.6 / 19					
19	66.5			5.3 / 18					
18	63		5.0 / 18	5.0 / 18					
17	59.5			4.6 / 17					
16	56.0		4.2 / 16	4.5 / 16	3.3 / 25				
15	52.5	1500 (246)		4.2 / 16				3.4 / 24.0	
14	49.0		3.4 / 14	4.1 / 15	3.3 / 20		3.0 / 25	3.1 / 24.0	3.0 / 25
13	45.5	1350 (221)		3.8 / 14			3.0 / 22.5		3.0 / 22.5
12	42.0		2.5 / 12	3.4 / 14	3.3 / 15		3.0 / 20	3.0 / 21.0	3.0 / 20
11	38.5	1200 (197)		3.1 / 13		2 / 25	3.0 / 17.5	3.0 / 17.5	3.0 / 17.5
10	35.0	1050 (172)	1.7 / 10	2.6 / 12	3.3 / 10		3.0 / 15	3.0 / 14.0	3.0 / 15
9	31.5	900 (148)		2.5 / 12		2 / 20	3.0 / 12.5		3.0 / 12.5
8	28.0	750 (123)		2.3 / 11			3.0 / 10	3.0 / 10.5	3.0 / 10
7	24.5			2.1 / 10	3.3 / 5	2 / 15	3.0 / 7.5	3.0 / 7.0	3.0 / 7.5
6	21.0	600 (98)		1.7 / 10			3.0 / 5		2.0 / 10.5
5	17.5	450 (74)				2 / 10	3.0 / 2.5	3.0 / 3.0	2.0 / 7.0
4	14.0	300 (49)		1.3 / 5	3.3 / 0	2 / 5	3.0 / 0	2.5 / 2.0	2.0 / 3.5
3	10.5			1.0 / 0	2.0 / 0	2 / 0	2.0 / 0	2.0 / 0.0	1.5 / 0
2	7.0	150 (24)							1.0 / 0
1	3.5								

RAMP protocol — PER 30 SEC, MPH / % GR (3.0 MPH throughout except lower stages):

3.0 / 25.0, 3.0 / 24.0, 3.0 / 23.0, 3.0 / 22.0, 3.0 / 21.0, 3.0 / 20.0, 3.0 / 19.0, 3.0 / 18.0, 3.0 / 17.0, 3.0 / 16.0, 3.0 / 15.0, 3.0 / 14.0, 3.0 / 13.0, 3.0 / 12.0, 3.0 / 11.0, 3.0 / 10.0, 3.0 / 9.0, 3.0 / 8.0, 3.0 / 7.0, 3.0 / 6.0, 3.0 / 5.0, 3.0 / 4.0, 3.0 / 3.0, 3.0 / 2.0, 3.0 / 1.0, 3.0 / 0, 2.5 / 0, 2.0 / 0, 1.5 / 0, 1.0 / 0, 0.5 / 0

BALKE-WARE protocol — % GRADE AT 3.3 MPH, 1 MIN STAGES:

26, 25, 24, 23, 22, 21, 20, 19, 18, 17, 16, 15, 14, 13, 12, 11, 10, 9, 8, 7, 6, 5, 4, 3, 2, 1

restricts movement less than the standard limb placement procedure. During the exercise test, at least three ECG leads (representing lateral, inferior, and anterior views) should be monitored continuously. A 12-Lead ECG should be recorded in the latter part of each stage, and more often if an abnormal reading or clinical symptoms are observed. During exercise testing, the ECG is used to evaluate the presence of conduction defects, atrial and ventricular arrhythmias, as well as myocardial ischemia. Patients referred for exercise testing are likely to be taking medications that can have significant effects on the ECG and hemodynamic responses. The most common medications are beta blockers and calcium channel-blocking agents, which attenuate heart rate at rest and during exercise. In part, because of the effects of these medications, age-predicted maximal heart rate should not be used as a test endpoint. Blood pressure should be assessed at rest as well as during the last minute of each stage of testing, and more frequently if hypotension or hypertension is apparent. Normally, SBP increases with increases in workload. Values exceeding 200 mmHg are not uncommon. However, when the SBP exceeds 250 mmHg, the test should be terminated [1]. The DBP normally stays the same or increases slightly during exercise. The fifth Korotkoff sound is frequently heard to 0 mmHg in some young, healthy individuals. When the DBP exceeds 115 mmHg, the test should be terminated [1]. If the SBP falls with increased workload, the blood pressure should immediately be taken again; if SBP decreases >10–20 mmHg, the test should be terminated, particularly if symptoms are present [1].

When measured, oxygen consumption (VO_2) and other ventilatory variables provide important information about cardiopulmonary function. Maximal oxygen consumption (VO_2max or VO_2peak) is the most common and, generally, the most useful measurement derived from gas exchange data during an exercise test. VO_2max defines the upper limits of cardiorespiratory function (i.e., the ability to increase heart rate, stroke volume, and oxygen extraction by active muscles). The clinical importance of an objective and accurate measurement of exercise capacity is underscored by studies on ▶ prognosis in patients with heart disease. In a review of the literature, exercise capacity was selected most frequently as a significant determinant of survival [3]. In ▶ heart failure patients, peak oxygen consumption (VO_2max) is one of the best predictors of survival and is widely used to determine the timing of cardiac transplantation. Although VO_2max is most accurately determined by measuring expired gases directly, the technology to do so is not always available. Equations that can be used to predict

VO_2max (also expressed as METS by dividing VO_2 by 3.5) for walking, running, arm and leg ergometry, as well as stair stepping have been described [1]. These equations were developed from experiments that used primarily young, healthy subjects during steady-state exercise; therefore, their use in other populations may result in significant errors in the prediction of VO_2max. Many factors such as age, functional capacity, disease status, medications, and use of handrail support can affect the accuracy of predicting VO_2. Ventilatory and gas exchange variables should be monitored continuously during exercise since they may be useful in determining maximum exertion and endpoints of testing. Symptoms, deconditioning, and/or unwillingness to tolerate fatigue may prevent the patient from reaching maximal levels; when these factors arise, it may be more appropriate to use the term VO_2peak. Although breath-by-breath measurements of VO_2 and other gas exchange parameters are now widely available on modern systems, they should be reserved for specific research applications. Peak exercise values based on 30-s averages represent an acceptable balance between precision and variability and are the most commonly used sample in the literature [3].

Symptoms and perception of effort should be assessed during exercise to help ensure patient safety and to optimize the diagnostic information yield. In order to make a valid assessment of subjective variables during exercise, the exercise professional must explain the scoring scale thoroughly prior to testing. For example, angina and ▶ dyspnea (the most common symptoms elicited during exercise testing) are each usually evaluated on a 4-point scale [2]. Patients should be encouraged to report all symptoms. In addition, they should be evaluated by the test administrator at least once during each stage of the exercise test for the presence of cardiopulmonary symptoms, such as angina and dyspnea. The combination of angina and an abnormal ST response during an exercise test is 98% predictive of significant CAD [4]. Moderately severe angina (grade III) and pain that would normally cause cessation of daily activities and/or nitroglycerin administration are indications to terminate exercise [1]. Dyspnea can be the predominant symptom in some patients with CAD, but it is more often associated with reduced left ventricular function or chronic obstructive pulmonary disease. In the former, it is usually accompanied by poor exercise capacity and can occur with an impaired SBP response. Dyspnea is appropriately quantified using a 4-point scale [1]. The rating of perceived exertion (RPE), when properly assessed during exercise, can be used to identify the endpoint of maximum effort. The Borg perceived exertion scale provides reproducible measures of effort and is generally not affected by medications, such as beta blockers [1]. An RPE should be obtained at least once during each stage of the exercise test.

The exercise test should include evaluation of the ECG, symptoms, and hemodynamic responses in recovery. Whether postexercise activities should be active or passive is a controversial issue. For diagnostic purposes, the supine position may be the most valuable immediately after exercise because it increases venous return, thereby increasing ventricular volume, myocardial wall stress, and consequently, myocardial oxygen consumption [2]. Several studies have shown that ST segment

Variable	Prior to exercise test	During the test	After exercise test
ECG	Monitored continuously; recorded supine position and posture of exercise	Monitored continuously; recorded during the last 15 s of each stage (interval protocol) or the last 15 s of each 2 min time period (ramp protocols)	Monitored continuously; recorded immediately post exercise, during the last 15 s of first minute of recovery and then every 2 min thereafter
HR[a]	Monitored continuously; recorded supine position and posture of exercise	Monitored continuously; recorded during the last 5 s of each minute	Monitored continuously; recorded during the last 5 s of each minute
BP[a,b]	Measured and recorded in supine position and posture of exercise	Measured and recorded during the last 45 s of each stage (interval protocol) or the last 45 s of each 2 min time period (ramp protocols)	Measured and recorded immediately post exercise and then every 2 min thereafter
Signs and Symptoms	Monitored continuously; recorded as observed	Monitored continuously; recorded as observed	Monitored continuously; recorded as observed
RPE	Explain scale	Recorded during the last 5 s of each minute	Obtain peak exercise value then not measured in recovery
Gas Exchange	Baseline reading to assure proper operational status	Measured continuously	Not needed in recovery

Exercise Testing. Fig. 2 Recommended monitoring intervals associated with exercise testing

abnormalities are enhanced in the supine position and that active recovery may attenuate these changes. ST segments observed 3–4 min into recovery may be helpful in detecting ischemia. Patients with symptom-limiting angina or dyspnea may have greater discomfort in the supine position and should be placed in a seated or semirecumbent position during recovery. A passive recovery in the standing position should be avoided due to potential complications associated with venous pooling. For a nondiagnostic test, such as when screening asymptomatic individuals, an active recovery at a low workload is more comfortable, is less likely to be associated with a hypotensive response, and may minimize the risk of dysrhythmia secondary to elevated catecholamines [2]. Regardless of the protocol, the recovery period should be monitored for at least 5 min. Blood pressure, ECG, and symptoms should be monitored and recorded at 1–2 min intervals. The recovery period should be extended to resolve symptoms or abnormal hemodynamic and/or ECG responses. A summary of the type and timing of measures that should be made during an exercise test are presented in Fig. 2.

Application

The majority of patients sent for exercise testing are referred for an evaluation of chest pain, most commonly to help make a diagnosis of CAD. Thus, the exercise test serves as a screen for further evaluation. Any screening test must be evaluated for its sensitivity and specificity for the condition being evaluated. Sensitivity is the percentage of tests that correctly identify that condition, in this case, CAD. Specificity is the percentage of tests that correctly identify individuals without CAD. The average reported sensitivity and specificity for ECG stress testing is 67% and 70%, respectively [5]. Sensitivity and specificity are inversely related. In addition, they vary with the population tested, the definition of the disease, and the criteria used for an abnormal test. A variety of factors can cause false-positive or false-negative test responses and should be evaluated before the exercise test. A false-positive test (an abnormal response in an individual without disease) will decrease specificity. A false-negative test (a normal response in an individual with disease) causes the sensitivity to be reduced. When a false-positive or false-negative response is suspected, an alternative diagnostic procedure may be indicated, such as an exercise or pharmacologic echocardiogram or radionuclide test.

Exercise testing is valuable in determining the prognosis, or probability of a given outcome of disease, of patients with cardiovascular disease [4]. Prognosis should be estimated because it provides information that can be useful for planning vocational and recreational activity and making important financial decisions. It is also useful for identifying additional interventions that may improve the outcome of therapy. An accurate estimation of risk can be obtaining by using any of a number of techniques to "score" exercise tests [3].

Radionuclide imaging complements the exercise ECG during exercise testing in known or suspected cases of CAD. It is particularly helpful with an equivocal exercise ECG or in patients who are likely to exhibit false-positive or false-negative responses. Nuclear imaging can be used to clarify the meaning of an abnormal ST segment response in asymptomatic individuals or the cause of chest discomfort. Patients with a positive exercise ECG and a positive radionuclide scan are 2.6 times more likely to have a subsequent event than patients with negative results [5]. Nuclear imaging of the coronary vessels is somewhat more sensitive and specific for CAD than the exercise ECG. The literature suggests that sensitivity and specificity of exercise thallium scintigraphy are 84% and 87%, respectively [5]. This modality also permits localization of ischemia, which is not possible with an ECG, and permits differentiation between fixed defects (representing myocardial infarction) and reversible defects (representing ischemia). Echocardiography is being used more often during exercise and pharmacologic testing. The diagnostic accuracy of echocardiography depends primarily on the methodology and as well as the clinical experience of the interpreter. The sensitivity and specificity of this technique are both approximately 85% [5].

Cross-References

▶ Ergometry

References

1. American College of Sports Medicine (2010) Guidelines for exercise testing and exercise prescription, 8th edn. Lippincott, Williams & Wilkins, Philadelphia
2. Brubaker P, Kaminsky L, Whaley M (2002) Coronary artery disease: essentials for prevention and rehabilitation programs. Human Kinetics, Champaign
3. Myers J (1996) Essentials of cardiopulmonary exercise testing. Human Kinetics, Champaign
4. Gibbons RJ, Balady GJ, Beasley JW, Bricker JT, Duvernoy WFC, Froelicher VF et al (2002) ACC/AHA guidelines for exercise testing: ACC/AHA 2002 guideline update for exercise testing: summary article. Circulation 106:1883–1892
5. Fletcher J, Balady G, Amsterdam E, Chaitman B, Eckel B, Fleg J et al (2001) Exercise standards for testing and training: a statement for healthcare professionals from the American Heart Association. Circulation 104:1694–1740

E

Exercise Training

Refers to habitual engagement in dynamic, whole-body exercise consisting of repeated skeletal muscle contractions and significantly increased metabolic rate. Examples include jogging/running, hiking, road or mountain cycling, rowing, and cross-country skiing. A variety of other physical activities are also relevant, however, such as soccer, ice hockey, figure skating, field hockey, and speed skating, among others. Thus, any activity that requires significantly increased metabolic and ventilation rates for extended periods of time during training or competition may be regarded as germane to this discussion. Regular physical aerobic exercise should be done daily, or at least 5–6 days a week, with an intensity of 70% of maximal exercise capacity during 30–45 min, alternatively, 20% can be covered with strength training. It thus can cut the risk for impaired glucose tolerance by half and the diabetes risk by up to three quarters. Endurance training is also recommended for patients with stable coronary artery disease. It increases exercise performance, improves the cardiovascular risk profile, reduces the cardiovascular complication rate, improves the myocardial perfusion, and also slows the progression of coronary artery disease. It is important to keep in mind that only moderate-intensity aerobic exercise augments the endothelium-dependent vasodilation in humans, whereas high-intensity exercise possibly increases the oxidative stress and risk for cardiovascular complications. It has further been demonstrated that exercise training, but not dietary lifestyle changes with food restriction, prevents endothelial dysfunction, although hyperglycemia, dyslipidemia, sensitivity to insulin, and abdominal fat content improved with both strategies.

Cross-References
▶ Cardiac Hypertrophy, Physiological
▶ Chronic Obstructive Pulmonary Disease
▶ Hypertension, Training
▶ Pulmonary System, Training Adaptation

Exercise Ventilation

▶ Pulmonary System, Performance Limitation

Exercise-Associated Functional Hypothalamic Amenorrhea

▶ Athletic Amenorrhea

Exercise-Associated Menstrual Disorder

▶ Athletic Amenorrhea

Exercise-Induced Adaptations

▶ Training, Adaptations

Exercise-Induced Airway Dysfunction

▶ Pulmonary System, Training Adaptation
▶ Pulmonary System, Performance Limitation

Exercise-Induced Asthma

Kai-Håkon Carlsen
Oslo University Hospital, Rikshospitalet, Deptartment of Paediatrics, University of Oslo, Norwegian School of Sport Sciences, Oslo, Norway

Synonyms
Exercise-induced bronchoconstriction; Exercise-induced bronchospasm; Indirect bronchial hyperresponsiveness to exercise

Definition
Exercise-induced asthma (EIA) and exercise-induced bronchoconstriction (EIB) are often used interchangeably but were recently defined with slightly different meanings: Exercise-induced asthma is defined by respiratory symptoms of bronchial obstruction and asthma occurring shortly after heavy exercise, whereas exercise-induced bronchoconstriction is defined as the reduction in lung function, forced expiratory volume in 1 s (FEV_1), occurring after a standardized exercise test [1]. EIB is seen as a measure of indirect non-specific bronchial hyperresponsiveness.

Mechanisms

Mechanisms of Exercise-Induced Asthma
Two hypotheses aim to outline the relation between physical activity and EIA: one relates to cooling of the airways

due to the increased ventilation during exercise, while the other hypothesis relates to increased water loss from the respiratory tract also caused by increased ventilation during exercise. Airway cooling caused by respiratory heat loss during the much increased ventilation due to physical exercise is thought to cause vasoconstriction in bronchial vessels followed by a secondary reactive hyperemia with resulting edema and airways narrowing in addition to nervous stimulation through the parasympathetic nerves [2, 3]. On the other hand, water loss is caused by the high ventilation rates of top athletes (up to >280 L/min) during exercise due to the saturation of the inhaled air with water. This results in increased osmolarity of the periciliary fluid lining the respiratory mucosal membranes. This is postulated to cause mediator release, increased airway inflammation, and bronchial constriction [4]. The use of inhaled mannitol to diagnose bronchial hyperresponsiveness further confirms this hypothesis [5].

Mechanisms of Asthma and Bronchial Hyperresponsiveness Occurring in Elite Athletes

An increase in BHR caused by highly intensive exercise was first demonstrated in Norwegian competitive swimmers after swimming exercise of 3,000 m [6] and later in young cross-country skiers during the winter season [7]. Heavy endurance training, especially when performed in an unfortunate environment, causes inflammation in the airway mucosal membranes, as shown by Sue-Chu et al. in bronchial biopsies from heavily training young skiers without asthma but with increased airway responsiveness to cold air [8, 9]. They found airway inflammation with lymphoid aggregates and increased tenascin expression (the thickness of the tenascin-specific immunoreactivity band in the basement membrane) in the skiers. Larsson showed that cold air inhalation increased the number of inflammatory cells in bronchoalveolar lavage [10]. Bernard and co-workers found that the time spent in swimming pools during early childhood was related to asthma development and markers of lung involvement as shown by increased serum levels of surfactant proteins [11] and reduced levels of Clara cell protein [12]. Also, respiratory tract infections increase bronchial responsiveness in actively training athletes [13]. The combination of heavy repeated exercise with an unfavorable environment, such as cold air in cross-country skiers and chlorine-containing humid air by swimmers, may thus be important for the development of asthma and bronchial hyperresponsiveness among top athletes.

Exercise Response

The typical response to exercise in individuals with EIA is shortness of breath, expiratory dyspnea, and objective signs of bronchial obstruction occurring shortly after a session of heavy physical exercise. EIA was previously thought to occur in 70–80% of asthmatics not receiving anti-inflammatory treatment [14]. However, in a more recent study, EIB was diagnosed after a standardized exercise test in 8.6% of a normal population of 10-year-old children and in 36.7% of the children with current asthma [15]. This change in reported occurrence of EIA may be due to the fact that many of the children with a diagnosis of asthma presently may have a milder asthma presentation than previously as a consequence of the heavily increased prevalence of asthma. However, Becker et al., reporting deaths linked to athletic performance over a 7-year period in the USA, illustrates the potential serious presentation of EIA. Out of 263 deaths related to athletic performance, 61 were due to asthma [16].

Diagnostics

The diagnosis of asthma is clinical and should be based upon history of symptoms, physical examination for the presence of bronchial obstruction, and variability in lung function spontaneously or due to bronchodilators. The term current asthma is used when at least one episode of asthma has occurred during the last year. An exact clinical history, examination with lung function measurements before and after inhalation of a β_2-agonist (requiring an increase in FEV_1 of 12%) and before and after a standardized exercise test such as treadmill run and/or a cold air inhalation test, and measurement of BHR by metacholine inhalation are parts of the diagnostic process. One important part of the diagnostic process is to follow up the patient to evaluate the treatment effect.

EIA may be diagnosed by exercise tests with a heavy exercise load recommended. A motor-driven treadmill may be employed with an inclination of 5.5%, rapidly increasing speed until a steady heart rate of approximately 95% of calculated maximum is reached, maintaining this for 4–6 min [17]. The running is performed with a room temperature of approximately 20°C and a relative humidity of approximately 40%. Lung function by FEV_1 is measured before running, immediately after cessation of running, and 3, 6, 10, 15, and 20 min after running. A fall of 10% is taken as a sign of EIB. Other tests used for the diagnosis of exercise-induced bronchoconstriction and BHR, especially in athletes, are eucapnic hyperventilation [18] and mannitol bronchial provocation, determining the inhaled dose causing a 15% decrease in FEV_1 [5].

Differential Diagnosis

There are several differential diagnoses to EIA, including poor physical fitness and other chronic disorders, like lung and heart disorders. One of the most common differential diagnoses is exercise-induced laryngeal inspiratory stridor or exercise-induced vocal cord dysfunction [19, 20]. Exercise-induced laryngeal stridor is more common among top trained adolescent female athletes. Audible inspiratory stridor during maximal exercise with a flattening of the maximal inspiratory flow volume curve [21] is typical, in contrast to EIA in which case expiratory dyspnea occurs after exercise. Other differential diagnoses in athletes include exercise-induced arterial hypoxemia [22] and swimming-induced pulmonary edema [23].

Cross-References

▶ Asthma Bronchiale

References

1. Carlsen KH, Anderson SD, Bjermer L, Bonini S, Brusasco V, Canonica W et al (2008) Exercise-induced asthma, respiratory and allergic disorders in elite athletes: epidemiology, mechanisms and diagnosis: part I of the report from the Joint Task Force of the European Respiratory Society (ERS) and the European Academy of Allergy and Clinical Immunology (EAACI) in cooperation with GA2LEN. Allergy 63(4):387–403
2. McFadden ER Jr (1990) Hypothesis: exercise-induced asthma as a vascular phenomenon. Lancet 335:880–883
3. Gilbert IA, McFadden ER Jr (1992) Airway cooling and rewarming. The second reaction sequence in exercise-induced asthma. J Clin Investig 90:699–704
4. Anderson SD, Daviskas E (1992) The airway microvasculature and exercise induced asthma. Thorax 47:748–752
5. Brannan JD, Koskela H, Anderson SD, Chew N (1998) Responsiveness to mannitol in asthmatic subjects with exercise- and hyperventilation-induced asthma. Am J Respir Crit Care Med 158(4):1120–1126
6. Carlsen KH, Oseid S, Odden H, Mellbye E (1989) The response to heavy swimming exercise in children with and without bronchial asthma. In: Morehouse CA (ed) Children and exercise XIII. Human Kinetics, Champaign, pp 351–360
7. Larsson K, Ohlsen P, Larsson L, Malmberg P, Rydstrom PO, Ulriksen H (1993) High prevalence of asthma in cross country skiers. BMJ 307(6915):1326–1329
8. Sue-Chu M, Karjalainen EM, Altraja A, Laitinen A, Laitinen LA, Naess AB et al (1998) Lymphoid aggregates in endobronchial biopsies from young elite cross-country skiers. Am J Respir Crit Care Med 158(2):597–601
9. Karjalainen EM, Laitinen A, Sue-Chu M, Altraja A, Bjermer L, Laitinen LA (2000) Evidence of airway inflammation and remodeling in ski athletes with and without bronchial hyperresponsiveness to metacholine. Am J Respir Crit Care Med 161(6):2086–2091
10. Larsson K, Tornling G, Gavhed D, Muller-Suur C, Palmberg L (1998) Inhalation of cold air increases the number of inflammatory cells in the lungs in healthy subjects. Eur Respir J 12(4):825–830
11. Bernard A, Carbonnelle S, Michel O, Higuet S, De Burbure C, Buchet JP et al (2003) Lung hyperpermeability and asthma prevalence in schoolchildren: unexpected associations with the attendance at indoor chlorinated swimming pools. Occup Environ Med 60(6):385–394
12. Lagerkvist BJ, Bernard A, Blomberg A, Bergstrom E, Forsberg B, Holmstrom K et al (2004) Pulmonary epithelial integrity in children: relationship to ambient ozone exposure and swimming pool attendance. Environ Health Perspect 112(17):1768–1771
13. Heir T, Aanestad G, Carlsen KH, Larsen S (1995) Respiratory tract infection and bronchial responsiveness in elite athletes and sedentary control subjects. Scand J Med Sci Sports 5:94–99
14. Lee TH, Anderson SD (1985) Heterogeneity of mechanisms in exercise-induced asthma. Thorax 40:481–487
15. Lodrup Carlsen KC, Haland G, Devulapalli CS, Munthe-Kaas M, Pettersen M, Granum B et al (2006) Asthma in every fifth child in Oslo, Norway: a 10-year follow up of a birth cohort study. Allergy 61(4):454–460
16. Becker JM, Rogers J, Rossini G, Mirchandani H, D'Alonzo GE Jr (2004) Asthma deaths during sports: report of a 7-year experience. J Allergy Clin Immunol 113(2):264–267
17. Carlsen KH, Engh G, Mork M (2000) Exercise-induced bronchoconstriction depends on exercise load. Respir Med 94(8):750–755
18. Dickinson JW, Whyte GP, McConnell AK, Harries MG (2006) Screening elite winter athletes for exercise induced asthma: a comparison of three challenge methods. Br J Sports Med 40(2):179–182
19. Landwehr LP, Wood RP 2nd, Blager FB, Milgrom H (1996) Vocal cord dysfunction mimicking exercise-induced bronchospasm in adolescents. Pediatrics 98(5):971–974
20. McFadden ER Jr, Zawadski DK (1996) Vocal cord dysfunction masquerading as exercise-induced asthma: a physiologic cause for "choking" during athletic activities. Am J Respir Crit Care Med 153(3):942–947
21. Refsum HE, Fönstelien E (1983) Exercise-associated ventilatory insufficiency in adolescent athletes. In: Oseid S, Edwards AM (eds) The asthmatic child in play and sports. Pitmann Books, London, pp 128–139
22. Powers SK, Williams J (1987) Exercise-induced hypoxaemia in highly trained athletes. Sports Med 4(1):46–53
23. Adir Y, Shupak A, Gil A, Peled N, Keynan Y, Domachevsky L et al (2004) Swimming-induced pulmonary edema: clinical presentation and serial lung function. Chest 126(2):394–399

Exercise-Induced Bronchoconstriction

Lower airway obstruction and symptoms of cough, wheezing, or dyspnea induced by exercise in individuals without asthma.

Cross-References

▶ Exercise-Induced Asthma

Exercise-Induced Bronchospasm

▶ Exercise-Induced Asthma

Exercise-Induced Cardioprotection

▶ Ischemia-Reperfusion Injury, Exercise-Induced Cardioprotection

Exercise-Induced Intestinal Hypoperfusion and Subsequent Intestinal Damage

▶ Ischemia-Reperfusion Injury

Exercise-Induced Muscle Damage

▶ Muscle Damage

Expiration

The process where the respiratory muscles relax and cause a decrease in the volume of the lungs. As a result, the intrapulmonary pressure increases and air flows out of the lungs to the atmosphere.

Extracellular Matrix

Michael Kjær
Institute of Sports Medicine and Centre for Healthy Ageing, Bispebjerg Hospital, University of Copenhagen, Copenhagen, Denmark

Synonyms

Collagen; Connective tissue; Matrix tissue; Supportive tissue

Definition

Extracellular matrix: The noncellular component of proteins and associated fluid, carbohydrates, fat, and electrolytes that surround all living cells. In relation to exercise science, the term is used for extracellular tissue within bone, cartilage, skeletal muscle, tendon, and ligaments, as these tissues are relevant for weight bearing and locomotion. The protein components are listed in Table 1 and interact closely with the cells present in the tissue to result in protein synthesis and degradation both under resting and under mechanically loaded situations.

Mechanotransduction: The overall tern for conversion of mechanical loading into an integrated biochemical in cells like fibroblasts, osteocytes, chondrocytes, smooth muscle cell and endothelial cells. In more detail, the term covers mechano-sensing which is the conformational and geometric changes of the cell, the mechanotransduction/conversion which is the occurrence of a biochemical signal (e.g., G-protein, tyrosin kinase, other kinase cascades, Ca^{++} activation, lipase activation) in response to mechanical loading, and finally the mechano-response, which is the integration of the biochemical signaling into an overall cellular behavior.

Basic Mechanisms

Matrix is the most important tissue in the body in order to connect and transform forces between cellular components, and the dominating substance in extracellular matrix is collagen, the most frequent molecule in the human body. Collagen molecules (300×1.5 nm) exists in 28 forms and has the characteristic triple helix motif with chains build of $(Glycine-X-Y)_n$ sequences. Collagens are commonly recognized as fibrillar ones (type I,II,III,V,XI, and others), where

Extracellular Matrix. Table 1 Extracellular matrix proteins ("Matrixome")

Collagen (Type I, II, III, IV . . . up to XXVIII)
Proteoglycanes (a) Leucine-rich repeat proteins (examples: Decorin, Biglycan, Fibromodulin, Lumican) (b) Large (examples: Aggrecan) (c) Membrane-associated (examples: Syndecan, Perlecan)
Glycoproteins (examples: Laminin, Tenascin, COMP, Fibronectin)
Growth and regulatory factors (examples: IGF-1, TGF-b, FGF, VEGF, NO, Prostaglandins)
Proteases (MMPs, TIMPs, ADAMTS)

they are structurally arranged in fibril (50–500 nm), fascicles (500–300 um), and fibers (100–600 um). Collagen does however also come as Fibril Associated Collagen with Interrupted Triple helix (FACIT) (type IX, XII and others), beaded filament forming ones (type VI), basal membrane–associated (type IV, VII, XV, XVIII), short chain collagen (VIII, X), and transmembrane ones (type XIII). In addition also collagen-like structures exist. Of relevance for exercise loading is especially the extracellular matrix in bone, cartilage, tendon, ligaments, and skeletal muscle, plus the obvious the matrix function in vessels. Whereas cartilage and bone are primarily subjected to compressive forces, tendon, ligaments, and intramuscular connective tissue are subjected primarily to tensile forces. Each of these tissues has their own characteristics. Bone is dominated by collagen type I and is mineralized, providing the special functional features of stiffness required by bone. For many years, bone has mainly been characterized by determination of its mineral content or density, whereas other features such as collagen content has been more difficult to assess, especially in vivo. This may limit our insight into full bone dynamics and the influence of physical activity. In cartilage, type II collagen is dominating (plus collagen XI), and the ability to bind water by the help of glucosaminoglycans (GAG) provides a structure that can absorb energy in association with joint loading with exercise. Tendons have primarily type I collagen (but also III and V), and, together with proteoglycans, the tendons can both transmit force efficiently (like the patella tendon) and can absorb and to a certain extent return elastic energy during loading (like the Achilles tendon). Finally, the ligaments primarily contain type I collagen together with elastin to provide flexibility. The different tissues have historically been studied for their biomechanical properties in relation to exercise, but tissue-wise the mentioned connective tissues have all been considered to be relatively inert with assumptions of having very long tissue protein turnover times [1]. The methods available to study these collagen-rich tissues in vivo have in the past been somewhat limited, and often findings were based solely on studies of cadaver tissue properties, or relied on cell culture work. With the present methodological developments and renewed interest for metabolic, circulatory and tissue protein turnover in collagen tissue such as tendon – in conjunction with a simultaneous determination of morphology and biomechanical tissue properties – a greater appreciation of a more dynamic tissue in relation to variations in mechanical loading. As an example, it has been shown that in response to mechanical loading the human tendon increases its blood flow, metabolic activity and substrate uptake (e.g., glucose) by three- to fourfold acutely associated with exercise (for references, please see [1]). It has been shown that relevant cells inside the extracellular matrix (e.g., fibroblasts) can sense mechanical loading and via integrin dependent mechanisms will convert these signals into biomechanical processes that will result in protein synthesis and tissue adaptation (mechanotransduction), and several of these mechanosensitive pathways (Rho-ROCK pathway, NFkappaB, MAP kinases, Calcium activated PKC) have been identified.

Matrix adaptation to loading involves several proteins, but the most mechanically important load-bearing structure in tendon tissue is collagen type I. Several indirect methods have been used so far to indicate changes of collagen turnover in connective tissue (pro-collagen mRNA or biosynthesis enzymes (P-4-H, GGT, LHy) in tissue, pro-collagen propeptides either in blood or in interstitial fluid). More directly, incorporation of labelled amino acid into the matrix has been used, and with the use of stable, non-radioactive tracers, in vivo studies can now be made in humans, provided that relevant tissue can be sampled. In human collagen containing tissues (bone, skin, tendon, skeletal muscle), it has more recently been shown that the fractional collagen synthesis rate in the basal state is from 0.02%/h to 0.05%/h equal to around 0.5–1% of the total collagen pool turned over every 24 h [1].

Exercise Intervention

Acute exercise has been shown to increase the fractional synthesis rate of collagen in the patella tendon from approximately 0.05%/h to around 0.10%/h within 24 h after exercise, showing a significant rise already after 6 h post exercise. Also in bone and skeletal muscle matrix a rise in collagen synthesis after acute exercise has been found. The determined values correspond to a collagen synthesis that on a 24 h level increases from around 1% at rest to 2–3% after exercise. The collagen synthesis rate remains elevated for at least 2–3 days after acute exercise. Similar to collagen synthesis, there is indication that protein degradation is activated after exercise, in that local levels of matrix metalloproteinases in tendon and muscle tissue are increased after acute exercise [1, 3].

Prolonged, repeated mechanical loading chronically elevates the collagen synthesis in tendon almost three- to fourfold, and, more recently, it has been shown that inactivity resulted in a decrease in protein synthesis of both collagen and myofibrillar protein of around 20–25%. If one takes the data on long-term adaptation toward training in both animal and human models, the increase in tensile strength of the structures is rather moderate (Table 2) and requires a long time [2, 4]. Conversely, just a few

Extracellular Matrix. Table 2 Function and adaptation of various tissues

Type of tissue	Ultimate strength (Tensile in MPa)	Training improvement (Max rise in strength) (%)	Inactivity fall in strength (Decrease after 3–4 weeks) (%)
Bone	50–200	5–10	30
Tendon	100	20	30
Ligament	60–100	20	30
Cartilage	5–10	5–10	30

weeks of inactivity has consistently been shown to reduce strength in all collagen rich tissue, and to lower bone mineral content in bone and reduce thickness of cartilage.

Unfortunately, it also recognized that tendons are unable to adapt to certain loading conditions and therefore end up with pathology, including so-called overuse injuries and complete tendon ruptures. Large variation exists in the tendon diameter along the length of both the human Achilles and patellar tendon. It is interesting to note that clinical conditions such as patellar and Achilles tendinopathy occur in the region with the greatest average stress for a given applied force, and the etiology may therefore be somehow related to the stress in the region. Furthermore, if in fact there is tendon hypertrophy in response to increased loading, there is some evidence that it may occur in a region specific manner. Animal data show that tendon may undergo both qualitative and hypertrophic changes in response to endurance type exercise, and humans' cross-sectional data suggest that habitual long distance running (>5 years) is associated with a markedly greater cross-sectional area of the Achilles tendon compared to that of non-runners [3]. A total training stimulus of ∼9 months of running in previously untrained young subjects did not result in tendon hypertrophy of the Achilles tendon. Cross-sectional data indirectly suggest that the ability of patellar tendon to adapt in response to habitual loading such as running is attenuated in women as evidenced by the similar tendon cross-sectional area, stiffness, and modulus in habitual runners and non-runners. Finally, it has recently been found that in athletes that load their two legs (and their patella tendons) differently, a significant difference in tendon size could be demonstrated, and loading was associated with thicker tendon [3]. Interestingly, despite marked changes in collagen synthesis with loading morphological changes of, e.g., the tendon are very minor which suggest that only a fraction of newly synthesized collagen is incorporated into mature tensile structures, or that exercise influences other structural proteins in the matrix that are not picked up by the present experimental methods.

An important regulating factor in collagen synthesis is the growth hormone (GH) – insulin-like growth factor 1 (IGF-1) axis, where in vitro data have shown a role for collagen formation. Although GH in skeletal muscle has been shown to exert an effect upon muscle growth in GH-deficient individuals, the effect of GH supplementation upon muscle protein synthesis is absent in both young and elderly humans, but IGF-1 is upregulated in several human connective tissues with exercise and is associated with increased collagen formation. Transforming growth factor beta 1 (TGF-b1) also plays a role in collagen synthesis with exercise. Both concentric and eccentric contractions rose expression of IGF-1, TGF-b1, and collagen in tendon, independent on type of contraction, which suggests a more prominent role for strain than for intensity of loading in signaling a growth factor release and subsequent increase in collagen formation in matrix dominated by fibrillar collagen [1, 3].

References

1. Kjaer M (2004) Role of extracellular matrix in adaptation of tendon and skeletal muscle to mechanical loading. Physiol Rev 84:649–698
2. Kjaer M, Krogsgaard M, Magnusson SP, Engebretsen L, Roos H, Takala T, Woo SL-Y (eds) (2003) Textbook of sports medicine – basic science and clinical aspects of sports injury and physical activity. Blackwell, Malden, p 802. ISBN 0-632-06509-5
3. Magnusson SP, Narici MV, Maganaris CN, Kjaer M (2008) Human tendon behaviour and adaptation, in vivo. J Physiol Lond 586(1): 71–81
4. Woo SL, Gomez MA, Woo YK, Akeson WH (1982) Mechanical properties of tendon and ligaments. The relationship of immobilization and exercise on tissue remodeling. Biorheology 19:397–408

Extracellular Matrix (ECM)

The sugar and protein gel outside of all cells that separates and connects our tissues together. Much of protein in the extracellular matrix is collagen the most prevalent protein in the body. The role of the ECM is diverse, and includes providing anchorage and support for cells, regulating communication between cells, storing cellular growth factors, and separating tissues from one another.

Extracellular Signal-Regulated Kinases (ERKs)

▶ Mitogen-Activated Protein Kinases

Extrinsic Falls Risk Factors

Falls risk factors outside of the individual, usually environmental factors such as uneven surfaces, poor lighting, slippery surfaces, and tripping obstacles.

Cross-References
▶ Fall, Risk of

F

Factor VIII/IX Deficiency

▶ Hemophilia

Failing Cardiomyocyte

▶ Cardiac Hypertrophy, Pathological

Fainting

▶ Orthostatic Intolerance

Fall

An unexpected event in which the participant comes to rest on the ground, floor, or lower level.

Cross-References
▶ Fall, Risk of

Fall Injury Prevention

▶ Fall Prevention
▶ Fall, Risk of

Fall Prevention

ANNE TIEDEMANN[1], CATHERINE SHERRINGTON[1],
DAINA L. STURNIEKS[2], STEPHEN R. LORD[2]
[1]Musculoskeletal Division, The George Institute for Global Health, University of Sydney, Sydney, NSW, Australia
[2]Falls and Balance Research Group, Neuroscience Research Australia, University of New South Wales, Sydney, NSW, Australia

Synonyms
Fall injury prevention; Preventing accidental falls; Preventing loss of postural balance; Preventing slips and trips

Definitions
According to the Kellogg International Working Group on the prevention of falls in the elderly, a *fall* is defined as "Unintentionally coming to the ground or some lower level and other than as a consequence of sustaining a violent blow, loss of consciousness, sudden onset of paralysis as in stroke or an epileptic seizure."

Characteristics

Falling in Older Age: Background
Population aging and the increased tendency to fall with age, present a major challenge to health care providers and health systems as well as for older people and their carers. Falls affect a significant number of older people worldwide, with over one third of community dwelling people aged 65 years and older falling one or more times every year. Falls can result in disability, loss of mobility, reduced quality of life, and fear of falling [1]. Most falls result in only minor injuries, however more serious consequences can include hip fracture, permanent disability, institutionalization, and death. With the worldwide proportion of people aged 65 years and older

Frank C. Mooren (ed.), *Encyclopedia of Exercise Medicine in Health and Disease*, DOI 10.1007/978-3-540-29807-6,
© Springer-Verlag Berlin Heidelberg 2012

expected to increase substantially in the years to come, this is a public health issue that demands attention.

The extensive published literature over the past 25 years provides a good understanding of the problem of falling in older age, including the factors that increase a person's risk of falling and the consequences of falls. There have also been many randomized controlled trials (RCTs) and systematic reviews conducted to explore the effectiveness of a range of fall prevention strategies. In this entry, we have utilized this high quality evidence to provide guidance on effective ▶ exercise prescription for the prevention of falls in older community-dwelling people.

Measurements/Diagnostics

Role of Exercise for Prevention of Falls

It is known that functioning of the sensorimotor systems that are involved in postural control decline with age, leading to an increased risk of falling. Falls are not random events and many can be predicted by assessing a number of risk factors. Some of these risk factors (e.g., reduced muscle strength and impaired balance and gait) can be improved with exercise, whereas others (e.g., poor vision, psychoactive medication use) require different, complementary intervention approaches.

There is good evidence that exercise can prevent falls in community dwellers. Exercise can prevent falls when delivered to the general community as well as to those at increased risk of falls. The recent Cochrane systematic review of interventions to prevent falls in community dwelling older people concluded that exercise interventions can reduce the risk and rate of falls in older people by 17–34%, depending on the type of program and measures used to assess effectiveness [2].

The role of ▶ physical activity (as opposed to structured exercise programs) in fall prevention is less clear. It is known that more active people have fewer falls and that this relationship persists after adjustment for other variables that are associated with falls. However, there is no evidence that simply providing advice with regard to being more active is an effective fall prevention strategy.

Other Interventions to Prevent Falls

Several other single interventions have been found to prevent falls, including home safety interventions in high risk people, psychoactive medication reduction, cataract surgery, the use of single lens rather than bi-, tri-, or multifocal glasses for outdoor mobility and the insertion of cardiac pacemakers for the small proportion of people who experience syncope and are diagnosed with the cardio-inhibitory form of carotid sinus hypersensitivity.

Multifactorial interventions include individual assessment and different combinations of the single interventions mentioned above, often including exercise. There is evidence that multifactorial interventions can reduce the rate of falls but due to their multidimensional nature, the specific factors that are most effective are yet to be conclusively determined.

The impact on the rate of falls of multiple and single interventions is similar and exercise as a single intervention appears to be one of the most cost-effective approaches to falls prevention [3]. Therefore, in the absence of contraindications, exercise should be considered a core fall prevention strategy for older people. In addition, people identified with additional risk factors not amenable to improvement through exercise should be referred for appropriate care. This entry focuses on the prescription and implementation of exercise as a key fall prevention strategy.

Exercise Prescription for Fall Prevention

Exercise programs that include exercises that challenge balance are more effective in preventing falls than programs that do not challenge balance [4]. These programs include: exercises conducted while standing in which participants aim to (1) stand with their feet closer together or on one leg, (2) minimize use of their hands to assist balance, and (3) practice controlled movements of the body's center of mass.

Tailoring to individual capability and safety need to be considered when prescribing the initial level of a balance exercise regimen. Once the balance task has been mastered in a stable manner without the need for upper limb support, the task should be progressed to increase the challenge to balance. Methods to increase the intensity and effectiveness of balance exercises over time include (1) using progressively difficult postures with a gradual reduction in the base of support (e.g., two-legged stand, semi-tandem stand, tandem stand, one-legged stand), (2) using movements that perturb the center of gravity (e.g., tandem walk, leaning and reaching activities, stepping over obstacles), (3) specific resistance training for postural muscle groups (e.g., heel stands, toe stands, hip abduction with added weights to increase intensity, unsupported sit to stand practice), and/or (4) reducing sensory input (e.g., standing with eyes closed, standing/walking on an unstable surface). Further challenge can be provided by the use of dual tasks, such as combining a memory task with a gait training exercise or a hand-eye coordination activity with a balance task. Some examples of exercises that challenge balance and are appropriate for older people to perform are included in Table 1.

Fall Prevention. Table 1 Balance challenging exercises suitable for prescription to older people and methods to progress exercise intensity

Baseline exercise	Progression
Graded reaching in standing	Narrower foot placement
	Reaching further and in different directions
	Reaching down to a stool or the floor
	Reaching for heavier objects
	Standing on a softer surface e.g., foam rubber mat
	Stepping while reaching
Stepping in different directions	Longer or faster steps
	Step over obstacle
	Pivot on non-stepping foot
Walking practice	Decrease base of support, e.g., tandem walk
	Increase step length and speed
	Walking on different surfaces
	Walking in different directions
	Walk around and over obstacles
	Heel and toe walking
Sit to stand	Do not use hands to push off
	Lower chair height
	Softer chair
	Add weight (vest or belt)
Heel raises	Decrease hand support
	Hold raise for longer
	One leg at a time
	Add weight (vest or belt)
Step ups- forward and lateral	Decrease hand support
	Increase step height
	Add weight (vest or belt)
Half squats sliding down a wall	Decrease hand support
	Hold the squat for longer
	Move a short distance away from the wall
	Add weight (vest or belt)
	One leg at a time

Information is also included about progression of exercise intensity over time.

Balance involves anticipatory and ongoing postural adjustments and is thus a coordination task. Activities such as aerobics, tennis, yoga, and dancing have not been evaluated for their effectiveness in preventing falls but as they require coordination practice they are likely to be beneficial in maintaining balance abilities for middle aged people and more able older people. For older people with poorer postural control, these activities may increase risk of falling so individually tailored exercises that safely challenge balance, such as those in the Otago Exercise Programme [5] should be prescribed.

Although the falls prevention literature emphasizes the importance of balance training, it is possible that strength training also plays a role in falls prevention, since lower limb muscle strength is an important risk factor for falls. Strength training may be particularly important for frail individuals, for whom increased strength is likely to result in improved function. Further research is needed to establish the direct benefits of strength training alone on risk of falls in older people.

There are also larger effects of exercise for falls prevention from programs that include a higher dose of exercise (e.g., a dose of more than 50 h of exercise, typically 2 × 1 h sessions per week for 6 months). Since benefits of exercise are rapidly lost when exercise is ceased, exercise programs should be ongoing or encourage people to continue undertaking exercise at the end of a formal program, as recommended by the American College of Sports Medicine.

Our recent systematic review and meta-analysis [4] found the inclusion of walking training in falls prevention programs was associated with a smaller effect on falls prevention. However, programs with and without walking training were effective in preventing falls. It is recommended that walking training be included in a program as long as it is not at the expense of balance training and as long as the individual participant is able to undertake such a program safely.

In summary, falls can be prevented by a range of exercise programs that target balance and provide ongoing exercise. These include the Otago Programme of home-based balance and strength training, group based-Tai Chi, and other group-based balance and strengthening exercise. Programs should be designed according to the needs of the target population to ensure they provide exercise that is challenging yet safe. Through this targeted approach the public health burden of falls and related injury may be reduced.

Special Considerations
People aged 85 years and over and those with chronic disease or functional limitations, are at a substantially increased risk of falls. Exercise programs for these groups must be

prescribed carefully to ensure they do not cause falls. There is evidence that falls can be prevented in people at increased risk of falls through well-designed exercise programs. Further research is needed to determine the optimal approach for preventing falls in people with specific medical conditions such as Parkinson's disease and stroke.

Exercise guidelines recommend an extended cool down period after physical activity for older people, to reduce the chance of hypotension, syncope or arrhythmias during the post-exercise recovery period. Dehydration is also more likely to occur in older people taking diuretics, so fluid intake is recommended before, during and after exercise.

Despite the evidence promoting its benefits, a major limitation of exercise as a public health intervention is low rates of participation. Consideration of factors that maximize uptake and participation in exercise programs by older people is important, such as moderate duration activity, program accessibility and convenience, emphasis on social aspects, strong leadership, and individually tailored exercise. Furthermore, it has been demonstrated that falls prevention programs that are labeled with a positive health message, such as "healthy aging," are likely to be more acceptable to older people than those which describe themselves explicitly as "falls prevention" programs.

References

1. Lord SR, Sherrington C, Menz HB, Close JCT (2006) Falls in older people: risk factors and strategies for prevention, 2nd edn. Cambridge University Press, Cambridge
2. Gillespie LD, Robertson MC, Gillespie WJ, Lamb SE, Gates S, Cumming RG et al (2009) Interventions for preventing falls in older people living in the community. Cochrane Database Syst Rev 15(2):CD007146. doi:10.1002/14651858.CD007146.pub2
3. Davis JC, Robertson MC, Ashe MC, Liu-Ambrose T, Khan KM, Marra CA (2010) Does a home-based strength and balance programme in people aged ≥80 years provide the best value for money to prevent falls? A systematic review of economic evaluations of falls prevention interventions. Brit J Sports Med 44(2):80–89
4. Sherrington C, Whitney JC, Lord SR, Herbert RD, Cumming RG, Close JCT (2008) Effective exercise for the prevention of falls: a systematic review and meta-analysis. J Am Geriatrics Soc 56:2234–2243
5. Robertson MC, Campbell AJ, Gardner MM, Devlin N (2002) Preventing injuries in older people by preventing falls: a meta-analysis of individual-level data. J Am Geriatrics Soc 50:905–911

Fall Risk Assessment

Encompasses two main approaches involving multifactorial and functional mobility assessment tools. *Multifactorial assessment* address a broad range of factors such as medication use, psychological status, acute/chronic illness, environmental hazards, fall history, sensory deficits, and mobility function. *Functional mobility assessment* of fall risk focuses on identifying functional movement and associated physiological factors that limit balance and gait stability, physical mobility, muscular strength and endurance, and speed of performance.

Fall, Risk of

MARK W. ROGERS[1], MARIE-LAURE MILLE[2,3]
[1]University of Maryland Claude D. Pepper Older American Independence Center, University of Maryland School of Medicine, Baltimore, MD, USA
[2]Université du Sud, Toulon–Var, La Garde, France
[3]Institut des Sciences du Mouvement, Aix–Marseille University & CNRS, UMR 6233, Marseille cedex 9, France

Synonyms

Fall Injury Prevention; Vulnerability to unintentional loss of balance

Definition

A ▶ fall has been defined as "an unexpected event in which the participant comes to rest on the ground, floor, or lower level" [1]. Hence, falls inextricably involve the ▶ loss of balance which occurs when the motion of the body center of mass with respect to the prevailing base of support exceeds certain spatial and temporal limits of stability. Falls are common events among older individuals aged 65 years or older. About 30% of community-dwelling people experience one or more falls per year with fall rates increasing beyond this age [2]. Older adults living in institutionalized settings have a higher fall risk than those living in their own homes. The causes, or risk factors, for age-associated falls are multivariate and numerous and often difficult to identify. Risk factors not only precipitate falls but also increase one's vulnerability to unintentional loss of balance which may impact functional mobility. Fall risk factors are numerous and may be broadly classified into the following categories: socio-demographic (e.g., advanced age, falls history), physiological and biomechanical (e.g., visual deficits, muscle weakness, poor reaction time), functional (e.g., balance and gait deficits), psychological (e.g., fear of falling), medical (e.g., use of multiple medications, orthostatic hypotension), and environmental (e.g., poor lighting, scatter rugs) [2]. This essay mainly focuses on ▶ risk of falling among community-dwelling older individuals living independently in their own homes or in retirement communities. However, there is often significant overlap in fall risk factors across different settings where falls frequently occur such as in supportive housing, acute care, and chronic care living environments.

Mechanisms

Although advanced age and a history of prior falls are strongly associated with fall risk, these socio-demographic factors provide no insights about the possible underlying causes. Medical factors best linked with falls (cognitive deficits, comorbid conditions) are similarly limited in explanatory value. However, medication use is well associated with falls especially polypharmacy and psychoactive substances that may impair neuromuscular coordination and other sensorimotor functions, perception, alertness, and judgment. Among the psychological risk factors strongly associated with falls, increased fear of falling likely predisposes many older individuals to adopt a more cautious or hesitant strategy of moving while upright. This strategy is characterized by antagonist muscle coactivation (joint stiffening) that complicates balance maintenance during everyday activities. While environmental hazards may be causal in some circumstances of falls, they do not generally appear to be a robust risk factor. This may reflect the interaction between an individual's level of mobility deficit and other risk factors with environmental factors [2]. Impairments in sensorimotor, neuromuscular, and biomechanical mechanisms contributing to limitations in balance and mobility are among the major risk factors for falls. Among these factors, impaired visual contrast sensitivity and depth perception, reduced somatosensation, muscle weakness, and slower reaction time are especially important risk elements. Although age-dependent changes in the control of standing stability discriminate between fallers and non-fallers, balance performance measures alone have generally shown limited ability to predict falls while performance on isolated multifactorial gait and whole-body mobility tests that better identify fall risk are less informative about the underlying causal factors of falls.

Because definitive identification of risk factors for falls remains unclear there is a pressing need for continued research aimed at better elucidating the causes of age-associated falls and their prevention. For example, in the balance domain, a protective stepping model involving motorized waist-pull-induced perturbations of standing balance has been used to identify impairments in neuromotor and biomechanical mechanisms predisposing older people to falls related to functional balance and locomotion performance [3]. Successfully stepping sideways as a protective response to imbalance is problematic for many older individuals. Lateral stepping responses are normally dependent upon high force, high-speed usage of hip abductor–adductor muscles to effectively move the limbs in the lateral direction with the correct timing and distance in order to prevent a fall from occurring. In community-living older adults, difficulties with protective stepping are characterized by the frequent use of multiple short recovery steps with dangerous collisions between the limbs when crossing one limb in front of the other to secure lateral balance. These studies revealed that lateral stepping patterns and hip abductor strength (joint torque) discriminate prospectively between fallers and non-fallers confirming that these inappropriate balance responses are even more common among older people who fall. These detrimental changes in lateral stepping patterns may result from neuromotor impairments in hip abductor–adductor joint moments of force (torques) that normally regulate lateral balance stability during standing, stepping, and walking. More comprehensive randomized controlled trials are needed to fully evaluate the predictive value of these risk factors and their influence on preventing falls when targeted in exercise intervention programs to prevent falls.

Exercise Response/Consequences

A recent Cochrane review [4] summarized the best evidence for effectiveness of interventions designed to reduce the incidence of falls in older people living in the community. It was concluded that, overall, exercise is an effective intervention to reduce the risk and rate of falls. Three different approaches to exercise interventions were found to be effective: multiple component group exercise, Tai Chi performed as a group exercise, and individually prescribed multiple component exercise performed at home (Fig. 1). Exercise modalities were classified according to The Prevention of Falls Network Europe Consensus exercise category taxonomy that includes gait/balance/functional training, strength/resistance training, flexibility training, 3D training (Tai Chi, dance, etc.), general physical activity, endurance. Exercise-only interventions comprised of two or more combined categories were more effective in reducing both the rate of falls and fall risk than single exercise approaches that mainly reduced the rate of falls but not fall risk.

A meta-analysis review [5] of exercise trials that reduced the rate of falls found greater relative effects for interventions that included exercises which highly

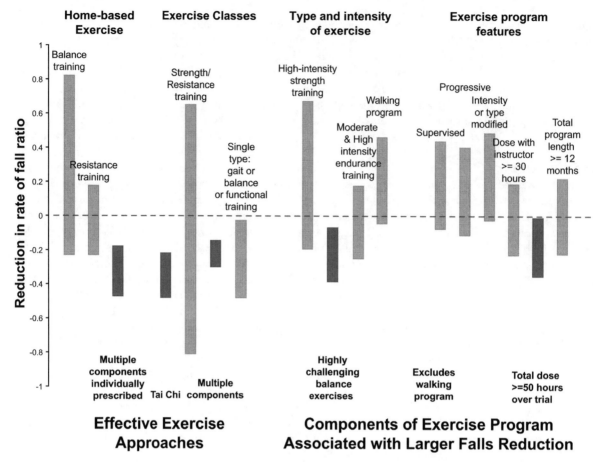

Fall, Risk of. Fig. 1 Fall rate ratio reduction for fall prevention exercise interventions, types of effective approaches, and important components of effective interventions. The reduction of fall rate ratio was calculated by subtracting one from the fall rate ratio calculated for various exercise approaches (data from reference [4]) with the types of effective approaches indicated. Important components of effective exercise programs are also presented (data from reference [5]). The rate of falls represents the number of fall over a specific period of time (often 1 year) and the rate ratio is the proportion of fall in the intervention group divided by the proportion of fall in the control group. It provides assessment of the efficacy of a fall prevention program. A negative value indicates that there were less falls in the intervention group and thus that the program is efficient in reducing falls. Since it is difficult to evaluate this value for an entire population, the figure presents the 95% confidence interval for the reduction of fall rate ratio. This indicates the degree of uncertainty associated with a sample estimate of this parameter where the wider the interval, the poorer the precision

challenged balance (exercises performed while standing with narrower base of support or on one leg, minimal use of upper limb support, and controlled movements of the body center of mass), used a higher dose of exercise (>50 h – twice weekly over 25 weeks), and did not include a walking program (Fig. 1). The inclusion of moderate to high-intensity muscle strength training was not associated with greater effects on fall reduction. Hence, it is likely that poor control of balance is a more potent risk factor for falls than diminished muscle strength. However, this finding may at least partially reflect a nonlinear relationship

between strength and falls whereby once the level of muscle strength is sufficient to avoid falls further gains in strength may not be beneficial to preventing falls [5]. Another viewpoint is that the use of muscle strengthening programs for fall prevention have traditionally emphasized training anterior–posterior compartment muscle groups that are mainly involved with maintaining balance in the sagittal plane, while there has been limited emphasis on strengthening muscle groups more directly involved with controlling balance in the frontal plane where older individuals are particularly vulnerable to losing balance.

Emphasis on devising exercise interventions that provide a high level of challenge to controlling standing balance to prevent falls such as high intensity induced step training, or through exposure to irregularities in the standing and walking terrain that progressively and unpredictably challenges functional balance stability would appear to offer a fruitful new direction for optimizing fall interventions focused on exercise. Importantly, such approaches should also take into account the need to train both proactive balance control which mainly accompanies planned voluntary movements and reactive balance control in response to unanticipated mechanical, sensory, or cognitive perturbations that may disrupt standing stability.

Diagnostics

The assessment of fall risk has utilized two main approaches involving multifactorial and functional mobility assessment tools [6]. Multifactor tools address a broad range of factors such as medication use, psychological status, acute/chronic illness, environmental hazards, fall history, sensory deficits, and mobility function. In contrast, functional mobility assessment of fall risk focuses on identifying functional movement and associated physiological factors that limit balance and gait stability, physical mobility, muscular strength and endurance, and speed of performance. Such diagnostic tools have shown moderate to good validity and reliability. In the community setting, functional mobility assessments using the 5 min walk, five-step test, and Functional Reach have shown high predictive value for identifying fall risk based on specificity and sensitivity. To date, there are a number of tests available to predict people at risk for falls but no single tool can be recommended for implementation in all settings or subpopulations. This gap in understanding paves the way for identifying currently unrecognized or little emphasized fall risk factors that may lead to the definition of new tests that might be more universal.

Acknowledgments

M.W.R. is supported by grants RO1AG029510, R01AG033607, and P30AG028747 from the US National Institutes of Health, National Institute on Aging.

References

1. Lamb SE, Jorstad-Stein EC, Hauer K, Becker C (2005) Development of a common outcome data set for fall injury prevention trials: the prevention of falls network Europe consensus. J Am Geriatr Soc 53:1618–1622
2. Lord SR, Menz HB, Sherrington C, Close JC (2007) Falls in older people. Risk factors and strategies for prevention, 2nd edn. Cambridge University Press, Cambridge
3. Hilliard MJ, Martinez KM, Janssen I, Edwards B, Mille M-L, Zhang Y, Rogers MW (2008) Lateral balance factors predict future falls in community-living older adults. Arch Phys Med Rehabil 89:1708–1713
4. Gillespie LD, Robertson MC, Gillespie WJ, Lamb SE, Gates S, Cumming RG, Rowe BH (2009) Interventions for preventing falls in older people living in the community. Cochrane Database Syst Rev (2): CD007146
5. Sherrington C, Whitney JC, Lord SR, Herbert RD, Cumming RG, Close JCT (2008) Effective exercise for the prevention of falls: a systematic review and meta-analysis. J Am Geriatr Soc 56:2234–2243
6. Scott V, Votova K, Scanlan A, Close J (2007) Multifactorial and functional mobility assessment tools for fall risk among older adults in community, home-support, long-term and acute care settings. Age Ageing 36:130–139

Fast Fourier Transform (FFT) Analyses

A widely used frequency domain analysis technique. The term applies to a class of algorithms used to covert (or "transform") a continuous series of some parameter as it varies over time into its the frequency components.

Fast Glycolytic Fibers

Also known as white fibers (Type II). They possess a low number of mitochondria and their major source of energy is through anaerobic metabolism. They have the lowest resistance to fatigue and they are the least efficient fiber type. However, their speed of contraction is the highest.

Fast Oxidative Fibers

Also known as intermediate fibers. They possess a moderate number of mitochondria and they obtain their energy through a combination of aerobic and anaerobic metabolism. Their resistance to fatigue and efficiency is moderate. Their speed of contraction falls between the slow fibers and the fast glycolytic fibers.

Fat

▶ Nutrition

Fat Mass or Body Fat

The total lipid content of the body, mainly located in adipose tissue.

Fat Metabolism

▶ Metabolism, Lipid

Fat Oxidation

▶ Metabolism, Lipid

Fat-Free Mass

Everything but the lipid content of the body, including mainly water, protein, bone and further solids.

Fatigue

PAAVO V. KOMI[1], CAROLINE NICOL[2]
[1]Neuromuscular Research Center, University of Jyväskylä, Jyväskylä, Finland
[2]Aix-Marseille Univ, UMR 6233, Marseilles, France

Synonyms

Functional impairments; Reduced force production capacity

Definition

As the purpose of the present entry in the Encyclopedia is to relate factors of fatigue during physical exercise, the major focus will be on neuromuscular fatigue. Neuromuscular fatigue is part of a complex and multifactorial phenomenon, which induces adaptation/maladaptation processes that are often experienced by both athletes and common individuals. In addition to the neuromuscular fatigue, other cause-and-effect models have been developed [1] such as : (1) cardiovascular/anaerobic; (2) energy supply/energy depletion; (3) muscle trauma; (4) biomechanical;

(5) thermoregulatory; (6) psychological/motivational; and (7) central governing theory. Neuromuscular fatigue should be considered in close relationship with these other models. From the several ways to define fatigue, we would support the following definition taken from Bigland-Ritchie and Woods [2]: "Any exercise-induced reduction in the ability to exert muscle force or power, regardless of whether or not the task can be sustained." Accordingly, the inability to continue a task is often termed "exhaustion" and considered as the culmination of these ongoing fatigue processes. As the space available for this entry is really limited, the reader is referred to Nicol and Komi [3] for more details.

As shown in Fig. 1, initiation of a voluntary movement is in itself rather demanding with regard to the several steps required until the final "command" reaches the muscles. Theoretically, the potential sites of impairments in Fig. 1a can take place anywhere from the voluntary motor centers in the brain to the contractile filaments in the single muscle fibers. In more general terms, the fatigue processes have been classified into two major categories and/or sites: peripheral and central (including supraspinal) fatigue. This is illustrated in Fig. 1b, which demonstrates these processes as revealed by motor nerve stimulation. Fatigue involves also pathways from the exercising muscles that "inform" the nervous system of the metabolic and mechanical states in the periphery (Fig. 1a). Thus, it is often very difficult to separate the central and peripheral components from each other. They are likely to occur simultaneously, depending on the specific situation. Task dependency is also a factor that has to be taken into consideration when dealing with fatigue [4]. The classical ergograph task is an example of the task dependency. If weights are lifted with eyes closed until exhaustion, the simple instruction to open the eyes allows the subjects to perform immediately 20–30% more extra work [5]. The reversed strategy (closing the eyes after reaching exhaustion with eyes opened) has no effect.

Mechanisms

Both development of fatigue and time to exhaustion are clearly dependent on the exercise intensity and on its mode (continuous or intermittent). To keep the focus on natural locomotion and possible fatigue effects, we need to define the basic form of muscle function. In most activities such as running, hopping, skiing, and throwing, the functional phases include the stretching of the preactivated muscles followed by their shortening. This is called stretch-shortening cycle [6]. SSC is a natural but complex activity, which in itself is often difficult to understand in

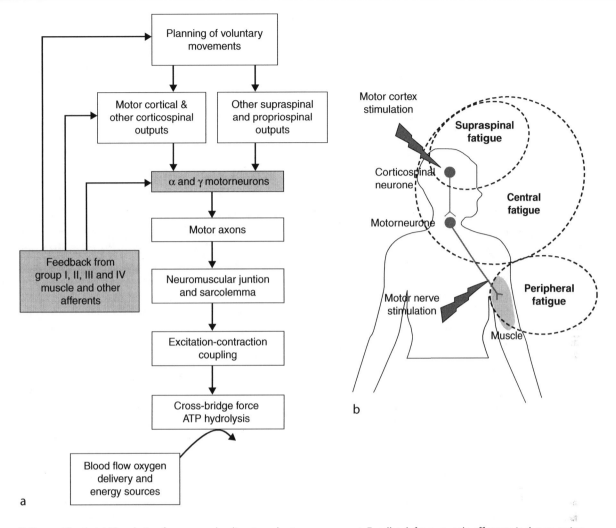

Fatigue. Fig. 1 (**a**) The chain of processes leading to voluntary movement. Feedback from muscle afferents is shown going to the motoneurons, the motor cortex, and premotor areas. (**b**) Division of muscle fatigue into peripheral and central fatigue by motor nerve stimulation. Supraspinal fatigue is a subset of central fatigue (From Nicol and Komi [3])

its all features. First, SSC is characterized by high impact forces that are often repeated over long durations (e.g., during a marathon). In fatiguing SSC exercises, the impact loads are repeated over time, stressing metabolic, mechanical, and neural components. Intensive and/or unaccustomed SSC type exercises may thus result in reversible ultrastructural muscle damage and delayed onset muscle soreness (DOMS). Secondly, the impact loads and the nature of stretches involved in the active braking phase of SSC are usually very fast, of short duration, and controlled simultaneously by reflex and central neural pathways. Thus, SSC fatigue model provides an excellent basis for studying neuromuscular adaptation to

exhaustive exercise, and it differs from pure isolated isometric, concentric, or eccentric type fatigue. Finally, the magnitude of metabolic stress is dependent on the velocity of stretch and on the coupling time between stretch and shortening. One practical example can be given here: as compared to marathon run, both free and traditional techniques of cross-country (X-C) skiing are characterized by long and relatively smooth braking phase. The repeated loading will consequently have greater stretch-induced effects in running than in X-C skiing [7]. In X-C, even when performed with the same intensity and duration as the marathon run race, the recovery processes from possible muscle damage take place much earlier, and the athletes are usually ready to repeat the 50 km race after a few days only. Marathon runners usually do not repeat the race so early. This emphasizes that SSCs, when repeated long enough and with high intensity cause reversible neural, structural, and functional disturbances, severity and duration of which are dependent on the nature of SSC task. Extending then the traditional fatigue thoughts to the SSC fatigue requires rearranging of the thinking of the possible mechanisms involved.

Exercise Response/Consequences

Intensive and/or unaccustomed forms of natural ground locomotion (SSC) induce various impairments of the neuromuscular function that are usually bimodal is nature (Fig. 2). This pattern is quite similar to the *bimodal recovery concept* of Faulkner et al. [8] after eccentric type exercise. After exhaustive forms of SSC, this bimodality is first characterized by large (20–40%) acute drops in maximal voluntary force, maximal activation, and stretch reflex response that may significantly influence the regulation of joint and muscle stiffness leading to reduced maximal running and jumping performances. This is followed after a few hours by a short-term "acute" recovery, which is in turn followed by a "delayed" functional reduction with a slow recovery that may last for 1–2 weeks. This delayed recovery phase is typically associated with delayed onset muscle soreness (DOMS) (Fig. 2), which influences also the muscle activation profiles (Fig. 1a). This bimodality concept is not always individually valid, however, especially if the exercise has not been exhaustive enough [9].

Diagnostics

The challenge lies in finding the origins and underlying mechanisms of this bimodal recovering process. Including both eccentric and concentric muscle actions, it is evident that natural forms of ground locomotion do stress the involved skeletal muscles both mechanically and metabolically.

From the bimodal nature of SSC fatigue recovery curve (Fig. 2), it is obvious that the immediate reductions in performance that recover within 2 h result from metabolic disturbances rather than from ultrastructural damage effects. That is, it is thought to be caused by the accumulation or depletion of metabolites or ions, either intra- or extra-cellularly, potentially combined with the effects of heat stress and dehydration. A decrease in muscle-tendon compliance might be expected as well to contribute to the dramatic reduction of the monosynaptic stretch reflex response and maximal SSC performance.

The delayed recovery presented in Fig. 2 is also complex in nature. When sufficiently exhaustive, SSC exercises may lead to reversible muscle damage, with subsequent inflammation/remodeling processes associated with delayed onset muscle soreness. In connection with these variables, the neural modifications are of considerable mechanistic interest. This is demonstrated by the parallelism between the central and peripheral neural and mechanical changes induced by SSC exercise. The observed inadequate neural drive is considered as an attempt of the neuromuscular system to protect the muscle-tendon unit from additional damage. The functional neural consequences and their coupling with muscle damage/remodeling induced by SSC exercise are illustrated in Fig. 3. Many studies suggest influence of exhaustive SSC exercise on the fusimotor-muscle spindle function as well as at the supraspinal level. Activation of small (III and IV) afferents is proposed as an attractive factor to cause presynaptic inhibition with subsequent reduction in the stretch reflex response, but also to result in inhibition and/or facilitation at the supraspinal level. Long-lasting structural and functional recovery may then prevent an individual from performing normal exercise routines for several days.

Finally, based on the reported SSC fatigue studies using maximal isometric and/or SSC testing tasks along the recovery period, it is emphasized that the SSC testing task may allow distinct examination and follow-up of the central and stretch reflex EMG changes. For instance, the maximal SSC tests confirmed the functional role of the stretch reflex EMG response. Even more meaningful are the submaximal SSC testing tasks as they may reveal different central

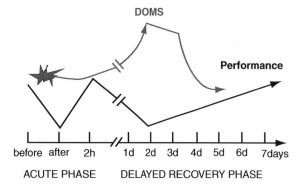

Fatigue. Fig. 2 Schematic presentation of the general trend of changes in performance and delayed onset muscle soreness (DOMS) after exhaustive SSC exercise (From Nicol and Komi [3])

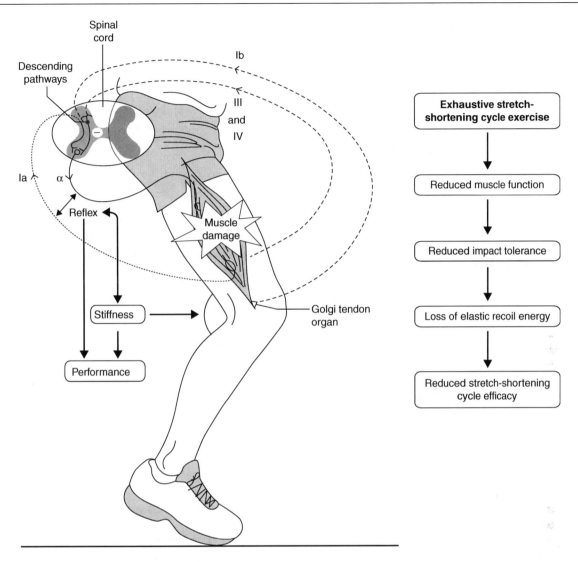

Fatigue. Fig. 3 Schematic representation of the possible interaction between neural pathways and the events of mechanical failure during the delayed recovery phase from exhaustive SSC exercise. Presynaptic inhibition pathway is not shown in this graph. When the muscle fatigues, it is characterized by reduced tolerance to repeated stretch loads, by a deterioration of elastic recoil, and increased work during the push-off phase, so that the same functional outcome can be maintained (From Nicol and Komi [3])

and reflex EMG adjustments in the acute and delayed recovery phases. As the SSC tasks involve several joints they also favor the examination of inter-muscular compensations.

References

1. Abbis C, Laursen P (2005) Models to explain fatigue during prolonged endurance cycling. Sports Med 35(10):865–898
2. Bigland-Ritchie B, Woods JJ (1984) Changes in muscle contractile properties and neural control during human muscular fatigue. Muscle Nerve 7:691–699
3. Nicol C, Komi PV (2011) Stretch-shortening cycle fatigue. In: Komi PV (ed) Neuromuscular aspects of sport performance. Blackwell, Oxford, pp 183–215
4. Enoka RM, Duchateau J (2008) Muscle fatigue: what, why and how it influences muscle function. J Physiol 586:11–23
5. Asmussen E, Mazin B (1978) A central nervous component in local muscular fatigue. Eur J Appl Physiol Occup Physiol 38(1):9–15
6. Komi PV (2000) Stretch-shortening cycle: a powerful model to study normal and fatigued muscle. J Biomech 33:1197–1206
7. Millet GY, Lepers R (2004) Alterations of neuromuscular function after prolonged running, cycling and skiing exercises. Sports Med 34:105–116

8. Faulkner JA, Brooks SV, Opiteck JA (1993) Injury to skeletal muscle fibers during contractions: conditions of occurrence and prevention. Phys Ther 73(12):911–921
9. Nicol C, Avela J, Komi PV (2006) The stretch-shortening cycle: a model to study naturally occurring neuromuscular fatigue. Sports Med 36:977–999

Fatigue Resistance

Ability to continue exercising at the desired intensity.

Fatty Acid Metabolism

▶ Metabolism, Lipid

Female Athlete Triad

ANNE B. LOUCKS
Department of Biological Sciences, Ohio University, Athens, OH, USA

Synonyms
The triad

Definition
As recently revised [1], the term "female athlete triad" refers to the physiological mechanisms by which energy availability affects menstrual function and bone mineral density (BMD). When sufficient energy is available, these mechanisms promote robust health in athletes, but when sufficient energy is not available, they may manifest clinically as eating disorders, functional hypothalamic amenorrhea (FHA), and osteoporosis. Each of these three clinical (symptomatic) conditions is now understood to comprise the pathological end of a spectrum of interrelated subclinical (asymptomatic) conditions between health and disease. Because an athlete can change her energy availability in a day, but effects on menstrual status may not become evident for a month or more, and effects on BMD may not be detectable for a year, an athlete at the pathological end of one spectrum may not exhibit symptoms of the other pathologies at the same time.

Characteristics

Consequences

Eating Disorders
Eating disorders are an Axis I type of clinical mental disorder. Among patients with eating disorders, 80% have additional Axis I disorders, such as depression, anxiety, mood disorders, and sexual disorders, and 70% have at least one Axis II type of long-lasting inflexible pattern of thought and action, such as narcissistic, obsessive-compulsive, paranoid and other so-called personality disorders. Axis III medical complications of eating disorders involve cardiovascular, endocrine, reproductive, skeletal, gastrointestinal, renal, and central nervous systems. Anorexia nervosa is an eating disorder characterized by restrictive eating in which an individual views herself as overweight and is afraid of gaining weight even though she is at least 15% below the expected weight for age and height. There is a sixfold increase in standard mortality rates in anorexia nervosa, and the rate of sustained recovery of weight, menstrual function, and eating behavior is only 33%.

Amenorrhea
Amenorrhea and other menstrual disorders occur more frequently in younger women, whose reproductive systems are more responsive to metabolic signals of low energy availability [2]. Amenorrhea is defined as the absence of menstrual cycles lasting more than 3 months. In primary amenorrhea, the age of menarche is delayed, and because menarche is occurring earlier, the defining age for primary amenorrhea was recently reduced from 16 to 15 years. Amenorrhea beginning after menarche is called secondary amenorrhea. Amenorrheic women are infertile, due to the absence of ovarian follicular development, ovulation, and luteal function. While recovering, however, they may ovulate before their menses are restored, resulting in an unexpected pregnancy, if a reliable form of birth control is not utilized. Hypoestrogenism in amenorrheic athletes is associated with impaired perfusion and oxidative metabolism in working muscle, elevated low-density lipoprotein cholesterol, vaginal dryness, and low BMD.

Osteoporosis
Women with low BMD and nutritional deficits or menstrual irregularities suffer more fractures than other women. The relative risk for stress fracture is two to four times greater in amenorrheic than eumenorrheic athletes. BMD declines as the number of missed menstrual cycles accumulates, and the loss of BMD may not be fully reversible.

Mechanisms

Figure 1 illustrates the full scope of the triad [1]. The triangle in the upper right corner of Fig. 1 represents the condition of healthy athletes who increase dietary energy intake to compensate for the energy cost of exercise. Thick arrows in this triangle illustrate how energy availability promotes bone health and development, both indirectly and directly. Indirectly, optimal energy availability maintains normal luteinizing hormone (LH) stimulation of the ovaries, preserving eumenorrhea and estrogen production, which restrains bone resorption. Directly, optimal energy availability also stimulates the production of metabolic hormones such as insulin, T_3, and IGF-I, which promote bone formation. As a result, BMD is often above average for the athlete's age.

The triangle in the lower left corner of Fig. 1 represents the condition of unhealthy athletes who exercise for prolonged periods without increasing energy intake, who severely restrict their diet, or who have clinical eating disorders. Thick arrows in this triangle illustrate how low energy availability impairs bone health and development indirectly by disrupting LH stimulation of the ovaries, inducing amenorrhea and removing estrogen's restraint on bone resorption, and directly by suppressing the metabolic hormones that promote bone formation. Bone mineral accrual has slowed or reversed for long enough to reduce BMD well below average for age, and one or more stress fractures may have already occurred.

The narrow arrows in Fig. 1 illustrate the spectrums of intermediate levels of energy availability, menstrual status, and BMD along which the population of athletes is distributed. Moderately or recurrently deficient energy availability may induce subclinical menstrual disorders and less severely suppress the hormones that govern bone turnover, and sufficient time may not yet have passed for BMD to decline below the expected range for age.

Pathogenesis

It is now clear that reproductive function and bone turnover are impaired in exercising women by low energy availability and not by low energy stores in the form of body fat or by the stress of exercise. Energy availability is defined conceptually as the amount of dietary energy remaining each day after exercise training for all other physiological functions, and is quantified for research, clinical, and management purposes as dietary energy intake minus exercise energy expenditure, normalized to energy-consuming tissue in units of kilocalories (or kilojoules) per kilogram of fat-free mass (kcal/kgFFM/day or kJ/kgFFM/day). Athletes reduce energy availability compulsively, intentionally, or inadvertently.

Athletes with eating disorders reduce energy availability compulsively as one manifestation of their mental illness. Other athletes reduce energy availability intentionally in rational pursuit of a realistically modified body size and composition through which they aim to qualify to participate or to improve performance in their chosen sports. Both of these groups may engage in prolonged exercise to expend energy, restrict their diets, practice disordered eating behaviors such as skipping meals,

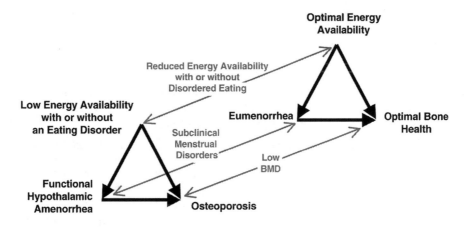

Female Athlete Triad. Fig. 1 Female athlete triad. The spectrums of energy availability, menstrual function, and bone mineral density along which female athletes are distributed (*narrow arrows*). An athlete's condition moves along each spectrum at a different rate, in one direction or the other, according to her diet and exercise habits. Energy availability, defined as dietary energy intake minus exercise energy expenditure, affects bone mineral density both directly via metabolic hormones and indirectly via effects on menstrual function and thereby estrogen (*thick arrows*) [1]

fasting, and vomiting, or use diet pills, laxatives, diuretics, and enemas. Other athletes reduce energy availability inadvertently as prolonged exercise suppresses appetite, and does so most extremely in those consuming the high-carbohydrate diet recommended to endurance athletes [3].

Corresponding reproductive and skeletal disorders also occur in undernourished male athletes, but less obviously because they do not menstruate, and in fewer numbers for reasons that may not be related to sports. Around the world, twice as many young women as men perceive themselves to be overweight *at every decile of body mass index.* The numbers actively trying to lose weight are even more disproportionate, and the disproportion *increases* as BMI declines, so that up to nine times as many lean women as lean men are actively trying to lose weight [4].

Diagnostics

Athletes presenting with one component of the triad should be tested for the others. Energy availability should be calculated from measures of energy intake, exercise energy expenditure, and fat-free mass, all of which can be made with sufficient accuracy by inexpensive commercial products. Because low energy availability can occur in the absence of clinical eating disorders, disordered eating behaviors, or even dietary restriction, eating disorders are not a necessary component of the triad. Therefore, diagnostic procedures and research protocols that require the presence of an eating disorder will miss cases and underestimate the prevalence of the triad, especially in sports requiring prolonged aerobic training. Athletes with and without eating disorders are distinguished by their degree of compliance with nutritional counseling and by the presence and absence of mental illness.

Similarly, diagnostic procedures and research protocols that rely on menstrual history surveys alone do not provide reliable information for detecting cases of the triad. Such surveys wrongly exclude very common subclinical reproductive disorders, such as luteal phase deficiency and anovulation, of which eumenorrheic athletes are completely unaware. Such surveys also wrongly include cases of amenorrhea caused by polycystic ovary disease and other diseases, the origin and treatment of which are completely unrelated to FHA. Therefore, amenorrhea should be diagnosed and menstrual function should be assessed by a physician employing an appropriate endocrine workup.

The International Society for Clinical Densitometry (ISCD) recommends that World Health Organization

(WHO) criteria for diagnosing osteoporosis in postmenopausal women on the basis of BMD alone should not be used in premenopausal women and adolescents because epidemiological data relating BMD to the subsequent occurrence of fractures is lacking in this population. The ISCD currently recommends that osteoporosis be diagnosed in adolescents only by the *combination* of age- and gender-adjusted BMD Z-scores below the expected range for age ($Z \leq -2.0$) *and* a history of fractures [5]. Osteoporosis can develop by failing to accumulate sufficient BMD during adolescence as well as by losing BMD in late adulthood. BMD should be monitored at annual or semiannual intervals in at-risk individuals to distinguish effects of diet and exercise from genetic variation.

Intervention

Prevention

Nutritional counseling is essential for preventing inadvertent low energy availability and for managing intentional modifications of body size and composition. Sports governing bodies and athletic organizations should also adopt policies and procedures to prevent harmful weight loss behavior.

Treatment

Research suggests that hormone replacement therapy provides no benefit and oral contraceptives delay and reduce the likelihood of restoring menstrual cycles in FHA patients without anorexia nervosa. Furthermore, pharmacological restoration of regular menstrual cycles does not normalize metabolic factors that impair bone formation, and no pharmaceutical agent approved for use in this population has been shown to fully restore BMD in women with FHA. Therefore, the first aim of treatment for the triad is to increase energy availability by increasing energy intake, reducing exercise energy expenditure, or both, according to the compliance of the affected athlete.

Athletes without eating disorders should be referred for nutritional counseling and management. In adults, menstrual cycles may be restored by increasing energy availability to more than 30 kcal/kgFFM/day (125 kJ/kgFFM/day) (i.e., resting metabolic rate), but a strong association between increases in BMD and increases in body weight suggests that energy availability may need to be increased to more than 45 kcal/kgFFM/day (185 kJ/kgFFM/day) (i.e., energy balance) in order to increase BMD. These energy availability thresholds may be higher in growing adolescents. Athletes who do not comply with recommended modifications of diet and exercise behavior should be restricted from training and competition and referred for psychiatric evaluation. Treatment for eating disorders includes psychotherapy in addition to nutritional counseling.

References

1. Nattiv A, Loucks AB, Manore MM, Sundgot-Borgen J, Warren MP (2007) American College of Sports Medicine position stand: the female athlete triad. Med Sci Sports Exerc 39:1867–1882
2. Loucks AB (2006) The response of luteinizing hormone pulsatility to five days of low energy availability disappears by 14 years of gynecological age. J Clin Endocrinol Metab 91:3158–3164
3. Stubbs RJ, Hughes DA, Johnstone AM, Whybrow S, Horgan GW, King N, Blundell J (2004) Rate and extent of compensatory changes in energy intake and expenditure in response to altered exercise and diet composition in humans. Am J Physiol Regul Integr Comp Physiol 286:R350–R358
4. Wardle J, Haase AM, Steptoe A (2005) Body image and weight control in young adults: international comparisons in university students from 22 countries. Int J Obes (Lond) 30:644–651
5. Rauch F, Plotkin H, DiMeglio L, Engelbert RH, Henderson RC, Munns C, Wenkert D, Zeitler P (2008) Fracture prediction and the definition of osteoporosis in children and adolescents: the ISCD 2007 pediatric official positions. J Clin Densitom 11:22–28

Female Athlete Triad-Associated Amenorrhea

▶ Athletic Amenorrhea

Fermentation

▶ Anaerobic Metabolism

Fiber Type

Fiber type is the term used to describe the categorical designation of skeletal muscle motor units or cells according to contractile response and biochemical properties. Each motoneuron innervates a collection of muscle cells that all have a common fiber type. In mammalian muscle, there are three primary fiber types (Slow, Fast oxidative and Fast fatigable), but four can be identified by myosin isoform determination: Type I, Type IIa, Type IIb and Type IIx. Human muscle does not have the Type IIb myosin isoform. Hybrid fibers exist, with complement of two (usually), or occasionally three myosin isoforms. The light chains of myosin also have fiber type associated isoforms. Considering hybrid fibers can have varying proportions of the constituent myosin isoforms, the concept of distinct fiber types may be obsolete. Distinguishing features of the fiber types include the following. Sag is present in fast-twitch motor units but not slow-twitch. Posttetanic potentiation is of greater magnitude in fast-twitch motor units than in slow-twitch units. Fatigability is greater in fast fatigable, less in fast fatigue resistant and least in slow-twitch motor units. Fast-twitch fibers have higher myosin ATPase activity than slow-twitch fibers, and this corresponds with a higher maximal velocity of unloaded shortening. Aerobic enzyme activity is greatest in slow-twitch fibers, intermediate in fast fatigue resistant fibers and least in fast fatigable motor units. However, this comparison does not work across species. For example, fast twitch (fatigue resistant) motor units of dog gastrocnemius muscle has a higher aerobic enzyme activity than cat soleus muscle. Myoglobin concentration corresponds with aerobic enzyme activity. Myoglobin gives muscle the red color, so red muscle is high in aerobic enzyme activity and white muscle is not.

The force-frequency relationship is also different between fast and slow-twitch muscle fibers or motor units. Fusion occurs at a lower frequency in slow-twitch fibers, so the half-maximal frequency is lower in slow-twitch and higher in fast-twitch fibers. This means the force-frequency curve is shifted to the left in slow-twitch motor units.

Motor unit size is also related to fiber type. The size of a motor unit relates to the number of muscle fibers innervated by the motoneuron. Slow-twitch motor units are small. Fast fatigue-resistant motor units are larger and the largest motor units are the fast-twitch fatigable units. This means that if you stimulate a single motoneuron with a single activating pulse, the twitch contraction will be small if the motor unit is slow-twitch and large if the motor unit is fast-twitch. The size principle of motor unit recruitment stipulates that during a graded isometric contraction, motor units will be recruited from the smallest to the largest.

Fibrinogen/Fibrin

Fibrinogen is a soluble (340 KDa) plasma glycoprotein synthesized by hepatocytes. It is a hexamer consisting of two sets of three different chains (α, β, and γ), linked to each other by disulphide bonds. The concentration of fibrinogen in plasma normally ranges between 1.5 and 4.0 g/L. Plasma fibrinogen levels are one of the main determinants of blood viscosity. Soluble fibrinogen is converted by thrombin into insoluble fibrin during blood coagulation. The conversion of fibrinogen to fibrin occurs in several steps. Initially, thrombin cleaves the N-terminus of the fibrinogen α and β chains to form fibrinopeptide A and B respectively. The resulting fibrin monomers polymerize to form protofibrils which in turn interact laterally to form fibrin fibers. Finally, the fibrin fibers associate to form the fibrin mesh. Fibrinogen per se can form bridges between platelets, by binding to their surface membrane glycoproteins; however, its major function in hemostasis is as the source of fibrin.

Fibromyalgia

A medical disorder characterized by chronic widespread pain and a heightened and painful response to pressure with unknown etiology.

Fibrosis

An increase in extracellular matrix deposition.

Fibrous Cap

A layer at the top (luminal site) of an arteriosclerotic plaque/lesion, like an upper shell, consisting of fibrous connective tissue and normally contains MΦ and smooth muscle cells, but may additionally contain collagen, elastin, foam cells and lymphocytes.

Fictive Locomotion

A reduced experimental animal preparation whereby the neural circuits in the spinal cord that generate the muscle activation patterns for locomotion are elicited, while the muscular targets of these centrally generated patterns remain quiescent and/or immobilized. This immobilization can be achieved by paralyzing or removing the muscles in the periphery without affecting the spinal circuits, by mechanically preventing movement through limb

fixation, or some combination of both methods. The sensory information coming from these muscles is also blocked from entering the spinal cord by surgical transection. This permits direct measurement of neuronal activity within the spinal cord to gain better understanding of the neural circuits controlling locomotion, which can be hampered by even small movement artifacts.

Field Potentials

Extracellular field potentials are local current sources or sinks that are generated by the activity of many cells. The EMG signal is a representation of the electric field potential generated by the depolarization of the sarcolemma (or cell membrane) of muscle fibers.

FINA

"Fédération Internationale de Natation Amateur" is the international organization that governed the following aquatic sports: competitive swimming, open water swimming, synchronized swimming, water polo, and diving.

Fluid Replacement

R. J. Maughan, S. M. Shirreffs
School of Sport, Exercise and Health Sciences, Loughborough University, Loughborough, UK

Synonyms
Dehydration; Rehydration; Water balance

Definition
Water is that largest single component of the human body, except in the extremely obese, and typically accounts for about 55–65% of total body mass. The rate of turnover of the body water pool is much higher than that of most other body components, with anything from about 2–5% being lost and replaced each day in sedentary individuals living in a temperate climate. The addition of heat or exercise stress, either singly or in combination, can increase daily turnover to an upper limit of about 20–30% of the pool. Water is lost from the lungs, through the

skin, via the sweat glands, and in urine and feces. Minerals and other solutes are lost in sweat, urine, and feces at varying concentrations. Water loss from the body is a continuous process, though the rate is constantly changing, but intake is episodic, so the body water content fluctuates over the course of the day. Homeostatic control mechanisms act to prevent excessive deviations from the euhydrated state, and in spite of the high turnover rates, body water content seldom deviates by more than 1–2% from the normal euhydrated state. Large losses of body water (5–10% of body mass) are clearly detrimental to some elements of both physical and mental performance. The point at which signs and symptoms are likely to become apparent is usually less than this, but is influenced by many factors. Greater levels of hypohydration may be tolerated without adverse effects at rest in a cold environment than during exercise in the heat.

Water loss from the lungs and through the skin is determined largely by the temperature and humidity of the environment, while sweat loss is dictated by the need to adjust the rate of evaporative heat loss in order to maintain body temperature. Sweat rates may exceed 3 l/h in some individuals. There is a certain obligatory minimum urine output – about 500 ml/day – that is necessary to eliminate excess solute, mostly in the form of the end products of protein metabolism or dietary cations (sodium and potassium), from the body. This will be influenced by various factors, including especially body size and the composition of the diet. Fecal water loss is generally small – about 200 ml/day – but can reach 1 l/h in severe infectious diarrhea.

Characteristics

Because water losses are largely outwith voluntary control, maintenance of water balance is achieved primarily by adjustment of intake. Dehydration results in an increase in circulating osmolality and sodium concentration, leading to an increased thirst sensation. A diuresis is invoked when body water content is high, usually as a result of excessive voluntary consumption, and urine output can exceed 1 l/h. A fall in plasma osmolality or plasma sodium concentration will suppress the release of antidiuretic hormone (ADH) from the pituitary, causing a reduction in the fractional reabsorption of water in the renal tubules. When plasma osmolality is high or blood volume is low, water is conserved by increasing tubular reabsorption.

Mechanism of Action

The ingestion of fluids during prolonged exercise can help maintain circulating blood volume, reducing cardiovascular strain and perceived exertion, and can also increase performance and reduce the risk of heat illness [1]. Ingested fluids have a number of effects in the mouth. The perception of temperature and taste may affect the desire for further ingestion, but may also have central nervous system effects, including effects on the perception of effort during exercise and the motivation to continue exercising. There is also some evidence that the carbohydrate content of drinks that are swilled in the mouth and then expectorated without swallowing can influence exercise performance, perhaps as a consequence of effects of the carbohydrate on receptors in the mouth.

There is little net absorption of water and solute in the stomach, so ingested fluids must first be emptied from the stomach before absorption can occur in the upper part of the small intestine [2]. In most exercise situations, fluid ingestion is of benefit only when the exercise is long enough to permit these processes to occur (i.e., longer than about 30–40 min), though possible benefits as a result of the act of drinking cannot be excluded. Ingested fluids should provide both water and carbohydrate as an energy source, and there may be benefits in some situations of providing electrolytes, especially sodium. Increasing the energy density of ingested drinks will slow gastric emptying: concentrated solutions will increase the rate of delivery of carbohydrate to the small intestine, but will slow the rate of water delivery. Glucose is actively absorbed at the brush border of the intestinal lumen and is cotransported with sodium: this solute flux increases water absorption by solvent drag but also by the creation of local osmotic gradients that favor net water uptake. Fructose is absorbed by a different pathway, and combinations of different sugars can help to maximize both water and carbohydrate availability. The use of disaccharides and maltodextrins can increase the carbohydrate content of drinks without an excessively high osmolality.

Strongly hypertonic drinks will cause a net secretion of water into the small intestine: this effect is transient, and is probably of little consequence at rest. During exercise, however, loss of water into the intestinal lumen will exacerbate any hypohydration and can also cause gastrointestinal symptoms that may adversely affect performance. The temperature of ingested fluids will influence their palatability and this is important when large volumes of fluid must be ingested over prolonged periods of time. Cool fluids generally promote greater intake when ad libitum consumption is allowed. Cool fluids will also act as a heat sink, helping to counter the rise in body temperature that normally occurs during exercise. Although this effect is relatively small, it may be important during hard exercise in the heat.

It is seldom the case that fluid ingestion during exercise matches the loss, so most athletes finish training and competition in a state of hypohydration. It is equally clear that athletes training hard on a daily basis in hot climates can effectively maintain their hydration status, so 24-h intake must match loss, and probably does so without conscious effort except when losses are unusually high. Restoration of water balance requires ingestion of sufficient fluid to match that lost as sweat plus an additional amount to meet ongoing urinary and other losses. Ingestion of plain water, however, will cause a prompt decrease in the sensation of thirst, even before volume losses have been replaced, and will also provoke a marked diuretic response. These responses occur because of the fall in plasma osmolality and plasma sodium concentration that follow ingestion of large volumes of plain water. Adding sodium to drinks will attenuate this fall, helping maintain the drive to drink and reducing the diuretic stimulus. If electrolyte losses are not replaced, water balance will not be fully restored, no matter how much fluid is consumed. The main electrolyte lost in sweat is sodium, and sodium concentrations in sweat are typically about 40–50 mmol/l, though the normal range extends from about 10–80 mmol/l. Replacement of the salt losses will normally be met by the salt content of foods and drinks consumed after training, but extra salt may be necessary when losses are at the upper end of the normal range.

Clinical Use

Fluid replacement is a key element of performance enhancement and can also reduce the risk of heat-related illness in endurance events. Fixed guidelines that prescribe set amounts of fluid are usually inappropriate: the optimum replacement regimen will depend on body mass, exercise intensity and duration, environmental conditions, clothing worn, and on individual variations in physiological function. Athletes should generally be encouraged to ingest sufficient fluid to restrict body mass loss to about 2% of initial mass. It should never be necessary to ingest so much fluid that body mass increases during an exercise session. Excessive fluid ingestion carries a risk of hyponatremia: while the risk is small, the consequences are potentially serious [3]. Charity runners in big city marathons should recognize that fluid replacement guidelines developed for serious runners are unlikely to apply to their situation. Plain water is often an appropriate beverage for fluid replacement during exercise, but addition of small amounts of carbohydrate, including glucose and perhaps also other sugars such as fructose, sucrose, and maltodextrins, as well as sodium, may confer additional performance benefits.

Diagnostics

Athletes should be encouraged to begin exercise well hydrated, and can assess their own hydration status based on urine frequency, volume, and color [4]. Laboratory assessment of urine osmolality or specific gravity can be used if available. Sweat loss can be estimated from change in body mass, with correction for fluid intake and urine output [5]. Sweat sodium loss can be estimated by collection and laboratory analysis of sweat samples: alternatively, "salty sweaters" can be identified by salt crusts on the skin and on dark clothing after training. Adequacy of a hydration strategy can be assessed from the change in body mass occurring during an exercise session. If body mass has fallen by more than about 2% of initial mass, it might be advisable to increase fluid on the next occasion where exercise is performed in similar conditions. If body mass had increased, too much fluid was consumed and less should be taken next time. The only caution on this last point would be if the individual had begun exercise in a seriously hypohydrated state: some weight gain would then be acceptable.

References

1. Sawka MN, Burke LM, Eichner ER, Maughan RJ, Montain SJ, Stachenfeld NS (2007) Exercise and fluid replacement. Med Sci Sports Exerc 39:377–390
2. Maughan RJ, Murray R (eds) (2000) Sports drinks: basic science and practical aspects. CRC Press, Boca Raton
3. Noakes TD (2003) Overconsumption of fluids by athletes. Br Med J 327:113–114
4. Armstrong LE (2007) Assessing hydration status: the elusive gold standard. J Am Coll Nutr 26:575S–584S
5. Maughan RJ, Shirreffs SM, Leiper JB (2007) Errors in the estimation of sweat loss and changes in hydration status from changes in body mass during exercise. J Sports Sci 25:797–804

Fluorescent Dye

A fluorescent dye is an important tool in the field of biochemistry and cell physiology. It contains in a molecule a functional group, the so-called fluorophore, which is able to absorb light of a specific wavelength. The photon energy is used to bring an orbital electron from its ground state to an activated state for a very short period of time (= excitation). Relaxation of the orbital electron to ground state is associated with the emission of photon light of a specific wavelength which is usually lower than the excitation wavelength. Fluorescent dyes can be used for several purposes, e.g., for the identification of cellular structures by labeling of structure specific antibodies, or the investigation of functional processes, such as monitoring intracellular ion concentrations with respect to location and time.

Foam Cells

MΦ/smooth muscle cells, having mLDL internalized via scavenger-receptors.

Fontan Circulation

Fontan circulation results from Fontan surgery which is a palliative operation for patients in whom a two ventricular repair is not feasible, such as in tricuspid atresia, pulmonary atresia with intact ventricular septum or various types of univentricular hearts. The surgical procedure involves diversion of the systemic venous return to the pulmonary artery, usually without the interposition of a subpulmonary ventricle.

Food

▶ Nutrition

Food Regimes for Active Individuals

▶ Athlete's Diet

Food Supplement

▶ Supplementation

Force-Frequency Relationship

The force of contraction of a muscle fiber, motor unit or whole muscle is dependent on the frequency of activation. This frequency dependence relates to the force-frequency relationship. If the force obtained during a tetanic contraction, where the frequency is applied long enough to allow development of a plateau of force, is plotted against frequency of stimulation, a sigmoidal relationship is obtained. That is, at low frequencies, force does not increase much as frequency is increased, but at a critical level, force will begin to increase substantially. At higher stimulation frequencies, force will reach a plateau of maximal force and any further increase in frequency will not result in an increase in force. The slope and the half-maximal stimulation frequency become defining characteristics of the force-frequency relationship. Fibre type, temperature and species under consideration are all factors that dictate these parameters of this relationship. Fatigue can diminish the force of contraction at any frequency, but low-frequency fatigue is defined by the selective depression of force when stimulation frequency is low. In fact, maximal force can be unchanged at a time when low-frequency fatigue selectively depresses low frequency forces. Activity dependent potentiation selectively increases active force at low frequencies of activation.

Frank–Starling Mechanism

Physiological phenomenon of working myocardium, where increased blood pressure stretches the ventricular wall, inducing more forceful heart contractions.

Free Ions

▶ Electrolytes

Free Radicals

A free radical is a very reactive chemical species because it has an unpaired, odd, electron in the outer shell. The half-life of most of these free radicals is very short and they can react very quickly with very important biological compounds such as lipids, proteins or DNA producing oxidative damage.

Cross-References

▶ Redox Status

Frequency Domain Analysis

Techniques that quantify the variation of a continuous sequence of data points by partitioning the overall variance into its frequency bands components. Techniques that "decompose" a complex wave form into its simpler frequency oscillation components. The data are displayed as a frequency spectrum and the "power" is the area under the spectral curve for a given frequency band. Hence, these methods are often also called power spectral density analysis techniques. The two most common frequency domain analysis approaches are fast Fourier Transform analysis (FFT) and autoregressive (AR) modeling.

Functional Capacity

Functional capacity refers to the capability of performing tasks and activities that people find necessary or desirable in their lives. This can be measured with an exercise stress test.

Functional Equivalence

The theory of Functional Equivalence of action execution and motor imagery predicts a similarity of these two conditions in neural terms. Both motor execution and motor imagery are associated with neural activation of the same motor and motor-related areas. This phenomenon of shared neural representations was named Functional Equivalence of motor execution and motor imagery.

Functional Flexibility

Players' ability to move their limbs over the full range of movement during actual match play or selected soccer-relevant activities (kicking, tackling, sprinting, change of directions, etc.).

Functional Hypothalamic Amenorrhea

Functional hypothalamic amenorrhea is the term used to describe amenorrhea typically seen in athletes as a result of an energy deficiency. The origin of the disorder resides in the hypothalamus and is characterized by decreased gonadotropin-releasing hormone pulsatility and decreased pulsatility of the gonadotropins, particularly luteinizing hormone, in the face of chronic hypoestrogenism. Levels of the ovarian steroids, estrogen and progesterone, are chronically suppressed.

Cross-References
▶ Female Athlete Triad

Functional Immaturity

This concept refers to the way of working of newborn neurons in the adult hippocampus, where the immature neurons may play some role before completing maturation and that such a role may be relevant for the hippocampal function, the contrary concept to the old view of immature functioning.

Functional Impairments

▶ Fatigue

Functional Overreaching

Short-term (up to approximately 2 weeks) decrease of performance following "overtraining" without severe psychological or other long lasting negative symptoms, which may eventually lead to an increased performance.

G

Gait Stabilization

▶ Locomotor Control

Gap Junctions

If tissue-forming cells are positioned close together as for example in epithelia, special cell–cell connections or junctions can be defined. In vertebrates four kinds of junctions occur:

- Tight junctions
- Adherens junctions
- Gap junctions
- Desmosomes

Cross-References

▶ Intercellular Signaling

Gas Exchange, Alveolar

PETER WAGNER
Department of Medicine, University of California, San Diego, CA, USA

Synonyms

Arterial blood gases; Arterial PCO_2; Arterial PO_2; Carbon dioxide output; Oxygen uptake

Definition

Alveolar gas exchange is the process by which O_2 is transferred from inspired air across the alveolar blood: gas barrier and into the pulmonary capillary blood. It also encompasses the opposite process of transfer of metabolically generated CO_2 from the pulmonary arterial blood across the blood: gas barrier into the alveolar gas and from there to the air. Alveolar gas exchange involves the transport of O_2 and CO_2 by ventilation, diffusion, and perfusion (blood flow).

Characteristics

Ventilation, diffusion, and perfusion are separate transport processes but they work in series as a "bucket brigade" passing O_2 molecules from the air to the alveolar gas (ventilation), then from the alveolar gas to the pulmonary capillary blood (diffusion), and finally from the capillary blood to the pulmonary veins, left heart, and on to the tissues (perfusion). For CO_2, the same processes work in reverse. Figure 1 depicts these processes.

Ventilation

Ventilation consists of alternating inspiration (from FRC) and expiration (back to FRC). Inspiration is accomplished by active contraction of respiratory muscles (diaphragm, inspiratory chest wall muscles) which expand the chest wall in all dimensions, thereby reducing intrapleural pressure, and causing the (elastic) lungs to passively inflate. Expiration at rest is normally passive, fueled by the stored elastic energy in the lung tissues provided by the prior inspiration (just as a stretched rubber band returns passively to its original position).

During exercise, greater inspiratory muscle nerve traffic leads to faster and deeper inspiration, while expiration is now accomplished by a combination of passive relaxation and active contraction of expiratory muscles (chest wall and abdomen). Accessory muscles of the shoulder girdle may further contribute during heavy exercise.

In health, exercise reduces end-expiratory lung volume to below FRC and increases end-inspiratory lung volume. Work of breathing rises disproportionately with increasing ventilation because both the elastic and resistive components are greater due to higher tidal volumes and flow rates respectively. Expiratory flow limitation from dynamic airway compression can occur at/near maximal ventilation, especially in older subjects, because of their decreased elastic recoil. Such flow limitation is common in patients with COPD even at light exercise.

As exercise intensity increases, alveolar ventilation (V_A) increases in proportion to metabolic CO_2 production

Frank C. Mooren (ed.), *Encyclopedia of Exercise Medicine in Health and Disease*, DOI 10.1007/978-3-540-29807-6,

The pathway for transport of O_2

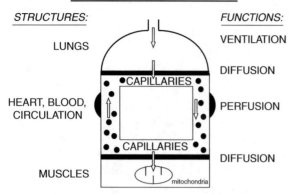

STRUCTURES: FUNCTIONS:

LUNGS   VENTILATION

                               DIFFUSION

HEART, BLOOD,   PERFUSION
CIRCULATION

                               DIFFUSION

MUSCLES

Gas Exchange, Alveolar. Fig. 1 Principal elements of the O_2 transport pathway. The lungs, heart, blood, vessels, and muscles together support the four main O_2 transport functions (pulmonary ventilation, alveolar-capillary diffusion, systemic perfusion, and muscle microvessel-mitochondria diffusion) which take place in an in series manner to deliver O_2 from the air to the muscle mitochondria

($\dot{V}_{CO_2}$), allowing alveolar P_{CO_2} (P_{ACO_2}) and therefore also arterial P_{CO_2} to remain normal at ~40 mmHg. The alveolar ventilation equation, which is a statement of conservation of mass, explains this result, as shown in Eq. 1 (k is a constant):

$$\dot{V}_{CO_2} = k \times \dot{V}_A \times P_{ACO_2} \qquad (1)$$

The same holds for O_2, as shown in Eq. 2, allowing alveolar P_{O_2} (P_{AO_2}) to also be maintained as $\dot{V}_{O_2}$ (O_2 uptake) rises. P_{IO_2} is inspired P_{O_2}.

$$\dot{V}_{O_2} = k \times \dot{V}_A \times [P_{IO_2} - P_{AO_2}] \qquad (2)$$

Strictly speaking, inspired and expired tidal volumes are different, but by only about 1%. This difference is ignored for clarity of presentation in Eq. 2, but can be taken into account. Because $\dot{V}_{CO_2}$ rises more than $\dot{V}_{O_2}$ from rest to exercise, and because ventilation is regulated primarily to keep P_{ACO_2} constant, P_{AO_2} rises even though P_{ACO_2} stays constant.

As blood lactate levels start to rise (at medium intensity exercise and above), there is additional ventilatory stimulus. Ventilation thus now rises faster than does $\dot{V}_{CO_2}$, and P_{ACO_2} begins to fall, P_{AO_2} rising further. Typically, at maximal $\dot{V}_{O_2}$, P_{ACO_2} is ~35 mmHg while P_{AO_2} is ~110 mmHg. Subjects capable of very high metabolic rates may not raise ventilation sufficiently, and may develop a small degree of hypercapnia.

Maximum minute ventilation ($\dot{V}_E$, the product of tidal volume and frequency) is normally in the range of 150–200 l/min. Maximal alveolar ventilation ($\dot{V}_A$, the product of [tidal volume-anatomic dead space] and frequency) rises to 95% of $\dot{V}_E$ as the anatomic dead space (the volume of gas in all of the conducting airways, usually ~150 ml) becomes an ever smaller percentage of tidal volume (~30% at rest falling to ~5% at peak exercise), as tidal volume rises from ~500 to ~3,000 ml. Respiratory frequency rises from ~15/min at rest to ~60/min at maximal effort.

Ventilation is not distributed equally to all alveoli. Gravitational and geometrical factors cause inequality in distribution, which becomes important in relation to the corresponding distribution of alveolar blood flow because the ratio of the two (ventilation/perfusion ($\dot{V}_A/\dot{Q}$) ratio) determines gas exchange. That said, the inequality is minor compared to that in respiratory diseases and usually affects gas exchange minimally.

Diffusion

All gases move across the alveolar wall (blood: gas barrier, Fig. 2 model plus EM) by passive diffusion. Direction of net movement of any gas across the barrier is dictated simply by its partial pressures on either side of the barrier, governed by Fick's law of diffusion – Eq. 3:

$$\dot{V}_{O_2} = D_L \times [P_{AO_2} - P_{capillary}O_2] \qquad (3)$$

Where $\dot{V}_{O_2}$ is instantaneous flow of O_2 at any position along the lung capillary, P_{AO_2} is alveolar P_{O_2} and $P_{capillary}O_2$ is P_{O_2} in the red cell at the same position along the capillary. D_L is the diffusing capacity of the barrier at that same position for O_2, and is assumed uniform along the entire capillary. Identical equations apply for all gases. D_L depends on the total alveolar-capillary network surface area, which determines the barrier diffusing capacity, D_M; the volume of blood in the capillaries (V_C); and on the reaction rate (θ) between O_2 and Hb as the former binds to the latter in the red cell, in accordance with Eq. 4 defined by Roughton and Forster [1]:

$$1/D_L = 1/D_M + 1/[\theta \times V_C] \qquad (4)$$

At rest in health, D_M and V_C are large enough that D_L is also large in relation to $\dot{V}_{O_2}$. In turn, this allows (P_{AO_2}-$P_{capillary}O_2$) (Eq. 3) to be negligible as the red cell reaches the end of its capillary transit, so that end capillary P_{O_2} equals P_{AO_2}. During exercise, D_L increases because greater perfusion pressure opens more capillaries and distends them, raising both D_M and V_C, but $\dot{V}_{O_2}$ rises more than does D_L. As a result, end capillary P_{O_2} may not reach P_{AO_2} during heavy and especially maximal

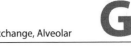

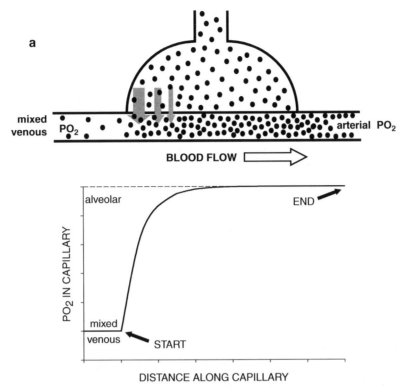

Gas Exchange, Alveolar. Fig. 2 Dynamics of alveolar-capillary diffusion. Due to high alveolar and low mixed venous PO_2, O_2 diffuses rapidly from alveolar gas into the capillary (**a** *top*, *arrows*) early in the red cell transit, resulting in a rapid rise in capillary PO_2 (**b** *lower*), where equilibrium with alveolar gas is reached well before the end of the capillary. Figure **b** is an electron micrograph of the blood gas barrier showing the very thin layer of cells and matrix separating alveolar gas from capillary blood

exercise (i.e., diffusion limitation develops), and arterial hypoxemia ensues. While this is uncommon in untrained subjects, it is seen ín ~50% of trained athletes [2] because of their higher cardiac output and correspondingly lower red cell capillary transit time. The effect is usually small but measurable, and by breathing a higher concentration of O_2, hypoxemia is easily corrected and maximal exercise capacity is immediately increased.

CO_2 obeys the same laws of diffusion, but because its diffusing capacity is about twice that of O_2, arterial hypercapnia from diffusion limitation has not been observed.

It turns out that diffusion limitation is determined by the ratio $D_L/(\beta \times \dot{Q})$, where β is the effective slope of the O_2Hb dissociation curve between the arterial and mixed venous P_{O_2}'s and $\dot{Q}$ is total pulmonary blood flow (in essence, cardiac output) [3]. All three variables increase with exercise, but D_L does not rise as much as does $\dot{Q}$ and so $D_L/(\beta \times \dot{Q})$ falls considerably. Moreover, the barrier component (D_M) of D_L is proportional to the solubility of O_2 in the water of the barrier, which at 0.003 ml/(dl.mm Hg) is some 67-fold less than β, (which during exercise is $\sim$0.2 ml/dl.mmHg) explaining why O_2 is so vulnerable to diffusion limitation during exercise. During exercise at altitude, β is even larger ($\sim$0.4) and thus diffusion limitation occurs in all subjects, significantly reducing ability to exercise.

Perfusion

Blood flow takes the O_2 added to the red cells by the above processes and moves those red cells around the body through the pumping action of the heart. The amount/minute of O_2 added to blood by diffusion from alveolar gas as blood passes through the lungs is given by Eq. 5:

$$\dot{V}_{O_2} = \dot{Q} \times [CendcapillaryO_2 - CvO_2] \qquad (5)$$

Where CaO_2 is systemic arterial and CvO_2 is mixed venous O_2 concentration. This equation, just like Eq. 2, simply expresses mass conservation for O_2. Just as for $\dot{V}_A$, and for the same reasons, $\dot{Q}$ is not uniformly distributed to the alveoli, and while there are some mechanisms that tend to match $\dot{V}_A$ to $\dot{Q}$, these are not perfect. Accordingly, the ratio $\dot{V}_A/\dot{Q}$ varies among the alveoli. This is important because when Eqs. 2 and 5 are considered together we have:

$$\begin{aligned} \dot{V}_{O_2} &= \dot{Q} \times [CendcapillaryO_2 - CvO_2] \\ &= k \times \dot{V}_A \times [P_{IO_2} - P_{AO_2}] \end{aligned} \qquad (6)$$

Or

$$\dot{V}_A/\dot{Q} = K \times [CendcapillaryO_2 - CvO_2]/[P_{IO_2} - P_{AO_2}] \qquad (7)$$

Importantly, this equation says that local P_{AO_2} is determined uniquely by the $\dot{V}_A/\dot{Q}$ ratio for a given makeup of inspired gas and mixed venous blood. Implicit in Eqs. 6 and 7 is the O_2Hb dissociation curve because $CendcapillaryO_2$ is the blood O_2 concentration corresponding to the alveolar P_{O_2}, P_{AO_2}. Therefore,

as local $\dot{V}_A/\dot{Q}$ ratio varies throughout the lung, so will P_{AO_2} (and P_{ACO_2}, for which identical equations hold). The end result is always impairment of gas exchange [4].

Impairment of gas exchange is conveniently assessed by the Alveolar-arterial PO_2 difference, $AaPO_2$. Dividing Eq. 1 by Eq. 2, we have:

$$\dot{V}_{CO_2}/\dot{V}_{O_2} = R = P_{ACO_2}/[P_{IO_2} - P_{AO_2}] \qquad (8)$$

where R is the respiratory exchange ratio. This is rearranged to yield:

$$P_{AO_2} = P_{IO_2} - P_{ACO_2}/R = P_{IO_2} - P_{aCO_2}/R \qquad (9)$$

because alveolar (P_{ACO_2}) and arterial (P_{aCO_2}) are essentially equal, so that:

$$AaPO_2 = P_{AO_2} - P_{aO_2} = P_{IO_2} - P_{aCO_2}/R - P_{aO_2} \qquad (10)$$

Equation 10 is the alveolar gas equation [5]. $AaPO_2$ is normally <10 mmHg at rest. It is not zero (as would happen in a perfectly homogeneous lung) because real lungs display $\dot{V}_A/\dot{Q}$ inequality as mentioned i.e., the $\dot{V}_A/\dot{Q}$ ratio is not everywhere the same. This causes arterial PO_2 to fall and $AaPO_2$ to increase. Exercise almost universally causes $AaPO_2$ to increase, frequently from $\sim$10 mmHg at rest to $\sim$30 mmHg on maximal exercise. The causes are variable combinations of $\dot{V}_A/\dot{Q}$ inequality and diffusion limitation, with a very small contribution from right to left shunting, exemplified in Fig. 3 [6].

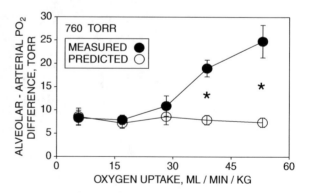

Gas Exchange, Alveolar. Fig. 3 The alveolar-arterial PO_2 difference ($AaPO_2$) in normal subjects at rest and increasing levels of exercise. *Solid circles* show the total $AaPO_2$. *Open circles* show that part of the $AaPO_2$ explained by ventilation/perfusion inequality. The difference is due to alveolar-capillary diffusion limitation, absent at rest and light exercise, but increasing with exercise intensity due to reduced capillary transit time (From [6])

Measurements/Diagnostics

Gas exchange during exercise is assessed in more than one manner. Total O_2 uptake ($\dot{V}O_2$) and CO_2 elimination ($\dot{V}CO_2$) by the lungs is determined by measuring ventilation and mixed exhaled concentrations of O_2 and CO_2 and applying Eqs. 1 and 2 to calculate $\dot{V}O_2$ and $\dot{V}CO_2$. Subjects must wear a noseclip and breath through a mouthpiece or use a tightly fitting face mask so exhaled gas can be accessed. Ventilation can be measured by (a) a timed collection of exhaled gas into a container and afterward measuring the volume collected/minute; (b) exhaling directly through a gas metering device such as a turbine or pneumotachograph. Exhaled O_2 and CO_2 levels can be determined by fuel cell (O_2), infrared meter (CO_2), mass spectrometer, or blood gas electrodes. PO_2 and PCO_2 in blood is measured by electrodes specific to each gas, and used with Eq. 10 to estimate $AaPO_2$.

References

1. Roughton FJW, Forster RE (1957) Relative importance of diffusion and chemical reaction rates determining rate of exchange of gases in the human lung with special reference to true diffusing capacity of pulmonary membrane and volume of blood in the lung capillaries. J Appl Physiol 11:290–302
2. Dempsey JA, Hanson PG, Henderson KS (1984) Exercise-induced arterial hypoxemia in healthy human subjects at sea level. J Physiol Lond 355:161–175
3. Piiper J, Scheid P (1981) Model for capillary-alveolar equilibration with special reference to O_2 uptake in hypoxia. Respir Physiol 46:193–208
4. West JB (1969) Ventilation/perfusion inequality and overall gas exchange in computer models of the lung. Respir Physiol 7:88–110
5. Rahn H, Fenn WO (1955) A graphical analysis of the respiratory gas exchange. American Physiological Society, Washington, DC
6. Wagner PD, Gale GE, Moon RE, Torre-Bueno JR, Stolp WB, Saltzman HA (1986) Pulmonary gas exchange in humans exercising at sea level and simulated altitude. J Appl Physiol 61:260–270

Gastroesophageal Reflux Disease

▶ Gastrointestinal Symptoms

Gastrointestinal Disorders

▶ Gastrointestinal Symptoms

Gastrointestinal Symptoms

FRANK C. MOOREN
Department of Sports Medicine, Justus-Liebig-University, Giessen, Germany

Synonyms

Gastroesophageal reflux disease; Gastrointestinal disorders; GERD

Definition

Exercise-induced gastrointestinal disorders have been recognized for some time. Despite their high incidence and great significance in clinical sport medicine, the gastrointestinal tract still remains on the periphery of research in this area of medicine [1]. Runners, in particular, frequently suffer from symptoms such as nausea and vomiting, reflux syndrome, or so-called runner's diarrhea, with microscopic or even macroscopic bleeding. Multiple factors are involved in these disorders, ranging from age and gender, quality and quantity of nourishment, and liquids intake, to training intensity and duration. The pathophysiological mechanisms underlying the origin of these disorders have not yet been fully elucidated.

Characteristics

In contrast to other organ systems such as heart, blood vessels, lung, or muscles, the GI tract has not been in the focus of exercise science studies during the recent years. This contrasts with the relevance of exercise-associated GI symptoms in the medical praxis. Questionnaire-based investigations during major sports events such as marathon runs reported an incidence of GI symptoms in up to 50% of endurance athletes. More than one third of these athletes complained that the symptomatology impaired their exercise performance. And, finally, about 5–6% of the athletes reported the more or less regular use of a GI tract–specific medication such as antacids, antidiarrheal drugs, etc. [2].

Symptoms and Variables

The incidence of exercise-induced gastrointestinal (GI) symptoms shows a relation to the sport type practiced. Long distance runners complain more often about discomfort of the lower GI tract, while sportsmen like bicyclists or rowers report more disorders of the upper GI tract. Leading symptoms of the upper GI tract are loss of appetite, nausea, heartburn, and vomiting. Abdominal cramping, urge to defecate, and diarrhea including microscopic/macroscopic bleedings are the major symptoms of exercise-induced alterations of the lower GI tract [3].

Several internal and external variables have been identified which have the potential to modify the exercise-associated gastrointestinal symptoms. Major factors are exercise intensity and duration which show a positive correlation to the symptomatology (Fig. 1). Further aggravating variables include nutritional aspects such as quantity and composition of food, and the time period between food intake and exercise start. Athletes should avoid a highly calorific diet as well as a protein- and fat-rich diet at least within the last 2 h before beginning to exercise. Furthermore, it has been reported that with respect to GI symptoms the use of plain water during exercise seems to be more comfortable than the use of sport drinks [4]. Hydration status is another important variable of exercise-induced GI symptoms as dehydration significantly aggravates the situation. Further variables include training status and age of the athletes. While the first point might address some kind of training adaptation of the GI tract, the latter fact points probably to the experience of the older sportsmen to cope better with the discomfort

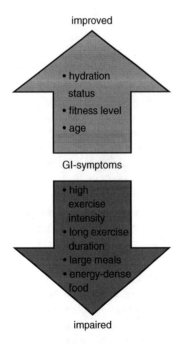

improved

- hydration status
- fitness level
- age

GI-symptoms

- high exercise intensity
- long exercise duration
- large meals
- energy-dense food

impaired

Gastrointestinal Symptoms. Fig. 1 Parameters known to improve (*green*) or to impair (*red*) exercise-associated gastrointestinal symptomatology/disorders

than unexperienced athletes. Some studies show a higher incidence of exercise-induced GI symptoms in women than in men. However, the case numbers seem to be too small in order to support actually a significant gender-specific effect. Finally, it has to be considered that many athletes use antiphlogistic drugs on a more or less regular basis, which are well known to have many side effects especially on gastrointestinal epithelia.

Clinical Relevance

Clinical and Diagnostic Findings

Important exercise-associated clinical findings include gastroesophageal reflux disease (▶ GERD) and diarrheas with/without bleedings. GERD usually is related to three factors – gastric acid secretion, functionality of the lower esophageal sphincter, and gastric motility. There are not many studies available about the effects of exercise on these factors. Older studies report an inhibition of exhausting exercise on basal and secretagogue-induced acid secretion. However, there are inconsistent findings between healthy athletes and athletes with gastric and/or duodenal ulcer. Similarly, the effects of exercise on esophagus motility vary. Recently, it could be shown that during an ergometer exercise corresponding to about 80% of VO2max the distal esophageal pressure decreased and peristaltic velocity increased. Gastric motility and emptying seem to depend on exercise intensity in a nonlinear way. During moderate exercise gastric emptying improves while at a threshold intensity of about 70–75% VO2max gastric emptying more and more decreases which is further aggravated during exercise in the heat and/or dehydration. Together, during exercise both lower tone of esophageal sphincter and reduced gastric emptying are important prerequisites for GERD [5]. Furthermore, the osmolality of sport drinks is a critical point as sugar concentrations of more than 10% are known to impair gastric emptying. Diagnostic tools for GERD include gastroscopy plus tissue biopsy in order to test for Helicobacter pylori, 24-h-esophageal pH monitoring, and esophageal manometry.

Diarrhea is defined as having more loose or liquid stools per day (>3 g/day) or as having more stool weight (>250 g/day) than is normal for that person. Diarrhea can be associated with any forms of bleeding from occult to macroscopic. It may result from an imbalance of the three processes: intestinal motility, absorption, and secretion. During exercise there is evidence that the various GI regions are differentially affected. In small intestine, moderate exercise of about 40–50% of VO2max already induces a frequency reduction of the migrating-motor complex and an increase of transit time. In contrast, some studies found a decrease of colonic transit time during exercise. In summary, this should result in a decrease of the mean oro-fecal transit time as it is more affected by the colonic than the small intestine transit.

Epithelial integrity is often compromised especially after long-term exercise as indicated by the detection of lipopolysaccharides in serum. But the LPS levels in serum often do not correlate with the clinical symptomatology. Another indicator of epithelial damage is the presence of fecal occult blood. Using a fecal occult blood test (FOBT) the incidence of exercise-associated microbleedings varied from 20% up to 80% after marathon and ultramarathon, respectively. Some case reports document also severe courses with radiologic and histologic signs of an ischemic colitis. Most cases, however, respond to conservative treatment and the need for operative intervention is extremely rare [6]. In case of recurrent diarrheal disease during/after exercise further clinical diagnostics in addition to endoscopic and radiologic approaches should include hydrogen breath tests for diagnosis of dietary disabilities such as lactose or fructose as well as bacterial overgrowth syndrome.

Pathophysiology

Some causal factors of exercise-related GI symptoms have been described in the previous section. However, there are even more under discussion, for example, the local release of neuroendocrine hormones such as vasoactive intestinal polypeptide, secretin, pancreatic polypeptide, and gastrin. In case of running associated dysfunctions also mechanical factors such as increased vertical bowel movements have been proposed. The most probable pathogenetic factor seems to be exercise-induced alterations of GI blood flow. With increasing sympathetic drive during exercise blood flow is shifted away from the GI tract predominantly toward contractile tissues and skin, which induces local and regional hypoxia and hyperthermia followed by reperfusion injury and oxidative stress. These findings are even more pronounced under hot environment or during dehydration.

Treatment Options

In case the diagnosis of exercise-related GI disorders has been confirmed several treatment options including training-specific and dietary aspects can be recommended. Initially, intensity of exercise and training bouts should be reduced. If GI symptoms disappear or diminish intensity and volume of the following training cycles should be gradually and carefully increased to allow for gastrointestinal adaptations. If this procedure interferes with the athlete's personal and seasonal objectives alternatively a change of exercise type can be considered. The so-called cross-training allows for relevant training stimuli while at the same time the gastrointestinal side effects may be avoided [7].

Dietary aspects focus on food quantity/quality and on the time point of food uptake before an exercise event. Usually the uptake of large meals before exercise enhances the probability of gastrointestinal discomfort. During phases of competition and high-intensity training the uptake of highly calorific diet should be avoided. However, in the meantime such a diet is helpful to enhance the intestinal absorptive capacity. Furthermore, it guarantees the optimization of glycogen pools and the supplementation with micronutrients. Specifically, the daily uptake of carbohydrates and proteins should amount to 7–12 g/kg body weight and 1.2–1.6 g/kg body weight, respectively. Percentage of fats should amount to at least 25% of whole food energy [8, 9, 11].

During competition the recommended carbohydrate uptake is about 30–60 g/h. There is no need for a higher dosage as this would exceed the limits of intestinal transport capacity [9]. Food known to be rich in dietary fiber should be avoided. The tolerance toward products of high-lactose content can be reduced during intensive exercise bouts. However, one should be aware that there exists a high degree of interindividual variations with regard to the dietary aspects.

Finally, the athlete should be aware of a balanced hydration status before exercise and an optimal fluid replacement during competition. The latter depends on exercise duration, environmental conditions, and individual aspects such as sweat rate, etc. Excessive fluid supplementation should be avoided in order to prevent exercise-induced hyponatremia. Therefore, fluid loss and uptake should be balanced that exercise-associated body weight changes of more than 2% are avoided [10].

With respect to the various sport drinks available athletes are asked to inform themselves about their composition and the individual taste and tolerance. Some drinks contain high concentrations of carbohydrates which may cause GI symptoms. Also fruit juices which are often diluted with water show great variations regarding the individual tolerance as the fruit acid can induce reflux symptoms.

Finally, many treatment options for prevention and therapy of exercise-associated GI disorders are quite similar for athletes and nonathletes. In case of GERD this includes the abstinence of food known to reduce lower esophageal sphincter such as chocolate, peppermint, onions, nicotin, coffee, etc. Moreover, a sleeping position with an elevated upper part of the body is recommended. Antacids, H2 antagonists, or proton pump inhibitors are used for pharmaceutical intervention. In case of exercise-induced diarrhea fluid replacement is suggested initially. Furthermore, drugs with motility-reducing effects such as loperamide can be used temporarily. Ischemic colitis usually requires an intravenous fluid replacement combined with the administration of antibiotics during severe courses of the disease.

References

1. de Oliveira EP, Burini RC (2009) The impact of physical exercise on the gastrointestinal tract. Curr Opin Clin Nutr Metab Care 12: 533–538
2. ter Steege RW, Van der Palen J, Kolkman JJ (2008) Prevalence of gastrointestinal complaints in runners competing in a long-distance run: an internet-based observational study in 1281 subjects. Scand J Gastroenterol 43:1477–1482
3. Peters HP, Bos M, Seebregts L, Akkermanns LM, van Berge-Henegouwen GP, Bol E, Mostered WL, de Vries WR (1999) Gastrointestinal symptoms in long-distance runners, cyclists, and triathletes: prevalence, medication, and etiology. Am J Gastroenterol 94:1570–1581
4. Peters HP, van Schelven FW, Verstappen PA, de Boer RW, Bol E, Erich WB, van der Togt CR, de Vries WR (1993) Gastrointestinal problems as a function of carbohydrate supplements and mode of exercise. Med Sci Sports Exerc 25:1211–1224
5. van Nieuwenhoven MA, Brouns F, Brummer RJ (1999) The effect of physical exercise on parameters of gastrointestinal function. Neurogastroenterol Motil 11:431–439
6. Cohen DC, Winstanley A, Engledow A, Windsor AC, Skipworth JR (2009) Marathon-induced ischemic colitis: why running is not always good for you. Am J Emerg Med 255:e5–e7
7. Murray R (2006) Training the gut for competition. Curr Sports Med Rep 5:161–164
8. Burke L, Kiens B, Ivy J (2004) Carbohydrates and fat for training and recovery. J sport Sci 22:15–30
9. Jeukendrup AE, Jentjens R (2000) Oxidation of carbohydrate feedings during prolonged exercise: current thoughts, guidelines and directions for future research. Sports Med 29:407–424
10. Coyle EF (2004) Fluid and fuel intake during exercise. J Sports Sci 22:39–55
11. Tarnopolsky M (2006) Protein and amino acid need for training and bulking up. In: Burke L, Deakin V (eds) Clinical sports nutrition, 3rd edn. Mcgraw Hill Medical, Sydney

Gene

A specific base sequence of DNA that provides the necessary information to direct the sequence of amino acids to be incorporated into a polypeptide. The human genome contains an estimated 30,000 genes.

Gene Doping

HIDDE J. HAISMA
Pharmaceutical Gene Modulation, Groningen Research Institute of Pharmacy, Groningen University, Groningen, The Netherlands

Synonyms

Genetic doping

Definition

Doping in sports has been defined by the World Anti-Doping Agency (WADA) as the "occurrence of one or more anti-doping rule violations" that have been further detailed in the World Anti-Doping Code [1]. Those rules include the presence of a prohibited substance or its metabolites or markers in an athlete's bodily specimen, the use or attempted use of a prohibited substance or method, refusal or failing to provide a doping control sample, violation of requirements regarding out-of-competition testing and athlete's availability, including failure to provide whereabouts information, tampering, or attempting to tamper with any part of doping control, possession of as well as trafficking in any prohibited substances and methods, and administration or attempted administration of a prohibited substance or method.

▶ Gene Doping is a prohibited method listed in The World Anti-Doping Code Prohibited List International Standard and is defined as follows:

Methods, with the potential to enhance athletic performance, are prohibited:
1. The transfer of cells or genetic elements (e.g., DNA, RNA)
2. The use of pharmacological or biological agents that alter gene expression

Peroxisome Proliferator Activated Receptor δ (PPARδ) agonists (e.g., GW 1516) and PPARδ-AMP-activated protein kinase (AMPK) axis agonists (e.g., AICAR) are prohibited [2].

Description

The elucidation of the complete human ▶ genome with approximately 35,000 different genes will lead to new possibilities for diagnosis and prevention of a wide variety of diseases. In addition, this knowledge may be used for the design of new therapeutics, based on the DNA sequence information. The rapidly increasing number of genetic therapies as a promising new branch of regular medicine has risen the issue whether these techniques might be abused in the field of sports [3]. Both the World Anti-Doping Agency (WADA) and the International Olympic Committee (IOC) have expressed concerns about this possibility. As a result, the method of gene doping has been included in the list of prohibited classes of substances and prohibited methods.

At this time, almost 200 genes have been identified that are associated with health and fitness. For example, some specific alleles of the ACE gene are associated with improved endurance. This ultimately allows for the selection of athletes ideally suited for a particular sport. Genetic screening at an early age may indicate the greatest potential for a specific child to develop into a top athlete and a specific training program may be designed. On the other hand, genetic screening of athletes may be used to select specific training methods to enhance or improve his or her genetic predisposition.

▶ Gene therapy is an approach to treating disease by either modifying the expressions of an individual's genes or correction of abnormal genes. By administration of DNA rather than a drug, many different diseases are currently being investigated as candidates for gene therapy. These include cystic fibrosis, cardiovascular disease, infectious diseases such as AIDS and cancer. For gene therapy, cells can be taken from the patient, modified in the laboratory, and then reintroduced, or a carrier ("vector") of the correct genetic material may be delivered directly into the patient. This vector can be (chemically modified) DNA or a virus, normally capable of causing disease, which has been modified to carry the required genetic information.

Genes encoding growth factors may be used to improve regeneration of sports-related injuries, including muscle injuries, ligament and tendon ruptures, meniscal tears, cartilage lesions, and bone fractures [4]. Other genes may possibly have an effect on athletic performance (Table 1) such as erythropoietin for increasing endurance or Insulin-like growth factor for improving muscle strength. In addition, gene modulating small molecules are being developed to indirectly increase gene expression. These include orally active small molecules in clinical development for the treatment of anemia and Id2 which is a small molecule-inducible modulator of PPARγ expression which affects endurance.

Clinical Use

Gene therapy is currently an experimental therapy delivered to patients in a well controlled setting. Recent clinical data show encouraging gene therapy results in major diseases: patients with x-linked severe combined immunodeficiency disease, adenosine deaminase

Gene Doping. Table 1 Gene doping genes

Gene	Effect
Endorphins	Decrease pain
EPO[a]	Increase hematocrit
IGF-1[b]	Increase muscle strength
PEPCK-C[c] or PPAR-delta[d]	Increase endurance
VEGF[e]	Increase blood flow

[a]Erythropoitin
[b]Insulin-like growth factor
[c]Phosphoenolpyruvate carboxykinase
[d]Peroxisome-proliferator-activated receptor
[e]Vascular endothelial growth factor

deficiency, chronic granulomatous disease or patients with hemophilia B. In addition, angiogenic gene therapy with vectors expressing the human vascular endothelial growth factor for the treatment of coronary artery disease, showed improvement in angina complaints.

The use of medicines by healthy people, gene therapeutics, or others always involves a certain risk. The risks involved in gene doping are several, and are related both to the vector used (DNA, viral) and to the encoded transgene. So far, clinical gene therapy studies have been relatively safe. Side effects from gene therapy that have been reported are mostly flu-like symptoms. There have been no reports on transfer of gene therapy vectors from treated patients to next of kin or to germ cells. Health risks related to the specific proteins used in gene doping are similar to those of other doping forms. People who unnaturally boost their Epo levels increase their chances of stroke and heart attack because adding red blood cells makes the blood thicker. Whereas the athletes using synthetic Epo today face similar risks, after a few weeks the risk subsides as Epo is cleared from the body and red blood cell production returns to normal levels. But if Epo would be delivered by gene therapy, the level and duration of Epo production is less controllable. The hematocrit level would be less manageable and could continue almost indefinitely, giving rise to pathological Epo levels. Other genes may give different health risks if the expression is not controlled. It may be envisioned that genetic growth hormone treatment with IGF-1 or VEGF may give rise to tumor development.

Detection of Gene Doping

A major concern in the athletic community, especially among doping control agencies, is that no one knows how easily gene doping can be detected, if at all.

The DNA which is used for gene transfer of the gene is of human origin, and therefore not different from that of the person applying gene doping. Many forms of genetic doping do not require the direct injection of genes in the desired target organ, i.e., the Epo gene may be injected into almost any site of the body to locally produce the Epo protein which will then enter the blood stream and stimulate the bone marrow. Only the (urine or blood) level of the protein may be indicative for doping abuse. In the case of Epo treatment, this might be detectable, because of the resulting increase in hemoglobin and hematocrit. However, genes may be turned on and off by taking specific medicines. Studies in monkeys have shown that Epo levels can be controlled in this way, resulting in desirable heamatocrit levels.

A possible solution to the problematic detection of gene doping is the use of RNA or protein markers, as indicators for disruption of normal physiology. ▶ Microarrays have been used to identify the effects of Tetrahydrogestrinone (THG) on the expression of the genes of the mouse genome in muscle. An anabolic steroid-specific signature was identified. RNA or protein signatures may be used to identify gene doping in the future. It will require the sampling and analysis at the level of the individual athlete's physiology over time. These techniques will require storage of samples at low temperatures and thus demands either on site testing or new handling regiments. With progress in RNA array and proteomic techniques, which allow the simultaneous screening of the expression of hundreds of proteins, this technique may become valuable for anti-doping testing.

References

1. World Anti-Doping Agency (2009) The world anti-doping code. http://www.wada-ama.org/Documents/World_Anti-Doping_Program/WADP-The-Code/WADA_Anti-Doping_CODE_2009_EN.pdf. (11-08-2009) 2010, Ref Type: Generic
2. World Anti-Doping Agency (2010) The 2010 prohibited list. http://www.wada-ama.org/Documents/World_Anti-Doping_Program/WADP-Prohibited-list/WADA_Prohibited_List_2010_EN.pdf. (11-08-2010), Ref Type: Generic
3. Haisma HJ, de Hon O (2006) Gene doping. Int J Sports Med 27(4):257–266
4. Huard J, Li Y, Peng HR, Fu FH (2003) Gene therapy and tissue engineering for sports medicine. J Gene Med 5(2):93–108

Gene Expression Profiling

Measurement of the activity of thousands of genes at once, to create a global picture of cellular functions.

Gene Therapy

Is an approach to treating disease by either modifying the expressions of an individual's genes or correction of abnormal genes. By administration of DNA rather than a drug, many different diseases are currently being investigated as candidates for gene therapy (American Society of Gene and Cell Therapy).

General Adaptation Syndrome

Hans Selye, who discovered the stress reaction, recognized that animals exposed to stress showed resistance to a variety of "nocuous" agents. This was a form of immunity, he thought, and he called it the general adaptation syndrome (GAS). GAS is virtually identical with the acute phase reaction. Indeed, APR is an acute host defense reaction mediated by the innate immune system.

Cross-References
▶ Acute Phase Reaction

General Fitness Training

General fitness training is an exercise training program designed to meet general health and fitness goals that involve increasing cardiovascular endurance, muscular strength, muscular endurance, flexibility, and improving body composition. This is typically achieved by performing aerobic exercise at 60–80% or maximum for 20–30 min/day; resistance exercise (e.g., 2–3 sets of 8–12 repetitions training major muscle groups), flexibility training (e.g., 3–5 static stretches held for 15–30 s), and eating a balanced diet to optimize body composition. People who participate in a general fitness program can typically meet nutritional needs following a normal diet (e.g., 1,800–2,400 kcals/day or about 25–35 kcals/kg/day for a 50–80 kg individual) because their caloric demands from exercise are not too great (e.g., 200–400 kcals/session).

Genetic Doping

▶ Gene Doping

Genetic Polymorphism

Genetic polymorphism is due to differences in the DNA sequence coding for a specific gene given rise to different traits. Thus, there may be several forms of DNA sequences at a locus within a population.

Genetics, Trainability

STEPHEN H. DAY, ALUN G. WILLIAMS
MMU Cheshire Sports Genetics Laboratory, Institute for Performance Research, Manchester Metropolitan University, Crewe, UK

Definition

Genetic influence on training describes the way in which human genetic variation influences the interindividual variability in the response of a variety of exercise ▶ phenotypes to standardized training programs. Current research continues to identify new associations between genetic variants and the magnitude of training responses to both endurance and resistance training programs.

Description

Precisely why differences in exercise performance are observed in individuals with similar training status, anthropometric measures, and social and cultural backgrounds is a matter that has intrigued exercise scientists for a significant amount of time. While environmental factors clearly have considerable importance, it is also known that genetic factors influence the way in which one responds to a given set of environmental stimuli. There is a substantial genetic influence on health-related fitness phenotypes. Early cross-sectional data indicated that, in monozygotic twins, maximal aerobic capacity (VO_{2max}) was subject to a heritable influence in excess of 90%, although this estimate has been revised to between 25% and 40%. The situation is less clear with regards to the genetic influence on strength and power performance. Cross-sectional studies have indicated that the heritable influence on lower limb muscle strength is within the range of 30% and 80%, depending on limb angle and velocity of contraction. More pertinent however is the heritability of the training response – particularly as training is widely prescribed for certain patient groups to improve disease prognosis, the general public to maintain health and competitive sportspeople alike. The heritability of the training response has been estimated at around 40–50% for VO_{2max} [1], which is relevant to endurance modalities. The heritability of the response to strength training has been estimated to be around 20% for 1RM arm, isometric and concentric strength [2], although more, larger studies are needed to confirm or adjust this initial estimate.

The molecular revolution in biomedical science, epitomized by the Human Genome Project, together with rapid advances in laboratory technologies, has brought the ability to examine genetic variation into the average biological laboratory. We now know that the human genome consists of approximately 21,000 protein-coding genes, although these sections only cover ~1.5% of the genome. The other ~98.5% includes many biologically functionally conserved noncoding elements. We know that all humans have a high degree of genetic similarity which is somewhere in excess of 99%, depending on how it is calculated. Nevertheless, variations in sequence and structural organization of the genome are at least partly responsible for the important interindividual differences seen in a wide range of biological phenotypes. Sequence variations occur approximately every 1,000 bp and in addition a typical person possesses approximately 100 copy number variations covering ~3 Mb of DNA. The vast majority of genetic variation is due to common variants, although the quantitatively fewer rare variants tend to have greater potential for major biological effects [3]. With this knowledge of the genome and genomic variation, exercise scientists now have the opportunity to precisely examine the genetic factors which confer superior physical performance on certain individuals. Primarily during the last 10 years, a considerable number of studies have examined the role of a variety of genetic polymorphisms on exercise phenotypes – as of April 2011, a Medline database search for articles under the MeSH terms "exercise" and "▶ genotype" returns 490 literature records. To date, over 250 DNA polymorphisms have been associated with some form of human physical performance or health-related fitness phenotype [4].

Genetic studies of elite athletes have generally not examined (for good practical reasons) the influence of genetic variation on the level of response which occurs following a controlled, standardized program of training. Therefore, the majority of the studies that have focused on genetic influence on training have examined subject populations that, initially at least, were relatively sedentary and certainly did not excel in competitive sport. Consequently, the majority of studies that have investigated genotype associations with exercise phenotypes provide evidence that is probably more applicable to exercise responses in a medicine or public health scenario than to elite sport. The next section will therefore briefly examine some selected polymorphisms which have been associated with the magnitude of the training response during either endurance or resistance training, when applied to relatively untrained individuals.

Genetics and Endurance Training

Endurance ability and related phenotypes are well-recognized as a predictor of all-cause mortality, as well as risk of certain diseases including various forms of cardiovascular disease and cancer. Research into the genetic influences on the responses to endurance training (which is commonly advised and prescribed for the maintenance of health and for the management of disease) is of interest to both researchers and practitioners. Identification of the relatively "good" and "poor" responders to endurance training, via genetics, would allow prescription of both exercise and pharmaceuticals to be better targeted.

One example of a genotype-phenotype association concerns the *ACE* I/D ▶ polymorphism. The I ▶ allele has been associated with a lower oxygen requirement for low-intensity exercise after training, although the importance of the *ACE* I/D polymorphism for other health-related phenotypes remains controversial. In another example, genetic polymorphisms associated with

calcineurin production and control have been associated with increases in cardiac output, stroke volume, and/or ejection fraction following endurance training. Single nucleotide polymorphisms (SNPs) in the *PPP3CC* and *PPP3R2* genes were associated with changes in the cardiovascular phenotypes.

Single polymorphisms will never be able to completely explain the heritable variability in training response for any exercise phenotype. Given the complexity of the human genome, and that exercise responses tend to involve multiple tissues and cell signaling pathways, it is more likely that polygenic effects are responsible for the variability observed. In the first ▶ genome-wide association study (GWAS) focusing on the change in VO_{2max} [5], 21 SNPs were identified which accounted for 49% of the variance in VO_{2max} trainability – a significant advance over any previous study. A "predictor SNP score" was calculated from the genetic data which distinguishes between individuals who show differing magnitudes of responses to training (Fig. 1). These extremely promising data require independent replication before these findings can be used for identification of high and low responders to endurance training in clinical or sport settings.

Genetics and Resistance Training

Muscle mass and strength, and their related phenotypes, have recently been confirmed as predictors of all-cause

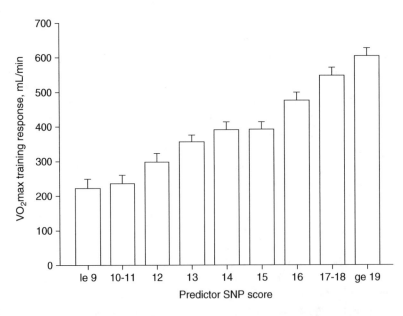

Genetics, Trainability. Fig. 1 The response of VO_{2max} to training in groups of individuals defined by a "predictor SNP score" derived from 21 polymorphisms identified via GWAS (Adapted from Figure 3 in Bouchard et al. [5])

mortality and also play major roles in the ability of older people to maintain functional ability and a high quality of life. Therefore, research into the genetic influences on the responses to strength training (which is increasingly being advised and prescribed for the maintenance of health and for the management of disease) is again of interest to both researchers and practitioners.

One example of a genotype-phenotype association concerns a repeat polymorphism in the promoter region of the *IGF1* gene. Carriers of the "192" allele have been shown to increase strength more in response to resistance training than the noncarriers. In another example, an R577X polymorphism in the *ACTN3* gene has been associated with changes in some skeletal muscle phenotypes following resistance training. Although still controversial, strength gains have been shown to be greater in women of XX genotype following resistance training. In a third example, polymorphisms in the *IL15* and *IL15RA* genes have been associated with the magnitude of increases in strength phenotypes during resistance training. There has been no GWAS conducted on the response to resistance training, nor indeed is there any other source of data to show that a panel of polymorphisms can predict a sizeable proportion of the interindividual variability in training response.

Application

Genetic analyses of athletes, based on strong evidence, could enable coaches to enhance their talent identification strategies, individualize training programs, and modify training load to minimize risk of injury. However, given the current stage of knowledge in exercise genetics, this appears premature and currently offers little in the way of tangible benefit to athletes and their coaches.

In the medical and public health domains, identification of patients whose condition may respond most from exercise (for example, via exercise training-induced reductions in hypertension, or exercise training-induced increases in the functional ability of muscle in older individuals) compared to those who would have a lesser response from exercise alone could enable more targeted exercise and pharmaceutical intervention strategies. Financial cost effectiveness, and the limiting of pharmaceutical interventions to those individuals who will not benefit substantially from the prescription of exercise alone, are both clearly attractive to health service providers. Fewer prescriptions of antihypertensive drugs and improved quality of life for older people are just two examples of the potential future applications of exercise genetics. For the moment, however, they remain aspirations – knowledge of exercise genetics is not yet ready to be

translated "from bench to bedside." One other important way that exercise genetics research may influence medicine is by providing insight regarding underlying molecular mechanisms. That insight can direct pharmaceutical research to specific processes and pathways that, ultimately, may produce drugs with the potential to treat patients regardless of genotype.

References

1. Bouchard C, An P, Rice T, Skinner JS, Wilmore JH, Gagnon J, Pérusse L, Leon AS, Rao DC (1999) Familial aggregation of VO₂max response to exercise training: results from the HERITAGE Family Study. J Appl Physiol 87:1003–1008
2. Thomis MAI, Beunen GP, Maes HH, Blimkie CJ, Van Leemputte M, Claessens AL, Marchal G, Willems E, Vlietinck RF (1998) Strength training: importance of genetic factors. Med Sci Sports Exerc 30:724–731
3. Lander ES (2011) Initial impact of the sequencing of the human genome. Nature 470:187–197
4. Bray MS, Hagberg JM, Pérusse L, Rankinen T, Roth SM, Wolfarth B, Bouchard C (2009) The human gene map for performance and health-related fitness phenotypes: the 2006–2007 update. Med Sci Sports Exerc 41:35–73
5. Bouchard C, Sarzynski MA, Rice TK, Kraus WE, Church TS, Sung YJ, Rao DC, Rankinen T (2011) Genomic predictors of maximal oxygen uptake response to standardized exercise training programs. J Appl Physiol 110:1160–1170

Genome

The complete genetic material of an organism, which includes both the chromosomes in the nucleus and the DNA in the mitochondria.

Genome-Wide Association Study (GWAS)

An approach to genomic research that does not begin with specific hypotheses about specific genes, but instead attempts to identify important variations in DNA sequence at any point in the genome.

Genotype

The genetic makeup of an individual. A person's genotype may refer to a single region of the DNA sequence or to several distinct regions of the DNA.

GERD

Gastroesophageal reflux disease.

Cross-References

▶ Gastrointestinal Symptoms

Geriatrics

A specialty of medicine focused on the health care of elderly people that aims to prevent and treat diseases and disabilities in older adults. Geriatrics involves ways to prevent or manage the diseases of aging. The field of "geriatrics" is also a specialty in nursing, dentistry, and physical therapy, and deals with the long-term health problems in older adults.

Gerontology

The study of the social, psychological, and biological aspects of aging. "Biogerontology" is concerned with the biological processes of aging and encompasses interdisciplinary research on the causes, effects, and mechanisms of biological aging. Gerontologists view aging from different perspectives, including chronological, biological, psychological, and social perspectives.

Cross-References

▶ Aging, Motor Performance

Giant Muscle Proteins: Titin/Nebulin

Julius Bogomolovas[1], Henk Granzier[2], Siegfried Labeit[1]
[1]Klinikum Mannheim GmbH Universitätsklinikum, Universitätsmedizin Mannheim, University of Heidelberg, Mannheim, Germany
[2]Department of Physiology and the Sarver Molecular Cardiovascular Research Program, University of Arizona, Tucson, AZ, USA

Synonyms

Connectin; Giant proteins

Definition

Titin

Titin, with up to 4.2 MDa, is the largest polypeptide chain discovered so far in nature [1]. While the titin polypeptide is easily overlooked by standard analytical procedures, titin is in fact an abundant component of vertebrate striated muscle (skeletal and heart muscle) where it comprises about 10% of the total proteome. In situ, the giant titin polypeptide chain spans entire half of the ▶ sarcomere. The N-terminus of titin is anchored in Z-discs whereas its C-terminal end is located at the M-line (see also Fig. 1, for review: [7]). Titin is extensively modular in structure. About 45% of titin consists of immunoglobulin-like (Ig), and 45% of fibronectin type III (Fn3) domain repeats. The remaining 10% of the molecule corresponds to specialized domains, including the so-called PEVK repeats (an element rich in proline (P), glutamate (E), valine (V), and lysine (K) residues) located in titin's elastic I-band region, the N2B unique sequence as a heart-specific domain with both elastic and signaling functions, and a serine/threonine kinase domain within the M-line titin region. Because titin molecules from adjacent half-sarcomeres[1] are connected within the Z-disc and in the M-line lattices by interactions with Z-disc and M-line proteins, respectively, titin forms a continuous filament system within the myofibril. This together with titin's intrinsic elasticity provides titin with a central role in muscle biomechanics.

Nebulin

Nebulin, after titin, is the second largest known polypeptide to date. This giant, 600–900 kDa sized, protein is expressed only in skeletal muscles [6]. A smaller 107-kDa nebulin-homologous protein, termed "nebulette," is found in cardiac muscle and encoded by a different gene [10]. Nebulin, like titin, is filamentous in structure: The nebulin filament is coextensive with the thin filament with its COOH-terminus being anchored in Z-disc and N-terminus interacting with tropomodulin at the end of I band. Like titin, the nebulin protein is extensively modular in structure. About 97% of nebulin consists of 35-residue alpha-helical actin binding motifs arranged in super-repeats with a sevenfold periodicity, thus matching the thin filament sevenfold repeat. Consistent with the idea that nebulin is critical for maintaining and regulating thin filament lengths, nebulin-knockout mice have shorter and less precise regulated thin filament lengths. A second hallmark of the nebulin-deficient sarcomeres is displacement of the Z-discs and the accumulation of the Z-disc derived nemaline bodies (both in the nebulin-knockout mouse models and in patients that have mutations in

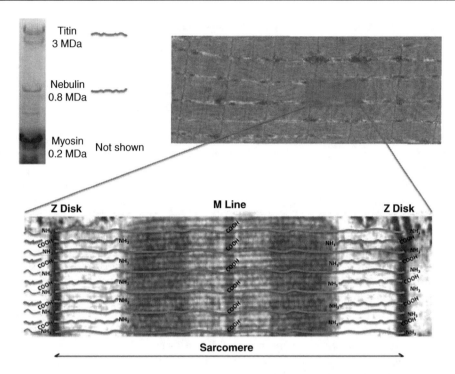

Giant Muscle Proteins: Titin/Nebulin. Fig. 1 In situ layout of the titin and nebulin filament systems within the sarcomere. *Upper right*: Ultrastructure of a myofibril as visualized by electron microscopy. *Bottom*: Blue and red indicate the span of titin and nebulin polypeptides with respect to Z-discs and M-lines in a single sarcomere. *Upper left*: On low percentage agarose gels, giant titin and nebulin polypeptides are detected far above myosin, consistent with their molecular weights, as predicted from sequencing studies

nebulin). These findings in human nemaline myopathy indicate importance of the nebulin in maintenance of the Z-discs and overall muscle homeostasis (for review: [8]).

Characteristics

Titin in Muscle Biomechanics

Functionally, titin elasticity is provided by its I-band region containing three different sequence elements, each of which has a different stiffness profile: At low stretch forces tandem arranged Ig domains that interact with each other weakly are stretched out. Upon further stretch, the PEVK repeats unfold. All striated muscles contain these two types of spring elements. In addition, the cardiac-specific N2B element provides a reserve element in heart to prevent overstretches. The inhomogeneous domain composition of titin's I-band region provides a complex sarcomere elasticity profile under the stretch that functionally operates more flexible than a homogeneous spring. In heart, these features of titin contribute to modulation of ▶ Frank–Starling mechanism in particular at the early diastole. The biomechanical properties of

titin are tailored to match the different physiological requirements of muscles. As an underlying mechanism operating long-term, titin's passive force is modulated by alternative splicing: Specific exon groups coding for PEVK or tandem Ig spring elements are skipped or included to adjust overall elasticity. Presumably faster adaptations are accommodated by posttranslational modification events: phosphorylation by protein kinases A and G (PKA and PKG) reduces and phosphorylations by protein kinase C increases titin-based stiffness. These three kinases phorphorylate at least in vitro specific motifs in titin's spring elements (for review: [3]). More recently, oxidative cross-linking of SH groups in titin's N2B elements has been found to enhance cardiac titin stiffness, a mechanism that could link together myofibrillar mechanics and ischemia [4]. Finally, not only modification of polypeptide itself, but also interaction of titin with other proteins can modify its biophysical parameters. Small heat shock protein ▶ αB crystallin interacts with N2B sequence of titin and stabilizes it [16]. In summary, a variety of mechanisms presumably operating under different time-scales and physiological states can adjust titin elasticity.

This indicates titin's central role in the regulation of muscle biomechanics.

Clinical Relevance

Titin Signaling

While titin is structurally a critical component for sarcomeric integrity, mutiple lines of evidence suggest signaling roles for titin. For example, a serine/threonine kinase domain located at the M-line spanning region of titin is likely involved in signaling processes. A dual activation including phosphorylation as well as mechanical stretch was proposed as prerequisites for the activation (for review: [2]). Stretch sensing by titin and transformation into an output signal may also be achieved by specific titin/ligand interactions (where binding to titin is predicted to occur to stretch-sensitive conformations). These titin/titin ligand complexes involved in muscle signaling and remodeling include, among others, muscle ring finger proteins (MuRFs), muscle-specific protease – calpain 3, muscle ankyrin repeat proteins (MARPs), and transcription modulators FHLs. Formation of these titin-based complexes was shown experimentally to be at least partially stretch modulated (for review: [5]).

An evolutionary conserved docking site for MuRFs (a family of E3 ubiquitin ligases) is located in a near proximity to the titin kinase domain. Physiologically, these proteins were identified to target muscle proteins to the ▶ proteosome degradation under catabolic conditions. It was shown that expression and localization of MuRF 1 and MuRF 2 are activity-dependent. However, the functional consequences of MuRF binding in near proximity to the titin kinase domain are not well understood.

Another titin-based myocellular signaling axis involves titin, muscle-specific protease – calpain 3, and muscle ankyrin repeat proteins (MARPs). The elastic N2A region of titin serves as a competitive docking platform for the MARP's and the protease. Upon eccentric exercise calpain 3 replaces MARP2 in N2A region, leading to the nuclear translocation where MARP2 promotes adaptive muscle response. This process malfunctions with catalytically inactive calpain 3 found to be the cause of human limb-girdle muscle dystrophy 2A. Mice lacing catalytically active calpain 3 develop muscle dystrophy with pathological susceptibility to the exercise-induced injury, mimicking the symptoms of human disease [11].

This signaling axis does not function isolated but rather involves other MARP family members. It was shown that MARP1 or CARP is a substrate of calpain 3 and the sarcomeric sequestration of CARP is promoted by the proteolysis of the protein, therefore altering the signaling potential of the CARP. The cross talk between titin CARP and calpain 3 could be more complex and far reaching: impaired binding of calpain 3 to N2A region of titin leads to severe muscle dysfunction and enormously high expression levels of CARP in mdm mice model (for review: [9]).

An additional titin-based stretch sensor is found in the heart. In heart, the so-called N2B spring region serves as an additional platform for stretch-regulated interactions. Two members of four and a half Lim domain (FHL) proteins, acting as transcriptional regulators, as well as the chaperone aB-crystallin are targeted to this region of titin under stress and strain conditions. Consistent with a role in stretch sensing, deletion of FHL1 rescues from pressure overload induced cardiac hypertrophy and subsequent heart failure [13]. Moreover, under physiological conditions myocardium of FHL1 knockout mice is more compliant and no increase in compliance is achieved by stimulating PKA activity. These data support a model that FHL1 bound to N2B region could physically prevent PKA-mediated titin phosphorylation, leading to an increased compliance [12].

Nebulin Signaling

Recent data indicate that nebulin similar as titin not only serves as a structural scaffold but has important signaling roles. For example, the ▶ IGF-1 signaling pathway, a major anabolic route mediating the induction of muscle hypertrophy, involves also nebulin. IGF-1 induces translocation and binding of ▶ N-WASP to the nebulin. This in turn induces the formation of the new thin filaments, and this event appears to be essential for the IGF-1-induced muscle hypertrophy [15]. In contrast to direct pro-anabolic signaling involving nebulin, the so far only discovered interaction between titin and IGF-1 involves suppression of catabolic agents. It was shown that activation of IGF-1 pathway leads to reduction of titin-associated ubiquitin ligase MuRF1 and therefore, this could block the muscle atrophy upon catabolic conditions [14]. In summary, nebulin has not only a central role as a structural component of the sarcomere, but recent data implicate nebulin in muscle homeostasis and as well as an active member of signaling networks.

Summary

In brief, both titin and nebulin are increasingly implicated as active players in muscle stress and exercise adaptations. An integrative understanding of their regulatory muscle functions will be incomplete without future research in cross talk between titin and nebulin itself and with the other myofibrillar filament components.

References

1. Bang ML, Centner T et al (2001) The complete gene sequence of titin, expression of an unusual approximately 700-kDa titin isoform, and its interaction with obscurin identify a novel Z-line to I-band linking system. Circ Res 89(11):1065–1072

2. Gautel M (2011) Cytoskeletal protein kinases: titin and its relations in mechanosensing. Pflugers Arch 462(1):119–134

3. Granzier HL, Labeit S (2004) The giant protein titin: a major player in myocardial mechanics, signaling, and disease. Circ Res 94(3):284–295

4. Grutzner A, Garcia-Manyes S et al (2009) Modulation of titin-based stiffness by disulfide bonding in the cardiac titin N2-B unique sequence. Biophys J 97(3):825–834

5. Hoshijima M (2006) Mechanical stress-strain sensors embedded in cardiac cytoskeleton: Z disk, titin, and associated structures. Am J Physiol Heart Circ Physiol 290(4):H1313–H1325

6. Labeit S, Kolmerer B (1995) The complete primary structure of human nebulin and its correlation to muscle structure. J Mol Biol 248(2):308–315

7. Labeit S, Kolmerer B et al (1997) The giant protein titin. Emerging roles in physiology and pathophysiology. Circ Res 80(2):290–294

8. Labeit S, Ottenheijm CA et al (2011) Nebulin, a major player in muscle health and disease. FASEB J 25(3):822–829

9. Laure L, Suel L et al (2009) Cardiac ankyrin repeat protein is a marker of skeletal muscle pathological remodelling. FEBS J 276(3):669–684

10. Moncman CL, Wang K (1995) Nebulette: a 107 kD nebulin-like protein in cardiac muscle. Cell Motil Cytoskeleton 32(3):205–225

11. Ojima K, Kawabata Y et al (2010) Dynamic distribution of muscle-specific calpain in mice has a key role in physical-stress adaptation and is impaired in muscular dystrophy. J Clin Invest 120(8):2672–2683

12. Raskin A, Sheikh F et al (2008) Mechanical role of FHL1 in modulating titin based passive tension poster session presented at: Research Expo 2008. La Jolla, CA

13. Sheikh F, Raskin A et al (2008) An FHL1-containing complex within the cardiomyocyte sarcomere mediates hypertrophic biomechanical stress responses in mice. J Clin Invest 118(12):3870–3880

14. Stitt TN, Drujan D et al (2004) The IGF-1/PI3K/Akt pathway prevents expression of muscle atrophy-induced ubiquitin ligases by inhibiting FOXO transcription factors. Mol Cell 14(3):395–403

15. Takano K, Watanabe-Takano H et al (2010) Nebulin and N-WASP cooperate to cause IGF-1-induced sarcomeric actin filament formation. Science 330(6010):1536–1540

16. Zhu Y, Bogomolovas J et al (2009) Single molecule force spectroscopy of the cardiac titin N2B element: effects of the molecular chaperone alphaB-crystallin with disease-causing mutations. J Biol Chem 284(20):13914–13923

Giant Proteins

▶ Giant Muscle Proteins: Titin/Nebulin

Gln

▶ Glutamine

Glucocorticoid

A hormone that bind to the glucocorticoid receptor (GR), and is associated with regulation of glucose and lipid metabolism as well as aspects of immune function.

Glucocorticoids (Inhaled for Asthma)

Inhaled steroids are the most potent and effective asthma medications to reduce airway inflammation. The regular use of inhaled steroids leads to better asthma control, fewer symptoms and flare-ups, and reduced need for hospitalization. Note that while inhaled steroids prevent asthma symptoms, they do not relieve asthma symptoms during and attack. Inhaled steroids need to be taken daily for best results. Some improvement in asthma symptoms can be seen in 1–3 weeks after starting inhaled steroids, with the best results seen after 3 months of daily use. As of 2011, the World Anti-Doping Agency allows the use of inhaled glucocorticosteroids. However, systemic use is prohibited and requires a Therapeutic Use Exemption.

Glucose

A monosaccharide sugar with a formula of $C_6H_{12}O_6$ and occurs widely in most plant and animal tissue. It is the principal circulating sugar in the blood and the major energy source of the body.

Glucose Intolerance

▶ Insulin Resistance

Glucose Transporters

Mark Hargreaves
Department of Physiology, The University of Melbourne, Melbourne, Australia

Synonyms
GLUT4

Definition

Glucose uptake into mammalian cells occurs by facilitated (energy-independent) diffusion, mediated by the GLUT (SLC2A) transport proteins. To date, 14 members of this transporter family have been identified in humans [1]. More detailed descriptions of these various proteins can be found in numerous reviews (see [1] for relevant references), but most attention has focused on the well-established transporters GLUT 1–4. GLUT1 has a wide tissue expression, but at high levels in the brain, erythrocytes, and endothelial cells, and plays a key role in basal glucose transport. GLUT2 is expressed at high levels in pancreatic β-cells, hepatocytes, and the basolateral membranes of kidney and intestinal epithelial cells. This, coupled with a high Km ($\sim$17 mM) for glucose, ensures rapid glucose transport between the extracellular space and the cytosol in those tissues. GLUT3 is the major glucose transporter in neuronal tissues. Finally, GLUT4 is found in adipose tissue and skeletal and cardiac muscle and has a fundamental role in mediating insulin-stimulated glucose uptake in all these tissues and contraction-stimulated glucose uptake in skeletal and cardiac muscle. Given its importance for these cellular processes in health and disease states characterized by insulin resistance, such as type 2 diabetes, it has been the most studied of the glucose transporters [1]. Alterations in both GLUT4 expression and its trafficking have been implicated in the pathogenesis of insulin resistance in various clinical conditions.

Given the importance of skeletal muscle for whole body glucose metabolism, and the well-known effects of acute and chronic exercise on the capacity of skeletal muscle to take up and metabolize glucose, there has been considerable research and clinical interest in the regulation of skeletal muscle glucose uptake during exercise, with a particular focus on GLUT4 [2].

Basic Mechanisms

Skeletal muscle glucose uptake occurs by facilitated diffusion and increases significantly in response to both insulin stimulation and contractile activity during exercise. Key sites of regulation include glucose delivery, sarcolemmal glucose transport by GLUT4, and intracellular glucose metabolism, following phosphorylation by hexokinase [2]. Although glucose transport is the rate-limiting step for glucose uptake at rest, the marked increase in sarcolemmal GLUT4 (translocation) that occurs in response to contractile activity removes it as a limitation during exercise [2]. That said, the lack of GLUT4 in skeletal muscle of transgenic mice completely abolishes exercise-induced skeletal muscle glucose uptake,

highlighting the fundamental role of GLUT4 and its translocation to the sarcolemma in glucose uptake during exercise. The molecular mechanisms responsible for the translocation from intracellular storage sites to the plasma membrane in response to insulin stimulation have been well studied [3]. Multiple steps in the insulin signaling pathway culminate in increased GLUT4 vesicle exocytosis to the plasma membrane, docking and fusion of GLUT4 vesicles, and increased plasma membrane GLUT4 levels [3]. The GTPase-activating protein TBC1D4, also known as AS160, has emerged as a key distal target linking insulin signaling with GLUT4 trafficking [3]. Of note, while the upstream signaling pathways mediating contraction-stimulated GLUT4 translocation remain to be fully elucidated (see later), they do appear to also engage with AS160 and this protein may be at the intersection of the insulin and contraction pathways [4].

Following isolation and characterization of the GLUT4 gene and its transcriptional regulatory regions in the early 1990s, there has been considerable investigation of the regulation of GLUT4 expression in health and disease [5]. A number of transcription factors can bind to the GLUT4 promoter including Sp1, CCAAT/enhancer-binding protein (C/EBP), myocyte enhancer factor 2 (MEF2), GLUT4 enhancer factor (GEF), MyoD, Kruppel-like factor 15, and thyroid hormone receptor α1 (TR α1), thereby modulating GLUT4 expression [5]. Of these, MEF2 and GEF binding appear to have a crucial role in skeletal muscle-specific GLUT4 expression. The effects of other transcription factors or coactivators, such as the nuclear respiratory factors NRF1 and NRF2 and peroxisome proliferator-activated receptor-γ coactivator-1α (PGC-1 α), on GLUT4 expression also appear to occur via induction of MEF2 [5]. MEF2 activity is inhibited by the transcriptional repressor histone deacetylase 5 (HDAC5). Phosphorylation of HDAC5 by upstream kinases such as AMPK-activated protein kinase (AMPK) results in nuclear export of HDAC5, removal of MEF2 inhibition, and increased GLUT4 expression.

Exercise Intervention

The translocation of GLUT4 to the sarcolemma is fundamental for the increase in skeletal muscle glucose uptake during exercise (Fig. 1), [6]. The molecular signals that result in this trafficking of GLUT4 vesicles in response to exercise have been the focus of considerable interest. A major reason for this is the observation that skeletal muscle glucose uptake is relatively normal in patients with insulin resistance, e.g., in patients with type 2 diabetes. Thus, identification of the "exercise signal" may lead to novel therapeutic strategies for managing insulin

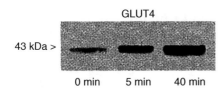

GLUT4

43 kDa >

0 min   5 min   40 min

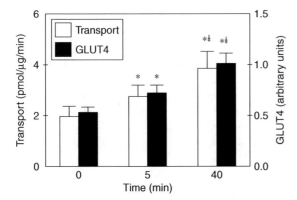

Glucose Transporters. Fig. 1 GLUT4 immunoblot (*top*) and mean glucose transport and GLUT4 protein content (*bottom*) in sarcolemmal vesicles from human muscle obtained before and after 5 and 40 min of cycling exercise at ~75% VO$_2$max. Values are means ± SEM, n = 9. * denotes different from 0, $P < 0.05$ (Reproduced from Kristiansen et al. [6]; Am. Physiol. Soc. used with permission)

resistance. That said, it is unlikely that such a strategy based on a specific signal(s) will fully recapitulate the pleiotropic effects of exercise. Most attention has focused on increased sarcoplasmic [Ca^{2+}], mediated via calcium-sensitive kinases such as Ca^{2+}-calmodulin dependent kinase (CaMK) and protein kinase C (PKC), and metabolic/energetic stress as sensed by AMPK [7, 8]. Other potential mediators of exercise-induced GLUT4 translocation include nitric oxide (NO), reactive oxygen species (ROS), and bradykinin [7, 8].

A major adaptation to regular exercise training is an increase in skeletal muscle GLUT4 expression and this partly contributes to the enhanced insulin action in the trained state. In recent years, it has been proposed that training adaptations may reflect the cumulative result of the responses to repeated, individual exercise sessions. In this regard, it has been observed that a single exercise bout increases GLUT4 gene expression, already at the end of exercise and during recovery. While GLUT4 mRNA levels usually return to basal levels within 24 h, they increase again with a repeated exercise bout and over time there is a progressive increase in GLUT4 protein expression with regular exercise training. The same signals that mediate GLUT4 translocation in response to acute

exercise, notably Ca^{2+} and metabolic/energetic stress, also appear to mediate exercise effects on GLUT4 expression. Phosphorylation of HDAC5 by AMPK and CaMK, indirectly via HDAC5 oligomerization with HDAC4 since HDAC4 is a CaMK substrate, results in nuclear export of HDAC5, reduced HDAC5-MEF2 association, and increased MEF2 DNA binding [9]. Together with p38 MAPK-mediated phosphorylation and activation of MEF2 activity, increased MEF2 binding results in increased GLUT4 transcription and ultimately translation [9]. Recently, we have observed that exercise training increases both skeletal muscle and adipose tissue GLUT4 protein levels in type 2 diabetes [10]. Given that adipose tissue GLUT4 expression is reduced in type 2 diabetes, this provides yet another reason to include regular exercise in the management of this and other metabolic conditions.

References

1. Thorens B, Mueckler M (2010) Glucose transporters in the 21st century. Am J Physiol 298:E141–E145
2. Wasserman DH (2009) Four grams of glucose. Am J Physiol 296:E11–E21
3. Huang S, Czech MP (2007) The GLUT4 glucose transporter. Cell Metab 5:237–252
4. Cartee GD, Funai K (2009) Exercise and insulin: convergence or divergence at AS160 and TBC1D1? Exerc Sport Sc Rev 37:188–195
5. Karnieli E, Armoni M (2008) Transcriptional regulation of the insulin-responsive glucose transporter GLUT4 gene: from physiology to pathology. Am J Physiol 295:E38–E45
6. Kristiansen S, Hargreaves M, Richter EA (1997) Progressive increase in glucose transport and GLUT-4 in human sarcolemmal vesicles during moderate exercise. Am J Physiol 272:E385–E389
7. Rose AJ, Richter EA (2005) Skeletal muscle glucose uptake during exercise: how is it regulated? Physiology 20:260–270
8. Jessen N, Goodyear LJ (2005) Contraction signaling to glucose transport in skeletal muscle. J Appl Physiol 99:330–337
9. McGee SL, Hargreaves M (2006) Exercise and skeletal muscle glucose transporter 4 expression: molecular mechanisms. Clin Exp Pharmacol Physiol 33:395–399
10. Hussey SE, McGee SL, Garnham A, Wentworth JM, Jeukendrup AE, Hargreaves M (2011) Exercise training increases adipose tissue GLUT4 expression in patients with type 2 diabetes. Diab Obes Metab 13:959–962

Glucose-Electrolyte Solution

A glucose-electrolyte solution (GES) is a water-based solution that typically contains 6–8% carbohydrate and electrolytes (e.g., sodium chloride, potassium, calcium, magnesium). Research indicates that ingesting GES prior to, during, and following exercise can help prevent dehydration and/or help athletes rehydration after exercise.

GLUT4

An insulin-sensitive glucose transporter found abundantly in skeletal muscle and adipose tissue. In the unstimulated state, GLUT4 largely resides within the cytosol of the cell. Upon stimulation with insulin, the GLUT4 protein translocates to cell surface membranes (e.g., plasma membrane and T-tubule). Once integrated in the membrane, glucose can enter the cell down its concentration gradient. Factors other than insulin (e.g., muscle contraction, hypoxia) can also trigger GLUT4 translocation to cell surface membranes.

Cross-References

▶ Glucose Transporters

Glutamine

L. M. Castell[1], P. Newsholme[2]
[1]University of Oxford, Green Templeton College, Oxford, UK
[2]School of Biomolecular and Biomedical Science, Conway Institute and Health Sciences Complex, University College Dublin, Dublin, Ireland

Synonyms

2-Amino-4-carbamoylbutanoic acid; 2-aminoglutaramic acid; Amide; D-Glutamine; Gln; Glutamine: $C_5H_{10}N_2O_3$; L-Glutamine

Definition

Glutamine ($C_5H_{10}N_2O_3$), the most abundant amino acid in the body, is endogenously synthesized from glutamate and NH_4^+ [9]. Glutamine has a variety of roles, for example, as a metabolic fuel, in the maintenance of acid–base balance, as a precursor for neurotransmitter synthesis such as glutamate and γ-amino butyric acid (GABA) and as a precursor for the antioxidant, glutathione. After protein digestion, individual amino acids travel via the hepatic vein to the liver and then, if not metabolized, to muscle where they can be used to produce glutamine in addition to becoming incorporated into new protein. Glutamine was originally classified as a nonessential amino acid. However, there is increasing evidence that glutamine becomes "conditionally essential" in specific conditions of stress.

Mechanism of Action

Glutamine is synthesized, stored, and released predominantly by skeletal muscle and, to a lesser extent, by adipocytes, liver, and lung: it is taken up by intestinal cells, such as enterocytes and colonocytes, by the kidney, liver, pancreatic islet cells, and by immune cells such as lymphocytes, macrophages, and neutrophils. During physiological stress such as exercise, an increase in the concentration of cortisol in the blood can initiate proteolysis of muscle proteins, transamination of amino acids to glutamate, synthesis of glutamine and increased release of glutamine. About 8–9 g of glutamine per day is released from the entire human musculature. In humans, the muscle concentration of glutamine is approximately 20 mM, compared to 0.7 mM in plasma. The rate of release across the plasma membrane, which occurs via a specific transporter, is controlled by the hormonal milieu and by chemical messengers such as cytokines. Cytokines may be released from cells of the immune system and can communicate with skeletal muscle. It has been demonstrated that the secretion of cytokines or cell surface activation markers is glutamine-dependent.

Glutamine is required by rapidly dividing cells and provides nitrogen for the synthesis of purine and pyrimidine nucleotides. These nucleotides are needed for the synthesis of new DNA and RNA, for mRNA synthesis and DNA repair. Work undertaken by Ardawi and Newsholme [1] showed a surprisingly high utilization of glutamine by resting, unstimulated human lymphocytes. Subsequent in vitro work in the same laboratory showed that, despite the presence of all other nutrients, only when glutamine was reduced did a decrease occur in the proliferative ability of human lymphocytes. Glutamine utilization was found to be similarly high in unstimulated or stimulated mouse macrophages and human monocytes. In vitro studies have demonstrated a small increase in the production of T-lymphocyte–derived cytokines (IL-1α, IL-6, and IL-10) in the presence of 1 mM glutamine.

Much novel research in the glutamine field, particularly in the contexts of muscle, immune and gut function, nutrition support, and exercise performance was initiated by Eric Newsholme, who died in March 2011.

Clinical Use

Early observations reported that the plasma concentration of glutamine (p[Gln]) was decreased in clinical situations such as major surgery, burns, starvation, and sepsis: these conditions are associated with impaired immune function. In particular, the (p[Gln]) is often greatly reduced in severe cachexia [10].

Muscle glutamine concentration can also be substantially reduced in various conditions. Roth et al. [14] observed a marked decrease (up to 80%) in patients with severe abdominal sepsis.

Glutamine Supplementation in Clinical Conditions

The first reported instance of glutamine feeding in humans was by Welbourne et al. [16]. They observed an increase in (p[Gln]) during alkalosis in patients with renal disease receiving enteral glutamine. Since then, glutamine, in either free or dipeptide form, has been administered parenterally or enterally to patients in intensive care after surgery, acute pancreatitis (AP), irritable bowel disease (IBD), etc., with different outcomes. Space precludes the discussion of more than a few studies, and the reader is referred to Castell [3] for some citations. Published studies have found effects of glutamine via the following:

Parenteral Nutrition

In an early study (1989), muscle glutamine loss was almost abolished and nitrogen balance increased with the provision of 12 g alanyl-glutamine dipeptide per diem after major surgery.

Griffiths et al. [7] undertook further analysis of data from their 1997 study and found that supplementation with glutamine-enriched total parenteral nutrition (TPN) had led to a decrease in both catheter-related and acquired infections in ICU patients.

Another early glutamine feeding study in a clinical setting was on bone marrow transplant patients. Among other findings, a decrease in infectious episodes and increased cell function was observed in the group receiving glutamine-enriched TPN as opposed to placebo.

In 2006, a large-scale study reported a decrease in infectious complications when supplementing ICU patients with a glutamine dipeptide (L-alanyl-glutamine) in TPN.

The role of glutamine in parenteral nutrition has recently been reviewed by Yarandi et al. [15].

Enteral Nutrition

In 1998, a decrease was observed in infectious morbidity in trauma patients given glutamine-enriched enteral nutrition.

A 2001 study compared the effect of a glutamine-rich with a non-glutamine-rich enteral formula on immunological parameters in 16 patients with AP. The recovery of immunological parameters was better and the time of disease recovery was shorter in the glutamine-treated group.

More recently, in a randomized controlled trial, a combination of arginine, glutamine, ω-3 fatty acids, and antioxidants was given enterally to 31 patients with severe AP: surprisingly, an increase in C-reactive protein was found in the study group compared with controls. Decreases reported from the same study in the length of ICU and hospital stay, and in the incidence of pneumonia and multi-organ failure, were not statistically significant.

Many clinical studies have reported that exogenous glutamine has beneficial effects on gastrointestinal function (see [3] for citations). A recent comprehensive review by Xue et al. [17] discusses the role of glutamine in nutritional modulation of gastrointestinal toxicity related to cancer treatments.

In in vitro studies, glutamine has been seen to enhance the bactericidal ability of neutrophils in samples after surgery and from burns patients.

There is still some difference of opinion as to whether enteral feeding, involving the provision of glutamine, is better for critically ill patients than parenteral nutrition [2]. However, one thing that can be said in favor of glutamine is that its supplementation in very high doses (as much as 0.6 g/kg bodyweight) has not been observed to have any deleterious effects on patients. This compares favorably with probiotics, which, in a large-scale random trial of a *Lactobacilli* and *Bifidobacterium* probiotic preparation, resulted in nine patients with severe acute pancreatitis in the supplement group (vs none in the placebo group) developing bowel ischemia which ultimately proved fatal for eight of them.

Glutamine continues to be recommended in many guidelines for clinical care of various patient groups, and such recommendations are supported by meta-analyses. To some, the science and logic of a positive role for glutamine appears irrefutable, and glutamine supplementation given routinely in clinical studies has often shown benefit in reducing infection risk. However, the design of some large studies has been poor. Such studies are best set up from the perspective of regarding glutamine as a nutritional agent rather than a drug: the importance of obtaining sound nutritional advice in this context cannot be over-estimated.

Glutamine and Heat-Shock Proteins

Glutamine has been reported to prevent atrophy of intestinal epithelial cells and to protect against sepsis via heat-shock proteins (HSP), in particular HSP70. Fehrenbach et al. [6] suggested a protective effect of

HSPs in leucocytes in athletes after endurance exercise. HSP70/72 are of particular importance in this role. Indeed, extracellular HSP72 stimulates cytokine activity, the "chaperokine" capacity of HSP72. The circulating concentration of HSP72 which increases after exercise also facilitates neutrophil activity [8]. Despite the considerable increase in circulating numbers of neutrophils after strenuous exercise, decreased neutrophil function has been observed in both runners and cyclists: more immature neutrophils will be recruited in such a situation, which will function less well than their mature counterparts.

There is increasing evidence from different studies that glutamine is important for HSP generation. Another role for glutamine was observed in a 1997 study showing that glutamine was utilized by rat neutrophils; a more recent study established the presence of glutaminase, the major enzyme for the degradation of glutamine, on the secretory granules of human neutrophils. Given this work, it is tempting to speculate that glutamine may have a role in increased HSP generation which is linked to neutrophil function.

Insulinotropic Actions of Amino Acids and the Essential Role of Glutamine

Under appropriate conditions, amino acids enhance insulin secretion from primary islet cells and beta cell lines. In vivo, L-glutamine and L-alanine are quantitatively the most abundant amino acids in the blood and extracellular fluids, closely followed by the branched chain amino acids (BCAA). However, individual amino acids do not evoke insulin-secretory responses in vitro when added at physiological concentrations, rather, combinations of physiological concentrations of amino acids or high concentrations of individual amino acids are much more effective. In vivo, amino acids derived from dietary proteins and those released from intestinal epithelial cells, in combination with glucose, stimulate insulin secretion, thereby leading to protein synthesis and amino acid transport in target tissues such as skeletal muscle [11].

While amino acids can potentially affect a number of aspects of beta cell function, a relatively small number of amino acids promote or synergistically enhance insulin release from pancreatic beta cells [12]. The mechanisms by which amino acids enhance insulin secretion are understood to rely primarily on: (1) direct depolarization of the plasma membrane (e.g., cationic amino acid, L-arginine); (2) metabolism (e.g., glutamine, leucine); and (3) co-transport with Na^+ and cell membrane depolarization (e.g., L-alanine). Notably, partial oxidation, for example, L-alanine, may also initially increase the cellular content of adenosine triphosphate (ATP)

impacting on K_{ATP} channel closure prompting membrane depolarization, Ca^{2+} influx, and insulin exocytosis. Additional mitochondrial signals may also be generated that affect insulin secretion and, in beta cells, the mTOR signaling pathway acts in synergy with growth factor/insulin signaling to stimulate mitochondrial function and insulin secretion [12]. Both rat islets and clonal BRIN-BD11 beta cells consume glutamine at high rates but, notably, while glutamine can potentiate glucose-stimulated insulin secretion and interact with other nutrient secretagogues, it does not initiate an insulin-secretory response [12]. In rat islets, glutamine is converted to γ-amino butyric acid (GABA) and aspartate and, in the presence of leucine, oxidative metabolism is increased. GABA may stimulate insulin but inhibit glucagon secretion, thus acting as an autocrine and paracrine regulator in the islets.

Glutamine in Exercise

The normal resting, fasting plasma concentration of glutamine (p[Gln]) is 0.5–0.7 mM, and athletes are generally associated with the upper end of this reference range. At 20 mM, muscle glutamine in humans is much higher than in blood.

Fasting, resting p[Gln] is decreased in athletes with unexplained underperformance syndrome. When studying elite athletes in training camp at moderate altitude a more marked decrease in p[Gln] was observed in those with the most severe illnesses. More recently, a similar observation was also reported in marines training in winter at higher altitudes (3,000–3,100 m).

The p[Gln] is increased in athletes after short-term exercise. However, in athletes after prolonged, exhaustive exercise such as a full marathon, the p[Gln] can be decreased by as much as 25%. This biphasic response of the p[Gln] to exercise was first reported by Poortmans et al. [13] and Decombaz et al. [5]. Two years later it was confirmed in a single study in athletes exercising on a treadmill for 3.75 h at 50% Vo_{2max}: the p[Gln] first increased during exercise but then decreased by 17% below pre-exercise levels after 3.75 h. A decrease in p[Gln] has been reported 5 h after repeated bouts of cycling for 1 h. In a recent study, a 30–35% decrease in glutamine was observed in Type I and II muscle fibers in humans after resistance exercise.

The post-exercise decrease in p[Gln] often tends to be concomitant with a decrease in circulating lymphocyte numbers, after a transient initial increase as part of the well-known leucocytosis observed after exhaustive exercise. Immune cell function is also decreased at this stage: for example, natural killer cell numbers and function can be depressed for up to 48 h after endurance exercise. A marked decrease in p[Gln] in triathletes at 2 h after prolonged exercise was paralleled by changes in lymphokine activated killer (LAK) cell activities. In recent studies, in moderately and exhaustively exercised rats, macrophages have been reported to utilize glutamine at a higher rate than in sedentary animals: phagocytosis was also increased in exercise compared with sedentary animals.

Interestingly, it has been reported in two studies that inactivity also produces a decrease in the p[Gln], for example, after 14 days of bed rest.

Glutamine Supplementation in Exercise

About 50% of dietary glutamine is utilized by the intestine. Nevertheless, the provision of a bolus dose of 0.1 g/kg glutamine as a drink after an overnight fast has resulted in a two fold increase in the p[Gln] within 30 min in humans.

Five studies have reported a decrease in the incidence of illness (particularly upper respiratory tract illness) in endurance athletes after an event following the provision of glutamine or glutamine precursors (BCAA). There was a decrease in the self-reported incidence of illness (43%) in 150 marathon runners taking 2×5 g glutamine versus placebo after a race; a similar decrease has also been observed in triathletes supplemented for 1 month prior to an event with BCAA versus placebo. The BCAA maintained the p[Gln], and the authors considered that this maintenance enabled an increased production of the cytokines IL-1, IL-2, TNF-α, and IFN-γ. The exercise-induced increase in plasma IL-6 has been well-documented: an augmentation of this response after 2 h cycling was shown to be due to glutamine or glutamine-enriched protein supplementation.

Glutamine and alanine, given in both dipeptide form and as free amino acids to rats, led to an increase in muscle glutamine in the soleus muscle before and after 6 weeks of swimming exercise. In addition, lower TNF-α during recovery, and a decrease in plasma creatine kinase (CK) was observed in the supplemented groups. This supports earlier findings, in which giving a supplement to athletes containing 12 amino acids during the recovery period resulted in an attenuation of both muscle soreness and damage, as well as lowered CK. A similar mixture has improved training efficiency in athletes. With all multi-ingredient supplement studies, it is difficult to ascertain which component might be responsible for the changes observed. However, several studies have found no effect of glutamine on some specific aspects of the immune system in exercise (see [3], for more details). In all these studies the p[Gln] was restored to, or maintained at or above the physiological level. In one study, neutrocytosis returned to normal in the glutamine group.

It has not yet been possible to demonstrate which aspects of exercise-induced immunodepression may be affected by restoring plasma glutamine to normal physiological levels, although there is increasing evidence implicating an effect on neutrophils [3]. Nevertheless, it remains possible that the consumption of glutamine-containing supplements after exercise may benefit immune function, and also post-exercise insulin secretion which could aid muscle recovery and repair.

The effect of glutamine on athletic performance is summarized in a short article by Castell et al. [4] in an A–Z series on nutritional supplementation in athletes, published by the British Journal of Sports Medicine.

Diagnostics

A low level of p[Gln] is likely to be a marker of cachexia in patients, and impaired immune function and/or vulnerability to opportunistic infections/infectious agents in athletes. Glutamine was not previously included in TPN because of problems of sterilization at high temperatures which causes glutamine to degrade to pyroglutamates. Thus, in many supplementation studies, the more expensive dipeptides such as L-alanyl-L-glutamine have been used because of their stability. However, with cold filtration having become feasible this is no longer such an issue.

Glutamine is not a banned substance and is not a drug. In powdered form dissolved in cold or lukewarm water, glutamine will appear in the blood stream within 15 min of ingesting a bolus dose, and will reach maximum concentration at approximately 30–40 min (the minimum amount of water which will dissolve 5 g glutamine is 160 ml). At rest, the ingestion of 5 g glutamine increases the p[Gln] about 2-fold for approximately 2h. Similar effects have been observed in a much more recent study, where 15 g glutamine was given together with carbohydrate and antioxidants. Tablets containing glutamine, on the other hand, take slightly longer to digest and thus to reach the circulation. Timing of both supplementation and the taking of samples is clearly very important. Most feeding studies take samples at sporadic intervals, giving little or no indication of what happens to cell functions or circulating concentrations of cells or supplement in the interim.

Glutamine Assays

Different glutamine assays can produce different data, and it is unwise to compare the absolute values of one research group with another unless they have used identical assays. For the enzymatic assays, using either asparaginase or glutaminase to start the reaction which converts glutamine to glutamate and NH_4^+, the "normal" value (given that there is a good deal of individual variation) is about 600 μM. Other assays can produce higher or lower values than this: for example, a bioassay using *E.coli*; high performance liquid chromatography (HPLC) due, perhaps, to poor resolution of co-eluting amino acids.

Pharmacological Doses

Glutamine has a very good safety record with no side effects reported even at quite high doses. Clinical studies routinely give pharmacological doses of glutamine (28 g/day in intensive care patients): occasionally this has been applied to exercise studies and healthy individuals. For example, 28 g per day was well tolerated for 14 days in healthy humans. Nevertheless, there is little point in healthy individuals consuming more than 0.2 g/kg bodyweight per day. Apart from any other considerations, excessive doses will simply not be absorbed.

References

1. Ardawi MSM, Newsholme EA (1985) Metabolism in lymphocytes and its importance in the immune response. Essays Biochem 21:1–44
2. Bongers T, Griffiths RD, McArdle A (2007) Exogenous glutamine: the clinical evidence. Crit Care Med 35:S545–S552
3. Castell LM (2003) Glutamine supplementation in vitro and in vivo, in exercise and in immunodepression. Sports Med 33:323–345
4. Castell LM, Newsholme P, Newsholme EA (2011) BJSM reviews: A-Z of nutritional supplements: dietary supplements, sports nutrition and ergogenic aids for health and performance Part 18. Brit J Sports Med 45(3):230–232
5. Decombaz J, Reinhardt P, Anantharaman K, von Glutz G (1979) Poortmans J R Biochemical changes in a 100 km run: free amino acids, urea and creatinine. Eur J Appl Physiol 41:61–72
6. Fehrenbach E, Niess AM, Schlotz E, Passek F, Dickhuth HH, Northoff H (2000) Transcriptional and translational regulation of heat shock proteins in leukocytes of endurance runners. J Appl Physiol 89:704–710
7. Griffiths RD, Allen KD, Andrews FJ, Jones C (2002) Infection, multiple organ failure and death in the ICU: influence of glutamine-supplemented parenteral nutrition on intensive care acquired infections and survival. Nutrition 18:546–552
8. Hinchado MD, Giralod E, Ortega E (2011) Adenoreceptors are involved in the stimulation of neutrophils by exercise-induced circulating concentrations of HSP72: cAMP as a potential "intracellular danger signal". J Cell Physiol. doi:10.1002/jcp. 22759
9. Krebs HA (1935) Metabolism of amino-acids: the synthesis of glutamine from glutamic acid and ammonia, and the enzymic hydrolysis of glutamine in animal tissue. Biochem J 29:1951–1969
10. Newsholme EA, Newsholme P, Curi R, Challoner DE, Ardawi M (1988) A role for muscle in the immune system and its importance in surgery, trauma, sepsis and burns. Nutrition 4:261–268
11. Newsholme P, Bender K, Kiely A, Brennan L (2007) Amino acid metabolism, insulin secretion and diabetes. Biochem Soc Trans 35:1180–1186
12. Newsholme P, Gaudel C, McClenaghan NH (2009) Nutrient regulation of insulin secretion and beta cell functional integrity. Advances in experimental biology and medicine book 'The Islets of Langerhans'. Adv Exp Med Biol 654:91–114
13. Poortmans JR, Siest G, Galteau MM, Houot O (1974) Distribution of plasma amino acids in humans during submaximal prolonged exercise. Eur J Appl Physiol 32:143–147
14. Roth E, Funovics J, Muhlbacher F et al (1982) Metabolic disorders in severe abdominal sepsis: glutamine deficiency in skeletal muscle. Clin Nutr 1:25–41
15. Yarandi S, Zhao YM, Hebber G, Ziegler TR (2011) Amino acid composition in parenteral nutrition: what is the evidence? Clin Nutrn Metabol Care 14:75–82
16. Welbourne T, Weber M, Bank N (1972) The effect of glutamine administration on urinary ammonium excretion in normal subjects and patients with renal disease. J Clin Invest 51:1852–1860
17. Xue H, Sawyer MB, Wischmeyer PE, Baracos VE (2011) Nutrition modulation of gastrointestinal toxicity related to cancer chemotherapy: from preclinical findings to clinical strategy. J Parenter Enteral Nutr 35:74–90

Glutamine: $C_5H_{10}N_2O_3$

▶ Glutamine

Glycation of Proteins

Nonenzymatic chemical modification of protein with physiologic sugars.

Glycemic Index

Some carbohydrates have a more profound effect on raising blood glucose and insulin than others; those that have a more marked effect are termed high glycemic index carbohydrates, while those with a more modest effect are termed low glycemic index carbohydrates.

Glycogen

A form of stored carbohydrate that occurs primarily in the liver and muscle tissue and is readily converted to glucose as needed by the body to satisfy its energy needs.

Glycogen Depletion

Decrease in muscle glycogen stores during the game. This phenomenon was reported to affect the ability to reiterate sprints during the final phases of the game and of being the agent of the so-called cumulative fatigues in soccer. A muscle fiber selective glycogen depletion was demonstrated with major effect on fast twitch fibers during the game. This may explain sprint performance impairment during the second half of a soccer game (cumulative fatigue).

Glycogen Loading

▶ Carbohydrate Loading

Glycogen Super-Compensation

▶ Carbohydrate Loading

Glycogen Synthase

An enzyme that is responsible for storage of glycogen in muscle.

Glycogenolysis

The biochemical breakdown or hydrolysis of glycogen to glucose.

Glycolysis

A metabolic process that breaks down glucose through a series of reactions to either pyruvic acid or lactic acid and release energy for the body in the form of ATP. The reactions take place in the cytoplasm and the free energy released is used for adenosine triphosphate (ATP) resynthesis. Pyruvate can either be further oxidized to carbon dioxide yielding big amounts of ATP but in low speed or it can be reduced to lactate and provide ATP faster but with lower efficiency. A control point of glycolysis is the enzyme that catalyses the third reaction. Exercise augments glycolysis in skeletal muscle by activating phosphofructokinase, among other mechanisms. Glycolysis is rapidly activated at the onset of exercise, particularly intense exercise, and is the predominant energy pathway during maximal intensity exercise of durations between about 30 s and 2 min. Glycolysis is always occurring, regardless of the exercise intensity, with the possible exception of extreme conditions in which fats and proteins are the only fuels being metabolized. A related term is "glycogenolysis" which refers to the breakdown of glycogen. Glycogen breakdown ultimately results in glucose-6-phosphate which feeds into the glycolytic pathway.

Cross-References
▶ Anaerobic Metabolism

GOLD Grade

Global Initiative for Chronic Obstructive Lung Disease = GOLD grading of COPD based on spirometry (www.goldcopd.com).

Cross-References
▶ Chronic Obstructive Pulmonary Disease

Golf Handicap Index

Method of statistical adjustment to allow competition among players with widely different skill levels.

G-Protein-Linked Receptors

Cell membrane bound receptor superfamily that response to an agonist stimulus by activating a protein called a G-protein which then activates an enzyme or opens an ion channel to produce the cellular response.

Graded Exercise Testing (GXT)

▶ Exercise Testing

Growth

ROBERT M. MALINA
Department of Kinesiology and Health Education,
University of Texas at Austin, Stephenville, TX, USA
Department of Kinesiology, Tarleton State University,
Stephenville, TX, USA

Definition

The "business of growing up" involves three interacting processes: physical growth, biological maturation, and behavioral development. The terms are often treated as having the same meaning. However, they refer to three distinct processes that characterize the daily lives of children and adolescents for approximately the first two decades of life.

Growth. Growth refers to the increase in the size of the body as a whole and of its parts. Thus, as children grow, they become taller and heavier, they increase in lean and fat tissues, their organs increase in size, and so on. Heart volume and mass, for example, follow a growth pattern like that for body weight, while the lungs and lung functions grow proportionally to height. Different parts of the body grow at different rates and different times. This results in changes in body proportions – relationship of one part of the body to another. The legs, for example, grow faster than the trunk during childhood; hence, the child becomes relatively longer-legged for his or her height.

Maturation. Maturation refers to progress toward the biologically mature state (maturity). It is an operational concept because maturity varies with body system. Studies of children and adolescents commonly focus on sexual and skeletal maturation, although other indicators are available. Maturation can be viewed in two contexts – timing and tempo. Timing refers to when specific maturational events occur, e.g., age at the beginning of breast development in girls, age at the appearance of pubic hair in boys and girls, age at maximum growth during the adolescent growth spurt or age at menarche. Tempo refers to the rate at which maturation progresses, e.g., how quickly or slowly the youngster passes through the adolescent growth spurt or sexual maturation. Timing and tempo vary considerably among individuals. When a child is seen at a single point in time, the focus is maturity status – where is he/she on the path to maturity?

Development. Development refers to the acquisition of behavioral competence, the learning of appropriate behaviors expected by society. It is a culture-specific concept. As children experience life at home, school, church, sports, recreation and other community activities, they develop cognitively, socially, emotionally, morally, and so on. They are learning to behave in a culturally appropriate manner.

Interactions. Growth, maturation, and development occur simultaneously and interact. The interactions influence skills and behaviors related to a sport or a sport discipline and also self-concept, self-esteem, body image, and perceived competence. The three processes and interactions also vary within and among individuals, especially during the adolescent growth spurt and sexual maturation.

Description

Growth in Body Size and Composition

The interval between birth and adulthood is commonly divided into age periods. The first year after birth (birth to the first birthday) is labeled infancy, which is followed by childhood. Childhood is usually subdivided into two phases, early and middle. The former approximates the "preschool" years, about 1 through 5 years of age. The latter approximates the "elementary school" years, about 5–6 through 10–11 years. The upper limit of middle childhood is arbitrary because it is followed by adolescence, which is variable in when it starts. Some fourth grade girls, for example, who are about 9–10 years of age, have already entered the early stages of adolescence. The termination of adolescence is also quite variable so that it is also difficult to specify when adulthood begins. Biologically, some girls are sexually mature by 12 years of age and some boys are sexually mature by 14 years of age; i.e., they are biologically adult. Yet, they are adolescents in the eyes of society. Adulthood is a socially defined concept, usually in the context of completing high school, and in some instances, completing college.

Height and weight are the two body dimensions most commonly used to monitor the growth of children and adolescents. With age, children are expected to become taller and heavier. Size attained at a given age (status) and rate of growth (progress) are usually monitored relative to growth charts which serve as a reference for evaluating the growth status (size attained) of individuals or samples of children and adolescents. Growth charts are available for many countries although the revised charts height and weight for American children from birth to 20 years of age [3] are widely used. These are based on nationally representative samples of American children and adolescents, and replace the earlier charts which were used internationally. The charts include several curves which indicate the distribution of heights and weights (percentiles) at a given age.

Height and weight increase gradually during childhood. By about 9–10 years in girls and 11–12 years in boys, the rate of growth in height begins to increase. This marks the beginning of the adolescent growth spurt, a period of rapid growth that is highly variable among individuals. With the onset of the growth spurt, the rate of growth increases until it reaches a peak (peak height velocity, PHV) or maximum growth in height during the adolescent spurt. It then gradually decreases and growth in height eventually stops. Girls, on average, start their growth spurts, reach PHV, and stop growing about 2 years earlier than boys. Nevertheless, when the growth spurt starts, when PHV is reached, and when growth stops are very variable among individuals.

The growth spurt in body weight begins slightly later than that of height. Body weight is a composite measure of many body tissues, but it is often viewed in terms of its lean (fat-free) and fat components. Thus, body weight = fat-free mass (FFM) + fat mass (FM). Major components of FFM are skeletal muscle and bone mineral. FFM has a growth pattern like that for body weight and experiences a clear adolescent spurt. FM increases more gradually during childhood and adolescence. Most other body dimensions follow a growth pattern similar to that for height and weight.

Biological Maturation

The maturity status and progress of children and adolescents are commonly viewed two ways: skeletally and sexually.

Maturation of the skeleton focuses on the bones of the hand and wrist, which generally reflect the remainder of the skeleton. An x-ray of the hand and wrist is needed to assess skeletal maturation. Protocols for assessing skeletal maturation vary, but are similar in principle and provide an estimate of skeletal age. Skeletal maturation is perhaps the best indicator of maturity status since it can be used from infancy though adolescence. It is also used along with height at a given age to predict adult height.

Sexual maturation is based on the development of secondary sex characteristics: breasts and pubic hair in girls and the testes and pubic hair in boys. Initial development of the breasts is the first physically apparent sign of sexual maturation in girls, followed by the appearance of pubic hair. The first overt sign of sexual maturation in boys, on average, is the initial enlargement of the testes, followed by the appearance of pubic hair. Each of these secondary sex characteristics goes through a series of changes as the individual passes through puberty to the mature state. Secondary sex characteristics are usually assessed by a physician at a clinical examination. Assessment requires invasion of the youngster's privacy at a time

of life when he/she is learning to cope with the physiological changes that are occurring during puberty. Monitoring of these characteristics requires utmost care and sensitivity to the youngster involved.

Age at menarche, the first menstrual period, is the most commonly used indicator of sexual maturity in girls; male puberty does not have corresponding overt, physiological event. Menarcheal status (i.e., has menarche occurred or not occurred) and age at menarche in individual girls can be obtained with a careful and sensitive interview. The average age at menarche in many populations varies between 12.5 and 13.0 years, although normal variation ranges from 9 to 17 years of age.

The timing of PHV is also an excellent maturity indicator, but 5–6 years of longitudinal observations that span about 9–15 years in girls and 10–16 years in boys are required for its derivation. Heights of an individual boy or girl are mathematically modeled to provide an estimate of age at PHV and the rate of growth at PHV. In many ways, it is a post facto maturity indicator. However, a protocol is available for predicting age at PHV from age, height, weight, sitting height, and leg length [9]. The protocol yields "maturity offset" – the time before or after PHV. Though potentially useful, the protocol is often uncritically applied and tends to yield a conservative estimate of age at PHV. It also does not work with female gymnasts and probably other samples of short children.

Application

Height and weight are frequently used in the form of the body mass index (BMI), weight divided by height squared (kg/m^2). After an increase in infancy, the BMI declines through early childhood. It reaches its lowest point at about 5–6 years of age, and then increases with age through childhood and adolescence, and into adulthood. Sex differences in the BMI are small during childhood, arise during adolescence, and persist into adulthood. The rise in the BMI after the low point at about 5–6 years of age has been labeled the "adiposity rebound."

Although the BMI is widely used as an indicator of overweight and obesity in public health surveys, its interpretation as an indicator of fatness in children and adolescents requires care. An elevated BMI is not necessarily indicative of fatness during childhood and adolescence. The BMI is reasonably well correlated with FM and percentage fat in heterogeneous samples of children and adolescents, but it is also well correlated with FFM. It has major limitations. Associations between BMI and fatness indicate a wide range of variability so that children with the same BMI can differ considerably in percentage fat and FM.

Sexual maturation and the growth spurt in boys are accompanied with marked gains in muscle mass and strength, and broadening of the shoulders relative to the hips. In girls, the two are accompanied by smaller gains in muscle mass and strength, by a widening of the hips relative to the shoulders, and by gains in fatness. The net result is sex differences in strength, body build, and body composition in late adolescence and young adulthood. Sexual maturation also influences behavioral development, e.g., increased self-consciousness, concern with weight gain in girls, relationships with the opposite sex, and so on.

Many functional parameters, e.g., aerobic power, muscular strength, and explosive power have their own adolescent growth spurts that may differ in timing and tempo relative to the adolescent growth spurt in body size.

Those working with children and adolescents in the context of sport and physical activity should be able to apply these general concepts of growth, maturation, and development to fit the needs of the youth in the program. Note, however, that the demands of sport are superimposed upon the processes of growth, maturation, and development which essentially represent a constantly changing base associated with inter- and intraindividual variation as youth progress from childhood into and through puberty and adolescence, and eventually into adulthood. A mismatch between the demands of a sport and those of growth, maturation, and development may be a source of stress among young athletes and perhaps between the youth athlete and adults. Several suggestions for dealing with changes in growth and maturation (and associated changes in performance and behavior) associated with the transition into and during the adolescent growth spurt and sexual maturation follow:

Be aware of individual differences. Variation within and between individuals in growth and maturation is the rule.

Avoid comments about body weight. Adolescents are very sensitive about their body weight, especially girls who in many cultures are taught that "thin is in."

Be careful in using body size as cut-points in sports. This especially affects late maturing youngsters who need to be reassured that they will eventually grow and mature and who need to be given the opportunity to participate and to keep working at improving skills.

Be aware of expected changes associated with growth and maturation. Examples:

Since growth in height occurs before growth in body weight and strength, there may be temporary periods during which a boy or girl may appear to "outgrow his/her strength." The youngster needs reassurance that his/her strength will eventually catch-up.

There may be intervals during which a skill may temporarily decline compared to performances prior to the growth spurt, or there may be intervals during which skills may not improve as quickly. These may be associated with rapid changes in body proportions during the adolescent growth spurt, or changes in body composition associated with sexual maturation. The legs, for example, experience their grow spurt before the trunk does, which temporarily alters the position of the center of gravity.

Changes in body composition and development of the hips, particularly in girls, also may influence performance. The adolescent girl needs to be nurtured through adolescence with reassurance and in a positive manner with appropriate instruction and practice in movement and sport-specific skills.

References

1. Kuczmarski RJ, Ogden CL, Grummer-Strawn LM, Flegal KM, Guo SS, Wei R, Mei Z, Curtin LR, Roche AF, Johnson CL (2000) CDC growth charts: United States. Advance data from vital and health statistics, no 314. National Center for Health Statistics, Hyattsville
2. Malina RM (1994) Physical growth and biological maturation of young athletes. Exerc Sport Sci Rev 22:389–433
3. Malina RM (1996) The young athlete: biological growth and maturation in a biocultural context. In: Smoll FL, Smith RE (eds) Children and youth in sport: a biopsychosocial perspective. Brown and Benchmark, Dubuque, pp 161–186
4. Malina RM (1998) Growth and maturation of young athletes: is training for sport a factor. In: Chang KM, Micheli L (eds) Sports and children. Williams and Wilkins, Hong Kong, pp 133–161
5. Malina RM, Beunen G (1996) Monitoring of growth and maturation. In: Bar-Or O (ed) The child and adolescent athlete. Blackwell Science, Oxford, pp 647–672
6. Malina RM, Bouchard C, Bar-Or O (2004) Growth, maturation, and physical activity, 2nd edn. Human Kinetics, Champaign
7. Mirwald RL, Baxter-Jones ADG, Bailey DA, Beunen GP (2002) An assessment of maturity from anthropometric measurements. Med Sci Sport Exer 34:689–694

Growth and Lactogenic Hormone (GLH) Family

Growth hormones, prolactins, and placental lactogens belong to this GLH family. GLH and type I cytokines share signal transduction (Jak/STAT pathway) and are capable of performing similar functions. GLH is heavily involved in physiology, reproduction, and also in the immune function. Residual prolactin alone can maintain vital bodily functions for 8 months in hypohysectomized rats.

Growth Cartilage

A type of cartilage that is located at three main sites in a growing child: the growth plates near the ends of the long bones, the cartilage lining the joint surfaces, and the point at which the major tendons attach to bone. Growth cartilage is present until the child stops growing and is more easily damaged from repetitive microtrauma.

Growth Factors

Proteins that stimulate the division and differentiation of cells which are important for regulating a variety of cellular processes. Growth factors include nerve growth factor, insulin-like growth factor-I, platelet-derived growth factor, and the interleukins.

Cross-References
▶ Neurotrophins

Guanidino Acid

An acid containing a guanidino group, which is characterized by three molecules of azote.

GXT

Cardiac (or graded) stress test.

Cross-References
▶ Ergometry

H

Habituation

▶ Cold

Hand Dominance

Hand dominance is the preference of one hand to perform fine and gross motor tasks, such as writing, cutting, or catching and throwing a ball.

Hand Preference

▶ Handedness

Handedness

ROBERT L. SAINBURG
Departments of Kinesiology and Neurology, The Pennsylvania State University, Pennsylvania, PA, USA

Synonyms
Hand preference; Motor lateralization

Definition
▶ Handedness, or motor lateralization, can be defined in a number of ways. In general, it refers to the tendency to prefer one arm for performance of many common tasks, such as writing, throwing, and cutting with scissors. The most common method to assess handedness is the questionnaire method. This method was originally validated by its ability to predict an individual's self-report as right- or left-handed. However, other methods have included assessment of the speed or accuracy of Peg-Board or drawing tasks, based on the idea that ▶ hand dominance is related to differences in performance between the hands. Overall, handedness can be defined by two criteria: First, the tendency to prefer one arm for the performance of most unilateral activities of daily living, and second, by the tendency of one arm to be more proficient in performing dexterous tasks. Unfortunately, a more specific definition has yet to be developed. Recent research has indicated that handedness is the result of ▶ neural lateralization, and that each arm might be specialized for different aspects of motor control.

Description

Neural Lateralization
Michael Gazzaniga and Roger Sperry [3] conducted research on split-brain patients that showed that each hemisphere is advantaged for different aspects of cognitive, language, and perceptual performance. For example, we now know that the left hemisphere in most individuals mediates semantic and lexicon features of language, while the right hemisphere is specialized for speech prosody, nonverbal communication, and specific types of visual spatial analysis. Gazzaniga proposed that the advantage of this organization might be to expand the circuits available for each function by reducing redundancy across the hemispheres, without requiring the evolutionary cost of expanding brain size. Gazzaniga's research on disconnection syndrome elegantly supported this view of neural lateralization, revealing specialization of each hemisphere for different, but often complementary functions. We are just beginning to understand how handedness might also be described by the specialization of each hemisphere for different aspects of motor control.

The Origin of Handedness
Right-handedness persists across cultures and time, a finding attributed to a variety of causes, including: in utero positional asymmetries, the side of feeding the mother chooses, preferences of adults for carrying children, and a bias in modeling eating, drawing, and writing behaviors. However, the idea that handedness might be culturally mediated is actually contradicted by the persistence of left-handers across cultures and time. David Wolman described a long history of religious, political, and social persecution that left-handers have endured over the ages

Frank C. Mooren (ed.), *Encyclopedia of Exercise Medicine in Health and Disease*, DOI 10.1007/978-3-540-29807-6,
© Springer-Verlag Berlin Heidelberg 2012

[12], arguing against a purely cultural origin for handedness. Vallortigara and Rogers [10] proposed that left-handedness might be attributed to evolutionary factors associated with game theory, in which left-handed genes might benefit from a right-handed population bias. For example, if a shoal of fish all turn right due to a population bias of the escape reflex, this may draw attention from the few "left-handers" who can escape unscathed. Thus, handedness is likely to be influenced by both biological and cultural factors.

Handedness has also been described as an artifact of lateralization in other systems, such as language [1]. According to this idea, left hemisphere lateralization for language leads to left hemisphere, and thus right hand, preference for language-related motor function, including manual gestures and writing. However, attempts to associate language and motor dominance have not been successful. Loring et al. [6] tested whether amobarbital injected into one carotid artery initially affects language function by anesthetizing the ipsilateral hemisphere. While most participants were left hemisphere dominant for language, some showed either no dominance at all, or right hemisphere dominance. The relationship between handedness and dominance was not strong enough to justify a causal relationship, a conclusion supported by later brain imaging studies. However, the strongest argument against the idea that language lateralization might determine motor lateralization is that Chimpanzees, as well as some other nonhuman primates, demonstrate strong individual handedness, as well as a substantial population level bias for right-handedness [5]. Thus, handedness neither seems a casual preference, nor an artifact of language lateralization.

A number of genetic models have fairly accurately predicted the distribution of handedness in families, communities, and monozygotic twins and their offspring. More direct evidence for a genetic determinant of handedness has been demonstrated in the form of a gene (LRRTM1) that increases the likelihood of being left-handed [2]. It is therefore likely that genetic factors lead to permissive conditions that require activity-dependent processes to facilitate development in a particular direction.

Behavioral Correlates of Handedness
Recent evidence suggests that each hemisphere/limb system might be differentially tuned to stabilize different aspects of task performance [8]. This hypothesis has been termed Dynamic Dominance, because of evidence that dominant arm control entails more efficient coordination of muscle actions with the complex biomechanical interactions that arise between the moving segments of the limb. While the nondominant arm has traditionally been viewed as a poorly controlled analog of the dominant arm, recent findings have revealed substantial advantages of this arm for positional stability, and for motor corrections to perturbations. This advantage is important for stabilizing an object that is acted on by the dominant arm. For example, when slicing bread, the dominant arm tends to control the knife while the nondominant arm stabilizes the loaf. This specialization is consistent with anthropological data that indicates that the specialized use of the "nondominant" arm for stabilizing objects evolved to support tool making functions in early hominids [7].

Application
Motor lateralization has direct implications for understanding motor deficits that result from central nervous system damage, such as ▶ stroke. Specifically, if each hemisphere is specialized for controlling different aspects of task performance, damage to one hemisphere should produce specific deficits in each arm. In support of this, studies in both animals and patients with unilateral brain damage have confirmed substantial deficits in the ▶ ipsilesional arm, following unilateral brain injury. Winstein and Pohl [11] showed that nondominant lesions produced slowing of the deceleration phase of rapid aiming movements, whereas dominant lesions produced slowing of the initial, acceleration phase of motion. Haaland and coworkers directly tested the idea that dominant hemisphere lesions produce trajectory deficits, whereas nondominant lesions produce deficits in the final position of targeted reaching movements [4]. In a series of studies, Schaefer and colleagues confirmed that lesions to the right hemisphere, in right handers, produced deficits in stabilizing functions in both arms, while lesions to the left hemisphere produced deficits in trajectory control (see [9]). In summary, deficits in stroke patients are differentially affected by unilateral stroke in a manner consistent with the idea that each hemisphere is better adapted for controlling different aspects of movement. Furthermore, these findings support the hypothesis that both hemispheres are necessary for accurate unilateral arm control.

References
1. Corballis MC (2003) From mouth to hand: gesture, speech, and the evolution of right-handedness. Behav Brain Sci 26(2):199–208, discussion 208–160
2. Francks C, Maegawa S, Lauren J, Abrahams BS, Velayos-Baeza A, Medland SE et al (2007) LRRTM1 on chromosome 2p12 is a maternally suppressed gene that is associated paternally with handedness and schizophrenia. Mol Psychiatry 12(12):1129–39

3. Gazzaniga MS (1998) The split brain revisited. Sci Am 279(1):50–55
4. Haaland KY, Prestopnik JL, Knight RT, Lee RR (2004) Hemispheric asymmetries for kinematic and positional aspects of reaching. Brain 127(Pt 5):1145–1158
5. Hopkins WD, Wesley MJ, Izard MK, Hook M, Schapiro SJ (2004) Chimpanzees (Pan troglodytes) are predominantly right-handed: replication in three populations of apes. Behav Neurosci 118(3):659–663
6. Loring DW, Meador KJ, Lee GP, Murro AM, Smith JR, Flanigin HF et al (1990) Cerebral language lateralization: evidence from intracarotid amobarbital testing. Neuropsychologia 28(8):831–838
7. Marzke MW (1997) Precision grips, hand morphology, and tools. Am J Phys Anthropol 102(1):91–110
8. Sainburg RL (2005) Handedness: differential specializations for control of trajectory and position. Exerc Sport Sci Rev 33(4):206–213
9. Schaefer SY, Haaland KY, Sainburg RL (2009) Hemispheric specialization and functional impact of ipsilesional deficits in movement coordination and accuracy. Neuropsychologia 47(13):2953–2966
10. Vallortigara G, Rogers LJ (2005) Survival with an asymmetrical brain: advantages and disadvantages of cerebral lateralization. Behav Brain Sci 28(4):575–589
11. Winstein CJ, Pohl PS (1995) Effects of unilateral brain damage on the control of goal-directed hand movements. Exp Brain Res 105(1):163–174
12. Wolman D (2005) A left hand turn around the world. Da Capo Press, Cambridge

HDL

▶ High-Density Lipoprotein

Health Behavior Theory(s) or Theoretical Framework(s)

Theory has been variously defined. The Oxford English Dictionary (online) defines a theory as a system of ideas, confirmed by observation or experiment, that explains a group of facts or phenomena. A range of theories and models has been used to specify variables that are believed to influence physical activity and other behaviors. Researchers test hypotheses derived from theories by examining associations among theoretically derived variables with behavior that help to "understand and predict" the behavior, and evaluating interventions that are designed to modify the influences that are believed to lead to behavior change. Interventions can be regarded as theory-based when the theory used to interpret findings has two characteristics: (1) first, it provides a clear account of hypothesized mechanisms or causal processes that generate behavior change, that is, it describes psychological processes accounting for the initiation, redirection or cessation of behavior achieved by the intervention; (2) second, the theory is supported by independent experimental work.

Improvements in both health behavior theory and intervention methods depend on each other. Indeed, when behavior change interventions consist of techniques based on empirically supported theory, then that theory provides an explanation of how the intervention works. Thus, theorists and interventionists need to treat a theory as a dynamic entity whose form and value rests upon it being rigorously applied, tested, and refined in both the laboratory and the field [1]. More experimental research is necessary to test behavioral theories, which should not be viewed as fixed entities, but should be further refined as well as integrated. To this end, greater advantage needs to be taken of the opportunities that interventions afford for theory testing and, moreover, the data generated by these activities need to stimulate and inform efforts to revise, refine, or reject theoretical principles.

References

1. Rothman AJ (2004) Is there nothing more practical than a good theory?: why innovations and advances in health behavior change will arise if interventions are used to test and refine theory. Int J Behav Nutr Phys Act 1(1):11–18

Health Benefits

Reduction in predicted future disease risk or improvement in morbidity and mortality.

Heart Abnormality

▶ Congenital Heart Disease

Heart Attack

▶ Coronary Heart Disease
▶ Ischemia-Reperfusion Injury, Exercise-Induced Cardioprotection

Heart Denervation

Separation of the heart muscle from its sensitive, sympathetic and parasympathetic nerves, resulting in absence of direct extrinsic nervous control of the heart function. Transplantation of a heart graft is a model of complete heart denervation at time of transplantation.

Heart Failure

Heart failure is generally defined as inability of the heart to supply sufficient blood flow to meet the body's needs. To compensate for the decreased cardiac output, a variety of deleterious pathophysiologic responses ensue.

Cross-References

▶ Cardiac Hypertrophy, Pathological

Heart Failure, Training

Andrew L. Clark
Hull York Medical School, Hull, UK

Synonyms

Cardiac rehabilitation; Chronic heart failure; Congestive heart failure

Definition

Exercise training for patients with stable chronic heart failure using aerobic exercise with the aim of improving exercise capacity, quality of life, and survival.

Pathophysiology

Definition of Heart Failure

Heart failure is defined as (1) the presence of symptoms compatible with a diagnosis of heart failure in the presence of (2) objective abnormalities of cardiac function. For the purposes of this section, I am going to discuss patients with *chronic* heart failure: there is no role for training patients with acute heart failure. Such patients should be admitted to hospital as an emergency.

Heart Failure, Training. Table 1 The New York Heart Association scale for symptoms in chronic heart failure

NYHA class	Exercise capacity
I	Unlimited
II	Limited at moderate exercise intensity
III	Limited at only mild exercise intensity
IV	Breathless at rest

1. The cardinal symptom of chronic heart failure is exercise intolerance. Exercise causes limiting breathlessness or fatigue. The exercise limitation is, indeed, the basis for the most widely used symptomatic classification of heart failure, the New York Heart Association classification (see Table 1).
2. The chronic heart failure syndrome is the net result of any sufficiently serious insult to the heart. In the Western world, overwhelmingly the commonest cause is ischemic heart disease with previous myocardial infarction resulting in myocardial damage. Depending upon the population studied, perhaps a third of patients have a dilated cardiomyopathy – that is, impaired myocardial function due to intrinsic muscle disease.

Diagnosis of Heart Failure

If heart failure is suspected on the basis of exertional breathlessness, particularly in a patient at risk, some form of cardiac imaging is essential. The most widespread method is echocardiography, but other techniques, such as cardiac magnetic resonance imaging or radionuclide imaging, may be used.

Most is known about patients with left ventricular systolic dysfunction. The severity of the dysfunction is often measured by the left ventricular ejection fraction, with the normal rage being above 50%. The importance of so-called "diastolic heart failure" in which patients have symptoms of heart failure but normal left ventricular ejection fraction is hotly debated.

Measuring Exercise

There is a large literature describing different techniques for measuring the subjective sensation of breathlessness, but most work on training in chronic heart failure starts from an appreciation of the changes seen to metabolic gas exchange on maximal incremental exercise. Patients have a reduced peak oxygen consumption (peak Vo_2) and an increase in the slope relating ventilation to carbon dioxide production (the Ve/Vco_2 slope), such that for any given level of carbon dioxide production, the ventilatory response is greater.

Origin of Symptoms

A common belief is that breathlessness is caused by "wet lungs" during exercise, and that fatigue is caused by poor skeletal muscle perfusion [1]. Perhaps surprisingly, there is very little relation between measures of left ventricular function at rest and exercise capacity in patients with chronic heart failure (see Fig. 1). The exercise metabolic gas exchange responses of patients are the same regardless of whether the patient is stopped by fatigue or breathlessness, raising the possibility that there is a common process underlying the symptoms.

The lungs are abnormal in two-thirds of patients with chronic heart failure; however, the arterial Pco_2 and Po_2 are normal during exercise (and, indeed, are, respectively lower and higher than in normal subjects toward peak exercise). It is unlikely that exercise is limited by abnormalities of lung function.

In contrast, skeletal muscle is abnormal, and becomes abnormal from a very early stage in the progression of chronic heart failure. Many of the changes seen are very similar to those seen in subjects who detrain (see Table 2).

Skeletal muscle bulk declines, and the muscle is weaker than normal as well as fatiguing more quickly. There are ultrastructural changes with a shift from type I (slow twitch, aerobic) toward type II (fast twitch, anaerobic) fibers. The capillary density of muscle declines and mitochondria are abnormal. The muscle is also metabolically abnormal with decreased levels of some enzymes of aerobic metabolism. During exercise, the muscle of patients develops early acidosis and a prolonged recovery of phosphocreatine during recovery.

There is a signal from exercising muscle to the central nervous system arising from ergoreceptors sensitive to work performed. Stimulation of the ergoreceptors causes an increase in ventilation, sympathetic activation, and vasoconstriction. The ergoreflex so defined is greatly enhanced in heart failure patients, and the more enhanced it is, the worse the exercise capacity and the greater the Ve/Vco_2 slope.

The importance of skeletal muscle in determining exercise capacity in chronic heart failure patients is seen in patients with severe left ventricular dysfunction who still have normal capacity. In contrast to symptomatic patients, they have normal skeletal muscle bulk and blood flow despite their cardiac abnormalities.

Therapeutic Consequences/Exercise Intervention

Treatment of Heart Failure

The standard treatment of heart failure is with agents blocking the consequences of neurohormonal activation; angiotensin converting enzyme inhibitors and beta-adrenoreceptor antagonists are the mainstays of treatment together with diuretics used to treat symptoms of fluid retention. However, these agents have inconsistent effects on exercise capacity, so that even when actively treated, patients still have symptoms of exercise limitation.

Older textbooks of cardiology prescribe "rest" as an important part of heart failure management. However, the similarities between musculature in heart failure and detraining, and the close relation between abnormal muscle and exercise capacity encourage the belief that exercise might, in fact, be beneficial.

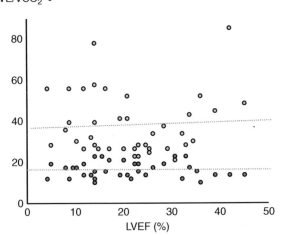

Peak VO$_2$ ●
VE/VCO$_2$ ○

Heart Failure, Training. Fig. 1 There is no relation between left ventricular function as assessed by ejection fraction and exercise performance measured by peak oxygen consumption or the slope of the relation between ventilation and carbon dioxide production

Heart Failure, Training. Table 2 Similarities between detraining and chronic heart failure

	Detraining	Heart failure
Heart rate	↑	↑
Exercise capacity	↓	↓
Muscle size	↓	↓
Muscle enzymes	↓	↓
Sympathetic	↑	↑
Renin:angiotensin	↑	↑
Heart rate variability	↓	↓

Training in Chronic Heart Failure

Formal studies of training started in the 1990s with a series of studies demonstrating an improvement in maximal aerobic capacity (peak Vo_2) of around 20% [2]. The changes occur without any major changes in central hemodynamics. Figure 2 shows a typical early study: in a crossover study, patients trained or rested in random order with improvements in exercise capacity during the training phase. Importantly, the training effect is proportional to compliance.

Subsequent studies have confirmed these results, with accumulated numbers representing thousands of patients. With training, there is an increase in peak Vo_2 and anaerobic threshold, accompanied by a decrease in the Ve/Vco_2 slope. The benefits of training persist as long as the training: if training stops, then exercise performance again declines.

Studies have repeatedly demonstrated an improvement in quality of life during training with patients reporting better health in general and fewer symptoms (and less breathlessness) in particular.

As a result of training, skeletal muscle gains in bulk and becomes more metabolically normal, with an increase in oxidative enzymes and a delay in the development of acidosis.

Other changes with training include a decrease in sympathetic nervous system activity and an increase in heart rate variability (low heart rate variability is an adverse prognostic feature). In addition, the activation of the immune system associated with the development of cardiac cachexia is reversed.

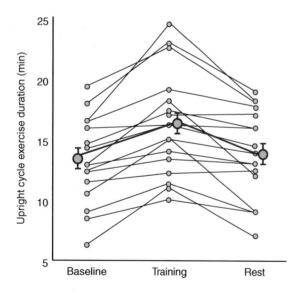

Heart Failure, Training. Fig. 2 The effects of exercise training on exercise performance after a period of training and after rest. Individual patients and mean times are shown

Level of Exercise

Most studies of exercise training in heart failure have used training stimuli of around 70% of previously determined peak heart rate. Further work has suggested that there is still a beneficial effect from more modest exercise, perhaps at around 50% of peak heart rate. The stimulus used is aerobic exercise: walking, cycling, and rowing. There is a theoretical concern that swimming may be dangerous for heart failure patients as total immersion results in a shift of fluid from the periphery to the thorax; however, formal studies have suggested that immersion is safe even in patients with quite severe left ventricular dysfunction.

For the training stimulus to be effective, it appears that 20 min, approximately three times a week, is adequate. Greater amounts of exercise lead to greater improvements.

Supervision of training is a difficult issue: perhaps 1% of the adult population has symptomatic heart failure due to systolic dysfunction with a further 1% having asymptomatic left ventricular dysfunction. It is clearly impossible to provide supervision for such a large number of people. Fortunately, exercise has been shown repeatedly to be safe in chronic heart failure patients, and while a supervised introduction to training is appropriate, patients can be encouraged to pursue their training unsupervised at home.

A common problem in heart failure patients is that of comorbidity. It is important to recognize that heart failure is a disease predominantly of the elderly, and most patients will have coincident conditions that limit exercise capacity. In turn, these may limit the ability of the patient to train.

In these circumstances, there is now some evidence that electrical muscle stimulation can be used to deliver a training stimulus effectively and lead to an improvement in peak Vo_2 [3]. Studies are ongoing to define its role in heart failure management more closely.

Effects of Training on Survival

Meta-analysis of early trials of exercise training suggested that there was a survival benefit from training. A large-scale trial (HF-Action) randomized 2,331 heart-failure patients (NYHA class II-IV, left ventricular ejection fraction $\leq 35\%$) to either an exercise program or to usual care [4, 5]. It is likely to be the largest study conducted in the field.

Among other results presented to date, HF-Action demonstrated an early and sustained improvement in quality of life. The safety of exercise training was confirmed.

The primary end point of the study was all-cause mortality and hospitalization, but this was "missed." However, all the secondary analyses were consistent with the hypothesis that exercise training increased survival. It is certainly safe with no increase in the risk of injury.

Part of the problem with such an open-label trial in contrast to a drug study is that it is impossible to prevent crossover: persuading reluctant patients to continue with training is difficult, as is dissuading the motivated patient from the control group from doing too much exercise. HF-Action will have underestimated the effects of training on survival.

Conclusions

All patients with chronic heart failure should be entered into a heart failure program, as such programs have been shown to improve survival. As part of the program, all patients should be offered exercise training: the training should be supervised initially, but thereafter can be safely carried out unsupervised at home.

Patients can be assured that training is safe, will improve quality of life, and exercise capacity. It may improve survival.

References

1. Clark AL, Poole-Wilson PA, Coats AJS (1996) Exercise limitation in chronic heart failure: the central role of the periphery. J Am Coll Cardiol 28:1092–1102
2. Coats AJS, Adamopoulos S, Meyer T, Conway J, Sleight P (1990) Physical training in chronic heart failure. Lancet 335:63–66
3. Banerjee P, Caulfield B, Crowe L, Clark AL (2009) Prolonged electrical muscle stimulation exercise improves strength, peak Vo_2 and exercise capacity in patients with stable chronic heart failure. J Cardiac Fail 15:319–326
4. O'Connor CM, Whellan DJ, Lee KL, Keteyian SJ, Cooper LS, Ellis SJ, Leifer ES, Kraus WE, Kitzman DW, Blumenthal JA, Rendall DS, Miller NH, Fleg JL, Schulman KA, McKelvie RS, Zannad F, Piña IL, HF-ACTION Investigators (2009) Efficacy and safety of exercise training in patients with chronic heart failure: HF-ACTION randomized controlled trial. JAMA 301:1439–1450
5. Flynn KE, Piña IL, Whellan DJ, Lin L, Blumenthal JA, Ellis SJ, Fine LJ, Howlett JG, Keteyian SJ, Kitzman DW, Kraus WE, Miller NH, Schulman KA, Spertus JA, O'Connor CM, Weinfurt KP, HF-ACTION Investigators (2009) Effects of exercise training on health status in patients with chronic heart failure: HF-ACTION randomized controlled trial. JAMA 301:1451–1459

Heart Period

The time interval between successive heart beats, the R-R interval on the electrocardiogram.

Heart Period Variability

▶ Heart Rate Variability

Heart Rate Variability

GEORGE E. BILLMAN
Department of Physiology and Cell Biology, The Ohio State University, Columbus, OH, USA

Synonyms

Heart period variability; R-R interval variability

Definition

▶ Heart rate variability is defined as the beat-to-beat variation in either heart rate or the duration of the R-R interval (▶ heart period) of the electrocardiogram (ECG) (Fig. 1) that occurs during a selected period of time (seconds to hours). A major component of this variability corresponds to respiration and is referred to as the ▶ Respiratory Sinus Arrhythmia (RSA). Thus, RSA is defined as periodic fluctuation in heart rate at the respiratory frequency such that heart rate increases (R-R interval shortens) during inspiration and decreases (R-R interval prolongs) during expiration.

Characteristics

Periodic fluctuations in the heart beat were first described by Rev. Stephen Hales over 200 years ago. By the early twentieth century, it became clear that these rhythmic changes in the heart rate at any given moment reflected the interactions between parasympathetic nerve fibers (activation decreases heart rate) and sympathetic nerve fibers (activation increases heart rate) on the pacemaker cells usually located in the sinoatrial node. Therefore, investigators began to evaluate the relationship between the beat-to-beat variation in heart rate and changes in cardiac autonomic neural regulation in both health and disease. A number of techniques have now been developed to quantify this beat-to-beat variability in order to provide indices of cardiac autonomic regulation [1, 2].

There are two primary approaches for the analysis of heart rate variability: time-domain and frequency-domain methods [1, 2]. The time-domain measures of this variability are easier to calculate but tend to provide less detailed information than the frequency-domain approaches. The time-domain methods employ either

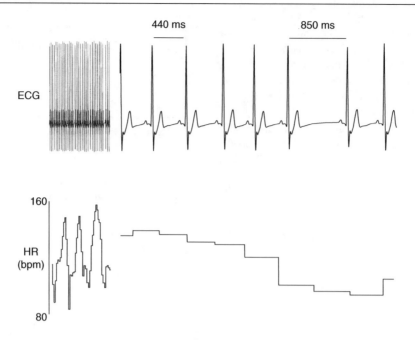

Heart Rate Variability. Fig. 1 Heart rate variability: representative electrocardiogram (ECG) recordings from a conscious dog that illustrate beat-to-beat variations in both R-R interval and heart rate

statistical or geometric approaches (Table 1). Each approach shares the common feature that either heart rate at any point in time (▶ instantaneous heart rate) or the intervals between successive normal beats are determined from a continuous ECG record. Only the normal QRS complexes are used for the calculation; that is, only beats that result from the normal electrical activation pattern (i.e., depolarization originating from the sinoatrial node) are included, any abnormal beats (arrhythmias) are excluded. Thus, the normal-to-normal (NN) interval (the interval between adjacent normal QRS complexes) or the instantaneous heart rate (heart rate calculated on a beat by beat basis) is determined and simple descriptive time-domain variables such as the mean NN interval, mean heart rate, and the range (longest NN minus the shortest NN) for a given time interval can be calculated. More detailed information is provided by the statistical analysis of a continuous sequence of normal beats (NN interval) for the time period of interest. Due to the ease of calculation, the standard deviation (i.e., the square root of the variance) of the NN interval (SDNN) is one of the most widely used time-domain indices of heart rate variability. This calculation measures the total variability that arises from both periodic and random sources (equivalent to total power as determined by frequency domain, spectral analysis). Other widely used statistical

time-domain calculations are listed in Table 1. A series of NN intervals can also be plotted to provide a geometric pattern of the variability. Measurement of the geometric pattern (the width of the distribution) or the interpolation of a mathematically defined shape such as a triangle is used to provide a measure of the heart rate variability (Table 1). One common nonlinear technique graphs the sequence of normal R-R intervals using Poincaré (return or recurrence mapping) plots, where the beat (n) is plotted against the next beat (n + 1). The resulting shape provides graphical display of the variability such that the greater the scatter the greater the variability.

Although time series approaches provide information about changes in the total variability, with one notable exception (see below), these techniques are less useful in identifying specific components of this variability. Beginning in the 1960s investigators applied techniques to partition the total variability in frequency components. Power spectral density analysis produces a decomposition of the total variance (the "power") of a continuous series of beats into its frequency components (i.e., how the power distributes as a function of frequency) [1, 2]. The spectral power for a given frequency can then be quantified by determining the area under the curve within a specified frequency range. The two most common spectral analysis approaches are fast Fourier transform analysis (FFT) and

Heart Rate Variability. Table 1 Heart rate variability measurements

Variable	Units	Definition
Time-domain measures		
a. Statistical		
SDNN	ms	Standard deviation of all normal R-R intervals
SDANN	ms	Standard deviation of the average normal R-R intervals calculated over short time periods (usually 5 min) for the entire recording period (usually 24 h)
RMSSD	ms	The square root of the mean squared differences between adjacent normal R-R intervals
SDNN index	ms	Mean of the standard deviations of the normal R-R intervals calculated over short time periods (usually 5 min) for the entire recording period (usually 24 h)
NN50		The number of pairs of adjacent normal R-R intervals that differ by more than 50 ms
pNN50	%	NN50 divided by the total number of normal R-R intervals X 100
b. Geometrical		
HRV triangular index		Number of normal R-R intervals divided by the height of the histogram of all the normal R-R intervals measured on discrete scale with bins of 1/128 s (7.8125 ms)
TINN	ms	Baseline width of the minimum square difference of triangular interpolation of the highest peak of the histogram of all normal R-R intervals
Frequency-domain measures		
Total	ms^2	Area under the entire power spectral curve (usually ≤ 0.40), variance of all normal R-R intervals
ULF	ms^2	Ultra low-frequency power (≤ 0.003 Hz)
VLF	ms^2	Very low-frequency power (0.003–0.0.04 Hz)
LF	ms^2	Low-frequency power (0.04–0.15 Hz)
HF	ms^2	High-frequency power (usually 0.15–0.40 Hz[a])
LFnu	nu	Normalized low-frequency power (LF/LF + HF)
HFnu	nu	Normalized high-frequency power (HF/LF + HF)
LF/HF		ratio of the low- to high-frequency power

nu normalized units
[a]HF is shifted to higher ranges (0.24–1.04 Hz) in infants and exercising adults

autoregressive (AR) modeling [1, 2]. FFT is based upon the assumption that a time series is composed of only deterministic components while with AR, the data are viewed as being composed of both deterministic and random components. For shorter duration recordings (2–5 min), three main peaks are often identified: very low frequency (VLF) <0.04 Hz, low frequency (LF), 0.04–0.15 Hz, and high frequency (HF) 0.15–0.4 Hz. It should be noted that in infants and in response to exercise, HF is shifted to higher frequency ranges (0.24–1.04 Hz). A fourth peak, ultra low frequency (ULF) 0.003–0.04 Hz is obtained during longer recording periods (24 h). The absolute power at a given frequency is reported as ms^2, but LF and HF power are often measured in normalized units (nu) obtained by dividing the frequency band of interest by total power minus VLF (in practice, since total power largely reflects the combination of VLF, LF, and HF; LF + HF is used as the divisor). Finally, the ratio of LF to HF (LF/HF, no units) has been used as an index of the sympathetic/parasympathetic balance. However, this concept has been challenged as there is considerable controversy concerning the relationship between these frequency components and a particular division of the autonomic nervous system [3–5].

One time-domain approach can also be used to partition heart rate variability within specific frequency bands, similar to those obtained by frequency-domain techniques. This method applies a moving polynomial filter to the heart period (R-R interval) time series to remove slow trends from the data. A specified band-pass filter is then applied to the detrended data to remove all variance outside of the target frequency band. The variance of the residual data set then provides an estimate of the heart rate variability within the target frequency band [2].

Although it is beyond the scope of the present essay to analyze extensively the strengths and weaknesses of the various indices used to measure heart rate variability, a brief discussion of some of the limitations with these techniques is merited. For a more detailed presentation, the reader is encouraged to read one or more of the review articles that eloquently address the technical issues concerning the heart rate variability and its relationship to cardiac autonomic regulation [1–5]. First and foremost, it must be emphasized that heart rate variability only provides an indirect assessment of cardiac autonomic activity and does not provide a direct measurement of either cardiac parasympathetic or sympathetic nerve activity. As a result, this relationship between heart rate variability and cardiac autonomic regulations is qualitative rather than quantitative in nature. In other words, a low or high amount of heart rate variability may reflect a decreased or increased cardiac autonomic regulation but

does not provide a quantification of the actual cardiac nerve firing rate. Furthermore, there is considerable debate as to the exact relationship between changes in cardiac autonomic activity and a particular branch of the autonomic nervous system. The LF (<0.15 Hz) and HF (>0.15 Hz) peaks, obtained by spectral analysis, are often assumed to correspond to cardiac sympathetic and cardiac parasympathetic neural activity, respectively [1–5]. However, accumulating evidence clearly demonstrates this assumption is naïve and greatly oversimplifies the complex nonlinear interactions between the sympathetic and the parasympathetic divisions of the autonomic nervous system [3–5]. This is particularly true with regard to the relationship between LF and cardiac sympathetic regulation [3–5]. Low-frequency power is reduced by selective parasympathectomy and cholinergic antagonists [3]. Furthermore, interventions that would be expected to increase cardiac sympathetic activity, such as acute exercise or myocardial ischemia, not only failed to increase low-frequency power but actually also provoked

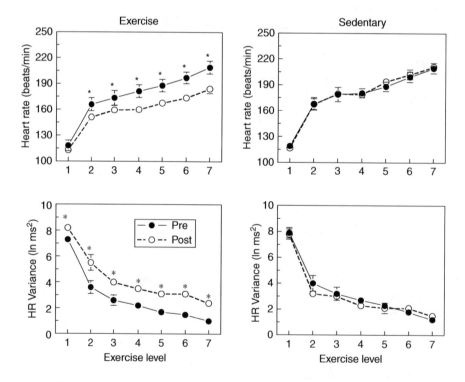

Heart Rate Variability. Fig. 2 Effect of exercise training on the heart rate and heart rate variability response to submaximal exercise. Exercise elicited significantly smaller increases in heart rate and smaller reductions in the high-frequency (0.24–1.04 Hz) component of R-R interval variance in the exercise-trained dogs (10 weeks of progressively increasing intensity, n = 9) as compared to animals that received a similar sedentary period (n = 7). * P < 0.01 pre- versus post-exercise training. Exercise levels: 1 = 0 kph/0% grade, 2 = 4.8 kph/0% grade, 3 = 6.4 kph/0% grade, 4 = 6.4 kph/4% grade, 5 = 6.4 kph/8% grade, 6 = 6.4 kph 12% grade, 7 = 6.4 kph/16% grade

significant reductions in this variable [3]. In a similar manner, sympathetic activity has also been shown to modulate the high frequency component of heart rate variability [3–5], albeit to a lesser extent than the parasympathetic influences on low-frequency power. Thus, heart rate variability data should be interpreted with appropriate caution.

Clinical Relevance

Heart rate variability has gained widespread acceptance as a clinical tool for the evaluation of cardiac autonomic changes in patients [3]. The term "heart rate variability" yields nearly 12,500 "hits" when placed in the PubMed search engine. A variety of cardiovascular risk factors and disease states have all been shown to reduce heart rate variability, including diabetes, smoking, obesity, hypertension, fetal distress, and heart failure [3]. Of particular interest, heart rate variability is reduced in patients recovering from a myocardial infarction, and further, those patients with the greatest reduction in this variable also have the greatest risk for sudden death [3].

Effect of Exercise

During an episode of exercise, heart rate variability decreases [3] with increasing exercise intensity, corresponding with the expected reductions in cardiac parasympathetic regulation (Fig. 2). Since endurance exercise training is well established to alter autonomic nervous system activity [3], one would predict that training should also elicit increases in heart rate variability suggestive of an increased cardiac parasympathetic regulation. Indeed, exercise training increased heart rate variability in patients recovering from myocardial infarction, and those patients with largest increases also exhibited the lowest mortality [3]. Similarly, exercise training significantly reduced the magnitude of tachycardia and the heart rate variability reduction elicited by either coronary artery occlusion or submaximal exercise (Fig. 2) in dogs with experimentally induced myocardial infarctions, an improvement that is absent in the sedentary group [3]. Interestingly, the exercise training prevented life-threatening changes in the cardiac rhythm (ventricular fibrillation) induced by myocardial ischemia in these dogs [3]. Finally, exercise training has also been shown to attenuate reductions in heart rate variability in patients with either hypertension or heart failure [3]. Thus, endurance exercise training can improve heart rate variability (consistent with an improved cardiac autonomic regulation) in patients with cardiovascular disease.

References

1. Task Force of the European society of Cardiology and the North American society of Pacing and Electrophysiology (1996) Heart rate variability: standards of measurement, physiological interpretation, and clinical use. Circulation 93:1043–1065
2. Berntson GG, Bigger JT, Eckberg DL, Grossman P, Kaufmann PG, Malik M, Nagaraja HK, Proges SW, Saul JP, Stone PH, van der Molen MW (1997) Heart rate variability: origins, methods, and interpretive caveats. Pyschophysiology 34:623–648
3. Billman GE (2009) Cardiac autonomic neural "remodeling" and susceptibility to sudden cardiac death: effect of endurance exercise training. Am J Physiol Heart Circ Physiol 297:H1171–1193
4. Eckberg D (1997) Sympathovagal balance: A critical appraisal. Circulation 96:3224–3232
5. Parati G, di Rienzo M, Castiglioni P, Mancia G, Taylor JA, Studinger P (2006) Point:Counterpoint: cardiovascular variability is/is not an index of autonomic control of circulation. J Appl Physiol 101:676–682

Heat Acclimation

▶ Heat Acclimatization

Heat Acclimatization

ZACHARY J. SCHLADER, TOBY MÜNDEL
School of Sport and Exercise, Massey University, Palmerston North, New Zealand

Synonyms

Heat acclimation; Heat adaptation

Definition

Heat acclimatization is a phenotypic adaptive response where physiological or behavioral changes occur that reduce the strain a person experiences when repeatedly exposed to the stress of a naturally hot climate. Examples include seasonal (e.g., summer) or geographical (e.g., tropical) adaptation. This should be compared to heat acclimation, which is an artificially induced adaptation to heat without other climatic components. Notably, acclimation and acclimatization are etymologically indistinguishable. Typically, heat acclimatization improves exercise tolerance in the heat resulting in a reduced incidence and severity of heat illness and an enhanced exercise performance. Short-term acclimatization occurs in days to weeks whereas long-term acclimatization (habituation) usually occurs after years of exposure to a hot climate.

Mechanisms

A sustained increase in core body temperature and sweating response are the two primary factors responsible for heat acclimatization. Current evidence suggests these two responses elicit the following adaptations: (1) a plasma volume expansion due to an increased concentration of plasma proteins and sodium and chloride retention, and (2) the regulation of the body core at a lower temperature. Additionally, the eccrine sweat gland is more active for a given core body temperature, and reabsorbs more sodium and chloride, which results in a greater efficiency of heat dissipation due to an increased difference in vapor pressure between the skin surface and air.

An increased plasma volume affords a greater stroke volume, lower cardiac frequency, and improved cutaneous blood flow and vasodilatory threshold. These all facilitate a more rapid transference of heat from the body core, or metabolically active tissue (muscle), to the periphery, thus improving non-evaporative heat loss. Increased and more efficient (dilute) eccrine sweating, especially when relative to (a reduced) core body temperature, enhances evaporative heat loss, which in turn reduces skin temperature, further improving non-evaporative heat transfer due to an increased core-to-skin temperature gradient.

Exercise Response/Consequences

Even before exercise begins, a heat acclimatized individual displays a lower resting core body temperature and cardiac frequency, and therefore the potential for increase (range) is greater during exercise. Hence, for a given exercise intensity cardiovascular strain – as evidenced by a lower cardiac frequency – is reduced. The core body temperature thresholds for cutaneous vasodilation and sweating are lowered, such that these occur at a lower body core temperature when compared to the unacclimatized state. Furthermore, the sweating response is more profuse with

sweat being more dilute. Together, these responses increase evaporative and non-evaporative heat loss and therefore reduce an individual's thermoregulatory strain for a given exercise intensity. Whole-body and muscle metabolism is altered such that in an acclimatized individual blood and muscle lactate accumulation and muscle glycogen utilization are reduced, and submaximal oxygen uptake is lower when exercise is performed in the heat. Following heat acclimatization, an individual is better able to match their thirst with their body's water needs. Combined with reduced sweat sodium and chloride losses and increased total body water content due to an increased blood (plasma) volume, "voluntary dehydration" is reduced. This becomes important as heat acclimatization increases sweating rate, and if this were not replaced then a greater degree of dehydration would ensue.

The aforementioned responses to exercise ensure that acclimatized individuals are less likely to suffer the detrimental effects of exercise-induced dehydration, hyponatremia, and hyperthermia. Furthermore, given the reductions in physiological strain, exercise capacity (duration) and performance are enhanced in the heat.

Diagnostics

As mentioned previously, the primary stimuli for heat acclimatization are a sustained increase in core body temperature and sweating response. Therefore while passive heat exposure and exercise in a cool or moderate climate result in some benefit, exercise in the heat is the most effective method of adaptation due to the combined exogenous (ambient) and endogenous (metabolic) heat loads. The process of acclimatization begins within the first few days of exercise in a hot environment and is normally complete within 7–14 days, depending on the individual (see Table 1). Although daily exposure is

Heat Acclimatization. Table 1 Range of days required for physiological adaptations to occur during exercise heat acclimatization

Adaptation	Days of heat acclimatization
	1 2 3 4 5 6 7 8 9 10 11 12 13 14
Decreased cardiac frequency	———
Plasma volume expansion	———
Decreased body core temperature	———
Decreased sweat [Na⁺, Cl⁻]	—————
Increased and earlier sweating	———————
Increased and earlier cutaneous vasodilation	———————

recommended, as long as no more than 2 or 3 days elapses between exposures acclimatization will continue but will require a greater total duration, i.e., 21–30 days. The mode of exercise is less important and might only be a consideration for athletes, but the process of acclimatization should be seen as separate to their specific training. Furthermore, when acclimating in an artificial environment such as a laboratory's heat chamber, only certain equipment may be available, e.g., cycle ergometer, treadmill, box step, etc. Exercise should be performed at an intensity exceeding 50% of an individual's maximal aerobic capacity (VO_2max) and while a continuous duration of 90–100 min appears optimal, with no beneficial effects of longer exposure, intermittent and higher-intensity exercise have shown to be effective as long as an elevated core body temperature and stimulation of sweating are maintained. Ambient temperature should ideally be warmer than skin temperature ($>30°C$) but if too hot might negatively impact on the ability to maintain the exercise. There is also a degree of specificity when comparing acclimatization between a hot-dry and hot-humid climate, and individuals should match the ambient humidity to that likely to be experienced. Although heat acclimatization in a dry climate offers an advantage when exposed to humid heat, there are differences in the physiological processes that lead to adaptation, such as a greater (maintained) sweat rate when acclimatizing in hot-humid conditions, most likely due to an inhibition of hidromeiosis.

Heat acclimatization is transient and will disappear if not maintained by repeat exposures. Although a reversible process, it takes greater time for the improved responses (cardiovascular, thermoregulatory, sudomotor) to decay. In general, 1 day of acclimatization is lost every 2 days away although maintenance or re-induction is possible via one additional exposure for every 5 days away. The rate of decay is affected by factors such as aerobic fitness and the number and frequency of heat exposures. Retention appears longer following dry heat acclimatization than humid heat, and the first adaptations to decay are those first developed, namely, cardiovascular responses.

While earlier research indicated that sex and age influenced the capacity to acclimatize, more recent studies have shown that when matched for physical and morphological characteristics, few differences exist between older and younger individuals or males and females. However, individuals with a higher aerobic fitness develop adaptations more quickly, and retain the effects for longer, than those less fit.

References

1. The Commission for Thermal Physiology of the International Union of Physiological Sciences (2001) Glossary of terms for thermal physiology. Jpn J Physiol 51:245–280
2. Nielsen B, Hales JRS, Strange S, Christensen NJ, Warberg J, Saltin B (1993) Human circulatory and thermoregulatory adaptations with heat acclimation and exercise in a hot, dry environment. J Physiol 460:467–485
3. Nielsen B, Strange S, Christensen NJ, Warberg J, Saltin B (1997) Acute and adaptive responses in humans to exercise in a warm, humid environment. Pflügers Arch Eur J Physiol 434:49–56
4. Armstrong LE, Maresh CM (1991) The induction and decay of heat acclimatisation in trained athletes. Sports Med 12:302–312
5. Pandolf KB (1998) Time course of heat acclimation and its decay. Int J Sports Med 19:S157–S160
6. Taylor NAS (2000) Principles and practices of heat adaptation. J Hum Environ System 4:11–22

Heat Adaptation

▶ Heat Acclimatization

Heat Illness

An array of disorders associated with an elevated ambient temperature and/or hyperthermia. These disorders include, but are certainly not limited to, heat cramps, heat exhaustion, heat syncope, heat oedema and heat stroke (exertional or classic). Heat stroke can be fatal and is therefore the most severe of the heat illnesses.

Heat Loss

Dry heat loss is the sum of heat flows or heat fluxes by radiation, convection, and conduction from a body to the environment. Evaporative heat loss refers to evaporative heat transfer from the body to the ambient by evaporation of water from the skin and the surfaces of the respiratory tract.

Heat Shock (Stress Response)

The mobilization, translocation, and activation of both constitutive heat shock proteins and the heat shock transcription factor which subsequently results in transcription of heat shock genes, accumulation of heat shock protein mRNA, and finally an increase in new cellular heat shock proteins. Although they do not induce exactly the same set of proteins, there is considerable overlap between proteins induced with heat shock and those resulting from other stressors, hence the more general term of stress response.

Heat Shock Proteins

KEVIN MILNE[1], EARL G. NOBLE[2]
[1]Department of Kinesiology, The University of Windsor, Windsor, ON, Canada
[2]Department of Kinesiology, The University of Western Ontario, London, ON, Canada

Synonyms
Molecular chaperones; Stress proteins

Definition
Heat shock proteins are important to the maintenance of cellular protein homeostasis, including de novo protein synthesis, intracellular protein trafficking, cell signaling, and cellular survival during stress. More recently, they have been recognized to have extracellular functions as immunomodulators, which include stimulation of both innate and adaptive immunity. Hence, heat shock or stress proteins have both intracellular and extracellular roles within the body. Heat shock proteins are categorized into families according to their molecular weights in kilodaltons (kDa), and span weight ranges from very small (<10 kDa) to very large (>100 kDa). Recently, an attempt has been made to standardize the nomenclature of the various human heat shock genes and protein families to account for the diversity in these proteins [2]. Heat shock proteins are found in every cell type thus far examined, and specialized forms exist in virtually every cellular location and organelle including the cytoplasm, nucleus, mitochondria, endoplasmic reticulum and even cell surfaces and in association with cells of the immune system. Further, although constitutively expressed, many of these proteins are highly inducible, such that most stresses that challenge the homeostatic environment of a cell also cause the transcription of heat shock genes and subsequent accumulation of heat shock proteins.

Basic Mechanisms
The first stimulus observed to elicit the heat shock response was an increase in temperature [5]. Subsequently, it was determined that nearly any stress which causes a disruption of the normal intracellular protein environment or cell integrity may cause induction of the intracellular stress response which includes mobilization and accumulation of heat shock proteins. For this reason, the heat shock response may be more generally referred to as the cellular stress response. These additional stimuli include oxidative stress, exposure to heavy metals, calcium transients, hypoxia, glucose deprivation, altered pH, mechanical deformation and activation of various cell cycling pathways [4]. Although slight variations may occur in the initiation of the stress response, at its root is the activation of the major and vital transcription factor for heat shock protein transcription known as the heat shock transcription factor, HSF. Although four major HSFs have been identified, the most important one in the activation of the cellular stress response in the majority of cells is HSF1. Cellular stresses, such as elevated temperature, may cause intracellular proteins to become denatured and expose hydrophobic residues (Fig. 1A1). Heat shock proteins complexed to HSF1 disassociate and bind to these denatured proteins, thereby freeing HSF1 (Fig. 1B) which can then trimerize with other HSF1 monomers, migrate to the nucleus, and, in conjunction with a series of phosphorylation events, bind to the heat shock element (HSE) of DNA (Fig. 1C), thus initiating the transcription of various heat shock genes and accumulation of HSP mRNA (Fig. 1D) for de novo HSP synthesis (Fig. 1E) [1]. While protein denaturation is typically a first step in this response, some stresses may also initiate or modify the heat shock response directly through various signaling cascades (Fig. 1A2). In either situation, the ultimate mobilization and synthesis of heat shock proteins promote cellular survival by protecting intracellular proteins from improper folding and/or aggregation until the stress subsides (Fig. 1F).

During de novo protein synthesis, partially completed proteins exiting the ribosome during translation may be held by HSPs (particularly HSPA8 or Hsc70) until they are completely synthesized, thereby providing them with the transient thermodynamic properties necessary to allow them to attain proper functional conformation. Additionally, HSPs may target proteins to intracellular locations where they can fold into their mature state. During stress, HSPs similarly bind to specific (often hydrophobic) regions of denatured proteins, protecting against improper folding and protein aggregation until the stress subsides. These actions are vital to the maintenance of the functional integrity of the cell, and without an adequate stress response, cells are susceptible to dysfunction or death after even minor stresses. Not surprisingly, the increased expression of heat shock proteins through either

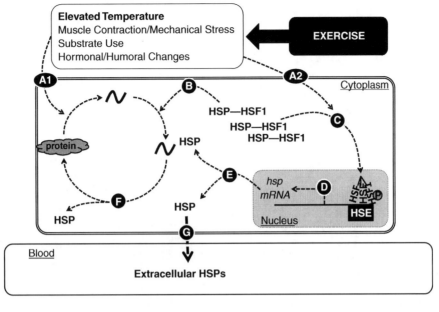

Heat Shock Proteins. Fig. 1 Graphical representation of the heat shock or cellular stress response to exercise. See text for details. *HSP* heat shock protein, *HSF1* heat shock transcription factor 1

genetic or physiological manipulation can be used to enhance the survival and function of cells, tissues and whole organs to what would normally be lethal stresses. This phenomenon is referred to as ▶ preconditioning. In particular, heat or ischemic preconditioning is a potent measure to fortify cells and organs against future stresses, and although there are other proteins and signaling pathways important to this preconditioning phenomenon, the accumulation of heat shock proteins is significant in this regard.

While the cytoprotective effects of HSPs have been well established, an exciting and rapidly evolving area of research is related to the observation that heat shock proteins may be released from live cells into the extracellular environment where they have distinct roles in inflammation and the immune response (Fig. 1G). These effects can be either local or remote, and the release can occur in the absence of cell damage or necrosis. For example, cultured embryonic cells, vascular smooth muscle cells, glial cells and blood mononuclear cells all possess mechanisms by which heat shock proteins are transported across the cell membrane. Moreover, certain immune cells and other tissues, including motor neurons and smooth muscle cells, possess receptors for extracellular heat shock proteins. The consequence of HSP binding to these receptors has yet to be completely unraveled, but release of proinflammatory or anti-inflammatory cytokines, activation or suppression of internal signaling pathways, and

initiation of a cellular stress response in the recipient cell are all potential outcomes. As a consequence, these observations suggest that these extracellular heat shock proteins possess roles as humoral messengers. Many of the intracellular heat shock proteins are involved in these immunomodulation and signaling roles, including mitochondrial Hsp60, inducible Hsp70, Hsp 27, and Hsp90. Importantly, HSPs and antibodies to HSPs found in extracellular fluids may be indicative of a reduced likelihood of various disease states or a susceptibility to these diseases. The role of these extracellular HSPs will undoubtedly be an important research focus in the immediate future.

Exercise Intervention

Physical exercise consists of many stressors to the biological system, including an elevation in temperature, and consequently, physical exercise is a potent stimulus to the heat shock response in a variety of cells and tissues [3]. Since the magnitude of both the temperature increase and the other stressors associated with exercise is typically greater with increasing exercise intensity, it is not surprising that in most tissues, the stress response to exercise is also intensity dependent (Fig. 2A). In fact, exercise bouts at or above the ▶ anaerobic threshold appear to be the most potent in inducing an accumulation of heat shock proteins in both animals and humans. However, it is important to note that different cell types may be more or less (e.g., Fig. 2B) responsive to the same relative

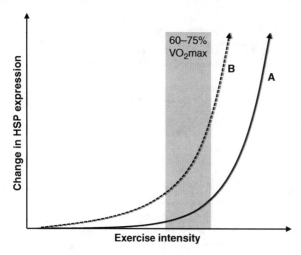

Heat Shock Proteins. Fig. 2 Typical accumulation of heat shock proteins in response to exercise of increasing intensity (A). Hypothetical example of a tissue, cell, or organism that has a lower exercise-related threshold for induction of the heat shock response. VO_{2max}, maximal oxygen uptake

exercise intensity and consequently exhibit different heat shock responses. Further, the intrinsic properties of different cell types as well as their proximity to other cells vary the responsiveness of any given organ or tissue to the stress of exercise. Nonetheless, an increase in exercise intensity will normally be sufficient to elicit the stress response in most tissues.

Both sex and age appear to modify the heat shock response to exercise such that, even though the ability to mount a significant response remains, the accumulation of heat shock proteins is diminished in females and the aged at the same relative exercise intensity following a single bout of exercise (e.g., Fig. 2A versus 2B). Importantly, multiple exercise bouts over the span of days or weeks (i.e., exercise training) may maintain the exercise-induced accumulation of heat shock proteins and, further, may eliminate the inhibitory effects of sex or age.

Similar to heat or ischemic preconditioning, the accumulation of heat shock proteins following exercise protects organs against subsequent stresses. In particular, the hearts of exercised animals, in which an accumulation of HSPA1 (Hsp70) has occurred, recover better after an ischemia–reperfusion insult. However, even within the heart, there are several different cell types that compose the functioning organ, and it has been shown that at least with heat preconditioning, the vasculature (i.e., endothelial and smooth muscle cells), more so than the cardiomyocytes per se, are the primary locations of heat

shock protein induction leading to cardiovascular protection. Even though the heart and skeletal muscle share many characteristics, intracellular increases of HSPs in specific muscle fibers are a common observation in skeletal muscle, and it has been shown that exercise-induced overexpression of HSPA1 (Hsp70) and genetically manipulated overexpression of HSPE (Hsp10) can prevent skeletal muscle damage and aid in the stability of important muscular ion channels.

Heat shock proteins are also increased in the plasma of exercising mammals. Although stress-related, these are not simply markers of damage (see above) since the likely site of damage (i.e., skeletal muscle) does not appear to be the origin of extracellular heat shock proteins during exercise. Rather, it appears that the hepaosplanchnic and brain regions and specific sites such as the endothelium are sources of these heat shock proteins. Similar to other tissues, temperature and metabolic substrate depletion appear to be the biggest stimuli for this release. Although extracellular proteins which result from exercise will clearly be found to have both immuno-modulatory and signaling functions, at present their roles are unclear.

In conclusion, exercise is a potent stimulus for the induction of both intracellular and extracellular heat shock proteins. Given the important protective and signaling roles of these ancient proteins, the activation of the cellular stress response may be a significant player in the beneficial effects of exercise.

References

1. Baler R, Dahl G, Voellmy R (1993) Activation of human heat shock genes is accompanied by oligomerization, modification, and rapid translocation of heat shock transcription factor HSF1. Mol Cell Biol 13:2486–2496
2. Kampinga HH, Hageman J, Vos MJ, Kubota H, Tanguay RM, Bruford EA, Cheetham ME, Chen B, Hightower LE (2009) Guidelines for the nomenclature of the human heat shock proteins. Cell Stress Chaperones 14:105–111
3. Locke M, Noble EG, Atkinson BG (1990) Exercising mammals synthesize stress proteins. Am J Physiol 258:C723–C729
4. Morimoto RI, Kroeger PE, Cotto JJ (1996) The transcriptional regulation of heat shock genes: a plethora of heat shock factors and regulatory conditions. Experientia 77:139–163
5. Ritossa F (1962) A new puffing pattern induced by temperature shock and DNP in *Drosophila*. Experientia 18:571–573

Heat Strain

▶ Thermoregulation

Hematopoietic Stem Cells

Hematopoietic stem cells are type of unspecialized bone marrow cells that renew themselves during the whole life through cell division and deliver the whole palette of differentiated blood cells.

Hemoglobin

Hemoglobin (Hb) – the O_2 transport protein of the erythrocytes – takes up O_2 in the lung and releases it in the respiring tissues. Furthermore, Hb buffers H^+ and binds CO_2 as carbamate. The normal Hb concentration ranges between 120 and 160 g/L blood in females and 140–180 g/L in males. Hb is a tetramer (molecular mass 64.5 kDa) of four subunits each composed of a heme (a porphyrin with a central Fe^{2+}) and a globin chain. The Fe^{2+} bonds with the four pyrroles of the porphyrin and the proximal histidine of the globin. At the sixth ligand site of the Fe^{2+}, O_2 can reversibly bind ("oxygenation," respectively, "desoxygenation"). Oxidation of Fe^{2+} to Fe^{3+} converts Hb to methemoglobin (hemiglobin), which cannot bind O_2. Also, Hb cannot bind O_2, when other ligands such as CO occupy the Fe^{2+} (carboxy-Hb). Because the absorption spectra of the Hb depend on the degree of oxygenation, venous blood appears darker (bluish-red) than arterialized blood. The spectral difference is used for clinical noninvasive study of blood oxygenation by pulse oximetry. Each two of the four globins of the Hb tetramer are always identical. Adult humans have mainly HbA (98%) that consists of two α and two β globin chains ($\alpha_2\beta_2$), which are composed of 141, respectively, 146 amino acids. Minor isoforms are HbA_2 (2%, $\alpha_2\delta_2$) and HbF (<1%, $\alpha_2\gamma_2$; fetal-type isoform). The globins of the Hb tetramer are connected by salt bridges, hydrogen bonds, and hydrophobic contacts, which dissolve on O_2 binding. This is called the transition from the T- (tense) to the R- (relaxed) structure. One mole of Hb can bind up to four moles of O_2. The percentage of the Hb that is oxygenated (O_2 saturation) depends on the prevailing O_2 partial pressure (pO_2). The binding of O_2 – first occurring at the $\alpha 1$ heme – causes a gliding of the Fe^{2+} into the plane of the porphyrin ring, a pulling at the proximal histidine and a rotation of the $\alpha 1\beta 1$ dimer relative to the $\alpha 2\beta 2$ dimer. Thus, the oxygenation of one Hb subunit produces a conformational change of the whole tetramer, and the other subunits gain an increased affinity for O_2. This explains as to why the Hb-O_2 binding curve is sigmoid (S-shaped). Its position – as a measure of the Hb-O_2 affinity – can be quantified by the P_{50}-value – the pO_2 producing 50% O_2 saturation. The P_{50} of arterial blood is 27 mmHg (3.5 kPa) at standard conditions (pH 7.40, pCO_2 40 mmHg, 37°C). The sigmoid shape of the Hb-O_2 binding curve has important consequences for the transport of O_2 in the blood. Even when the arterial pO_2 decreases (e.g., at high altitude) the O_2 saturation is still relatively high, because the Hb-O_2 binding curve is so flat in the upper part (at pO_2 60 mmHg, the arterial O_2 saturation is still 90%). On the other hand, the steep slope in the middle of the Hb-O_2 binding curve is advantageous with respect to the peripheral release of O_2. In venous blood the pO_2 is about 35 mmHg, if the curve were hyperbolic, less than 10% of the O_2 carried would be released at that pressure and tissue hypoxia could occur. In addition, the tetrameric structure of the Hb allows for allosteric reactions. The binding of H^+ and CO_2 to amino acids of the globins stabilizes the T-structure and reduces the Hb-O_2 affinity, thereby facilitating the release of O_2 (so-called Bohr effect). Conversely, the alkalization of the blood in the lung capillaries leads to an increase in the Hb-O_2 affinity, thereby facilitating the uptake of O_2. The T-structure of Hb is also stabilized by 2,3-bisphosphoglycerate (2,3-BPG), an intraerythrocytic metabolite of glycolysis. The binding of 2,3-BPG to the β globin chains strongly reduces the Hb-O_2 affinity, which favors the unloading of O_2 in the periphery. Pathophysiologically, two types of inherited deficiencies of the synthesis of Hb can be distinguished. In hemoglobinopathies, Hb variants with an abnormal amino acid sequence are synthesized. For example, in sickle cell disease glutamic acid in position 6 of the ß chain is mutated to valine (HbS). In thalassemias, the genetic defect results in a reduced rate of the synthesis of one of the globin chains. Another important clinical aspect relates to the diagnosis and follow-on of diabetics. HbA combines irreversibly with glucose, yielding glycated Hb, which is termed HbA_{1c}. The HbA_{1c} percentage (normally <6% of the total) is representative of the glucose level in the blood averaged over a longer time. An increased HbA_{1c} level is indicative of abnormally high glucose concentrations.

Hemoglobin Concentration

Hemoglobin mass in 100 ml (g/dl) or in 1 l (g/l). For example, 15 g/dl in a male subject.

Hemoglobin Mass (Hb-mass)

Absolute hemoglobin content of the body in gram. For example, 800 g in a male subject.

Hemophilia

FELIPE QUEROL[1,2], SOFIA PÉREZ-ALENDA[1,2], JOSÉ A. AZNAR[2]
[1]Department of Physiotherapy, University of Valencia, Spain
[2]Haemostasis and Thrombosis Unit, University Hospital La FE, Valencia, Spain

Hemophilia. Table 1 Clinical classification of hemophilia and characteristics of hemorrhages

Classification	Clotting factor in %	Clinical characteristics of hemorrhages
Severe	<1%	Frequent hemorrhages for no apparent reason
Moderate	1–5%	Frequent hemorrhages with minor trauma
Mild	>5%	Hemorrhages with serious trauma, dental procedure, or surgery
Over 40–50% of cases (as well as female carriers) do not usually suffer hemorrhages or require treatment, but vigilance is advisable if they undergo surgery		

Synonyms

Congenital coagulopathy; Exercise; Factor VIII/IX deficiency

Definition

Hemophilia is a recessive X-linked genetic disorder. It is characterized by spontaneous hemorrhagic lesions, which can be life-threatening if not promptly and adequately treated. Bleedings most often affect the musculoskeletal system, can lead to ▶ hemophilic arthropathy, and condition a poor quality of life, requiring specific hematological therapy and general care measures including physical activity and supervised sports practice.

The morbidity of this congenital coagulopathy and its socioeconomic importance justify, despite its limited incidence (1–2/10,000 of live births), the knowledge of this pathology. Without a prophylactic treatment, 100% of severe hemophiliacs will have musculoskeletal complications leading to irreversible damages and physical disability at early ages.

In western countries, genetic counseling is decreasing the incidence of hemophilia. Its inheritance pattern is characteristic: the woman carrying the defective gene passes the disease to her male children. The phenomenon of immigration and the spontaneous cases (de novo mutations) keep the prevalence. Nowadays the life expectancy of hemophiliacs is similar to that of the general population.

Hemophilia is classified into three degrees: *Severe, Moderate, and Mild* (Table 1). The severity of the problems is proportional to the level of active clotting factor, expressed in percentage (one international unit corresponds to 1%) [1].

Pathogenetic Mechanisms

Hemophilia is an alteration of the physiology of hemostasis and it involves a deficiency of clotting factors: VIII in hemophilia A or IX in hemophilia B.

Blood hemostasis comprises a variety of mechanisms aimed at preserving the integrity of the vascular tree to prevent blood loss. This includes *primary hemostasis* and *coagulation*. The first step is vasoconstriction of the damaged vessel. Secondly, platelets stick to the subendothelium through glycoprotein Ib, with intervention of the von Willebrand factor. Platelets are activated and start to aggregate (stick to one another) through glycoprotein IIb–IIIa. The key point in the mechanism of coagulation is the conversion of fibrinogen to fibrin by action of thrombin. Both in hemophilia A and B, there is a reduced production of thrombin, via the intrinsic pathway (because of factor VIII/IX deficiency), and a faulty inhibition of fibrinolysis, due to low activation of Thrombin Activatable Fibrinolysis Inhibitor (i.e., TAFI).

The most important physiopathologic effect is joint bleeding – the hemarthrosis. Bleeding episodes in muscles and joints start at childhood (before 2 years of age) in 100% of severe hemophiliacs, if not appropriately treated (Fig. 1). The usual inflammation following a hemorrhage in the musculoskeletal system leads to severe alterations of musculoskeletal structures, affecting joint motion and strength. Its treatment requires immobilization and joint rest, which entails a dysfunction that aggravates the problem, since its functional recovery increases the risk of re-bleeding. In short, it is a serious and complex problem requiring a specific therapy with a triple approach: hematological, orthopedic, and rehabilitationist.

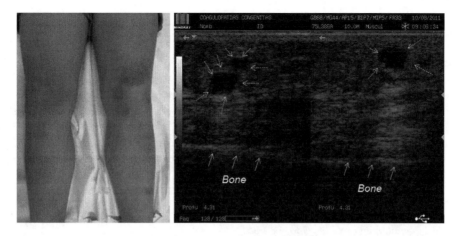

Hemophilia. Fig. 1 Hemophilic child showing many hematomas produced by simple rubbing or minor contusion. On ecography, the *dashed arrows* show the blood collectors and their situation more or less close to the bone

The first hemarthrosis already determines changes in the chondrocyte and the onset of synovitis. The synovial fluid loses its physical and chemical properties, with the presence of proteolytic enzymes product of the degradation of blood. Iron deposits play a part in the inflammatory hyperplasic reaction, as well as the intra-articular pressure increased by the antalgic contracture of acute hemarthrosis. The damage of articular surfaces starts in the subchondral bone tissue; trabecular resorption entails subsidence of the cartilage, under the action of joint load (areas of maximum damage). The articular interline is modified, with widening of the epiphysis. Articular destruction leads to residual arthropathy, which sets in during child growth (Fig. 2).

The progression of hemophilic arthropathy in the child (if not adequately treated) is similar to degenerative osteoarthritis in adults. A 15-year-old youth can have suffered complete joint destruction and be severely disabled.

Exercise Intervention/Therapy

Hematological treatment alone is not sufficient to prevent and treat musculoskeletal bleeding. Indeed, the combination of this treatment and a sedentary lifestyle in such patients often leads to problems associated with inactivity, such as decreased strength, worse balance and coordination, as well as an increased risk of overweight. These problems promote instability and changes to the joint loads, thus leading to the appearance of new bleeds and increased joint damage. Likewise, in acute cases, if the rest period required after hemarthrosis is not accompanied by

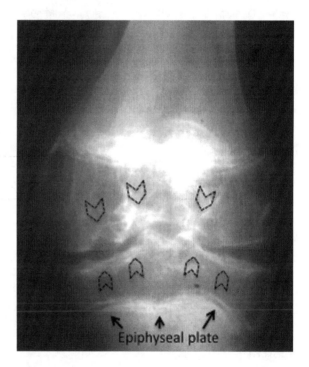

Hemophilia. Fig. 2 X-ray image of a hemophilic arthropathy in a child. Note the significant degeneration of the articular surface

the correct physiotherapeutic treatment, a vicious circle of inactivity, which leads to new bleedings and finally hemophilic arthropathy and loss of function, rapidly sets in these patients [2].

Consequently, the treatment of hemorrhages in the musculoskeletal system of the hemophilic patient includes:

1. Basic measures of local hemostasis: immobilization and cold therapy in affected joints.
2. Factor replacement treatment: infusions of the deficient clotting factor (VIII or IX), as promptly as possible.
3. Physiotherapy management of neuromusculoskeletal dysfunction: treatment of the articular system, neural system, and muscle system.

On the other hand, the prevention of musculoskeletal injuries in hemophilia includes physical exercise and sport: physical activity, regular training, and practicing a suitable sport help hemophiliacs to develop the basic motor skills required for sports such as coordination, flexibility, cardiorespiratory capacity, and strength. All these skills help keep the musculoskeletal system in good health. The benefit of regular physical exercise and sport for hemophilic patients also includes psychosocial aspects like higher self-esteem and socialization, which lead to a better quality of life [3].

People with hemophilia can practice physical exercise and sport as long as their clotting factor activity (natural or increased by regular therapeutic replacement of factor VIII or factor IX) minimizes the risk of bleeding and provides reliable control of any bleeds that occur. If these conditions are fully met, the equally important aspects of training the musculoskeletal system can be tacked at no added risk [4].

The essential requirements to practice physical exercise or sports are [4]:

- A factor VIII or IX clotting activity above 15%. This level is sufficient to prevent bleeds.
- Practice sporting activities as a hobby or leisure sport with regular training sessions performed without causing fatigue, ideally two to three times per week, for not more than 1 h in each case.
- Compliance with the following basic principles, validated by sports scientist:
  - Warm-up routine before starting any sporting activity.
  - Cool-down routine with stretching of the exposed muscles after finishing the sporting activity.
  - Never go beyond your physical limits or train to the point of exhaustion. Take plenty of breaks to automatically lower your risk of injury and overstrain.
  - Technical mastery of the sporting discipline. A higher risk of bleeding is for unpracticed beginners in some sports.
  - Modify the sporting activity to suit the environmental conditions (weather, terrain,…) and your physical and mental conditions.

There are different classifications of recommended and not recommended sports for hemophilic patients. One of these subdivides them into contact, minimal contact, and non-contact on the basis of the probability of contact or collision. Examples of the first group include football, basketball, water polo, handball, hockey, ice hockey, boxing, and rugby, whereas the second group includes kayaking, canoeing and various forms of skating, with swimming, tennis and badminton falling into the third category. Other classifications based on the incidence of injuries (high, medium, or low risk) are also used. Thus, the recommended sports for hemophiliacs are usually those considered to be non-contact or with a low risk of injury, such as swimming, table tennis, golf, cycling, kayaking, canoeing, badminton, boule, curling, and bowling. Swimming is considered the ideal leisure activity for people with hemophilia. The great advantage of swimming is the reduction of vibration and gravity. The buoyancy effect eases the strain on the muscles and joints.

Although such classifications can be used as a guide, they are not wholly appropriate or sufficient to definitively suggest which sport a hemophilic patient should practice, as contact is not the only cause of injuries in this type of patient. Indeed, sports with a low incidence of injuries can also result in severe or very severe injuries in this population on occasions. A biomechanical study of the sport or physical exercise, a physical aptitude test, and an orthopedic analysis of the patient should be performed in order to help to choose the appropriate preventive physiotherapy and sport. Thus, preventive physiotherapy could counteract any deficiencies encountered, such as musculotendinous shortening, synovitis, or muscular atrophy. This strategy, together with the appropriate orthopedic modifications, should prepare the patient to practice the sport in question, thereby minimizing the risk of injury. On the other hand, organized sports programs should be encouraged as opposed to unstructured activities, where protective equipment and supervision may be lacking [3].

Hence, the patient should consult with a specialist team (e.g., physician, physiotherapist) before engaging in sports activities to discuss appropriateness, protective gear, and prophylaxis prior to the activity. However, we cannot forget that the choice of sports should reflect an individual's preference and local customs [5, 6].

Table 2 shows details of some of the recommended sports for hemophilic patients, as well as the most frequent

Hemophilia. Table 2 Sports in hemophilia: risks of frequent injuries and mechanisms of injury

Sport	Risk rating[a]	Most frequent injuries	Mechanism of injury	Preventive orthotic devices
Swimming	Low	Hemarthrosis in shoulder and elbow	Poor technique: inadequate body roll and subaquatic stroke in front crawl and backstroke	None
		Bruising on fingers or hands	Colliding with other swimmers or with the swimming pool lane lines	
		Fallings	Slipping on wet surfaces outside the pool	
Golf	Low	Contracture in the low back and lesion in shoulder girdle	Swinging without actually hitting the ball	Stabilization with elbow-caps
		Bruising and sprains on the arm	Bad swing	
Table tennis	Low	Ankle sprain	Ankle twist	Stabilizing ankle support or bandage
		Fallings	Slip	Trainers with nonslip sole
Freestyle dance and ballroom dance	Low	Fallings	Uncontrolled high-speed turns	Suitable footwear
		Ankle sprain		Stabilizing ankle support or bandage
Kayaking	Low	Acute injuries are strange	Poor technique and/or poor physical condition	Stabilizing elbow support or bandage
		Risk of overuse in shoulder joints and flexors in the upper arm. Contractures in spinal muscles		
Snorkeling	Low	Bruising	Beaten with rocks and coral	None
		Hemarthrosis in the ankle	Fins too long	
Tennis	Medium–low	Ankle sprain	Slip	Suitable footwear
		Fallings	Stepping on a ball	Stabilizing ankle support or bandage
		Overuse injuries in the forearm and shoulder in the dominant arm and lower back area	Repetitive movements	Elbow-caps
Cycling	Medium–Low[b]	Fallings: bruises, sprains, and fractures in the shoulder girdle and wrist, trauma head	Fall on one side, shot out of the bicycle	Helmet
		Hemarthrosis in the ankle	Falling with feet caught in automatic pedal or foot strap	
		Contractures of muscles in the back	Forward-flexed position in mountain and road bike	

[a]Risk rating applies to beginners or advanced amateurs. The risk for competitive athletes is usually higher
[b]The risk is minimal when pedaling an exercise bike at home. Risk is minimized by choosing easy even grounds and rides of no more than 1 h or 1 h and a half. Beginners must avoid automatic pedals or pedals with foot straps

injuries (especially acute injuries), main mechanisms of injury, and basic orthotic devices for prevention in each of them.

As we have seen, although sport is not completely risk-free, the appropriate choice of sport should mean that the benefits, including both emotional and social well-being as well as the obvious physical effects, outweigh the risks for patients with hemophilia. For this reason, the consensus regarding the suitability of including sports in the overall handling of hemophilia is widespread today.

Consequences

Untreated patients with hemophilia can be at high risk from even apparently trivial hemorrhagic processes. Musculoskeletal bleeds are by far the most common in hemophilic patients, with hemarthrosis, hematomas, and synovitis being the most frequent musculoskeletal injuries [5, 7].

Hematoma

It is defined as a morbid swelling of clotted blood within the tissue (Fig. 3) and is classified as superficial and deep (muscular). In hemophilia, the hemorrhage stops when the tissue pressure rises to the point of compressing the damaged vessel, but, in the most severe cases, this same pressure can be a cause of acute compartment syndrome (i.e., a space-occupying lesion that compresses neighboring structures, with the resulting risk of muscle ischemia, nerve damage, and possible aftereffects).

A muscle hematoma may encapsulate, and the vascularization of its capsule can cause continuous re-bleedings, which may even affect the nearby bone cortical, invading it and leading to a hemophilic pseudo-tumor of catastrophic consequences (Fig. 4).

Hemarthrosis

The rupture of blood vessels, in the sub-synovial plexus, leads to an intra-articular hemorrhage (Fig. 5), which only stops when the intra-capsular pressure raises and consequently compresses the bleeding vessel. According to the physiopathologic principles of resorption, as the pressure decreases a new episode of hemorrhage occurs, due to the impossibility of completing the hemostatic process, and, if no factor replacement therapy is administered, a vicious circle of difficult solution sets in.

Clinical symptoms start with the patient experiencing certain "sensations" called "aura," which prognosticate the

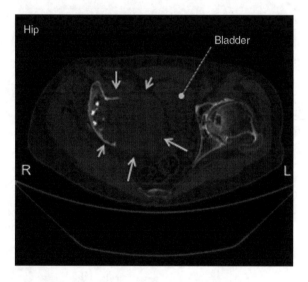

Hemophilia. Fig. 4 Hemophilic pseudotumor: the *arrows mark* the pseudotumor that is inserted into the bone, destroying and displacing the bladder

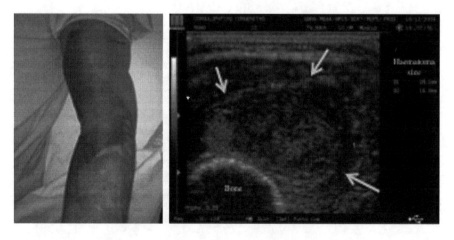

Hemophilia. Fig. 3 Muscle hematoma in a hemophilic patient. Clinical and ultrasound image

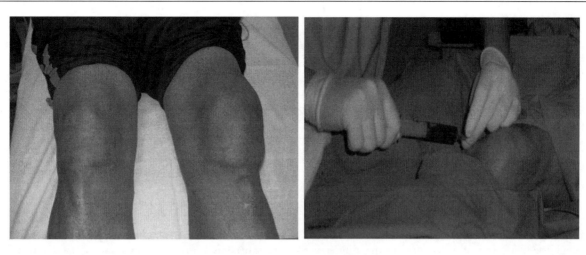

Hemophilia. Fig. 5 Hemarthrosis in a *left* knee in hemophilic patient. Arthrocentesis

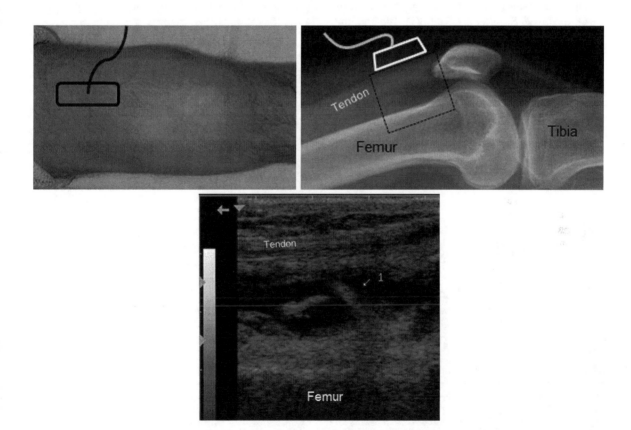

Hemophilia. Fig. 6 Synovitis in the knee of a hemophilic patient: note in the ultrasound image synovial villous (*1*) that occupies the interior of the joint

hemarthrosis. Then, a progressive inflammation sets in, with its classic characteristics: heat, redness, pain, swelling, and loss of function. The member adopts an antalgic posture, pain is described as highly intense, and physical examination reveals a swollen joint and exacerbation of the inflammatory signs.

Synovitis

Inflammation of the synovial membrane that lines the joint (Fig. 6). The process starts with an irritant synovial hyperplasia, aimed at facilitating the resorption of intra-articular blood. In acute hemarthrosis, blood resorption entails a decrease in intra-capsular pressure which in turn reopens the bleeding vessel. Recurrent episodes of synovitis lead to synovial hypertrophy, which in its first phase (pigmented synovitis) will predispose to re-bleeding (rich vascularization and fragility of new vessels), and the final step is arthropathy.

Hemophilic Arthropathy

When the first hemarthrosis occurs, the main difference with non-hemophilic individuals lies in the deficiency of coagulation that maintains the hemorrhage and modifies the physiopathology of the degenerative process of arthropathy. In short, immediately after the beginning of the effusion, its resorption through the synovial membrane starts; the synovium itself, due to its rich vascularization, and as internal pressure decreases, keeps producing the effusion. Chemical and physical factors play a part in the process, which is aggravated by disuse muscle atrophy, thus modifying joint mechanics and completing the circle of arthropathy (Fig. 7).

The musculoskeletal committee of the World Federation of Hemophilia (WFH) provides recommendations for the diagnosis and assessment of arthropathy. Table 3 shows a summary of the data required for its physical examination.

The prevention of these conditions constitutes the concept of prophylaxis for hemophilic arthropathy, which involves: (1) Replacement therapy of factor VIII/IX, (2) Physiotherapy, and (3) Physical exercise and/or sport to maintain a good physical condition.

As we have seen, although sport is not completely risk-free, the appropriate choice of sport should mean that the benefits, including both emotional and social well-being as well as the obvious physical effects, outweigh the risks for patients with hemophilia. For this reason, the consensus regarding the suitability of including sports in the overall handling of hemophilia is widespread.

Briefly: to stay in good health condition, hemophilic patients require factor replacement therapy, physiotherapy, physical activity, and sports.

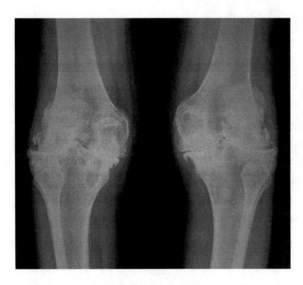

Hemophilia. Fig. 7 Hemophilic arthropathy: note the significant destruction of bone

Hemophilia. Table 3 Clinical data for evaluation of hemophilic arthropathy, according to the criteria of the World Federation of Hemophilia

Items of "Scores"	Description
Swelling	Volume of the joint, assessed by perimeter measurement (tape measure) in the articular interline
Atrophy	Volume of the muscle, evaluated by perimeter measurement in the muscle belly (using anatomical references)
ROM and contracture	Joint range of motion, in degrees (scores correspond to percentages of effective range and percentages of joint range for the contracture)
Axial deformity	Varus/valgus angle
Instability	Concept combining ligamentous instability, loss of range of motion, and strength
Crepitus	Joint cracking with movement
Pain	Pain at rest or with movement
Strength	Strength score according to Kendall's criteria
Orthosis	Use of orthotic devices in activities of daily living
Gait	Gait criteria

References

1. White GC II, Rosendaal F, Aledort LM, Lusher JM, Rothschild C, Ingerslev J, Factor VIII and Factor IX Subcommittee (2001) Definitions in hemophilia. Recommendation of the scientific subcommittee on factor VIII and factor IX of the scientific and standardization committee of the International Society on Thrombosis and Haemostasis. Thromb Haemost 85:560
2. Wittmeier K, Mulder K (2007) Enhancing lifestyle for individuals with haemophilia through physical activity and exercise: the role of physiotherapy. Haemophilia 13:31–37
3. Querol F, Pérez-Alenda S, Gallach JE, Devís-Devís J, Valencia-Peris A, González LM (2011) Haemophilia: exercise and sport. Apunts Med Esport 46(169):29–39
4. Kurme A, Seuser A (2006) Fit for life. A guide to fitness, games, sports and dance for people with haemophilia, 2nd edn. OmniMed, Haumburg
5. World Federation of Hemophilia (2005) Guidelines for the management of hemophilia. World Federation of Hemophilia, Montreal. http://www.wfh.org/2/docs/Publications/Diagnosis_and_Treatment/Guidelines_Mng_Hemophilia.pdf (28-07-2011)
6. Mulder K (2006) Exercises for people with hemophilia. World Federation of Hemophilia, Montreal. http://www.wfh.org/2/docs/Publications/General_Guides/Exercise_Guide_med.pdf (28-07-2011)
7. World Federation of Hemophilia (2004) What is hemophilia? World Federation of Hemophilia, Montreal. http://www.wfh.org/2/docs/Publications/General_Guides/Hemophilia_Booklet_Eng.pdf (28-07-2011)

Hemorheology

▶ Blood Rheology

Hemorrhagic Stroke

Focal brain hemorrhage leading to acute neurological injury; usually arises from rupture of small arteries or arterioles.

Hemostasis

Stavros Apostolakis[1,2], Gregory Y. H. Lip[1]
[1]Haemostasis Thrombosis and Vascular Biology Unit, University of Birmingham Centre for Cardiovascular Sciences, City Hospital, Birmingham, UK
[2]Department of Cardiology, Democritus University of Thrace, Alexandroupolis, Greece

Synonyms

Clotting; Coagulation; Thrombus formation

Definition

Hemostasis (or haemostasis) is a complex biochemical process that is activated to prevent bleeding. The product of hemostasis is a thrombus: a solid mass consisting mainly of platelets and ▶ fibrin that forms locally in a vessel. Hemostasis is mediated by an enzymatic cascade that leads to the activation of the serin protease, thrombin. Thrombin catalyzes the formation of fibrin. Fibrinolysis is the opposite process wherein a fibrin clot is enzymatically resolved. Hemostasis is regulated by activators and inhibitors that normally sustain a fine balance.

Characteristics

The conventional model of coagulation consists of two distinct initiation cascades: the intrinsic (or contact activation) pathway and the extrinsic (or tissue factor) pathway (Fig. 1). The two pathways merge at the level of factor Xa to a common cascade. The slower intrinsic clotting pathway depends on circulating coagulation factors such as factors IXa and factor VIIIa. The more rapid extrinsic pathway is activated when blood is exposed to an extravascular stimuli, mainly tissue factor (TF).[1, 2] Nevertheless, it is now believed that TF and its ability to complex with activated factor VII is the primary initial step of hemostasis in vivo [1, 2].

Tissue factor is expressed on perivascular pericytes and fibroblasts and is exposed to the circulation in cases of vascular injury. Activated factor VII (fVIIa), a serine protease that normally circulates in blood in low concentration, binds to TF. The TF/fVIIa complex activates factor X. Activated factor X (fXa) produces thrombin by the enzymatic cleavage of two sites on the ▶ prothrombin molecule. Thrombin in turn acts as a serine protease that converts soluble ▶ fibrinogen into insoluble strands of fibrin. Thrombin further catalyzes numerous coagulation-related reactions [1, 2].

There are two inhibitors that regulate TF-triggered pathways: Tissue factor pathway inhibitor (TFPI) neutralizes fXa when it is in a complex with TF-fVIIa. Antithrombin (AT), a serine protease inhibitor, neutralizes the initially formed fXa but also activated forms of other coagulation factors and, to a lesser extent, thrombin. Thus, coagulation proceeds only when high enough levels of TF are exposed to overcome the activity of the natural inhibitors [1, 2].

Circulating platelets contribute to thrombus formation at the site of vascular injury. They adhere to subendothelial collagen-▶ von Willebrand factor (vWF) via their glycoprotein receptors. Thrombin generated by the extrinsic pathway is capable of activating adherent

Coagulation and Fibrinolysis

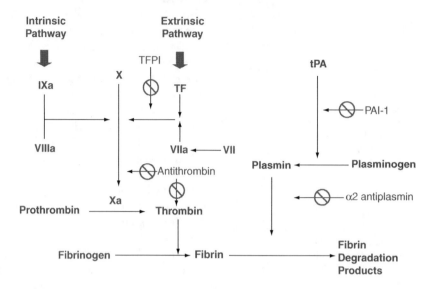

Hemostasis. Fig. 1 The conventional cascade of coagulation. The model consists of two separate triggering cascades: the intrinsic and extrinsic pathways, which ultimately merge at the level of Factor Xa. Formations of fXa and thrombin are regulated by natural inhibitors such as the tissue factor pathway inhibitor (TFPI) and antithrombin (AT). Fibrinolysis is activated to dissolve the fibrin-rich thrombus. The key step in fibrinolysis is activation of plasminogen by tissue plasminogen activator (tPA). Fibrinolysis is regulated by the natural inhibitors: plasmin activator inhibitor-1 (PAI) and α2 antiplasmin

platelets. Thrombin-activated platelets play a pivotal role in the processes of hemostasis in several ways: Platelet receptors bind to factor XI, and they also localize factor VIII to the site of endothelial disruption. Furthermore, mediators of hemostasis are released from platelet granules upon platelet activation. Moreover, key components of coagulation are concentrated on the activated platelet surface to locally generate thrombin more efficiently.

Finely balanced with coagulation, fibrinolysis is the process by which a fibrin-rich thrombus is degraded. The activation of the fibrinolytic system results in the conversion of the proenzyme plasminogen to the active enzyme plasmin. Plasmin degrades fibrin thrombi, resulting in the release of a variety of fibrin degradation products, including ► D-dimers. Plasminogen is activated by two types of activators: tissue plasminogen activator (tPA) and urokinase plasminogen activator (uPA). tPA-mediated plasminogen activation is mainly involved in the dissolution of fibrin in the circulation while u-PA binds to a specific cellular receptor resulting in enhanced activation of cell-bound plasminogen. Inhibition of the fibrinolytic system may occur either at the level of plasmin, by a2-antiplasmin, or at the level of the plasminogen activators, by plasminogen activator inhibitors (PAI-1 and PAI-2) [2].

Clinical Relevance

Imbalance between hemostasis and fibrinolysis is known to have clinical and prognostic relevance in cardiovascular disease [3–5]. Moreover, epidemiological data have demonstrated an explicit and strong relationship between physical activity and reduced risk for cardiovascular events. However, little and commonly conflicting data are available regarding the effects of exercise on hemostasis. Discrepancies of data on hemostasis and exercise may be explained by methodological variations, including use of different exercise protocols, use of different analysis techniques or study designs and most importantly the assessment of different populations. Most data come from population based cross sectional studies and few small scale interventional studies or prospective randomized control trials. Prothrombin time (PT), activated partial thromboplastin time (APPT), and thrombin time (TT) have been extensively used as overall measures of blood coagulability in initial reports. Plasma levels of coagulation factors and ex vivo assessment of hemostatic and fibrinolytic properties have been assessed in more recent studies. Both acute effects of exercise and long-term effects of regular training on hemostasis have been studied in healthy individuals and patients with cardiovascular disease.

Imminent Postexercise Effects

There is general agreement that hemostasis is affected by exercise and the overall effect has been associated with the intensity of exercise. Mild to moderate exercise seems to affect beneficially the balance between fibrinolysis and coagulation, while intensive exercise has been associated with an increase in plasmin formation, accompanied by a concomitant increase in markers of blood coagulation. The duration of exercise seems to also influence its effects on hemostasis. Endurance exercise such as marathon running was followed by an activation of blood coagulation, as indicated by the formation of thrombin and subsequently fibrin [5]. However, it seems that coagulation is activated in lesser extent than fibrinolysis making the overall effect of endurance exercise favorable. Moreover the pro-coagulant effect of endurance exercise –if any- has not been correlated with increased incidence of adverse cardiovascular events in long-term follow-up of middle aged marathon runners [5].

The mechanisms underlying modification of hemostasis by exercise have been also investigated. Exercise of varied intensity and duration has been associated with plasma levels and activity of coagulation factors. Increases in factor VIII activity and antigen have been reported acutely post exercise and positively associated with the intensity of exercise. The mechanism underlying exercise mediated effects on factor VIII are still obscure. It may be either due to the activation within the circulation or due to the overexpression of factor VIII [2, 3]. The stimulus responsible for exercise-induced increases in factor VIII seems to be mediated through the activation of b-adrenergic receptor pathway. Plasma fibrinogen levels are one of the main determinants of whole-blood viscosity and play a pivotal role in the blood clotting mechanism. Exercise has been shown to affect fibrinogen plasma concentration. However results are conflicting. Both significant increases and significant decreases have been reported while a number of studies reported no significant effects of exercise on plasma fibrinogen [2, 3].

It is generally accepted that intense exercise induces significant activation of fibrinolysis as a consequence of the release of both tissue and urinary -type plasminogen activators. Tissue-type plasminogen activity and antigen levels have been shown to increase significantly following both endurance and resistance exercise. This increase seems also to be intensity dependent. This hyperfibrinolysis is transient, although there are conflicting data regarding the duration of this phenomenon post exercise [3–5].

Exercise significantly affects inhibitors of fibrinolysis. Reduced levels of PAI-1 activity have been observed post endurance exercise. Resistance exercise also produced a similar reduction. As it is the case with tPA response, the PAI-1 response to exercise is related to the training intensity. Increased levels of D-dimer have been also reported post exercise supporting the concept of attenuated fibrinolytic activity.

Exercise seems to affect platelet count and function. Strenuous exercise results in an increased platelet count. Nevertheless, attempts to relate exercise to changes in platelet activation adhesion and aggregation have produced conflicting results. A number of studies reported increased platelet activation and aggregation both in healthy individuals and patients with chronic coronary artery disease. Exercise-induced activation of platelets was attributed to anaerobic metabolism since activation of platelets seems to be more pronounced in exercise above the anaerobic threshold. Catecholamines seem to be the common pathway for enhanced platelet aggregation. Nevertheless, several studies reported reduced platelet aggregation post exercise. As a result, it is not possible to draw conclusions regarding the influence of acute exercise on platelet function [2, 3].

Long-Term Effects of Exercise

Physical training in post myocardial infarction patients seems to suppress blood coagulability. This is constantly demonstrated by studies assessing different markers of hemostasis and fibrinolysis, including APTT and resting levels of FVIII after several weeks of physical training.

Epidemiological studies have reported a favorable association between physical training and plasma fibrinogen levels both in healthy individuals and patients with cardiovascular disease.

The effect of physical training on parameters of blood fibrinolysis has been further assessed. Exercise rehabilitation programs have been shown to result in significant reductions in PAI levels in cardiovascular patients but not in healthy controls. Three months of detraining seems to reverse the favorable reduction in PAI activity. Enhanced fibrinolysis in response to exercise seems to be related to the training status of the individual as suggested by the higher tPA release and lower tPA/PAI complex after exercise in physically trained subjects compared with untrained individuals. Therefore, rehabilitative exercise programs affect fibrinolysis favorably in cardiac patients [2, 3].

The effects of regular training on platelet function have not been sufficiently assessed, and many reported results are controversial. Exercise training in healthy individuals was associated with a decrease in resting and post exercise platelet adhesiveness and aggregation. These favorable effects seem to be transient and disappear with detraining [2, 3].

In conclusion, the available evidence suggests that acute exercise causes activation of blood coagulation, acceleration of blood fibrinolysis with a beneficial overall effect. Alterations in platelet number and function have been also observed acutely post exercise; however the exact effect and its clinical significances are still obscure. Regular training attenuates fibrinolysis and suppresses blood coagulability especially in the state of cardiovascular disease. Thus, the overall outcome of regular moderate exercise in hemostasis seems beneficial, with maximum effect observed in those that mostly need it. Nevertheless, these observational data should be further examined, and available studies should be replicated in different healthy and diseased populations.

References

1. Tanaka KA, Key NS, Levy JH (2009) Blood coagulation: hemostasis and thrombin regulation. Anesth Analg 108:1433–1462
2. Lee KW, Lip GYH (2003) Effects of lifestyle on hemostasis, fibrinolysis and platelet reactivity. Arch Intern Med 163:2368–2392
3. El-Sayed MS, Sale C, Jones PG, Chester M (2000) Blood hemostasis in exercise and training. Med Sci Sports Exerc 32:918–925
4. Hegde SS, Goldfarb AH, Hegde S (2001) Clotting and fibrinolytic activity change during the 1 h after a submaximal run. Med Sci Sports Exerc 33:887–892
5. Siegel AJ, Stec JJ, Lipinska I, Van Cott EM, Lewandrowski KB, Ridker PM, Tofler GH (2001) Effect of marathon running on inflammatory and hemostatic markers. Am J Cardiol 88:918–920

Hepatic Glucoregulation

Activity of the liver to achieve glucohomöostasis by concerted regulation of glycogenolysis and gluconeogenesis and delivery of glucose into circulation.

Hepatitis B

Hepatitis B virus infection is highly prevalent in some parts of the world where acquisition of the virus is often perinatal and then often leads to a chronic disease state. Those with chronic hepatitis B infection, often have relatively high levels of infectious virus in their blood as well as other fluids. Hepatitis B virus is believed to be 100 times more transmissible than HIV, and 10 times more transmissible than hepatitis C. The most efficient routes of transmission for hepatitis B are sexual intercourse, parenteral exposure, and to a lesser degree, mucosal contact with infected blood and blood products. The perinatal route from mother-to-child remains a common form of transmission in high-prevalence regions. Hepatitis B is resistant to alcohol, some detergents and has been shown to be present on some environmental surfaces for over 7-days. A safe and effective vaccine is available to prevent hepatitis B infection and it is now recommended in the universal child-immunization schedule as well as for adults who may be at higher-risk of exposure or disease due to occupational and lifestyle exposures as well as co-morbid diseases.

Cross-References

▶ Blood-Borne Infections

Hepatitis C

Prevalence data from 1999 to 2002, suggests that 1.6% of the population in the United States has been infected with hepatitis C. Worldwide prevalence rates are similar to the U.S. with the exceptions of several countries where there may be higher rates of infection within certain groups. Hepatitis C transmission occurs almost exclusively through the parenteral route and it therefore poses a significant risk among drug users and others who share needles. In past decades, prior to the recognition of this pathogen, significant segments of the population worldwide may have been exposed and infected iatrogenically from transfusions and the reuse of needles during medical care and mass vaccination campaigns. Although initially felt to be rare and difficult to prove, recent data now suggest that sexual transmission appears to play a role in transmission, especially among certain populations such as those who are co-infected with HIV. Perinatal acquisition has also been documented to occur in hepatitis C infection to a lesser degree than in hepatitis B.

Cross-References

▶ Blood-Borne Infections

Hepcidin

Hepcidin is a 25-amino-acid peptide hormone with responsibility for iron homeostasis. Its name is based on the facts that is produced in the liver (hep-) and that it has bacteriocidic properties ("-cidin" for "killing"). Hepcidin binds to the cell-surface iron export protein ferroportin, thereby causing its internalization and proteolytic degradation. Thus, hepcidin prevents the iron export from cells. In the gut, the loss of basolateral ferroportin leads to retention of iron in the intestinal epithelium. In iron-recycling macrophages, the loss of ferroportin prevents the release of iron liberated from the hemoglobin of engulfed erythrocytes. As a result, the level of plasma iron decreases. Hepcidin production increases primarily in conditions of iron overload, hypoxia or inflammation (stimulated by interleukin 6). The production of hepcidin ceases normally, when the plasma level of iron is below normal. This results in an increase in ferroportin activity, and iron uptake in the intestinal tract is augmented. At the cellular level lack of iron causes an iron-responsive element-binding protein to stabilize mRNA molecules translating transferrin receptors. Upon the expression of these receptors, transferrin, the iron (Fe^{3+}) transport protein in blood plasma, can bind to the membrane and deliver the iron to the cell. The increased activity of hepcidin in inflammation likely supports the innate immune reaction against invading pathogens, because these depend on iron for survival. On the other hand, the increased production of hepcidin restricts the iron availability in inflammatory diseases, thus contributing to the pathophysiological condition known as the "anemia of chronic disease" (ACD).

Cross-References
▶ Erythropoiesis

High Altitude

▶ Hypoxia, Focus Hypobaric Hypoxia

High Blood Pressure

Systolic blood pressure >140 mmHg.

Cross-References
▶ Hypertension
▶ Hypertension, Physical Activity
▶ Hypertension, Training

High Elevation

▶ Altitude, Physiological Response

High Energy Phosphate Bonds

An energy-rich phosphate linkage present in adenosine triphosphate (ATP), phosphocreatine (PCr), and certain other biological molecules.

High-Density Lipoprotein (HDL)

Is a lipoprotein whose primary apoprotein is apoA1. There is structural and functional heterogeneity and distinct HDL species, but they all share the common characteristic of serving as the primary actor in atheroprotection. HDL has well described anti-inflammatory, antithrombotic, antioxidant properties and serves primarily as the scavenger particle that mediates reverse cholesterol transport.

High-Intensity Aerobic Interval Training

Often performed as brisk uphill walking or running at intensities close to maximal heart rate (90–95%) or VO_{2max} (80–90%) for approximately 4–5 min, whereas the recovery periods consist of walking or "jogging" at considerably lower intensities (50–60% of the intensity during the high-intensity interval) for approximately 2–4 min.

High-Intensity Exercise

▶ Oxygen Partial Pressure (PO_2), in Heavy Exercise

High-Intensity Submaximal Interval Training

▶ Endurance Training

High-Intensity Training

▶ Interval Training

High-Intensity Training Young Athletes

▶ Children, in Competitive Sports

Hippocampus

A brain region that plays a critical role in learning and memory, and in which neurons degenerate in Alzheimer's disease.

HIV

W. Todd Cade, Kevin E. Yarasheski
Program in Physical Therapy and Department of Medicine, Washington University School of Medicine, Saint Louis, MO, USA

Synonyms

Acquired immune deficiency syndrome (AIDS); HIV-associated lipodystrophy; HIV-related cardiometabolic complications; Human immunodeficiency virus (HIV)

Definition

Human immunodeficiency virus (HIV) is a lentivirus capable of inserting its genetic material into the host cell nuclear DNA; a process that facilitates viral replication even in nondividing cells. HIV targets host immune cells (CD4$^+$ T-lymphocytes, macrophages, ▶ dendritic cells), where it integrates into the host DNA, replicates, produces new virion particles that infect and reduce CD4+ T-cell number. Advanced HIV disease results when many CD4+ T-cells are destroyed; this defines the Acquired Immune Deficiency Syndrome (AIDS). In AIDS, host immune function is severely compromised and inadequate to protect against common ▶ pathogens. The host becomes susceptible to common opportunistic infections and cancers that are typically fatal. Worldwide, ~40 million

people are living with HIV/AIDS, including ~18 million women and ~2.3 million children. HIV prevalence is the highest in sub-Saharan Africa (~12%); prevalence is lower in Westernized countries (e.g., US and Europe ~1%) and in Middle Eastern countries (<0.1%). HIV is transmitted through mucosal membranes exposed to infected blood, semen, or vaginal secretions. HIV can be transmitted during homosexual and heterosexual contact, blood transfusion, shared needles among intravenous drug users, during childbirth (mother-to-child transmission), and breast-feeding. Currently, there is no vaccine or cure for HIV infection. HIV infection is a risk factor for several endocrine, metabolic, anthropomorphic, and cardiovascular disorders that can reduce the quality and quantity of life.

There are many ▶ antiretroviral medications that effectively inhibit HIV replication by acting at different steps in the HIV life cycle (Fig. 1) and slow the progression from HIV infection to AIDS. These drugs are classified by their mode of action: HIV entry (CCR5 – CXCR4) inhibitors, HIV fusion inhibitors, non-nucleoside analogue reverse transcriptase inhibitors (nNRTI), nucleotide analogue reverse transcriptase inhibitors (NtRTI), nucleoside analogue reverse transcriptase inhibitors (NRTI), HIV integrase inhibitors, and HIV aspartyl protease inhibitors. Newer anti-HIV medications and regimens are being developed and are needed to reduce pill burden, drug resistance, and toxicities.

When available and properly prescribed, highly active antiretroviral therapy (HAART) reduces HIV-related mortality and morbidity rates so effectively that HIV infection has become a chronic manageable infection that can be controlled for many years. With the introduction of HAART (1995–2001), mortality from HIV decreased by ~70%. Life expectancy for HIV infected people with well-controlled viremia and immune status can exceed 30 years; much longer than in the pre-HAART era. Nowadays people living with HIV die more frequently from injury, cancer, heart disease, or drug abuse than from AIDS. Many HIV infected adults treated with HAART will attain 70–80 years of age; long enough to develop typical age-associated comorbidities. Some evidence suggests that HIV infection and HAART result in an accelerated or premature aging phenotype characterized by immune, cognitive, and physical frailty.

Pathogenic Mechanisms

Approximately 50% of people living with HIV and treated with HAART will develop insulin resistance/type 2 diabetes mellitus, ▶ hypertriglyceridemia, ▶ hypercholesterolemia,

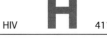

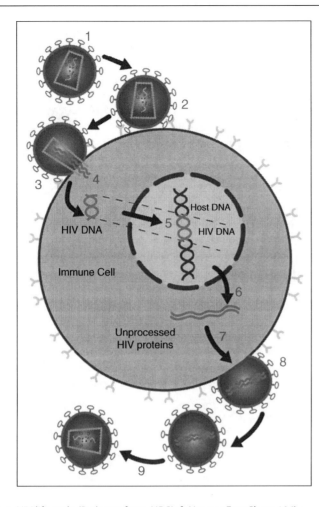

1. Viral particle (HIV virion)

2. **Binding-** viral particle binds to immune cell surface receptors (CD4 and a co-receptor; CCR5 or CXCR4)

3. **Fusion-** lipid membranes fuse; viral particle contents (viral RNA) enter immune cell.

4. **Reverse transcription-** viral RNA is reverse transcribed into viral DNA.

5. **Integration-** viral DNA integrates into host nuclear DNA.

6. **Transcription-** with cell replication, viral DNA is transcribed into viral proteins.

7. **Viral assembly-** viral proteins are joined and processed.

8. **Budding-** proteases cleave and activate viral proteins that are extruded from and encapsulated in immune cell lipid membrane.

9. **Maturation-** final protease processing of viral proteins to form mature infective virion.

HIV. Fig. 1 HIV life cycle (Redrawn from AIDSInfoNet.org Fact Sheet 106)

low high-density lipoprotein levels, elevated serum free fatty acid levels, central adiposity, peripheral ▶ lipoatrophy, or ▶ osteopenia/▶ osteoporosis. These conditions are frequently termed the HIV Lipodystrophy Syndrome or the HIV Metabolic Syndrome. The molecular mechanisms for these complications are not clear. The complications are associated with many potentially interrelated factors, including: intracellular molecular mechanisms driven by replicating HIV; a chronic proinflammatory, prooxidant state associated with chronic viral infection; rapid immune reconstitution after initiating HAART (increased CD4+ and CD8+ T-cell populations); certain antiretroviral drug toxicities (e.g., HIV protease inhibitors inhibit glucose transport efficiency and alter lipid/lipoprotein processing and partitioning pathways; thymidine nucleoside analogue reverse transcriptase inhibitors block ▶ mitochondrial polymerase γ, mitochondrial

biogenesis, and adipogenesis); genetic background (genotype); coinfection with other sexually transmitted diseases (hepatitis, cytomegalovirus); and lifestyle/behavioral factors such as tobacco/drug abuse, physical inactivity, poor nutritional choices. This cluster of complications mimics "▶ The Metabolic Syndrome" that is common among the general population, and associated with increased cardiovascular disease (CVD) risk, morbidity, and mortality. In fact, HIV infected adults have twice the risk for myocardial infarction and stroke than the general population. Myocardial contractility and function are also worse in HIV infected adults than in the general population.

Insulin Resistance and Diabetes. In age- and body mass index-adjusted analyses, the prevalence and incidence of type 2 diabetes was 4–5 times higher in HIV infected men than in HIV-seronegative men. By age, diabetes prevalence was 11% in HIV infected men <40 years old and 3% in HIV-seronegative men <40 years old. Diabetes prevalence was 18% in HIV infected men ≥40 years old and 13% in HIV-seronegative men ≥40 years old. Potential mechanisms for insulin resistance and diabetes in people living with HIV include: physical inactivity; antiretroviral drugs that block tissue glucose transport; virus- and drug-related factors that increase free fatty acid levels and lipid accumulation (lipotoxicity) in muscle, liver, heart; and thymidine nucleoside analogue reverse transcriptase inhibitor-induced mitochondrial toxicity that impairs substrate processing by the mitochondria.

Dyslipidemia. Prior to HAART, hypertriglyceridemia was common and it was attributed to elevated de novo hepatic lipogenesis. In the current HAART era, hypertriglyceridemia, low high-density lipoprotein and elevated total cholesterol levels were reported in ~27% of HIV infected adults taking HIV protease inhibitors, ~23% of those taking a non-nucleoside analogue reverse transcriptase inhibitors, and ~10% in those only taking a nucleoside analogue reverse transcriptase inhibitor. These rates increase among HIV infected people with central adiposity or peripheral lipoatrophy. Potential mechanisms for HIV-related dyslipidemia include: antiretroviral drugs that block triglyceride clearance; proinflammatory processes that increase hepatic synthesis of very low density lipoproteins and increase lipolytic rate.

Adipose Tissue Accumulation and Peripheral Lipoatrophy. The most common alteration in body adiposity among people living with HIV is peripheral adipose wasting or lipoatrophy. It can occur independently or in conjunction with trunk adipose accumulation (central adiposity). Lipoatrophy is linked to the duration of use of thymidine nucleoside analog reverse transcriptase inhibitors and certain HIV protease inhibitors. Trunk adiposity is frequently caused by visceral adipose accumulation, and is associated with increased risk for diabetes and cardiovascular disease. Potential mechanisms for HIV lipoatrophy include: antiretroviral drugs that inhibit adipocyte differentiation and adipogenesis, perhaps by altering mitochondrial function, and HIV or antiretroviral drug-induced activation of lipolysis. Potential mechanisms for HIV lipohypertrophy include: physical inactivity, excessive energy intake, and HIV or antiretroviral drugs that dysregulate lipid partitioning or utilization.

Osteopenia and Osteoporosis. The prevalence is 35–50% among HIV infected adults taking HAART. HIV-related osteopenia is characterized by decreased bone formation and increased bone resorption. HIV osteopenia and osteoporosis have been associated with increased visceral adiposity, chronic T-cell activation, antiretroviral drug-induced mitochondrial toxicity, lower body weight, corticosteroid use, and antiretroviral drugs that impair kidney function.

Exercise Intervention/Therapeutical Consequences

The availability of HAART and improved clinical care has increased life expectancy among HIV infected people. But, they are living longer to experience common endocrine, metabolic, anthropomorphic, and cardiovascular complications that are associated with advanced age, but especially responsive to aerobic and resistance exercise-training programs. In the general population, the benefits of a physically active lifestyle for controlling CVD risk factors (insulin resistance, diabetes, dyslipidemia, hypertension, central adiposity, autonomic dysfunction, low aerobic capacity) and CVD progression are well documented. Many HIV infected adults are sedentary, have low aerobic capacity, develop CVD risk factors, and live long enough to develop atherosclerosis. HIV infected people with insulin resistance/diabetes other CVD risk factors are well suited to benefit from a physically active lifestyle.

Aerobic Exercise Training in HIV

Several studies have examined the effects of short-term (<6 months), moderate intensity (50–70%) aerobic (constant and interval) exercise training on cardiorespiratory, immune and psychological outcomes in people living with HIV. Overall, it appears that aerobic exercise training is immunologically and virologically safe; it does not reduce CD4+ T-cell number or increase plasma viremia (HIV RNA copies/mL). It is generally recognized that aerobic exercise training is safe for those with well-controlled or mildly symptomatic HIV infection.

The benefits of aerobic exercise training for people living with HIV include: improved oxygen consumption, peak work rate, and ventilatory threshold. Specific exercise training levels that have been studied in HIV ranged from moderate (50–85% HR max or 50–80% VO_{2peak}) to intense (75–85% HR max or 75–85% VO_{2peak} and one study 50% difference between anaerobic threshold and VO_{2peak}), mostly occurring 3x/week for durations of 5–24 weeks. All training intensities and durations were effective in increasing aerobic fitness and it appears that individuals with HIV can safely participate in and respond to standard aerobic exercise-training recommendations (e.g., American College of Sports Medicine).

Limited data from middle-aged, HIV-infected adults suggest that aerobic exercise training improves cardiovascular risk parameters including a reduction in serum triglycerides and cholesterol, and a reduction in body adiposity, although not all studies report improvements in dyslipidemia. Aerobic exercise training appears to reduce trunk and total adipose content in adults and children. Caloric restriction-induced weight loss combined with an aerobic exercise-training program may aid in adipose tissue loss in HIV infected adults. Two reports indicate that aerobic exercise-training-induced weight loss and adipose tissue loss improve insulin sensitivity or glycemic control in HIV infected adults. Combining aerobic exercise training with other safe and effective interventions (oral lipid-lowering, glucose-lowering, or antihypertensive medications) may provide greater metabolic and cardiovascular benefits in HIV infected adults, but additional research is required.

Perceived quality of life and psychological state are lower in people with HIV compared to the general population. Aerobic exercise training appears to improve psychological status, measures of depression, quality of life, and the perception of overall health in people living with HIV. Aerobic exercise training may be a useful adjunctive therapy to improve psychological well-being and overall health perception in persons living with HIV.

Unfortunately, adherence/compliance with regular aerobic exercise-training programs is low among people living with HIV. Novel motivational methods that create tangible incentives for adhering to aerobic exercise-training regimens among HIV infected people are required.

Resistance Exercise Training in HIV

Progressive isometric and isotonic resistance exercise training (i.e., weight training) does not adversely affect immune or virologic status in HIV infected adults, and it has been used to increase muscle protein mass, improve muscle strength and function, reduce adiposity, and improve cardiovascular disease risk.

The benefits of progressive resistance exercise training for people living with HIV include: improved muscle mass and strength, reduced serum triglycerides, and when combined with aerobic exercise training, reduced serum cholesterol concentrations and reduced body adiposity. Peak oxygen consumption, a strong predictor of future cardiovascular morbidity and mortality in the general population, was improved in HIV infected adults after progressive resistance exercise training. When combined with metformin, an insulin sensitizing medication, resistance exercise training decreased thigh muscle adipose content, which is a predictor of insulin resistance in HIV infected and diabetic people.

Summary

HIV infection is a chronic manageable condition. In countries where highly active antiretroviral therapy is available, HIV morbidity and mortality have dramatically declined. However, longer life expectancy with HIV translates into several endocrine, metabolic, and anthropomorphic complications that increase cardiovascular disease risk in people living with HIV and taking highly active antiretroviral therapy. HIV infection is an independent risk factor for cardiovascular disease. The etiology for these cardiometabolic complications is complex, multifactorial and interrelated. Interventions that target chronic inflammation and modifiable behavioral/lifestyle factors (e.g., physical activity, nutrition, tobacco/drug/alcohol cessation) are safe, reasonable and effective in HIV infected people, but additional research should focus on using multidisciplinary approaches to discover the underlying pathogenesis and targeted treatments for these complications. Similar to the general population, combined aerobic and resistance exercise-training programs appear to be effective non-pharmacologic treatments for managing HIV metabolic, endocrine, anthropomorphic, cardiovascular complications, and for improving quality of life. Regular aerobic and resistance exercise-training recommendations can follow established guidelines (American College of Sports Medicine, American Heart Association) and should be included as part of routine clinical care for HIV infected people.

Cross-References

- ▶ AIDS, Exercise
- ▶ Blood-Borne Infections

References

1. Grinspoon S, Carr A (2005) Cardiovascular risk and body fat abnormalities in HIV-infected adults. N Engl J Med 352:48–62
2. Grinspoon SK, Grunfeld C, Kotler DP, Currier JS, Lundgren JE, Dube MP, Lipshultz SE, Hsue PY, Squires K, Schambelan M, Wilson PWF, Yarasheski KE, Hadigan CM, Stein JH, Eckel RH (2008) State of the Science Conference. Initiative to decrease cardiovascular risk and increase quality of care for patients living with HIV/AIDS executive summary. Circulation 118:198–210
3. Martinez E, Visnegarwala F, Grund B, Thomas A, Gibert C, Shlay J, Drummond F, Pearce D, Edwards S, Reiss P, El-Sadr W, Carr A, and for the INSIGHT SMART study group (2010) The effects of intermittent, CD4-guided antiretroviral therapy on body composition and metabolic parameters. AIDS 24:353–363
4. The Strategies for Management of Antiretroviral Therapy Study Group, El-Sadr WM, Lundgren JD, Neaton JD, Gordin F, Abrams D, Arduino RC, Babiker A, Burman W, Clumeck N, Cohen CJ, Cohn D, Cooper D, Darbyshire J, Emery S, Fätkenheuer G, Gazzard B, Grund B, Hoy J, Klingman K, Losso M, Markowitz N, Neuhaus J, Phillips A, and Rappoport C (2006) CD4+ count-guided interruption of antiretroviral treatment. N Engl J Med 355:2283–2296

5. Yarasheski KE, Roubenoff R (2001) Exercise treatment for HIV-associated metabolic and anthropomorphic complications. Exerc Sport Sci Rev 29:170–174
6. Yarasheski KE, Cade WT, Overton ET, Mondy KE, Hubert S, Laciny E, Bopp C, Lassa-Claxton S, Reeds DN (2011) Exercise training augments the peripheral insulin sensitizing effects of pioglitazone in HIV-infected adults with insulin resistance and central adiposity. Am J Physiol Endocrinol Metab 300:E243–E251

HIV-Associated Lipodystrophy

▶ HIV

HIV-Related Cardiometabolic Complications

▶ HIV

Hoffman Reflex

The Hoffman reflex refers to the monosynaptic reflex when it is evoked experimentally by applying a long duration (1 ms), low intensity electrical stimulus to a peripheral nerve to preferentially activate la afferents. Afferent input to the a-motor neuron pool will recruit a portion of the pool dependent upon its intrinsic excitability and summed synaptic input. The amplitude of the EMG response recorded from the muscle provides an indication net spinal excitability.

Homeostasis

Maintenance of the physiological status quo, usually referring to the rested condition, but during exercise applying to a new balance during steady state submaximal exercise.

Cross-References

▶ Thermoregulation

Homotope

Epitope means antigenic determinant for adaptive immunity. Innate immune receptors are constant, as are the germ-line genes that encode them. Consequently they must recognize antigens that never change (evolutionarily conserved) and such antigens must be cross-reactive (homologous). *Homotope* is a short term for *homologous epitope*. An analogous term in the literature is *pattern recognition* which implies that similar structures are recognized (e.g., homologous patterns).

Hormesis

Chronic exposure to low-dose toxins can result in increased tolerance to higher doses and protection from stress.

Hormones

Chemical substances produced in one part or organ of the body that initiate or regulate the activity of an organ or group of cells in another part. The term "hormone" originally applied to substances secreted by endocrine glands and transported via the bloodstream to target organs, but has been applied more broadly to substances having similar actions but not produced by special glands. Some common hormones include growth hormone, parathyroid hormone, follicle stimulating hormone, and luteinizing hormone.

Hormones Regulating Vascular Tone and Body Fluids

▶ Renin-Angiotensin Mechanism

Human Growth Hormone (hGH)

hGH is a peptide hormone growth factor that is assumed to be misused in sports to accelerate recovery and increase muscle mass, especially when coadministered with anabolic androgenic steroids.

Human Immunodeficiency Virus (HIV)

▶ HIV

Huntington's Disease

An inherited fatal neurodegenerative disorder characterized by the progressive degeneration of neurons that control body movements.

Cross-References
▶ Neurodegenerative Disease

Hybrid Fiber

A muscle fiber type containing multiple myosin heavy chain isoforms.

Hydroxyapatite

Calcium and phosphate mineral that makes up the main inorganic component of bone.

Hypercholesterolemia

High blood levels of cholesterol. Cholesterol is carried in the circulation by lipoproteins; low density lipoproteins (LDL) are associated with greater, and high-density lipoproteins (HDL) are associated with lower cardiovascular disease risk.

Hypercytokinemia

An uncontrolled, excessive production of cytokines. Cytokines have strong bioactivity, so if they are leaked into blood circulation, they may influence fever, sickness, and immunomodulation. If the production of cytokines results in a positive feedback loop, further increasing cytokine production a "cytokine storm" ensues and this is a hallmark of the systemic inflammatory response syndrome (SIRS).

Hyperglycemia

Blood glucose measured above 11 mmol/L (4–11 mmol/L is the normal range). Beside the corner stone of physical exercise blood glucose control is of major importance. The relevance of an adequate blood glucose control has been underscored in several epidemiologic studies, which have shown that hyperinsulinemia is an independent risk factor for cardiovascular disease. Furthermore correction of insulin resistance is clearly important in the management of type 2 diabetes. Patients with type 2 diabetes treated with metformin, which decrease hyperinsulinemia and insulin resistance, had a 30% reduction in microvascular disease events compared with those given conventional therapy. Although there was only a trend toward a reduction in macrovascular complications, epidemiologic analysis showed a statistically significant effect of HbA1c lowering with an approximate 14% reduction in all-cause mortality and myocardial infarction for every 1% reduction in HbA1c. Beside an adequate control of diabetes, measured by glycosylated hemoglobin levels, also the duration of diabetes and pathologic high levels of glycosylated hemoglobin predict cardiac events and mortality in patients with diabetes. Although numerous studies have demonstrated the beneficial effect of glycemic control on microvascular complications, fewer studies have shown a reduction in cardiovascular events with good glycemic control alone. Overall it has been shown a significant lower incidence of cardiovascular events in patients whose level of glycosylated hemoglobin was <7% of total hemoglobin. In patients with newly diagnosed type 2 intensive treatment of hyperglycemia over a 10-year period leads to an absolute reduction in the risk of myocardial infarction. Vice versa the same way insulin resistance may contribute to endothelial dysfunction, defects in NO-mediated vasodilatation may contribute to insulin resistance as suggested by some authors. This observation is in the context of some clinical trials, which showed that an angiotensin-converting enzyme inhibitor and a statin, besides improvement of endothelial function, slowed the progression of CAD and cardiovascular death and prevented the onset of type 2 diabetes in high-risk patients by approximately 30% and 35%, respectively.

Hyperlipidemia

▶ Lipid Metabolism Disorders

Hyperplasia

Hyperplasia occurs as a consequence of cell division resulting in an increased number of cells in a tissue. It differs from hypertrophy, where cell number remains constant, but tissue size increases. Skeletal muscle development is initiated through a process of hyperplasia e.g., the proliferation of myoblasts. However, during human embryogenesis the number of fibers is set at approximately 6 months of gestation and any further muscle growth occurs as a process of hypertrophy. Hyperplastic responses in other tissues occur as a consequence of the demands placed upon a tissue or an organ and are a normal physiological response to demand – e.g., glandular hyperplasia of the uterine wall and breast during pregnancy. Hyperplastic growth is tightly regulated, which is in contrast to neoplastic growth which underpins tumor formation and is governed by aberrant or even uncontrolled survival and therefore proliferation of genetically mutated cells. A good example of this inappropriate growth (neoplasia) is provided by the human prostate cancer cell line LNCaP in which the tumor suppressor PTEN, a protein tyrosine phosphatase inhibitor of the PI3Kinase pathway is mutated, allowing inappropriate survival and therefore ultimately proliferation of these cells.

Hypertension

Linda S. Pescatello
Department of Kinesiology U-1110, Human Performance Laboratory, Neag School of Education, University of Connecticut, Storrs, CT, USA

Synonyms
Antihypertensive effects of exercise; Essential hypertension

Definition
▶ Hypertension is a significant global public health issue.
▶ High blood pressure (BP) (systolic BP [SBP] >140 mmHg) results in 7.6 million deaths (13.5% of total deaths) and 92 million ▶ disability adjusted life years (DALYs) (6.0% of total DALYs) worldwide [1]. Much of the disease burden attributed to high BP occurs in middle-aged people and those with ▶ pre-hypertension. Table 1 contains the Joint National Commission's BP classification scheme. Due to its significant public health burden, the prevention, treatment, and control of hypertension have become a global health priority.

Characteristics
Endurance exercise is recommended as essential lifestyle therapy for the primary prevention, treatment, and control of hypertension [2]. An evidenced based review on exercise and hypertension has been published by the American College of Sports Medicine (ACSM) [3]. The 25 evidence based statements made in this position stand are shown in Table 2. The authors concluded that aerobic exercise training lowers BP an average of 5–7 mmHg in the majority of people with hypertension, with the greatest BP reductions seen in those with the highest resting BP. Although not as well researched, the BP reductions resulting from resistance exercise training are less than those from endurance exercise training. In addition, the antihypertensive effects of exercise are less when measured under ambulatory conditions than those assessed by auscultation in the

Hypertension. Table 1 Blood pressure classification for adults aged 18 and older [a,b,c,d] [2]

JNC VI blood pressure category	JNC VII blood pressure category	Systolic blood pressure (mmHg)		Diastolic blood pressure (mmHg)
Optimal	Normal	<120	and	<80
Normal	Pre-hypertension	120–129	and	80–84
High Normal	Pre-hypertension	130–139	or	85–89
Stage 1 hypertension	Stage 1 hypertension	140–159	or	90–99
Stage 2 hypertension	Stage 2 hypertension	160–179	or	100–109
Stage 3 hypertension	Stage 2 hypertension	≥180	or	≥110

[a]Produced from Chobanian et al. [2]
[b]Not taking antihypertensive drugs and not acutely ill. When the systolic and diastolic blood pressure categories vary, the higher reading determines the blood pressure classification. For example, a reading of 152/82 mmHg should be classified as Stage 1 hypertension and 170/116 mmHg should be classified as Stage 3 hypertension. In addition to classifying stages of hypertension on the basis of average blood pressure levels, clinicians should specify presence or absence of target organ disease and additional risk factors. This specificity is important for risk classification and treatment
[c]Optimal blood pressure with respect to cardiovascular risk is below 120/80 mmHg. However, unusually low readings should be evaluated for clinical significance
[d]Based on the average of two or more readings at each of two or more visits after an initial screen

Hypertension. Table 2 American College of Sports Medicine (ACSM) exercise and hypertension position stand evidence statements [3]

Section heading	Evidence statement	Evidence category [a]
Exercise BP and the prediction of hypertension and CVD morbidity and mortality	• Exercise BP contributes to the prediction of future hypertension in persons with normal BP	C
	• The prognostic value of exercise BP regarding CVD complications depends on the underlying clinical status and hemodynamic response and is therefore limited	D
Exercise BP benefits	• Higher levels of physical activity and greater fitness at baseline are associated with a reduced incidence of hypertension in white men; however, the current paucity of data precludes definitive conclusions regarding the role of gender and ethnicity	C
	• Dynamic aerobic training reduces resting BP in individuals with normal BP and in those with hypertension	A
	• The decrease in BP with aerobic training appears to be more pronounced in those with hypertension	B
	• Aerobic training reduces ambulatory BP and BP measured at a fixed submaximal work load	B
	• BP response differences among individual studies are incompletely explained by the characteristics of the training programs, that is, the weekly exercise frequency, time per session, exercise intensity and type of exercise	B
	• Dynamic exercise acutely reduces BP among people with hypertension for a major portion of the daytime hours	B
	• Resistance training performed according to the ACSM guidelines reduces BP in normotensive and hypertensive adults	B
	• Limited evidence suggests static exercise reduces BP in adults with elevated BP	C
	• Limited evidence suggests resistance exercise has little effect on BP for up to 24 h after the exercise session	C
	• There are currently no studies available to provide a recommendation regarding the acute effects of static exercise on BP in adults	None
	• Regular endurance exercise reduces BP in older adults as it does in younger persons	B
	• Limited evidence suggests PEH occurs in older adults	C
	• Endurance and resistance training do not reduce BP in children and adolescents	B
	• Endurance exercise training reduces BP similarly in men and women	B
	• Limited evidence suggests acute endurance exercise reduces BP similarly in white men and women	C
	• Currently no convincing evidence exists to support the notion ethnic differences exist in the BP response to chronic exercise training	B
	• Currently no convincing evidence exists to support the notion ethnic differences exist in the BP response to acute exercise	C
Exercise recommendations	• For persons with high BP, an exercise program that is primarily aerobic based is recommended	A
	• Resistance training should serve as an adjunct to an aerobic-based program	B
	• The evidence is limited regarding frequency, intensity, and duration recommendations; nonetheless, the antihypertensive effects of exercise appear to occur at a relatively low total volume or dosage	C
	• Limited evidence exists regarding special considerations for those with hypertension	D

Hypertension. Table 2 (continued)

Section heading	Evidence statement	Evidence category [a]
Mechanisms	• Neural and vascular changes contribute to the decreases in BP that result from acute and chronic endurance exercise	C
	• Emerging data suggest possible genetic links to acute and chronic exercise BP reductions	D

Reprinted with permission by Pescatello et al. [3]

BP blood pressure, *CVD* cardiovascular disease, *PEH* postexercise hypotension

[a]Evidence category weighting description, *A* highest to *D* lowest

laboratory. Although data are limited, age, gender, and ethnicity do not alter the BP response to endurance exercise training.

Clinical Relevance

The ▶ exercise prescription (ExR$_x$) for lower BP consists of the *F*requency (how often), *I*ntensity (how hard), *T*ime (how long), and *T*ype (what modality) of physical activity or *FITT*. The BP reductions that result from endurance exercise training occur rapidly after just three sessions, and after short amounts (durations as short as 10 min) and low exertion levels (intensities equivalent to an enjoyable walking pace) of exercise [4]. Therefore, the ACSM ExR$_x$ for those with high BP is as follows [3]:

Frequency: Aerobic exercise on most, preferably all days of the week; resistance exercise 2–3 day per·week as a supplement to aerobic exercise.

Intensity: ▶ Moderate intensity, aerobic exercise (i.e., 40–<60% of maximum oxygen consumption [VO$_2$max]) supplemented by resistance training at 60–80% of the one repetition maximum (1-RM).

Time: 30–60 min·day^{-1} of continuous or intermittent aerobic exercise. If intermittent, perform a minimum of 10 min bouts accumulated to total 30–60 min·day^{-1} of exercise. Resistance training should consist of at least one set of 8–12 repetitions.

Type: The primary emphasis should be placed on aerobic activities such as walking, jogging, cycling, and swimming. Resistance training using either machine weights or free weights may supplement aerobic training. Such training programs should consist of 8–10 different exercises targeting the major muscle groups.

Special considerations for those with hypertension when exercising include:

- If resting SBP >200 mmHg and/or DBP >110 mmHg, do not exercise. When exercising, it is prudent to maintain SBP ≤220 mmHg and/or DBP ≤ 105 mmHg.

- Beta-blockers and diuretics may adversely affect thermoregulatory function and cause hypoglycemia in some individuals. In these situations, educate patients about the signs and symptoms of heat intolerance and hypoglycemia, and the precautions that should be taken to avoid these situations.

- Beta-blockers, particularly the nonselective types, may reduce submaximal and maximal exercise capacity primarily in patients without myocardial ischemia. Consider using perceived exertion to monitor exercise intensity in these individuals.

- ▶ Antihypertensive medications such as α blockers, calcium channel blockers, and vasodilators may lead to sudden reductions in postexercise BP. Extend and monitor the cool-down period carefully in these situations.

- Many individuals with hypertension are ▶ overweight or obese. ExR$_x$ for these individuals should focus on increasing caloric expenditure coupled with reducing caloric intake to facilitate weight reduction. See the American College of Sports Medicine's Guidelines for Exercise Testing and Prescription eighth edition for additional information on ExR$_x$ guidelines and recommendations for those who are overweight and obese [5].

- A majority of older persons will have hypertension. See Thompson et al. [5] for additional information on ExR$_x$ guidelines and recommendations for older adults.

- The BP lowering effects of aerobic exercise are immediate, a physiologic response referred to as ▶ postexercise hypotension [3]. To enhance patient adherence, educate patients about the acute or immediate BP lowering effects of exercise.

- For individual with documented episodes of ischemia during exercise, the exercise intensity should be set (≥ 10 beats·min^{-1}) below the ▶ ischemic threshold.

- Avoid the ▶ Valsalva maneuver during resistance exercise training.

References

1. Lawes CMM, Vander Hoorn S, Rodgers A (2001) Global burden of blood-pressure-related disease. Lancet 371:1513–1518
2. Chobanian AV, Bakris GL, Black HR, Cushman WC, Green LA, Izzo JL Jr, Jones DW, Materson BJ, Oparil S, Wright JT Jr, Roccella EJ and the National High Blood Pressure Education Program Coordinating Committee (2003) Seventh report of the joint national committee on prevention, Detection, evaluation, and treatment of high blood pressure. JNC 7- complete version. Hypertension 42:1206–1252
3. Pescatello LS, Franklin BA, Fagard R, Farquhar W, Kelly GA, Ray CA (2004) American College of Sports Medicine position stand. Exercise and hypertension. Med Sci Sports Exerc 25:533–553
4. Pescatello LS (2005) Exercise and hypertension: recent advances in exercise prescription. Curr Hypertens Rep 7:281–286
5. Thompson W, Gordon N, Pescatello LS (eds) (2009) American College of Sports Medicine. ACSM's guidelines for exercise testing and prescription, 8th edn. Lippincott, Williams and Wilkins, Baltimore

Hypertension, Physical Activity

R. H. FAGARD
Hypertension and Cardiovascular Rehabilitation Unit, Hypertension Unit, University of Leuven K.U. Leuven, U.Z. Gasthuisberg, Leuven, Belgium

Synonyms

Essential hypertension; Exercise; High blood pressure; Training

Definition

Hypertension is defined as a systolic blood pressure of ≥140 mmHg or a diastolic blood pressure of ≥90 mmHg, or both, based on multiple blood pressure measurements, taken on separate occasions, in the sitting position, by use of a mercury sphygmomanometer or another calibrated device [1]. Hypertension is an important health problem because its prevalence amounts to ~25% in population-based studies and is associated with increased incidence of all-cause and cardiovascular mortality, sudden death, stroke, coronary heart disease, heart failure, atrial fibrillation, peripheral arterial disease, and renal insufficiency. In addition, hypertension is often associated with other cardiovascular risk factors such as obesity, dyslipidemia, and glucose intolerance and causes target organ damage such as left ventricular hypertrophy, microalbuminuria, and vascular stiffness. Therefore, high blood pressure should not be considered in isolation but in the context of an overall cardiovascular risk stratification model in which risk factors, target organ damage, and associated clinical conditions are taken into account, and in which patients are classified as having low, moderate, high, or very high risk [1].

Pathogenesis

Hypertension is a multifactorial "disease" in which genetic and environmental/lifestyle factors play an important role, including sodium, alcohol, and caloric intake, stress, and physical inactivity. There is indeed evidence from cross-sectional epidemiological studies that physical inactivity is involved in the pathogenesis of hypertension, and longitudinal observational studies found that physical activity or fitness are inversely related to the later development of hypertension [2]. Therefore, physical activity plays an important role in the prevention and control of high blood pressure.

Many studies have analyzed the relationship between physical activity and blood pressure. In some studies, physical fitness was estimated from an exercise test; other studies used questionnaires and sometimes an interview relating to the subject's physical activity at work, at leisure time, or both. It is accepted by most authors that the estimation of physical activity by questionnaire and interview is a poor but nevertheless useful and possibly the best available tool. Furthermore, the relationships between results of physical fitness tests and physical activity pattern by interview or questionnaire are of a low order. In general, therefore, the methodology to estimate physical activity lacks accuracy. In addition, there are several confounding variables that might affect the relationship between physical activity and blood pressure. Some of these such as age, weight, or indices of body fatness can be accounted for in the analysis. Others such as self-selection are hardly controllable. Indeed, "fit" subjects may have lower blood pressures and choose a more active lifestyle, whereas subjects with higher blood pressures may suffer from cardiovascular diseases resulting in a lower degree of physical activity. Another problem is that the level of physical activity is low in most Western societies, which may hamper the finding of an association with blood pressure.

Whereas several studies did not observe significant independent relationships, others reported inverse relationships between blood pressure and either habitual physical activity or physical fitness. The difference in blood pressure between the most and the least physically active or fit usually amounted to no more than about 5 mmHg [2].

Training/Exercise Response

Exercise Training and Blood Pressure: Longitudinal Intervention Studies

It remains difficult to ascribe differences in blood pressure within a population to differences in levels of physical activity or fitness because of the potentially incomplete statistical correction for known confounders and because of the possible influence of confounding factors which were not considered or which cannot be taken into account, such as self-selection. Therefore, longitudinal intervention studies are more appropriate to assess the effect of physical activity and training on blood pressure. Most investigators assessed the effect of dynamic aerobic endurance training on blood pressure, others applied resistance exercises. Blood pressure was most often measured in resting conditions or in response to stress, particularly during exercise testing, and also by use of ambulatory monitoring techniques. Meta-analyses of randomized controlled intervention studies concluded that regular dynamic endurance training at moderate intensity significantly reduces blood pressure. A recent meta-analysis [3] involved 72 trials and 105 study groups. After weighting the number of participants, training induced significant net reductions of resting and daytime ambulatory blood pressure of, respectively, 3.0/2.4 mmHg (P < 0.001) and 3.3/3.5 mmHg (P < 0.01). The reduction of resting blood pressure was more pronounced in the 30 hypertensive study groups (−6.9/−4.9) than in the others (−1.9/−1.6) (P < 0.001 for all). Systemic vascular resistance decreased by 7.1% (P < 0.05), plasma norepinephrine by 29% (P < 0.001) and plasma renin activity by 20% (P < 0.05). Body weight decreased by 1.2 kg (P < 0.001), waist circumference by 2.8 cm (P < 0.001), percent body fat by 1.4% (P < 0.001) and the HOMA-index of insulin resistance by 0.31 units (P < 0.01); HDL-cholesterol increased by 0.032 mmol.L^{-1} (P < 0.05). There was no convincing evidence that the blood pressure response depended on training intensity between ~40% and ~80% of maximal aerobic power.

In a recent meta-analysis of randomized controlled trials [4], "resistance" training at moderate intensity was found to decrease blood pressure by 3.2 mmHg for systolic blood pressure (P = 0.10) and by 3.5 mmHg (P < 0.01) for diastolic blood pressure. The meta-analysis included nine studies designed to increase muscular strength, power, and/or endurance, and all but one study involved dynamic rather than purely static exercise. In fact, few sports are characterized by purely static efforts. However, only three trials in the meta-analysis reported on patients with hypertension, so that knowledge on resistance training is limited in this condition.

Recommendations

Diagnostic Evaluation

Diagnostic procedures comprise a thorough individual and family history, physical examination, including repeated blood pressure measurements according to established recommendations, and laboratory and instrumental investigations, of which some should be considered part of the routine approach in all subjects with high blood pressure, some are recommended, and some are indicated only when suggested by the core examinations [1]. In the exercising patient, the pre-training screening evaluation mainly depends on the intensity of the anticipated exercise and on the patient's symptoms, cardiovascular disease risk, and associated clinical conditions, and may include echocardiography, exercise testing, ECG Holter monitoring, etc. For example, the indication for exercise testing depends on the patient's risk and on the sports characteristics [5, 6]. In patients with hypertension about to engage in hard or very hard exercise (intensity ≥60% of maximum), a medically supervised peak or symptom-limited exercise test with ECG and blood pressure monitoring is warranted. In asymptomatic men or women with low or moderate added risk, who engage in low-to-moderate physical activity (intensity < 60% of maximum), there is generally no need for further testing beyond the routine evaluation. Asymptomatic individual patients with high or very high added risk may benefit from exercise testing before engaging in moderate-intensity exercise (40–60% of maximum) but not for light or very light activity (<40% of maximum). Patients with exertional dyspnea, chest discomfort, or palpitations need further examination, which includes exercise testing, echocardiography, Holter monitoring, or combinations thereof.

A major problem with exercise testing in a population with a low probability of coronary heart disease and in subjects with left ventricular hypertrophy is that the majority of positive tests on electrocardiography are falsely positive. Stress myocardial scintigraphy or echocardiography, and ultimately coronarography, may be indicated in cases of doubt. There is currently insufficient evidence that the blood pressure response to exercise should play a role in the recommendations for exercise in addition to blood pressure at rest. However, subjects with an excessive rise of blood pressure during exercise are more prone to develop hypertension and should be followed up more closely. Finally, physicians should be aware that high blood pressure may impair exercise tolerance.

Treatment

Exercising patients should be treated according to the general guidelines for the management of hypertension [1]. Appropriate non-pharmacological measures should be considered in all patients, that is, moderate salt restriction, increase in fruit and vegetable intake, decrease in saturated and total fat intake, limitation of alcohol consumption to no more than 20–30 g ethanol/day for men and no more than 10–20 g ethanol/day for women, smoking cessation, and control of body weight. Antihypertensive drug therapy should be started promptly in patients at high or very high added risk for cardiovascular complications. In patients at moderate or low added risk, drug treatment is only initiated when hypertension would persist after several weeks or months despite appropriate lifestyle changes. The goal of antihypertensive therapy is to reduce blood pressure to at least below 140/90 mmHg, to lower values if tolerated in all hypertensive patients and to below 130/80 mmHg in diabetics and other high or very high risk conditions.

Current evidence indicates that patients with white-coat hypertension, that is, high blood pressure in the office and normal blood pressure out of the office, do not have to be treated with antihypertensive drugs, unless they are at high or very high risk, but regular follow-up and non-pharmacological measures are recommended [1]. Also, subjects with normal blood pressure at rest and exaggerated blood pressure in response to exercise should be followed up more closely.

Several drug classes can be considered for the initiation of antihypertensive therapy: diuretics, beta-blockers, calcium channel blockers, angiotensin converting enzyme inhibitors, and angiotensin II receptor blockers [1, 6]. However, diuretics and beta-blockers are not recommended for first-line treatment in patients engaged in competitive or high-intensity endurance exercise. Diuretics impair exercise performance and capacity in the first weeks of treatment through a reduction in plasma volume, but exercise tolerance appears to be restored during longer-term treatment; nevertheless, diuretics may cause electrolyte and fluid disturbances, which are not desirable in the exercising patient. Beta-blockers reduce maximal aerobic power by on average 7% as a result of the reduction in maximal heart rate, which is not fully compensated by increases of maximal stroke volume, peripheral oxygen extraction, or both.

Furthermore, the time that submaximal exercise can be sustained is reduced by ~20% by cardioselective beta-blockers and by ~40% by nonselective beta-blockers, most likely as a result of impaired lipolysis. Calcium channel blockers and blockers of the renin-angiotensin system are currently the drugs of choice for the exercising hypertensive patient [6] and may be combined in case of insufficient blood pressure control. However, the combination of an angiotensin converting enzyme inhibitor and an angiotensin II receptor blocker is not advocated for the treatment of hypertension. If a third drug is required, a low-dose thiazide-like diuretic, possibly in combination with a potassium sparing agent, is recommended. There is no unequivocal evidence that antihypertensive agents would impair performance in "resistance" sports.

Recommendations for Sports Participation

Recommendations for participation in sports in patients with hypertension are based on the results of the evaluation and on the risk stratification and with the understanding that the general recommendations for the management of hypertension are observed, as described above and provided that the clinical condition is stable [6]. Recommendations may be restrictive in patients who aim to engage in competitive sports or hard or very hard leisure-time sports activities meant to substantially enhance performance. However, most recreational physical activities are performed at low-to-moderate intensity. Dynamic sports activities are to be preferred, but low-to-moderate resistance training is also not harmful and may even contribute to blood pressure control. In case of cardiovascular or renal complications, the recommendations are based on the associated clinical conditions.

Finally, all patients should be followed up at regular intervals, depending on the severity of hypertension and the category of risk. In addition, all exercising patients should be advised on exercise-related warning symptoms, such as chest pain or discomfort, abnormal dyspnea, dizziness, or malaise, which would necessitate consulting a qualified physician.

Acknowledgment
The authors gratefully acknowledge the secretarial assistance of N. Ausseloos.

References
1. The Task Force for the Management of Arterial Hypertension of the European Society of Hypertension (ESH) and of the European Society of Cardiology (ESC) (2007) 2007 guidelines for the management of arterial hypertension. J Hypertens 25:1105–1187

2. Fagard RH, Cornelissen V (2005) Physical activity, exercise, fitness and blood pressure. In: Battagay E, Lip GYH, Bakris GL (eds) Handbook of hypertension: principles and practice. Taylor & Francis, Boca Raton, pp 195–206

3. Cornelissen VA, Fagard RH (2005) Effects of endurance training on blood pressure, blood pressure regulating mechanisms and cardiovascular risk factors. Hypertension 46:667–675

4. Cornelissen VA, Fagard RH (2005) Effect of resistance training on resting blood pressure: a meta-analysis of randomized controlled trials. J Hypertens 23:251–259

5. Pescatello LS, Franklin B, Fagard R, Farquhar WB, Kelley GA, Ray CA (2004) American college of sports medicine position stand: exercise and hypertension. Med Sci Sports Exerc 36:533–553

6. Fagard RH, Björnstad HH, Børjesson M, Carré F, Deligiannis A, Vanhees L (2005) European society of cardiology study group of sports cardiology recommendations for participation in leisure-time physical activities and competitive sports for patients with hypertension. Eur J Cardiovasc Prev Rehabil 12:326–331

Hypertension, Training

FABIO MANFREDINI, ROBERTO MANFREDINI
Department of Biochemistry and Molecular Biology, Section of Biochemistry of Physical Exercise Center Biomedical Studies Applied to Sport, Vascular Diseases Center, University of Ferrara, Ferrara, Italy

Synonyms

Arterial hypertension; Essential hypertension; Exercise training; High blood pressure; Physical training; Primary hypertension; Sports training

Definition

According to the Medical Subject Headings (MeSH) 2010 dictionary (http://www.ncbi.nlm.nih.gov/mesh), the term "hypertension" refers to persistently elevated systemic arterial blood pressure. Based on multiple readings (blood pressure determination), hypertension is currently defined as systolic pressure consistently greater than 140 mmHg or diastolic pressure consistently greater than 90 mmHg.

At minimum, three sets of blood pressure (BP) measurements taken over a 3-month interval are necessary before the term hypertension can be applied. Hypertension is associated with at least doubling of the long-term risk of cardiovascular mortality. The recommendations from the Sixth Joint National Committee on Prevention, Detection, Evaluation, and Treatment of High Blood Pressure (JNC-6) considered BP levels (systolic/diastolic) <120/<80 mmHg as optimal, <130/<85 mmHg as normal, between 130 and 139 mmHg systolic and 85 and 89 mmHg diastolic as high-normal, and >140/90 mmHg

as hypertension. Since several studies have shown a significant increase in the risk of cardiovascular events over time in the high-normal group, the JNC-7 report [1] stratified this group, defining levels above 120/80 mmHg as prehypertension and above 140/90 mmHg as hypertension. This was based on evidence that prehypertensive individuals have a higher chance of developing hypertension than those with a normal BP (<120/80 mmHg) at all ages. However, the European Society of Hypertension (ESH)–European Society of Cardiology (ESC) Guidelines [2] elected not to use the JNC-7 terminology due to three considerations. First, there is little reason to join the normal and high-normal groups as patients with high-normal BP had an increased risk of developing hypertension compared to subjects with normal BP. Second, guideline writers feared that use of the term prehypertension would create anxiety among patients and/or requests for unnecessary physician visits or examinations. Finally, the prehypertension population represents a highly diverse category, characterized by both subjects in no need of any intervention as well as subjects with a high- or very-high-risk profile.

The term "training," as in exercise or physical training, refers to repetitive movements or actions aimed at inducing physiologic adaptations to improve specific skills influencing performance of activities or factors contributing to a higher physical fitness level. A training program is based on the proper selection of intensity, time, and type of exercise. It should be specific for the activity and the muscles involved and adapted to gender, age, individual capabilities, and fitness level. It can be progressive, with periodization aimed at obtaining a peak performance with phases of overload and periods of recovery.

Pathogenetic Mechanisms

Pathogenetic mechanisms of arterial hypertension are multiple, including:

1. *Endothelial dysfunction*: Capacity of endothelial cells to produce either relaxing (e.g., nitric oxide) and constricting (e.g., endothelin) substances.
2. *Genetic predisposition*: Multiple genes plus environmental factors.
3. *Hemodynamic factors*: For example, changes in cardiac output, peripheral resistance, and heart rate.
4. Hyperactivity of the sympathetic nervous system.
5. *Renin-angiotensin mechanism*: In particular, activation of *local* rather than *general* RAA systems may give rise to a series of angiotensin II–mediated, unfavorable mechanisms.
6. *Sodium retention*.

7. *Vascular hypertrophy*: For example, altered pressor mechanisms, abnormal hypertrophic response to pressure, and increased humoral agents.

Exercise Intervention/Therapeutical Consequences

Exercise training is considered a nonpharmacological intervention; its acute and chronic effects can prevent and manage hypertension. If higher levels of fitness are associated with a reduced incidence of hypertension, exercise has a direct effect on lowering BP. The key points outlined in the literature [3–6] are summarized below:

1. A single bout of dynamic exercise may evoke a prolonged decrease of arterial BP below basal levels (postexercise hypotension).
2. Frequent bouts of exercise accumulated over a time period, rather than vigorous and prolonged periods of exercise, are able to induce training adaptations associated with a significant decrease of both systolic and diastolic BP. For hypertensive patients, 30–60 min/day of continuous exercise, or three to six bouts of 10 min of intermittent exercise, should be performed on most days of the week at low to moderate intensity, corresponding to 40–60% of maximal oxygen uptake or to an intermediate level on the Borg scale of perceived exertion. Further increases in intensity or in exercise time per week, especially for older or less fit subjects, may not add significant benefits, increase cardiovascular and orthopedic risks, and reduce training program compliance.
3. Different modes of exercise training are effective. Aerobic training with activities involving the continuous use of multiple muscle groups (walking, jogging, running, or cycling) is recommended to lower BP in adults. Resistance training is also efficacious for reducing resting BP in adults; however, for hypertensive patients, the association with aerobic training is recommended. Different types of exercise (Qigong, T'ai Chi) have also been investigated as nonpharmacological means for reducing BP.
4. The antihypertensive action of exercise training is multifactorial. Even if exercise training yielded positive effects on cardiac structure, exercise-induced BP reduction is mainly related to a decrease in peripheral vascular resistance and changes in vessel diameter, according to Poiseuille's law. These changes derive from alterations in the sympathetic nervous system activity, from improvements in endothelial function, and from structural vascular adaptations, with the possible influence of genetic factors.

Physical training, activating the autonomic nervous system activity during each bout of exercise, contributes to regulate its overactivity typical of hypertensive patients. The training effect causes a decreased sympathetic outflow, with a lower norepinephrine release rate and decreased plasma levels. Exercise-induced muscle adaptations also improve insulin sensitivity and reduce the activation of the sympathetic nervous system associated with hyperinsulinemia and insulin resistance. Training also limits the responsiveness of the peripheral vasculature to adrenergic receptor stimulation by norepinephrine and lowers the levels of endothelin-1, a potent vasoconstrictor. These BP-lowering effects on endothelial function are accompanied by exercise training–enhanced local vasodilator activity; they are also partly dependent on the properties of nitric oxide (NO) to regulate vascular tone. Training increases blood flow and shear stress, stimulates endothelial NO synthase mRNA and protein expression, and improves the balance between antioxidant and pro-oxidant factors. These factors increase NO availability in the vascular smooth muscle, particularly in larger vessels with greater capacities for NO production and endothelium-dependent vasodilatation. This effect mainly occurs in subjects with impaired endothelial function, such as patients with ► coronary artery disease, hypertension, and dysmetabolism. Vascular adaptations occur rapidly; changes in the vessel function are observed during the first phases of training. Vascular remodeling follows the advanced phases of training, with enlargement of the vessel luminal diameter and a decrease in peripheral resistance. However, these improvements can regress without adequate stimulation. Training may also induce an angiogenic response, producing new vessel and muscle capillary growth, with a possible BP-lowering effect. Finally, an interaction between training effects and genetic factors favoring these adaptations might also play a role, with some genes identified as possible contributors to the antihypertensive effect.

According to the literature, the effect of training adaptations on BP reduction is favorable [3–6]. Following aerobic exercise in trials lasting 3–24 or more weeks, an average reduction in systolic BP of 3.84 mmHg and in diastolic BP of 2.58 mmHg was observed, independent of mode, frequency, or intensity of exercise; gender; or change in body weight. The BP-lowering effect is more marked in hypertensive than in normotensive subjects. Similarly, following resistance exercise programs, studies have reported BP decreased an average of 3 mmHg, with no difference between conventional or circuit resistance training protocols.

Training-induced BP reductions may seem irrelevant from the clinical point of view; however, the effect is more pronounced in subjects with higher baseline BP levels, and the impact of this reduction on the general population is relevant in terms of cardiovascular disease morbidity and overall mortality.

As is true for any therapy, exercise-based therapy requires precautions as well as specialized skills. Cooperation between physicians and physical training experts is critical; each patient's level of risk must be estimated, and, when necessary, a preliminary medical evaluation or an assessment for exercise tolerance has to be performed. Finally, personnel must be expert in developing an "exercise prescription" and be able to tailor a safe, effective training program based on the patient's capabilities and designed for long-term adherence.

References

1. Chobanian AV, Bakris GL, Black HR et al (2003) The seventh report of the joint national committee on prevention, detection, evaluation, and treatment of high blood pressure. The JNC 7 report. JAMA 289:2560–2572
2. Mancia G, De Backer G, Dominiczak A et al (2007) 2007 Guidelines for the management of arterial hypertension: the task force for the management of arterial hypertension of the European Society of Hypertension (ESH) and of the European Society of Cardiology (ESC). J Hypertens 25:1105–1187
3. Pescatello LS, Franklin BA, Fagard R, Farquhar WB, Kelley GA, Ray CA, American College of Sports Medicine (2004) American College of Sports Medicine position stand. Exercise and hypertension. Med Sci Sports Exerc 36:533–553
4. Whelton SP, Chin A, Xin X, He J (2002) Effect of aerobic exercise on blood pressure: a meta-analysis of randomized, controlled trials. Ann Intern Med 136:493–503
5. Green DJ (2009) Exercise training as vascular medicine: direct impacts on the vasculature in humans. Exerc Sport Sci Rev 37:196–202
6. Manfredini F, Malagoni AM, Mandini S, Boari B, Felisatti M, Zamboni P, Manfredini R (2009) Sport therapy for hypertension. Why, How, How much? Angiology 60:207–216

Hyperthermia

A thermal state in which core body temperature is elevated above its range specified as the normal active state of the species. Hyperthermia may be a regulated response (e.g., during fever) or forced if heat production exceeds the capacity for heat loss, such as during muscular work (exercise).

Hypertriglyceridemia

High blood levels of triglycerides ($\geq$150 mg/dL or $\geq$1.7 mmol/L). The most abundant lipid species in the circulation. It is a risk factor for atherosclerosis and pancreatitis (at extremely high levels >1,000 mg/dL or >11 mmol/L).

Hypertrophy

Hypertrophy is the term used to describe the growth or increase in size (cross sectional area) of skeletal muscle as a whole or of the individual fibers. Age, growth, exercise, nutrition and hormones can all affect the rate and extent of hypertrophy. Current interest focuses on the potential means for increasing hypertrophic responses to exercise through the consumption of carbohydrates and amino acids in the early post-exercise state, although controversy exists regarding the generalization of these data. Myofiber hypertrophy occurs when the overall rate of protein synthesis outweighs protein degradation. Fundamentally, this can be achieved in one of two ways, firstly, to enable increased cross sectional area, new myonuclei from resident satellite cells can be recruited to the fiber, thereby facilitating de novo protein synthesis. Alternatively, the absolute amount of contractile material which is produced by resident nuclei already within the fibers may be increased. It is likely that a combination of both mechanisms prevails. The signals driving muscle hypertrophy are as varied as the muscle contraction itself (via activation of the FAK signalling pathway), local hormonal responses to the exercise (via IGF-mediated phosphatidyl-inositol-3 kinase, Akt and mTOR signalling) or changes in Calcium abundance and phospholipase activities. Ultimately, it must be remembered that there is a variable response to exercise with regards to muscle hypertrophy, suggesting a genetic potential for this response.

Hypobaric Hypoxia

▶ Altitude, Physiological Response
▶ Hypoxia, Focus Hypobaric Hypoxia

Hypobaropathy

▶ Acute Mountain Sickness

Hypohydration

The state of having a body water content that is less than normal.

Hypomagnesemia

Hypomagnesemia (or hypomagnesaemia) is an electrolyte disturbance characterized by an abnormally low blood concentration of magnesium. Reference ranges in serum are 0.73–1.06 mmol/L and 0.77–1.03 mmol/L for men and women, respectively. Hypomagnesemia is often associated with other electrolyte disturbances such as hypokalemia (40%), Hypophosphatemia (30%), or hypocalcaemia (23%). Hypomagnesemia does not necessarily indicate a status of magnesium deficiency as serum magnesium levels represent only about 1% of the body's magnesium pools. Therefore hypomagnesemia can be present without magnesium deficiency and vice versa. Hypomagnesemia results from an imbalanced relation of magnesium uptake and excretion. An inadequate uptake may result from dietary mistakes and diseases such as malabsorption, chronic diarrhea, etc. An enhanced loss of magnesium can be found after chronic administration of diuretics. Moreover, an enhanced turnover of magnesium such as under conditions of chronic stress or training process may result in hypomagnesemia.

Hyponatremia, Exercise Associated

Nancy J. Rehrer[1], Lawrence E. Armstrong[2], Gemma A. McLeod[1]
[1]School of Physical Education and Department of Human Nutrition, University of Otago, Dunedin, New Zealand
[2]Human Performance Laboratory, University of Connecticut, Storrs, CT, USA

Synonyms

Electrolyte disorder; EAH

Definition

Hyponatremia is defined clinically as a serum or plasma [Na+] of <130 mmol/L with mild hyponatremia being defined as 130–135 mmol/L, the latter being typically asymptomatic. Hyponatremia, particularly <125 mmol/L, can result in nausea, dizziness, vomiting, and, as the severity increases, seizures, confusion, and disorientation from cerebral edema and/or respiratory distress from pulmonary edema and even coma or death. It is also recognized that the rate of decrease may be more important to the development of symptoms than the absolute value. A decrease in [Na+] of 7–10% over 24 h can precipitate symptomology, even when the absolute value falls within the "mild range" [1].

Characteristics

Introduction to Issues and Risk Factors Associated with Exertional Hyponatremia

Over a number of years, a lively debate has ensued regarding causes and risk factors associated with exertional, or exercise associated, hyponatremia (EAH) [2]. Although at times this discussion has been less than amicable, fuelled by accusations of inappropriate recommendations resulting from commercial interests, it has resulted in a flurry of research and data from which to gauge varying theoretical perspectives. Epidemiological data from numerous endurance events compiled over 20 years implicates beverage consumption in excess of fluid losses as the main risk factor. This is typically determined by gain in body mass over the course of an event. However, it is recognized that some loss of mass will occur during endurance events that does not indicate hypohydration [3], due to some net loss with substrate metabolism and possibly to a stored water buffer (with glycogen and due to plasma volume expansion typically observed in the regularly training individual) such that a maintenance of body mass may also indicate hyperhydration.

The 2007 EAH Consensus Panel recognized, in addition to excessive drinking behavior and weight gain during exercise, the following risk factors: low body weight, female sex, slow running or performing pace, event inexperience, nonsteroidal anti-inflammatory agents, high availability of drinking fluids, >4 h exercise duration, unusually hot conditions, and extreme cold temperature [1]. The effects of sodium intakes in ameliorating or precipitating hyponatremia are less clear. Dependent upon the level of fluid replacement or overhydration, sodium intake can affect the rate of change in [Na+].

A great deal of emphasis for prevention has been placed upon fluid intake volumes (availability of drink stations; sports drinks advocates overselling hydration message; and less-well-trained, slower competitors having more time to drink); yet mechanisms altering excretion of water and sodium are equally important and are known to be greatly influenced by exercise, environment, and training status.

The context within which recommendations are being made must also be borne in mind. The EAH Consensus Statement had the sole purpose to reduce or eliminate the morbidity and mortality due to EAH. To this end, it may be justified to advise error on the side of hypohydration, since symptomatic hyponatremia is less common during dehydrating exercise, as even the saltiest sweat is hypotonic with respect to extracellular fluid and plasma [Na+] concentration increases without replacement of fluid. However, when making recommendations concerning fluid ingestion to competitive sportsmen and sportswomen, the performance implications of these recommendations and their interpretation should be considered. The magnitude of hypohydration, as evidenced by relative body mass decrease, that will result in a performance decrement is not identical for everyone in every situation. Environmental temperatures, type of exercise, and individual differences all can influence if, and at what point, performance will be impacted. At increasing environmental temperatures, the lesser the body mass decrease will be tolerated. Very short-lasting, interval, or low-intensity events in which heat generation and cardiac output are low will be less affected, if at all. High-intensity, moderately long-lasting or very long-lasting events with high heat production and cardiac output will be more affected by body mass decrease. Based upon experimental data, Coyle [4] has put forward a theoretical model juxtaposing environmental temperature on body mass change and the expected relative performance decrease. The point at which body mass decrease will result in a decrement in performance ranges from ~2% to ~3%. As was alluded to earlier, not all mass loss reflects a decrease in net fluid balance, and thus some loss in mass should be expected in endurance events, dependent upon intensity and length and thus substrate metabolism. An additional consideration, which Coyle also highlights, is the reduction in energy needed for locomotion with decreasing mass, particularly in weight-bearing sports. It may be that the performance decrement associated with a slight decrease in fluid balance (and body mass) might be offset by a reduced cardiac output and energetic demand.

Magnitude and Effect of Sweat Losses on Plasma Sodium

Sweat rates vary across sports in different environmental conditions in men and women. In women, sweat losses ranging from 0.7 or 0.8 $L \cdot h^{-1}$ (basketball indoor training, soccer outdoor training, cycling in cool and mild environments) to 1.5 $L \cdot h^{-1}$ (10 km run in a mild environment) have been described. Men typically have higher sweat rates, ranging from 0.7 $L \cdot h^{-1}$ (soccer training, cycling 40 km in a mild environment) to 1.8 $L \cdot h^{-1}$ (10 km run, Australian football in mild environments) or 2.1 $L \cdot h^{-1}$ (soccer training in a hot environment). Among the highest published sweat rates, a female rower experienced a 2.3 $L \cdot h^{-1}$ loss during training, and a male tennis player 3.4 $L \cdot h^{-1}$ during competition.

Sweat analyses, utilizing a whole-body rinse technique, present the following ranges for electrolyte concentrations: sodium, 13–47; chloride, 13–38; and potassium, 2–5 $mmol \cdot L^{-1}$. When considering the contribution of sweat electrolytes to symptomatic EAH, both sweat rate and sweat electrolyte concentration are important factors. Published EAH simulations, for example, indicated that fluid overload is the primary etiologic factor during marathon events (42.1 km), but that overdrinking relative to sweat rate is not a prerequisite for EAH during longer events such as Ironman triathlons. During these latter events, an athlete with a high but normal sweat sodium concentration can experience a sufficient whole-body sodium deficit that results in a hypovolemic hyponatremia. This simulation is supported by field observations of ultra-endurance athletes who experience a body mass loss (−2 to −10%) concurrent with a plasma sodium level of 130 $mmol \cdot L^{-1}$ or less.

Effect of Salt Intake on Plasma Sodium

The kidneys, under influence of several hormonal modulators, excrete or conserve sodium, which is one of the main mechanisms of fluid balance correction. Urinary excretion of sodium ranges from 20 to 200 mmol/L and is highly dependent upon dietary intake, and is quickly adjusted upward with increasing intake. The response to an acute low sodium intake following a chronic high-salt diet is less well studied, particularly when coupled with substantial salt loss and high water turnover. This may be the case for many endurance athletes who follow a typical "western" diet and then participate in a long-lasting (ultra) endurance event during which salt intake is very low. It is possible that the chronic high-sodium diet has a carry-over effect on kidney function which dampens an appropriate response to low plasma sodium. Studies following the response of soldiers previously on high- and low-salt diets support this.

During endurance exercise, the acute effects of sodium intake on plasma sodium vary substantially. These varied results are due to widely differing conditions, in terms of rate and total volume of fluid intake and losses (and thus net fluid balance), intensity and duration of exercise, and possibly training status. With euhydration or moderate hyperhydration (< −1% to +3% body mass change), depending on the concentration of the salt in the beverage, plasma sodium concentration change can be influenced by the sodium content. However, all sports drinks have a sodium concentration less than that of plasma. Therefore, if a volume of beverage is consumed in excess of losses, plasma sodium concentration will decrease; however, the rate of that decrease can be ameliorated dependent upon the sodium content of the beverage. For example, if 2.4 L of a fluid containing 18 mmol·L^{-1} is consumed during 2 h of exercise, plasma sodium concentration can be 4 mmol·L^{-1} greater than when a similar amount of water is ingested. Therefore, if exercise is long enough, and fluid ingestion rate is above that of fluid loss, hyponatremia will still occur; by increasing the sodium intake symptomatic hyponatremia can, however, be delayed.

Post-race (re-)hydration strategies can also influence fluid balance and plasma sodium. Particularly during ultra-endurance events over multiple days, with large sweat losses, not replacing sodium results in a gradual decrease in total body water over the course of the event. After a dehydrating event, if fluids are provided without sodium a delay occurs in returning to normal water balance, due to a greater urine production. In some instances, vigorous sodium-free fluid ingestion (above the capacity of urinary excretion) has resulted in post-race hyponatremia.

Influence of Exercise on Water Diuresis

Research in the 1930s demonstrated that blood flow to the kidneys, glomerular filtration rate, and diuresis are decreased with intensive exercise, and if that exercise is in the heat, there is a further reduction. This may be a contributing factor to the preponderance of hyponatremia with over-hydration during endurance exercise. Accordingly, when water is consumed in excess of needs at rest, there is a larger range of fluid overload that can be compensated via diuresis than during exercise. During exercise, particularly in the heat, the reduction in the rate of water clearance can result in hyponatremia with a lesser degree of fluid overload.

The decrease in blood flow is increased with increasing relative intensity. Therefore untrained individuals may have blood flow to the kidneys and associated decrease in urine production decreased to a greater extent than those trained, since, at a given velocity, they would be exercising at a higher relative intensity. This could contribute to the observation that untrained individuals are more susceptible to hyponatremia.

Hyponatremia Without Fluid Overload

Numerous studies have shown that EAH can occur without fluid overload. In situations of heavy sweat loss, the losses, if only compensated with sodium-free beverage, can also result in a dilutional hyponatremia, the extent of which can be modified, if not avoided, by ingesting sodium at a level to approximate losses. In some situations of extensive sweat and sodium loss, there may be a negative fluid balance accompanied by dilutional hyponatremia when a large portion, although not all, of the fluid loss is replaced with water. In this situation, osmoreceptors and baroreceptors may be in conflict, and due to a prioritization on blood pressure, a low plasma sodium concentration may not necessarily result in an increase in free water clearance. In this situation, vasopressin (AVP) release may not be inhibited. There is some evidence to suggest that "inappropriate" AVP release plays a role in the development of EAH [1]. In the above scenario, it is questionable if this is "inappropriate" or simply a case of prioritization of perfusion pressure over osmolarity.

Montain has developed a mathematical model to evaluate the effects of different drinking behaviors on hydration status and plasma sodium concentration (factoring in body mass, body composition, sweat sodium concentration, running speed, weather conditions, and beverage sodium content) which demonstrates the relative proportional effect of each factor in the development of hyponatremia and concludes that hyponatremia can occur with dehydration [5].

Clinical Relevance

In line with increasing prevalence and awareness of hyponatremia and the difficulty in prescribing one fluid regimen for all sports participants, recent guidelines regarding fluid consumption during exercise from sports medicine organizations have been modified and take into account individual needs. Recommendations are less prescriptive in terms of rates of fluid intake and advocate athletes to weigh themselves to assess needs in a particular event in particular conditions and, in any instance, avoid gaining weight during an event. The most recent recommendations also acknowledge that even maintaining weight can represent hyperhydration, and losing weight (i.e. negative fluid balance) can coexist with EAH. However, the most serious clinical outcomes occur in athletes who consume and retain a large volume (e.g., 8–10 L) of hypotonic fluid. It is also acknowledged that the point at which body mass decrease results in an endurance performance decrement is not the same for all athletes and may vary from > ~2% to > ~3%, in warm and cool conditions, respectively.

Chronically, consuming sodium above the daily physiological requirement, prior to prolonged endurance exercise, may establish a hormonal milieu (e.g., a low plasma aldosterone level) which encourages sodium excretion. Consuming sodium acutely during training sessions or endurance events can delay symptomatic EAH to a minor extent.

References

1. Hew-Butler T, Ayus JC, Kipps C, Maughan RJ, Mettler S, Meeuwisse WH et al (2008) Statement of the Second International exercise-associated hyponatremia consensus development conference, New Zealand, 2007. Clin J Sport Med 18(2):111–121
2. Noakes TD, Speedy DB (2006) Case proven: exercise associated hyponatraemia is due to overdrinking. So why did it take 20 years before the original evidence was accepted? [see comment]. Br J Sports Med 40(7):567–572
3. Maughan RJ, Shirreffs SM, Leiper JB, Maughan RJ, Shirreffs SM, Leiper JB (2007) Errors in the estimation of hydration status from changes in body mass. J Sports Sci 25(7):797–804
4. Coyle EF (2004) Fluid and fuel intake during exercise. J Sports Sci 22(1):39–55
5. Montain SJ, Cheuvront SN, Sawka MN (2006) Exercise associated hyponatraemia: quantitative analysis to understand the aetiology. Br J Sports Med 40(2):98–105, discussion −6

Hypoperfusion

Decreased tissue blood flow.

Hyposthenuria

Excretion of urine of low specific gravity, due to inability of the tubules of the kidneys to produce concentrated urine.

Hypothalamic-Pituitary-Cortisol Hypothesis

Prolonged stress causes cortisol to be released into the bloodstream; elevated levels of cortisol has been linked to depression.

Hypothalamus-Pituitary-Adrenal (HPA) Axis

The hypothalamus regulates vital bodily functions. In the hypothalamus, corticotropin-releasing hormone (CRH) and vasopressin (VP) are produced, which stimulate the adrenocorticotropic hormone (ACTH) in the pituitary gland. VP also stimulates prolactin. The CRH-ACTH-glucocorticoid (from the adrenal) axis stimulates innate immunity and suppress adaptive immunity. VP is able to maintain immunocompetence during homeostasis as it stimulates both ACTH and prolactin and these hormones maintain both innate and adaptive immunity in a physiologically balanced condition.

Hypoxemia

▶ Hypoxia, Focus Hypoxic Hypoxia

Hypoxia, Focus Hypobaric Hypoxia

LOUISE ØSTERGAARD[1], MAX GASSMANN[1,2]
[1]Zurich Center for Integrative Human Physiology (ZIHP), Institute of Veterinary Physiology, University of Zürich, Zürich, Switzerland
[2]Universidad Peruana Cayetano Heredia, Lima, Peru

Synonyms
High altitude; Hypobaric hypoxia; Low oxygen

Definition
With increasing ▶ altitude there is an exponential decrease in oxygen partial pressure that parallels the reduction in atmospheric density. This means that at sea level total air pressure is 760 mmHg (or 101 kPa) whereas at the top of Mt. Everest (8,848 m), it drops to 253 mmHg (or 34 kPa). As oxygen constitutes approximately 21% of the total atmospheric pressure, the oxygen partial pressure (pO_2) is then 160 mmHg and 53 mmHg at sea level and Mt. Everest, respectively. At the roof of the world this results in an extremely small pressure difference and therefore oxygen exchange is severely hindered. Obviously, this represents the most extreme condition but even at altitudes above 1,500 m the cardiovascular, respiratory, and metabolic systems are affected. This is characterized as hypobaric hypoxia, reflecting that the low oxygen tension is paralleled by low atmospheric pressure. Another aspect of low oxygen tension is normobaric hypoxia, meaning that at sea level, with normal atmospheric pressure, the body can still experience oxygen partial pressure alterations, caused either by reduced oxygen delivery or malfunction of cellular utilization. This situation can affect either a particular tissue or even the whole body (Fig. 1).

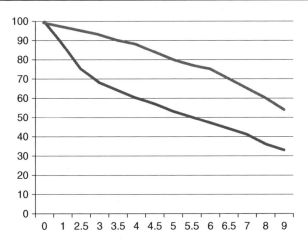

Hypoxia, Focus Hypobaric Hypoxia. Fig. 1 *Lower line*: The decrease in oxygen partial pressure (pO_2) measured as %, where sea level (0 m) is 100%, at increasing altitudes up to 8,848 m (Mt Everest). *Upper line*: The corresponding values of the arterial blood's oxygen saturation (SO_2)

Mechanisms

The following parameters are important for determining the response to diminished oxygen availability and utilization; (a) ▶ pulmonary ventilation, (b) ▶ gas exchange, (c) ▶ oxygen diffusion capacity, (d) transport to the tissues, and (e) mitochondrial consumption.

Hypoxia causes a reduction in the inspired pO_2, which in turn lowers the alveolar partial pressure of oxygen (PAO_2), leading to a drop in the diffusion driving pressure across the alveolar–capillary barrier. The consequence is a reduction in both, the arterial partial pressure of oxygen (PaO_2) and the arterial oxygen saturation (SaO_2), resulting in less oxygen being delivered to the tissues. The main effect of acclimatization is therefore to restore the amount of oxygen delivered to the tissues (DO_2). DO_2 is defined as the product of cardiac output (Q) and arterial oxygen content (CaO_2).

The peak oxygen consumption, or VO_2max, reflects the individual's capacity for aerobic work and is defined as the volume of oxygen consumed during maximal exercise. This parameter is therefore also a measure for muscle metabolism. At altitude where oxygen uptake is limited, an initial drop in CaO_2 is experienced, but following acclimatization, that is, adaptation to lower oxygen tension, this is almost completely restored, even at maximal exercise. On the other hand, VO_2max is only slightly improved with altitude acclimatization. Consequently, other mechanisms must be responsible for the limited oxygen consumption at altitude.

Several mechanisms are activated during acclimatization to high altitude [1, 2], especially in the pulmonary circulation. This includes ventilation and gas exchange but also oxygen transport in the systemic circulation as well as in the muscles play a role. Finally, the mitochondrial function is emerging, too, as a significant player.

When oxygen tension drops, peripheral chemoreceptors such as the carotid body will sense the lower supply of oxygen and react by stimulating an increase in ventilation. This response, called the hypoxic ventilatory response (HVR), is activated within minutes and will increase over a few weeks before reaching a plateau. During exercise the HVR is even further augmented. The effects of HVR include an increase in arterial oxygen content and a left shift of the hemoglobin O_2 dissociation curve due to hyperventilation, leading to augmented oxygen saturation (Fig. 2).

This will of course help, at least partly, to restore the oxygen delivery to the muscles and thereby the VO_2max.

Another factor that will augment the oxygen-carrying capacity of the blood is the increase in hemoglobin (Hb) content. This is achieved through two processes: a fall in the plasma volume and increased production of red blood cells. When exposed to hypoxia, on of the first physiological reactions is to increase the release and synthesis of ▶ erythropoietin (Epo) [4], a hormone synthesized by the kidneys. As soon as 1 h after hypoxic exposures, an increase in renal Epo mRNA has been shown, whereas the maximal circulating plasma concentration of Epo is observed after approximately 48 h. After this time, the plasma's Epo content will decline even with continued hypoxia. Epo has several functions, the most known being the stimulation of the bone marrow to release increased amounts of red blood cells. This will in turn increase the oxygen-carrying capacity of the blood and also a decrease in cardiac output. The result is therefore augmented oxygen transport to the tissue, longer time for the tissue to extract oxygen from the blood, and an increase in VO_2max and thereby maximum exercise capacity.

A final, and thus limiting, step is the delivery of oxygen to the muscle mitochondria. The diffusion of oxygen to the mitochondria relies on the oxygen pressure gradient, meaning that mitochondrial PO_2 must be lower than capillary PO_2. This is the case under exercise but with hypoxia this gradient is obviously smaller due to less available oxygen. This is termed diffusion limitation and therefore measures to increase the PO_2 gradient are necessary. As mentioned, this is attained by increasing ventilation, by a shift in the oxygen dissociation capacity and with chronic hypoxia, an increase in Hb. This works for

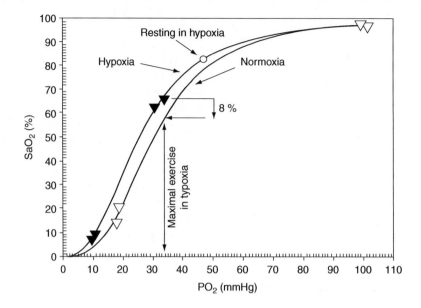

Hypoxia, Focus Hypobaric Hypoxia. Fig. 2 Impact of hypoxia–hyperventilation on the hemoglobin dissociation curve. Effect of severe acute hypoxia on the O_2 dissociation curve of the Hb during exercise in normoxia (*white triangles; fine line*) and hypoxia (*black triangles; thick line*). Note the *left* shift caused by hyperventilation and its impact on SaO_2 at maximal exercise in hypoxia. Points on the graph represent the mean arterial or femoral venous values for each condition in nine subjects. (PO_2 values corrected for blood temperature) [3]

small mass, but not for whole-body exercise under hypoxia, where a decrease in VO_2max and exercise capacity is observed.

Important players in the response to hypoxia are the hypoxia sensitive transcription factors. Upon activation, the transcription factor will translocate from the cytoplasm to the nucleus, bind to target genes and initiate transcription. Epo expression was previously used to study hypoxia-responsive transcription factors and this led to the identification of the hypoxia-inducible factor (HIF)-1 [5]. Besides Epo, close to 200 validated HIF target genes such as glycolytic enzymes, proteins involved in angiogenesis or cell proliferation, transcriptional regulation, and others have been identified. Notable is the fact that HIF rarely upregulates just one target gene in a given pathway, but rather coordinates the response of all necessary steps. A direct role for HIF in gene adaptation to exercise has also been proposed.

Exercise Response/Consequences

The consequences of long-term exposure to hypoxia are lower exercise capacity, fatigue, and weakening of the muscles. As the exercising muscle requires increasing oxygen supply relative to the exerted work, and in view that muscle homeostasis in general is dependent on a constant transfer of adequate oxygen, the efficiency of the oxygen delivery system is therefore essential. Thus, when oxygen is limited, the working muscle needs to shift to anaerobic metabolism. As this is much less efficient, a reduction in exercise capacity will result.

It would be expected, since acclimatization restores PaO_2 and DO_2, that also VO_2max and exercise capacity would be restored, but it has been demonstrated that this assumption is not true. Acute exposure to hypoxia leads to a predictable reduction in ► VO_2 max, which is proportional to the reduction in CaO_2 but as this is not the case during chronic hypoxia, other mechanisms must be contributing. It was demonstrating by Lundby and colleagues [6] that the a reduction in leg blood flow and subsequent fall in oxygen conductance, defined as an estimation of muscle diffusion capacity, is the main factor for the lack of a restoration of VO_2max after acclimatization. Blood flow to the legs was decreased by approximately 25% after 8 weeks at 5,250 m due to blood being diverted to other tissues such as the brain, myocardium, and respiratory muscles. This is most likely a consequence of a shift in the balance between vasoconstricting and vasodilating mechanisms in chronic hypoxia.

Other factors are also worth considering in this setting, whether it is for competition at high altitude or high altitude training, including for instance the development of acute mountain sickness (AMS), high altitude pulmonary edema (HAPE) and high altitude cerebral edema (HACE). This will usually occur at altitudes above 2,500 m and can cause headache, nausea, loss of appetite, fatigue, weakness, and sleep disturbance and can, in worst case, be fatal if not treated. A reduction in immunity is also reported under both hypoxia and intense exercise, causing the athlete to be more prone to developing infections and a slower recovery from injuries. Longer exposures to hypoxia can also inflict a strain on the heart, as the pulmonary pressure will increase and thereby also the workload of the right ventricle. Also with prolonged exposures is the risk of dehydration and, more severe, weight loss and muscle wasting. Therefore an optimized time frame is necessary for athletes competing or training at high altitude.

Diagnostics

The increase in Epo and red blood cell mass is obviously one of the reasons that the "Live high – train low" regime has been widely used by athletes in the hope to "naturally" increase this "endogenous doping" hormone and thereby augment VO_2max. The rational behind this is that by living at altitude (hypoxic conditions) oxygen delivery and utilization should be increased whereas the "low" training ensures maximal intensity, which is otherwise reduced under hypoxia.

Despite this, the field is highly controversial with reports of both beneficial effects, in terms of a higher VO_2max, which was directly correlated with an increase in hematocrit [7] to no effects at all. It should be noted, that large individual differences are observed in terms of the onset and duration of red blood cell production and in addition, very few studies have investigated the long-term effects. An important factor is that red blood cells rapidly undergo destruction when they are no longer needed. Therefore, the initial increase in red blood cell mass and subsequent in VO_2max can be rather short-lived.

References

1. Jose AL (2009) Calbet and Carsten Lundby. Air to muscle O_2 delivery during exercise at altitude. High Alt Med Biol 10(2):123–134
2. Martin D, Windsor J (2008) From mountain to bedside: understanding the clinical relevance of human acclimatisation to high-altitude hypoxia. Postgrad Med J 84:622–627
3. Calbet JA, Boushel R, Radegran G, Sondergaard H, Wagner PD, Saltin B (2003) Determinants of maximal oxygen uptake in severe acute hypoxia. Am J Physiol Regul Integr Comp Physiol 284: R291–R303
4. Jelkmann W (2003) Erythropoietin. J Endocrinol Invest 26(9):832–837
5. Fandrey J, Gassmann M (2009) Oxygen sensing and the activation of the hypoxia inducible factor 1 (hif-1)–invited article. Adv Exp Med Biol 648:197–206
6. Lundby C, Sander M, van Hall G, Saltin B, Jose A, Calbet L (2006) Maximal exercise and muscle oxygen extraction in acclimatizing lowlanders and high altitude natives. J Physiol 573(2):535–547
7. Levine BD, Stray-Gundersen J (1997) "Living high-training low": effect of moderate-altitude acclimatization with low-altitude training on performance. J Appl Physiol 83:102–112

Hypoxia, Focus Hypoxic Hypoxia

Luigi Varesio[1], Michele Samaja[2]
[1]Laboratory of Molecular Biology, Giannina Gaslini Institute, Genova, Italy
[2]University of Milan – San Paolo, Milan, Italy

Synonyms

Anoxia; Dysoxia; Hypoxemia; Ischemia; Oxygen deficiency

Definition

▶ Hypoxia is generally defined as a condition of deficiency in the amount of oxygen (O_2) reaching the tissues. The most common way to express the amount of O_2 is through the O_2 tension or PO_2, which is calculated as:

$$PO_2 = \frac{(BP - P_{H_2O}) \times \%O_2}{100}$$

where BP represents the barometric pressure, PH_2O represents the water vapor tension (47 mmHg at 37°C), and $\%O_2$ is the molar fraction of O_2 in inspired air. A low PO_2 may thus stem from two sources: either low BP, as at high altitude, which leads to "▶ hypobaric hypoxia," or low $\%O_2$, as in several pathological situations, commonly referred to as "hypoxic hypoxia." Usually, the term hypoxia is not based on an absolute criterion (in this sense, all the body cells are always "hypoxic" with respect to the atmosphere), but rather to any situation whereby the amount of O_2 reaching the tissues is less than that normally found under physiological conditions. Indeed, O_2 is continuously taken up by the cell to sustain oxidative phosphorylation, the basic pathway that provides biological energy to the organism, thus introducing the concept of "O_2 flux" to supply the required amount of O_2 to tissues/cells. Whenever such supply becomes reduced, tissues experience "tissue hypoxia" or "dysoxia." Such reduction may therefore be the consequence of several factors: hypobaric hypoxia, increased metabolic needs (as for example during inflammation and exercise), disruption of the architecture of the vessels reaching the tissues (as for example during the development of fast growing tumors)

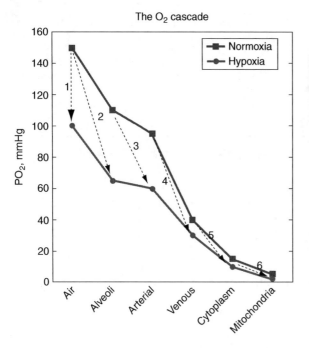

Hypoxia, Focus Hypoxic Hypoxia. **Fig. 1** Representation of the O_2 cascade during the flow of O_2 from the atmosphere to the mitochondria at sea level (normal O_2 content) and a hypothetical situation of hypoxia corresponding to roughly one third reduction in O_2 supply. Adequate supply of O_2 to the last compartment depends on the maintenance of the gradient at each step. There are six steps where inadequate O_2 flow may result into hypoxia: (*1*) Low air PO_2 due to exposure to high altitude or hypoxic chambers; (*2*) low alveolar PO_2 due to respiratory failure (emphysemas, asthma, lung tumors, bronchial obstruction); (*3*) low arterial PO_2 due to poor pulmonary perfusion and right-to-left heart shunt (congenital heart diseases); (*4*) low venous PO_2 due to blood O_2 transport failure (abnormal O_2 transport, variant Hb, anemia, low cardiac output, high O_2 demand); (*5*) low cytoplasm PO_2 due to poor O_2 diffusion from blood to cell (low tissue perfusion, altered diffusion geometry, tumor angiogenesis); (*6*) low mitochondria PO_2 due to inability to use O_2 for biochemical blocks, inhibition, or poisoning

and others. Figure 1 gives a summary of the physiological and pathological conditions that may lead to hypoxia.

There are several instances where the O_2 supply to tissues is altered. The term "hypoxia" is sometimes improperly attributed to any of them, but there are subtle differences with dramatically different phenotypes as shown in Table 1.

Hypoxia, Focus Hypoxic Hypoxia. **Table 1** Various forms of hypoxia and correlated pathologies

Name	Explanation or experimental situation	Correlated pathologies
Chronic hypoxia	Prolonged O_2 supply/demand unbalance without interruption, typical of decreased tissue perfusion for altered geometry of O_2 diffusion from capillary to cell	Chronic obstructive pulmonary disease, congenital heart disease, cancer-derived anemia, blood O_2 carrying failure, CO poisoning, high altitude
CH with repetitive reoxygenation	Animals housed in hypoxic chambers that are opened for cleaning and animal feeding	Some cases of immature capillary network with pulsing perfusion changes
Intermittent hypoxia	Repetitive hypoxic events either induced or innate	Obstructive sleep apnea, sickle cell anemia crises, asthma, immature capillary network with pulsing perfusion changes

Basic Mechanisms

Molecular O_2 is the preferred oxidizing substrate in almost every form of life on the Earth. Severe and/or prolonged hypoxia unavoidably leads to an array of dysfunctions that include impaired biological energy production and ability to maintain the homeostasis of ions, cell swelling, and death. The body has the ability to adapt, to a certain degree, to this potentially lethal condition through changes that reduce the strain imposed by hypoxia. Phenotypic adaptation is also termed "▶ acclimatization." The body and the cells adapt to the various forms of hypoxia by establishing some degree of compensation at several levels [1]:

1. *Ventilatory.* Hypoxic stimulation of chemoreceptors causes an immediate increase of alveolar ventilation. The consequent washout of large quantities of CO_2 initially reduces arterial CO_2 tension ($PaCO_2$) and increases arterial pH (pHa). Subsequently, whereas the chemoreflexogenic hyperventilatory response remains unchanged, pHa tends to return to near normal levels as a consequence of HCO_3-loss through the kidney.

2. *Circulatory.* Hypoxia increases circulatory efficiency by at least three mechanisms: (1) immediate increase in cardiac output, followed by a return to near normal levels in a few days; (2) increase of tissue capillarity; (3) increase the red cell concentration of 2,3-diphosphoglycerate, which decreases hemoglobin (Hb)-O_2 affinity thereby enhancing O_2 delivery to tissue.

3. *Hemopoietic.* Hypoxia stimulates kidney production of the hormone ▶ erythropoietin that stimulates spleen and bone marrow to increase their production of red blood cells. This leads to two main consequences: (1) progressive increase of circulating Hb over a period of several months, (2) faster replacement of relatively "old" red blood cells by "young," fresh red blood cells with more favorable O_2 transport characteristics.

4. *Metabolic.* This mainly includes the switch from the aerobic to ▶ anaerobic metabolism (e.g., glycolysis). The ▶ anaerobic metabolism is less efficient but markedly spares O_2, which becomes available for other purposes. The long-term sustainability of the aerobic-to-anerobic switch is questionable because of the progressive intracellular accumulation of waste products as lactate and acidity.

5. *Vascular.* Hypoxia has two contrasting effects on vasculature: pulmonary vessels contract and systemic vessels dilate. Pulmonary vasoconstriction helps shunting blood away from poorly ventilated regions thereby improving total ventilation, and is mediated by closure of one or several of the K^+ voltage-gated channels. In contrast, systemic vessels dilation, mediated in part by the K_{ATP} channels of vascular myocytes, improves the perfusion and the oxygenation of hypoxic tissues.

6. *Transcriptional.* Hypoxia is perceived, at a cellular level, through O_2 sensor relays operating inside the cell and leading to the activation of transcriptional activators contributing to the establishment of the hypoxic phenotype [2]. Hypoxia-inducible factor 1 (HIF-1) is critical for the adaptation of mammalian cells to oxygen deprivation. It is composed of a constitutively expressed β subunit and two HIF-α subunits (HIF-1α and HIF-2α), which are tightly regulated by oxygen concentrations. The α-subunit is rapidly degraded in the presence of oxygen by a pathway involving hydroxylation of proline residues and binding to the product of the tumor suppressor gene von-Hippel Lindau (VHL), which targets HIF-1 for ubiquitylation and proteasomal degradation. With oxygen becoming limiting, HIF1α can no longer be hydroxylated and degraded and rapidly accumulates,

translocates to the nucleus where, upon dimerization with HIF-1β, binds to hypoxia responsive elements present in regulatory regions of HIF-1 target genes. Other ▶ transcription factors, such as NF-κB, ATF-425, Egr-126, Ets-127 are also involved in the hypoxic regulation of gene expression. AP-1 was recently identified as a hypoxia-inducible transcription factor. The prolonged activation of AP-1 by hypoxia may depend on HIF-1α, providing an example of cooperative interaction between these two transcription factors in the transactivation of target genes.

Many adaptation mechanisms are intimately intertwined and recruited at the same time. For example, exploitation of the pathways 1–5 is strictly dependent on transcriptional mechanisms, which in turn tend to be inactivated by feedback mechanisms. Adaptation to hypoxia might result in "maladaptation" if the recruitment of some mechanism becomes excessive and the body overreacts to hypoxia. For example, Andean high-altitude dwellers apparently respond "too much" to hypoxia in terms of red blood cells production. This leads to a situation of polycythemia whereby high blood viscosity offsets the benefits of increased O_2 transport and causes chronic mountain sickness.

Exercise Intervention

Training and PO_2

The notion that exercise training is an excellent way to reduce the probability to suffer from cardiovascular disease is well established. However, exercise training exposes skeletal and cardiac muscle to repetitive hypoxic challenge because tissue PO_2 decreases progressively in proportion to exercise intensity. This hypoxic situation, caused by increased energy demand, favors O_2 diffusion from capillary to mitochondria and elicits several responses that involve O_2-sensitive potassium channels, mitogen-activated protein kinases, nitric oxide synthase, endoplasmic reticulum stress, and antioxidant activities [3]. The targets of these adaptations, improvement of O_2 availability to hypoxic cells, and injury prevention are met at multiple levels, including growth of vascular endothelium, control of apoptosis and sprout of angiogenesis, and erythropoiesis. Thus, hypoxia serves two synergistic purposes: optimizing O_2 availability and signaling for tissue remodeling. These targets are particularly relevant in a preventive medicine perspective, i.e., cardioprotection.

High Altitude

Exposure to high altitude is the best available paradigm for hypobaric hypoxia. In fact, the O_2 fraction in the atmosphere is stable at 20.93% irrespectively of altitude and latitude, but BP decreases progressively with altitude as for the equation:

$$P = P_0 e^{-Mgh}/RT$$

where P0 is BP at sea level, M is the average molecular weight of gas molecules, g the acceleration of gravity, and h the height. The consequent BP decrease leads to a progressively lower PO_2 in inspired air and therefore in all the body's districts as indicated in Fig. 1. On the summit of Mt. Everest (8,848 m), PO_2 can be as low as 52 mmHg, one third of the PO_2 at sea level posing a major challenge to humans departing from sea level.

Exercise at Altitude

Exercising at altitude becomes clearly an inducer of greater hypoxia because cells perceive exercise as an inducer of hypoxia. Several reports point at the deleterious effects of maximal exercise at altitude. For example, the Olympic games at Mexico City ($>$2,000 m altitude) were associated with poor performance, especially for disciplines requiring aerobic exercise. The quest for climbing Mt. Everest represents another paradigm to describe the situation encountered when exercising in hypoxia. One of the first attempts to climb Mt. Everest in 1924 ended in tragedy at 300 m from the summit. After this attempt, many climbers reached the summit while breathing pure O_2, but only in 1981 Mt. Everest was climbed without additional O_2: the last 300 m took 57 years to be climbed.

Hypoxic Training

Despite the adverse effects led by hypoxia on performance in endurance athletes, training in hypoxia might become an elective practice to boost physical performance in view of important sea-level competitions: when athletes train for several weeks at altitudes $>$2,400 m, simultaneous adaptation to hypoxia and to training might yield hitherto unsuspected favorable effects. However, for obvious safety and practical reasons, other paradigms might become of wider and easier applicability without causing discomfort. First, altitude training can be simulated through use of simulation tents or mask-based hypoxicator systems where BP is kept the same, but %O_2 is reduced. Second, athletes may sojourn for variable times at high altitude while training at lower altitudes ("live high, train low") [4], thereby combining the effects of hypoxia adaptation and training without distress: the recruited molecular pathways turn out to be useful when athletes travel to competitions at lower altitudes by giving them a competitive advantage. Third, intermittent hypoxia is emerging as a noninvasive, drug-free technique to improve performance and well-being [5]. Briefly, an intermittent hypoxia session consists in a few minutes interval of breathing low %O_2 as alternated with ambient air over a 45- to 90-min session per day. Intermittent hypoxia delivers a non-damaging training-like stimulus that triggers adaptation without adverse effects. Intermittent hypoxia can be beneficial not only for boosting athletic performance, but also for the treatment of a wide range of degenerative diseases including chronic heart and lung diseases, hypertension, asthma, chronic bronchitis, iron-deficiency anemia, lack of energy, and fatigue. Furthermore, intermittent hypoxia is predicted to replace the endogenous mechanisms of cardiovascular protection that are absent in people who cannot exercise, as for example elder or tetraplegic persons.

References

1. Samaja M (1997) Blood gas transport at high altitude. Respiration 64:422–428
2. Simon MC, Liu L, Barnhart BC, Young RM (2008) Hypoxia-induced signaling in the cardiovascular system. Annu Rev Physiol 70:51–71
3. Sica A, Melillo G, Varesio L (2011) Hypoxia: a double-edged sword of immunity. J Mol Med 89:657–665
4. Wilbur RL (2007) Live high + train low: thinking in terms of an optimal hypoxic dose. Int J Sports Physiol Perform 2:223–238
5. Levine BD, Stray-Gundersen J (2005) Point: positive effects of intermittent hypoxia (live high:train low) on exercise performance are mediated primarily by augmented red cell volume. J Appl Physiol 99:2053–2055

Hypoxia Markers

Hypoxia markers are surrogate endogenous or chemical markers of tumor oxygenation (e.g., hypoxia-inducible factor HIF-1α).

Hypoxia, Training

MICHAEL VOGT, FABIO BREIL, HANS HOPPELER
Department of Anatomy, University of Bern, Bern, Switzerland

Synonyms

Altitude training; Hypoxic, training

Definition

Since the 1968 Olympic Games which were held in Mexico City at an altitude of 2,300 m, ▶ altitude training has become popular among coaches, athletes, and scientists to prepare for competition at altitude and to increase exercise performance at sea level. It was observed that maximal oxygen consumption (VO₂max) and exercise performance are compromised at altitude. For endurance athletes living near sea level and untrained subjects, a decrease in VO₂max has been observed already at relatively low altitudes between 300 and 800 m. This ▶ altitude sensitivity is different between individuals and genders [16]. Our data show that VO₂max fell on average by 0.9% for every 100 m above an altitude of 1,100 m, which is similar to the decrement shown in other studies [11].

On the other hand exposure to moderate altitude (2,000–3,000 m) for several weeks was shown to increase hemoglobin mass and thus oxygen-carrying capacity, whereas effects on exercise performance are controversial [2]. To boost the oxygen-carrying system while minimizing possible adverse effects of chronic altitude exposure, the "▶ live high – train low" model was introduced. This method employs chronic hypoxic exposure at altitudes of around 2,500 m to increase hemoglobin mass interspersed by low-altitude training, where adequate exercise intensity and mechanical loads to muscles can be better attained. The advantages and limitations of this altitude training concept are discussed elsewhere [2].

The alternative "▶ live low – train high" training concept (sometimes denoted as intermittent hypoxia training), which employs hypoxic conditions only during the individual training sessions, stems from the observation that permanent exposure to severe hypoxia (i.e., residency at altitudes around 5,000 m and higher for example at Mt. Everest base camp) leads to considerable deterioration of skeletal muscle tissue.

In view of sizeable muscle loss and mitochondrial deterioration with prolonged exposure to high altitude, it was reasoned that chronic exposure to hypoxia might be detrimental to muscle tissue due to some hypoxia-dependent decrease in muscle protein synthesis, a reduction in the overall exercise intensity or mechanical load at altitude. These contentions led to experiments and training programs which applied hypoxia only during the training sessions, thus maximizing the hypoxic stimulus on muscle during activity, but allowing subjects to spend the remaining time in normoxia in order to optimize muscle recovery.

Mechanisms

The general consensus seems to be that the "live low – train high" model produces training effects similar but not identical to those seen after normoxic training. The rationale for using hypoxia during exercise sessions is to increase the "metabolic" stress on skeletal muscle tissue. Hypoxic training protocols have been expected to induce adaptive results beyond those achieved under normoxia, increasing the cellular disturbance, and thus the adaptive stimulus, in particular in muscle tissue. Several studies assessed the effects of hypoxic training on muscle tissue [7] which will be summarized in this section.

Muscle Oxidative Capacity

Endurance performance is limited by the capacity to transport oxygen from the lungs to the working muscles, and to consume that oxygen in muscle mitochondria, which can be easily estimated from maximal oxygen consumption (VO₂max). The effect of training in hypoxia on muscle oxidative capacity is controversial. While most studies found increased mitochondrial density or citrate synthase activity, others did not. Again these studies differed greatly in regard to subject training state, training duration and intensity, and simulated altitude. Although a final conclusion on the effects of hypoxic training on muscle oxidative capacity in hypoxia cannot be drawn, it seems that exercise intensity plays an important role.

Muscle Glycolytic Capacity

In vitro experiments have shown that hypoxia induces upregulation of glycolytic enzymes. It can therefore be assumed that training in hypoxia affects anaerobic muscle performance. Training competitive triathletes 120 min per day for 10 days at a simulated altitude of 2,500 m, Hendriksen et al. found positive effects of hypoxia training on anaerobic power (Wingate test) compared to normoxic training [6]. mRNAs coding for enzymes of the glycolytic pathway (phosphofructokinase), glucose transport (GLUT4), and pH regulation (MCT1, CA3) were upregulated in previously untrained subjects or in endurance athletes after 6 weeks of training in hypoxia [17]. Although increased enzyme activity of phosphofructokinase was found, effects of hypoxia training on glycolytic pathways are inconclusive.

Oxygen Supply to the Muscle

Oxygen supply to muscle cells is facilitated by a more extensive branched capillary bed. There is good evidence that training in hypoxia increases the number or density of capillaries. These results are in accordance with enhanced gene expression of vascular endothelial growth factor

(VEGF) found after several weeks training in hypoxia. At least for previously untrained subjects, exercise intensity seems to determine the effectiveness of hypoxic training, since training at high (but not low) intensity improved VEGF mRNA concentration and capillary density [15].

Oxygen Transport and Storage Within the Muscle

Myoglobin is able to carry and store oxygen in muscle cells. Endurance training, sprint training, and resistance training in normoxia have all failed to induce changes to muscle myoglobin concentration in humans. However, in elite cyclists, a high correlation was shown between cycling performance and muscle myoglobin content [3]. High myoglobin concentration could facilitate oxygen supply when training or competing at altitude. Terrados et al. [14] had untrained subjects train one leg in a hypobaric hyp-oxia chamber (simulated 2,300 m) and the other leg under sea-level conditions. Both legs performed 30-min sessions at 65% of pre-training normoxic maximal power output, three to four times per week for 4 weeks. In the hypoxically trained leg, time to fatigue was improved significantly more than in the normoxically trained leg. Moreover, the hypoxic-trained leg showed a significantly larger increase in citrate synthase activity and an increase in myoglobin concentration. In agreement with this finding, we found an increase in myoglobin mRNA concentration after 6 weeks of hypoxic training but only when training was performed at a high intensity [15, 17]. In conclusion there is some, but not completely conclusive evidence of increased muscle myoglobin concentration demonstrated in humans after training, hypoxia being dependent on exercise intensity.

Muscle Contractility

The Na^+–K^+-ATPase pump is an important enzyme which regulates trans-sarcolemmal sodium and potassium gradients, membrane excitability, and thus contractility. Na^+–K^+-ATPase pump activity is very adaptable in skeletal muscle, being increased with physical training, but reduced with inactivity. In hypoxia studies using both the "live low – train high" and "live high – train low" models, a decrease of Na^+–K^+-ATPase pump activity has been observed [5]. The reasons for this are unclear, but it is remarkable that in the study of Green [5], citrate synthase activity (oxidative capacity) was increased while Na^+–K^+-ATPase pump activity decreased in the hypoxic training group. These results indicate that training in hypoxia might be detrimental to muscle contractility.

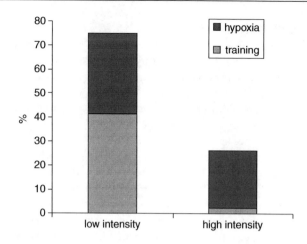

Hypoxia, Training. Fig. 1 Global molecular response of genes coding for metabolic pathways, oxygen sensing, oxygen transport, and stress proteins after 6 weeks of training in hypoxia or normoxia at two different exercise intensities. Probes were taken from *M.vastus lateralis* of previously untrained subjects in a resting state (From Vogt et al. 2001, for further details see [15])

Oxygen Sensing and Molecular Response

Hypoxia is perceived to magnify the metabolic stress in muscle tissue. We note that the transcription factor HIF-1 is seen as a key player in the response to hypoxia in most tissues [13]. HIF-1 is known to function as a master regulator of many genes of erythropoesis, angiogenesis, pH regulation, and glycolysis. On the other hand, there is also some recent evidence which questions the importance of HIF-1 in the regulation of hypoxia-induced adaptive responses in humans, as well as in animals [8]. It should be considered that many other players can influence oxygen-related adaptive processes in muscle tissue. We can present evidence that in muscle a more pronounced transcriptional response of metabolic genes is observed after training in hypoxia, independent of intensity and training state [15, 17], which could at least in part be related to changed levels of the regulatory α-subunit of HIF-1 (see also Fig. 1).

Exercise Response

One of our recent reviews published in 2008 [7] analyzed key functional data from studies in which only exercise sessions were carried out in hypoxia, and which included a control group training in normoxia. We reported data from 9 studies on trained subjects and 12 done on previously untrained subjects [7]. Since then, two additional hypoxia training studies on trained athletes and two on healthy active subjects have been published.

A common feature of virtually all studies on "live low – train high" is that hypoxic exposure only during exercise sessions is not sufficient to induce changes in hematological parameters. Likewise, in the studies reviewed by Hoppeler et al. [7], there were no changes in maximal blood lactate concentration or heart rate between hypoxic and normoxic training conditions.

Performance at Sea Level

Collectively, "live low – train high" studies have failed to yield a clear picture of this training concept's effects on VO_2max, peak power output during incremental testing or time trial performance. Only five of 11 studies on trained subjects and nine of 14 on untrained subjects were able to show an additional benefit of hypoxic training [7]. The studies on trained athletes showed additional improvements in VO_2max, maximal power output, anaerobic performance during Wingate testing, time trial or time to exhaustion performance, and running economy. In previous untrained subjects, additional functional benefits of hypoxia compared to normoxic training were found for VO_2max, maximal power output, hypoxia ventilatory response (HVR), time to exhaustion, and risk for cardiovascular disease. Some cautioned against the use of hypoxic training due to potentially harmful effects on the training processes.

There is no clear trend among the studies on "live low –train high" as to differential effects of the severity or the duration of hypoxia exposure and training intensities [7]. In untrained subjects, the main stimulus seems simply to be the introduction of exercise to a previously sedentary lifestyle. With regard to the functional results, it appears to be of minor importance whether exercise is carried out in normoxia or hypoxia. Four studies on untrained subjects used exercise training at the same absolute intensity in normoxia and hypoxia. While some showed a larger improvement with exercising at the same absolute workload in hypoxia than in normoxia, others showed similar results for training in normoxia and hypoxia regardless of whether exercise was carried out at the same relative or absolute workload.

A closer look at the studies with trained subjects reveals that one important requisite for positive effects is that hypoxic training sessions should not overstress the athletes. Hypoxic training bouts in these studies often comprised only a small fraction of the total training load.

Performance at Altitude

There is a general lack of data comparing performance in normoxia and hypoxia. Only a small number of hypoxic training studies tested performance in hypoxia. This is unfortunate, since important competitions are sometimes held at altitudes above 2,000 m (i.e., in soccer, cross-country skiing, mountain biking). Four of seven studies [16] reported generally larger performance gains measured at altitude for subjects who trained at altitude. In one study that failed to show a performance improvement at altitude after hypoxic training, it was supposed that the hypoxic training was too stressful for the athletes and induced a state of overreaching. Despite the lack of functional improvement in either experimental or control training groups, this study reported a significant increase in oxygen saturation during exercise at simulated altitude after hypoxic training. Additional support for a potential benefit of hypoxic training on competition at altitude comes from studies that estimated hypoxic ventilatory response (HVR) after hypoxic training. All found positive effects on HVR only after hypoxic training, whereas HVR was unchanged or reduced after normoxic training.

Although there is some evidence that hypoxic training is beneficial for competition at altitude, it is currently difficult to make specific recommendations until more data on performance in hypoxia after hypoxic training become available. Of note, nonetheless, is that HVR showed positive effects of hypoxic training. One could, therefore presume that athletes preparing for competition at altitude may profit from simulated hypoxic training sessions, in particular if other means of acclimatization are unavailable.

Muscle Hypertrophy and Strength

With prolonged exposure to extreme altitude, muscle mass and oxidative capacity are lost [16]. Furthermore the hypertrophic response of resistance training under chronic hypoxic conditions seemed to be significantly lower compared to normoxia [9]. On the other hand, it is known that low-intensity resistance training with vascular occlusion (kaatsu training) induces muscle hypertrophy and strength improvement. This effect was attributed to be facilitated by the local tissue hypoxia induced during kaatsu training. It is plausible to postulate that muscle hypertrophy could also be induced by applying systemic hypoxic environment, a hypothesis which was only tested by a few studies. Recently, young and active subjects were assigned to a typical 6-week high-intensity resistance training program (70% 1RM, 10 repetitions) of elbow flexion and extension, either in hypoxia or in normoxia [10]. It was found that resistance training in a hypoxic environment improves strength and muscle hypertrophy more effectively than training under normoxic conditions. Friedmann et al. applied a 4-week low-intensity resistance training program (30% 1RM,

25 repetitions) in hypoxia and normoxia [4]. They found no indications that low-resistance/high-repetition training in hypoxia is superior to equivalent normoxic training. Being far away from conclusive, it might be speculated that resistance training in hypoxia has additional effects but only when intensity is high enough and recovery take place in a normoxic environment.

Hypoxia Training and Health Benefits

Beside the effects of the hypoxic stimuli on exercise performance, there is some evidence that intermittent hypoxia training might have clinical implications. Bailey et al. trained physically active subjects either in normoxia or in normobaric hypoxia (F_iO_2: 16%) [1]. After both conditions, concentrations of free fatty acids, total cholesterol, HDL-cholesterol, and LDL-cholesterol were decreased. The concentration of homocysteine, an amino acid implicated in coronary mortality, was reduced by 11% after hypoxic training only. Furthermore, maximal systolic blood pressure was reduced after hypoxic training, indicating a hypotensive effect of hypoxic training possibly mediated by morphological changes in the endothelium. From these results, the authors concluded that hypoxic training might be beneficial for patients with cardiovascular diseases.

Diagnostics

Training in hypoxia according to the "live low – train high" model is applied, for instance, by cross-country skiers when performing on-snow training sessions on

Hypoxia, Training. Table 1 "Live low – train high" training protocols

Protocol:	Intermittent intensity	Intermittent hypoxia	Threshold training I	Threshold training II	Low intensity training	Combined LH/TL – TH
Method:	Change between high and low intensity in hypoxia	Series of 5 min training in hypoxia and 5 min rest in normoxia	Constant load at "respiratory compensation point"	Constant load at "respiratory compensation point"	Low to moderate intensity – high-volume hypoxia training	14 h/days exposure at 3,000 m in combination with sessions at 2,200 m
Duration:	3–6 weeks	3–6 weeks	3–6 weeks	3–6 weeks	1–2 weeks	3 weeks
No. of sessions:	2–3 per week	2–3 per week	2 per week	3–5 per week	6–7 per week	4 per week
Duration per session at altitude	30–40 min	60 min	Week 1,2:2 × 10 min / Week 3,4: 2 × 15 min / Week 5,6: 2 × 20 min	30 min	90–120 min	In total: 4–5 h/week
Intensity:	Switch between: 2 min @ 90–95% Hf_{max} / 3 min @ 75–80% Hf_{max}	90–95% Hfmax	85–90% Hf_{max}	85–90% Hf_{max}	75–80% Hf_{max}	Low to high intensity
Altitude:	2,500–3,000 m natural or artificial	3,000–5,000 m artificial	2,500–3,000 m natural or artificial	3,000–3,500 m natural or artificial	2,000–3,000 m natural or artificial	3,000 m/2,200 m natural or artificial
Additional endurance training:	Low-intensity endurance training in normoxia	Low-intensity endurance training in normoxia	Low-intensity endurance training in normoxia	None	None	Regular training at or near sea level
Target group:	Athletes	Athletes	Athletes	Untrained subjects	Athletes	Athletes

a glacier (around 2,500–3,500 m) during their summer training camps. It is also used by athletes to acclimatize for competition at altitude or to increase sea level exercise performance. The implementation of "live low – train high" has been used in endurance sports and in sports where high levels of aerobic and anaerobic metabolism are important for energy provision (e.g., downhill skiing, soccer, hockey, etc.). Our work and that of others show that different training protocols have evolved, which are described in detail in Table 1.

Different methodologies have been established to utilize the hypoxia stimuli to increase fitness and performance in athletes. A recent meta-analysis indicates that "live low – train high" and "live high – train low" produce ~1% performance enhancements in sub-elite and elite athletes, respectively [2]. Being aware that a wide range of training intensities, frequencies, and severity of hypoxia make a pooling of hypoxia training results problematic, the benefit of these procedures seems to be rather small. Only one recent control-group-designed study examined the effectiveness of combining both "live low – train high" and "live high – train low" (LH/TL + TH) [12]. For a total of 3 weeks, trained middle distance runners spent 14 h/day in an altitude chamber (3,000 m), performed four sessions/week at a simulated altitude of 2,200 m at different intensities, and maintained their normal training near sea-level altitude. Although performance in 3-km time trial run was only marginally improved, combined LH/TL + TH elicited increases in physiological capacities (VO$_2$max, Hb$_{mass}$) which were greater compared to LH/TL or TH alone [12].

The access to natural hypoxia is not universal. Natural settings at high altitude (hypobaric hypoxia; glacier training of cross country or alpine skiers) have the advantage that training tasks can be carried out in a sport-specific manner. Disadvantages may include travel and expenses. When training at altitude, descents should be as rapid as possible to enable immediate recovery in a normoxic environment.

Different altitude simulation systems are commercially available. These systems allow exposure to normobaric hypoxia during either rest or exercise. These devices allow simulated altitudes above 5,000 m. Safety aspects must be considered when exposing untrained subjects or athletes to this artificial environment. The advantage of altitude simulation devices is that the climatic conditions and the level of hypoxia can be precisely adjusted and regulated. An obvious disadvantage is that use of altitude simulation systems requires a stationary training situation, in which the exercise task can often not be performed in a sport-specific way, a potential problem for technically complex sports.

Acknowledgment

The authors gratefully acknowledge year long support of the Swiss National Science Foundation, the University of Bern, the Swiss Federal Sports Commission, Swiss Olympic, and Swiss Ski.

References

1. Bailey DM, Davies B, Baker J (2000) Training in hypoxia: modulation of metabolic and cardiovascular risk factors in men. Med Sci Sports Exerc 32(6):1058–1066
2. Bonetti DL, Hopkins WG (2009) Sea-level exercise performance following adaptation to hypoxia: a meta-analysis. Sports Med 39(2):107–127
3. Faria IE (1992) Energy expenditure, aerodynamics and medical problems in cycling. An update. Sports Med 14(1):43–63
4. Friedmann B, Kinscherf R, Borisch S, Richter G, Bartsch P, Billeter R (2003) Effects of low-resistance/high-repetition strength training in hypoxia on muscle structure and gene expression. Pflugers Arch 446(6):742–751
5. Green H, MacDougall J, Tarnopolsky M, Melissa NL (1999) Downregulation of Na + −K + −ATPase pumps in skeletal muscle with training in normobaric hypoxia. J Appl Physiol 86(5): 1745–1748
6. Hendriksen IJ, Meeuwsen T (2003) The effect of intermittent training in hypobaric hypoxia on sea-level exercise: a cross-over study in humans. Eur J Appl Physiol 88(4–5):396–403
7. Hoppeler H, Klossner S, Vogt M (2008) Training in hypoxia and its effects on skeletal muscle tissue. Scand J Med Sci Sports 18(Suppl 1): 38–49
8. Mason S, Johnson RS (2007) The role of HIF-1 in hypoxic response in the skeletal muscle. Adv Exp Med Biol 618:229–244
9. Narici MV, Kayser B (1995) Hypertrophic response of human skeletal muscle to strength training in hypoxia and normoxia. Eur J Appl Physiol Occup Physiol 70(3):213–219
10. Nishimura A, Sugita M, Kato K, Fukuda A, Sudo A, Uchida A (2010) Hypoxia increases muscle hypertrophy induced by resistance training. Int J Sports Physiol Perform 5(4):497–508
11. Robergs RA, Quintana R, Parker DL, Frankel CC (1998) Multiple variables explain the variability in the decrement in VO$_2$max during acute hypobaric hypoxia. Med Sci Sports Exerc 30(6):869–879
12. Robertson EY, Saunders PU, Pyne DB, Gore CJ, Anson JM (2010) Effectiveness of intermittent training in hypoxia combined with live high/train low. Eur J Appl Physiol 110(2):379–387
13. Semenza GL (2001) HIF-1 and mechanisms of hypoxia sensing. Curr Opin Cell Biol 13(2):167–171
14. Terrados N, Jansson E, Sylven C, Kaijser L (1990) Is hypoxia a stimulus for synthesis of oxidative enzymes and myoglobin? J Appl Physiol 68(6):2369–2372
15. Vogt M, Puntschart A, Geiser J, Zuleger C, Billeter R, Hoppeler H (2001) Molecular adaptations in human skeletal muscle to endurance training under simulated hypoxic conditions. J Appl Physiol 91(1):173–182
16. Vogt M, Hoppeler H (2010) Is hypoxia training good for muscles and exercise performance? Prog Cardiovasc Dis 52(6):525–533
17. Zoll J, Ponsot E, Dufour S, Doutreleau S, Ventura-Clapier R, Vogt M, Hoppeler H, Richard R, Fluck M (2006) Exercise training in normobaric hypoxia in endurance runners. III. Muscular adjustments of selected gene transcripts. J Appl Physiol 100(4): 1258–1266

Hypoxia-Inducible Factors

Adaptation of cells to low O_2 pressure (pO_2) leads to a series of responses mediated by specific hypoxia-inducible transcription factors (HIFs). The HIF system operates in all nucleated cells of the organism. HIFs are heterodimeric protein complexes (about 200 kDa) consisting of an O_2-labile α-subunit and a stable β-subunit. HIF-1β is also involved in xenobiotic reactions, as it is identical to the "aryl hydrocarbon receptor nuclear translocator" (ARNT). Three different isoforms of HIF-α have been described (HIF-1α, HIF-2α, HIF-3α). In hypoxia, the O_2-labile HIF-α subunits are preserved and translocated from the cytoplasm into the nucleus, where they dimerize with HIF-1β. Supported by co-activators (CBP/p300), the transactivating HIF-α/β complexes bind to specific DNA sequences in the promoter or enhancer region of O_2-dependent genes (HIF-binding sites). Some of the translational products of the HIF-responsive genes increase the O_2 supply of hypoxic tissues, namely, erythropoietin (Epo), which stimulates the production of red blood cells, and vascular endothelial growth factor (VEGF), which stimulates angiogenesis. Others improve the cellular glucose supply (glucose transporters, GLUTs) or adapt the cellular metabolism to hypoxia (glycolytic enzymes). Over 100 HIF target genes have already been identified. The relative activity of the different HIFs appears to be tissue-specific. HIF-1 is particularly important with respect to glycolysis, while HIF-2 stimulates *Epo* transcription. HIF-3 is thought to inhibit gene expression. The HIFs are inactive in normoxia because of O_2-dependent enzymatic hydroxylation and subsequent proteolysis of their α-subunit. Three HIF-α prolyl hydroxylases (PHD-1, -2, and -3) initiate proteasomal degradation while an asparaginyl hydroxylase (factor inhibiting HIF, FIH) causes functional loss of the C-terminal transactivation domain of HIF-α. Because of their O_2-dependence and their HIF controlling function the HIF-α hydroxylases are considered biological O_2 sensors. In addition to O_2 and 2-oxoglutarate, the HIF-α hydroxylases require Fe^{2+} and ascorbate as cofactors. Products of glycolysis can act as endogenous inhibitors of HIF hydroxylases, which may lead to sustained activation of HIFs in cancer cells. Hence, both pharmacological and genetic interventions that increase HIF activity and such lowering of itare of therapeutic interest. On stabilization of HIF, the production of Epo increases, which is of benefit in anemia. Stimulation of HIF-dependent gene expression accelerates angiogenesis for possible application in ischemic diseases. Actually, 2-oxoglutarate analogs have emerged as promising tools for stimulation of erythropoiesis and angiogenesis in preclinical and clinical trials (so-called HIF-stabilizers). Furthermore, HIF activation augments cell proliferation, wound healing, and distinct inflammatory reactions. HIF suppression, on the other hand, is potentially beneficial to prevent tumor angiogenesis and tumor cell adaptation to hypoxia.

Hypoxic Training

▶ Hypoxia, Training
▶ Training, Altitude